Jillian Smith

NMS

National Medical Series for Independent Study

Surgery

NMS

National Medical Series for Independent Study

Surgery

Sixth Edition

Bruce E. Jarrell, MD

Professor
Department of Surgery
University of Maryland School of Medicine
Baltimore, Maryland

Stephen M. Kavic, MD

Associate Professor
Department of Surgery
Program Director
Residency in General Surgery
University of Maryland School of Medicine
Baltimore, Maryland

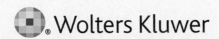

Wolters Kluwer

Philadelphia • Baltimore • New York • London
Buenos Aires • Hong Kong • Sydney • Tokyo

Acquisitions Editor: Tari Broderick
Product Development Editor: Amy Weintraub
Editorial Assistant: Joshua Haffner
Marketing Manager: Joy Fisher-Williams
Production Project Manager: Priscilla Crater
Design Coordinator: Terry Mallon
Manufacturing Coordinator: Margie Orzech
Prepress Vendor: Absolute Service, Inc.

Sixth Edition

Library of Congress Cataloging-in-Publication Data

NMS surgery / [edited by] Bruce E. Jarrell, Stephen M. Kavic. — Sixth edition.
  p. ; cm. — (National medical series for independent study)
National medical series surgery
Includes index.
ISBN 978-1-60831-584-0
I. Jarrell, Bruce E., editor. II. Kavic, Stephen M. (Stephen Michael), editor. III. Title: National medical series surgery. IV. Series: National medical series for independent study.
  [DNLM: 1. Surgical Procedures, Operative—Examination Questions. 2. Surgical Procedures, Operative—Outlines. 3. General Surgery—methods—Examination Questions. 4. General Surgery—methods—Outlines. WO 18.2]
  RD37.2
  617.0076—dc23
                                                                                      2015010501

We both thank the many mentors who have advised us each throughout our careers. We are forever indebted to them.

I wish to thank my wife, Leslie, and my wonderful children for all of their support during my career, and for their understanding during the writing of the many editions of NMS Surgery – BEJ

Dedicated to my loving wife Jennifer and to my lovely daughter Emily – SMK

Foreword

It is with tremendous pride that I introduce the sixth edition of *NMS Surgery*. This work has occupied a central role in the education of a generation of medical students. The outline format makes it a superb reference for those learning the basics of surgery and a thorough review for those who already practice our art.

The current edition has special significance to the University of Maryland School of Medicine. Dr. Jarrell is the Chief Academic and Research Officer and Dean of the Graduate School. He also was my predecessor as Chair of the Department of Surgery. Dr. Kavic is the current program director of our surgery residency. The chapter authors and contributors include a virtual directory of our trainees and faculty. It is a privilege to be associated with these esteemed educators.

I am continually impressed by the talents of the surgeons and surgeons-in-training at the University of Maryland. That quality is reflected in the following chapters. I know that you will enjoy this edition as much as I take pride in it.

Stephen T. Bartlett, MD
Peter Angelos Distinguished Professor of Surgery
Chair
Department of Surgery
Surgeon-in-Chief
University of Maryland Medical System
University of Maryland School of Medicine
Baltimore, Maryland

Preface

Welcome to the sixth edition of *NMS Surgery*.

This book aims to build on the legacy of the previous five editions. We have retained much of the organization and format from the last versions. At the same time, we have strived to make this volume more readable.

It is an increasing challenge to limit content in the face of rapidly expanding surgical knowledge. As in previous editions, the text is not meant to be all-inclusive but rather serves as an introduction for the student of surgery. All of the chapters have been thoroughly reviewed, rewritten, and updated to reflect the current state of the art in surgery.

There are dramatic differences in the format of this volume. Perhaps most importantly, each section now begins with "Chapter Cuts and Caveats," which are some of the most important principles worthy of the reader's attention. Within each chapter, we have added "Quick Cuts," which are highlights that have been brought out separately from the text. In addition, we have added a new section at the end, "Grade A Cuts," which are pairings that highlight associations in surgical thinking.

For the tremendous work put into this edition, we are indebted to the authors. Their high-quality and frequently punctual contributions have made our jobs as editors pleasant. We are also grateful to the editorial team at Wolters Kluwer for their guidance and support throughout the process.

The sixth edition of *NMS Surgery* is written primarily for students and residents in general surgery, but practicing surgeons as well as physicians in other specialties will no doubt find it a useful reference. We hope that all readers will find that the book represents a declaration of the state of surgical art in 2015.

—Bruce E. Jarrell, MD
—Stephen M. Kavic, MD

Contributors

William R. Alex, MD, FACS
Cardiothoracic Surgery
Riverside, California

H. Richard Alexander, MD, FACS
Professor of Surgery
University of Maryland School of Medicine
Baltimore, Maryland

Andrea C. Bafford, MD, FACS
Assistant Professor of Surgery
University of Maryland School of Medicine
Baltimore, Maryland

Emily Bellavance, MD, FACS
Assistant Professor of Surgery
University of Maryland School of Medicine
Baltimore, Maryland

Hugo Bonatti, MD, FACS
General and Minimally Invasive Surgery
Easton, Maryland

Cherif Boutros, MB, CHB, MSc, FACS
Associate Professor of Surgery
University of Maryland School of Medicine
Baltimore, Maryland

Jonathan Bromberg, MB, PhD, FACS
Professor of Surgery
Chief
Division of Transplantation
University of Maryland School of Medicine
Baltimore, Maryland

Brandon Bruns, MD, FACS
Assistant Professor of Surgery
University of Maryland School of Medicine
Baltimore, Maryland

Laura S. Buchanan, MD, FACS
Assistant Professor of Surgery
University of Maryland School of Medicine
Baltimore, Maryland

Whitney Burrows, MD, FACS
Assistant Professor of Surgery
University of Maryland School of Medicine
Baltimore, Maryland

Clint D. Cappiello, MD
Resident in Surgery
University of Maryland Medical Center
Baltimore, Maryland

Kenneth M. Crandall, MD
Resident in Neurosurgery
University of Maryland Medical Center
Baltimore, Maryland

Robert S. Crawford, MD, FACS
Assistant Professor of Surgery
University of Maryland School of Medicine
Baltimore, Maryland

Peter E. Darwin, MD
Professor of Medicine
University of Maryland School of Medicine
Baltimore, Maryland

Jose J. Diaz, MD, FACS
Professor of Surgery
Chief
Division of Acute Care Surgery
University of Maryland School of Medicine
Baltimore, Maryland

Garima Dosi, MD
Fellow in Vascular Surgery
University of Maryland Medical Center
Baltimore, Maryland

Richard N. Edie, MD, FACS
Cardiothoracic Surgery
Philadelphia, Pennsylvania

Steven Feigenberg, MD
Professor of Radiation Oncology
University of Maryland School of Medicine
Baltimore, Maryland

Jessica Felton, MD
Resident in Surgery
University of Maryland Medical Center
Baltimore, Maryland

James S. Gammie, MD, FACS
Professor of Surgery
Chief, Division of Cardiac Surgery
University of Maryland School of Medicine
Baltimore, Maryland

Jinny Ha, MD
Resident in Surgery
University of Maryland Medical Center
Baltimore, Maryland

Natasha Hansraj, MD
Resident in Surgery
University of Maryland Medical Center
Baltimore, Maryland

Andrea Hebert, MD
Resident in Otolaryngology
University of Maryland Medical Center
Baltimore, Maryland

Tripp Holton, MD, FACS
Assistant Professor of Surgery
University of Maryland School of Medicine
Baltimore, Maryland

Helen G. Hui-Chou, MD
Fellow in Plastic Surgery
University of Maryland
Johns Hopkins University
Baltimore, Maryland

Ajay Jain, MD, FACS
Associate Professor of Surgery
State University of New York Upstate Medical University
Syracuse, New York

Steven B. Johnson, MD, FACS, FCCM
Professor and Chairman
Department of Surgery
University of Arizona
Phoenix, Arizona

Jessica Joines, MA, MGC
Instructor of Medicine
University of Maryland School of Medicine
Baltimore, Maryland

Stephen M. Kavic, MD, FACS
Associate Professor of Surgery
Program Director
Residency in General Surgery
University of Maryland School of Medicine
Baltimore, Maryland

Edwin Kendrick, MD
Fellow in Vascular Surgery
University of Maryland Medical Center
Baltimore, Maryland

Susan B. Kesmodel, MD, FACS
Assistant Professor of Surgery
University of Maryland School of Medicine
Baltimore, Maryland

Mark D. Kligman, MD, FACS
Assistant Professor of Surgery
University of Maryland School of Medicine
Baltimore, Maryland

Andrew Kramer, MD, FACS
Associate Professor of Surgery
University of Maryland School of Medicine
Baltimore, Maryland

Natalia Kubicki, MD
Resident in Surgery
University of Maryland Medical Center
Baltimore, Maryland

Katherine G. Lamond, MD, FACS
Assistant Professor of Surgery
University of Maryland School of Medicine
Baltimore, Maryland

Matthew Lissauer, MD, FACS, FCCM
Associate Professor of Surgery
Rutgers Robert Wood Johnson Medical School
New Brunswick, New Jersey

Daniel E. Mansour, MD
Resident in Surgery
University of Maryland Medical Center
Baltimore, Maryland

Daniel Medina, MD, PhD
Resident in Surgery
University of Maryland Medical Center
Baltimore, Maryland

Mayur Narayan, MD, MPH, MBA, FACS
Assistant Professor of Surgery
University of Maryland School of Medicine
Baltimore, Maryland

Silke Niederhaus, MD, FACS
Assistant Professor of Surgery
University of Maryland School of Medicine
Baltimore, Maryland

John A. Olson Jr, MD, PhD
Professor of Surgery
Chief
Division of General Surgery and Surgical Oncology
University of Maryland School of Medicine
Baltimore, Maryland

Natalie A. O'Neill, MD
Resident in Surgery
University of Maryland Medical Center
Baltimore, Maryland

D. Bruce Panasuk, MD, FACS
Chief of Surgery
Wilmington VA Medical Center
Wilmington, Delaware

Jonathan P. Pearl, MD, FACS
Assistant Professor of Surgery
University of Maryland School of Medicine
Baltimore, Maryland

Srinevas K. Reddy, MD, FACS
Surgical Oncology and Hepatobiliary Surgery
Minneapolis, Minnesota

Daniel Reznicek, MD
Resident in Urologic Surgery
University of Maryland Medical Center
Baltimore, Maryland

Ernest L. Rosato, MD, FACS
Professor of Surgery
Director
Division of General Surgery
Thomas Jefferson University
Philadelphia, Pennsylvania

Francis E. Rosato Jr, MD, FACS
General and Minimally Invasive Surgery
Pennington, New Jersey

Charles A. Sansur, MD
Assistant Professor of Neurosurgery
University of Maryland School of Medicine
Baltimore, Maryland

Rajabrata Sarkar, MD, FACS
Professor of Surgery
Chief
Division of Vascular Surgery
University of Maryland School of Medicine
Baltimore, Maryland

Joseph R. Scalea, MD
Transplant Surgery Fellow
University of Wisconsin
Madison, Wisconsin

Thomas Scalea, MD, FACS
Professor of Surgery
Physician-in-Chief
R Adams Cowley Shock Trauma Center
University of Maryland School of Medicine
Baltimore, Maryland

Max Seaton, MD
Resident in Surgery
University of Maryland Medical Center
Baltimore, Maryland

Devinder Singh, MD, FACS
Associate Professor of Surgery
University of Maryland School of Medicine
Baltimore, Maryland

Alexis D. Smith, MD
Resident in Surgery
University of Maryland Medical Center
Baltimore, Maryland

Robert Sterling, MD
Assistant Professor of Surgery
Johns Hopkins University School of Medicine
Baltimore, Maryland

Eric Strauch, MD, FACS
Associate Professor of Surgery
University of Maryland School of Medicine
Baltimore, Maryland

Oliver Tannous, MD
Resident in Orthopedic Surgery
University of Maryland Medical Center
Baltimore, Maryland

Julia Terhune, MD
Resident in Surgery
University of Maryland Medical Center
Baltimore, Maryland

Douglas J. Turner, MD, FACS
Associate Professor of Surgery
University of Maryland School of Medicine
Baltimore, Maryland

Keli Turner, MD
Resident in Surgery
University of Maryland Medical Center
Baltimore, Maryland

A. Claire Watkins, MD
Resident in Cardiothoracic Surgery
University of Maryland Medical Center
Baltimore, Maryland

Ronald J. Weigel, MD, PhD, MBA, FACS
Professor and Chair of Surgery
University of Iowa
Iowa City, Iowa

Niluka A. Wickramaratne, MD
Resident in Surgery
Virginia Commonwealth University
Richmond, Virginia

Jeffrey S. Wolf, MD
Associate Professor of Otolaryngology—Head and Neck Surgery
University of Maryland School of Medicine
Baltimore, Maryland

Contents

Part II: Thoracic Disorders

Part III: Vascular Disorders

Part V: Breast and Endocrine Disorders

Part VI: Special Subjects

Part VII: Surgical Subspecialties

Introduction
Chapter Cuts and Caveats

Part I

CHAPTER 1

Principles of Surgical Physiology:

◆ Management of sick patients requires resuscitation, with the goal of restoration of perfusion. Quickly and accurately finding the source of the clinical deterioration and fixing that problem is crucial; otherwise, the resuscitation will ultimately fail to allow adequate oxygen delivery.

◆ Shock is the state of physiologic decompensation resulting in inadequate tissue perfusion (oxygen demand outstrips oxygen supply).

◆ Ultimately, no one formula best determines postoperative fluid and electrolyte management.

◆ High insensible losses (both evaporative losses and leakage into the third space) occur during and after surgical procedures that involve open body cavities; that are invasive and open many tissue planes; that are prolonged; that are associated with sepsis, inflammatory conditions, and ischemia of organs; that result in hypotension; and that are done in emergent settings.

◆ Hyperkalemia must be treated aggressively to avoid life-threatening arrhythmias. The best emergent treatment is IV bicarbonate and IV insulin and glucose, which moves potassium intracellularly and lowers serum levels. IV calcium is also useful by affecting the threshold for action potential and decreasing cardiac membrane excitability.

◆ Adequate oxygenation is assessed by more than blood pressure and pulse. It is also monitored by assessing markers of tissue perfusion (urine output and renal function), oxygenation (chest x-ray and lung auscultation for signs of pulmonary edema, blood oxygenation, and other measures), serum electrolyte levels, pH, arrhythmias, mentation, external signs of hydration state, hematocrit, and the patient's overall appearance.

◆ When evaluating a patient who is clinically deteriorating, always prioritize the evaluation of diagnoses in your differential that will lead to the fastest and greatest deterioration.

◆ New anemia in a postoperative patient is surgical bleeding until proven otherwise. Packed RBC transfusion provides excellent physiologic support but has side effects including allergic reactions and the potential for infectious transmission—*treat blood like a drug*! Clerical error is the most common cause for transfusion reaction.

◆ Enteral nutrition is preferred in most patients. The risk of central venous catheters outweighs nutritional benefits for short-term supplementation if nutritional support is needed for less than 1 week. Low albumin levels correlate with mortality.

◆ Patients with inadequate oxygenation or increased work of breathing should have ventilatory support: *When in doubt, intubate.*

CHAPTER 2

Essentials of General Surgery:

◆ For wound infections: Abscess must be drained, necrotic tissue must be debrided, crepitus suggests a necrotizing gas-forming infection demanding that the wound be opened, foreign bodies (including tubes or drains) must be removed, and enteric leak must be controlled.

- Systemic antibiotics are not the primary treatment for wound infections.
- Perioperative antibiotics given to patients with clean-contaminated wounds (which are usually closed primarily) reduce the incidence of wound infections and the subsequent risk of hernia.
- Any condition that interferes with the four phases of wound healing (hemostasis, inflammation, proliferation, and remodeling) will impair the rate of healing and the final wound strength. Both local and systemic factors have an effect.
- Local factors: Wounds should be free of bleeding, hematoma, gross contamination, and necrotic tissue; wound edges should be free of tension; and local tissue should be healthy and well vascularized.
- Systemic factors that impair wound healing: metabolism, poor nutritional state, zinc and vitamins A and C deficiency, presence of infection, hypoxia, low-flow states, smoking, poorly controlled diabetes, obesity, collagen vascular diseases, and renal and liver failure
- Medications: systemic glucocorticoids, some chemotherapeutic and immunosuppressive drugs, and angiogenesis inhibitors
- Postoperative fevers may result from the 5 W's: wound, water, wind, walking, and wonder drugs.
- Surgical site infections are a major source of morbidity and are most commonly due to skin flora (especially *Staphylococcus*).
- Nonhealing GI fistulas may result from FRIEND (foreign body, radiation, inflammation, epithelialization, neoplasia, distal obstruction) and often respond to nonoperative management.

CHAPTER 3

Medical Risk Factors in Surgical Patients:

- Assessment of medical risk for invasive surgical procedures includes a thorough history, physical, and laboratory examination.
- Patients with cardiac conditions are at increased risk for cardiac complications following noncardiac surgery, and standardized classification systems help stratify risk. Functional capacity more than 4 METs predicts a low risk of postoperative cardiac events. Elective surgery should be postponed at least 4 weeks following *acute* cardiac events or revascularization.
- All patients should be assessed for the degree of risk for venous thromboembolic events, and prophylaxis with heparin is appropriate for most surgical patients.

CHAPTER 4

Life-Threatening Disorders: Acute Abdominal Surgical Emergencies:

- When evaluating a patient for acute abdominal pain, first determine whether the patient has a surgical abdomen on examination, judged by a distressed patient with pain that is severe and generalized and associated with rebound or guarding. Clinical judgment is supplemented by radiographic studies, such as extraluminal peritoneal free air, and laboratory studies, such as findings supportive of ischemia, inflammation, acute hemorrhage into the peritoneal cavity, or infection. If the judgment of a surgical abdomen is made, immediate intervention after resuscitation is indicated.
- GI hemorrhage necessitates localizing the bleeding and formulating a plan to control it before surgery. Identifying the source of bleeding in the operating room by evaluating the external surface of the GI tract is very difficult.
- To manage a significant GI hemorrhage, balancing three problems simultaneously becomes necessary: volume resuscitation, coagulation defect correction, and identification and control of the site of hemorrhage. Transfusion of blood and blood products may be critical in managing all three problems. Transfusion beyond several units results in increased morbidity and mortality because blood and its products have many potential side effects, such as transfusion reactions with anaphylaxis and hemolysis, infectious agent transmission, and immune suppression, among others.
- Location can indicate common pathology: RUQ suggests the biliary tree; RLQ, the appendix; and LLQ, the sigmoid colon.

Chapter 1

Principles of Surgical Physiology

Steven B. Johnson and Matthew Lissauer

 FLUID AND ELECTROLYTES

Normal Body Composition

I. **Body water:** Water accounts for 50%–70% of body weight (the higher percentage in young people, thin people, and man—the lower percentage in older people, obese people, and women). Body water is divided into various intracellular and extracellular compartments (Fig. 1-1).

   A. **Two-thirds rule:** This is a simple method of approximating compartment volume because of the variation among patients and within the same patient. Total body water comprises slightly less than two-thirds body weight.

   B. **Plasma volume:** Using the above rule, ~5% of body weight is plasma volume (e.g., 3.5 L for a 70-kg male). Plasma is ~60% of the blood volume (if the hematocrit is 40%); therefore, the 70-kg male has 5 L of blood.

II. **Electrolyte composition:** Electrolytes determine the amount of water that exists in any one space at any time, and their concentrations and compositions differ between intracellular and extracellular spaces due to ion pumps (principally Na^+/K^+ ATPase), as shown in Table 1-1. Change in osmotic pressure in one compartment causes water to redistribute from the other compartments to regain equilibrium.

   A. **Intracellular (principal osmotic cation is potassium):** has higher concentration of osmotic and oncotic (protein) particles than the extracellular compartment, thus allowing water to flow into the cell, creating turgidity

   B. **Extracellular (principal osmotic cation is sodium):** Interstitial and plasma composition is nearly but not quite identical.

Water and Electrolyte Maintenance

I. **Water:** Required amount depends on the person's weight, age, gender, and illness.

   A. **Water calculation methods**

      1. **Amount of body water excreted**

         a. Most water lost from the body is through urine production; generally, 0.5 mL/kg/hr is the minimum needed to excrete the daily solute load.

 Quick Cut
The compartments are important because calculating fluid losses, blood losses, and amount of resuscitation needed is key to ensuring patients' survival.

 Quick Cut
Two-thirds rule: Total body water = (slightly less than) two-thirds total body weight.

 Quick Cut
Of total body water, two thirds is intracellular and one third extracellular (three fourths = interstitial and one fourth = intravascular).

 Quick Cut
Water follows electrolytes across cell membranes to equilibrate osmolality.

 Quick Cut
Adequate urine output is ½ mL/kg/hr, or about 250 mL/8 hr in adults.

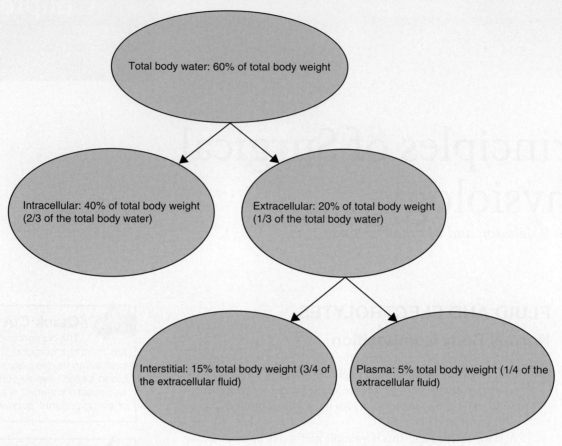

Figure 1-1: Water compartments.

Table 1-1: Electrolyte Composition of Various Water Compartments

Electrolytes	Intracellular Compartment	Extracellular Compartment
Anions		
Sodium (Na$^+$)	10 mEq/L	142 mEq/L
Potassium (K$^+$)	140 mEq/L	4 mEq/L
Chloride (Cl$^-$)	4 mEq/L	103 mEq/L
Bicarbonate (HCO$_3^-$)	10 mEq/L	28 mEq/L
Phosphate (PO$_4^{3-}$)	75 mEq/L	4 mEq/L
Sulfate (SO$_4^{2-}$)	2 mEq/L	1 mEq/L
Calcium (Ca^{++})	<1 mEq/L	5 mEq/L
Magnesium (Mg^{++})	18 mEq/L	2 mEq/L
Organic acids	—	5 mEq/L
Various proteins	40 mEq/L	1 mEq/L

b. The next highest daily water loss is insensible loss (i.e., sweat, respiration, stool), which is estimated as 600–900 mL/24 hr.

c. Minimal water maintenance for a 70-kg man: (70 kg × 0.5 mL/kg/hr × 24 hours) + 750 mL/24 hr + 1,590 mL/24 hr. (Again, this is the minimum and does not take into account any excess loss such as fever, which will increase the insensible loss.)

2. **Body weight:** This method is often used for pediatric patients because their body weights vary widely; estimations are 100 mL/kg/day or 4 mL/kg/hr for the first 10 kg of body weight, 50 mL/kg/day or 2 mL/kg/hr for the second 10 kg of body weight, and 20 mL/kg/day or 1 mL/kg/hr for each additional kilogram of body weight.

3. **Given amount of water per kilogram of body weight:** The value used for this method is generally 35–40 mL/kg/day, adjusted higher or lower based on age (older adults often require only 15 mL/kg/24-hr maintenance due to higher fat/lower muscle mass).

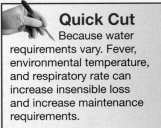

Quick Cut
Remember the shortcut for estimating fluid maintenance: The first 20 kg of weight = 60 mL/hr and then 1 mL/kg/hr above that, so a 60-kg person = 100 mL/hr.

B. **Evaluating maintenance rates:** Patients not only have different maintenance needs, but replacing water or removing excess water may also be of concern (see I C 1). Simple methods in the *noncritically* ill population to monitor adequacy of fluid administration include the following:

1. **Urine output variations:** If urine output is high (i.e., >1 mL/kg/hr), then less water may be required; if urine output is low, more water may be required, or further assessment may be necessary.

2. **Tachycardia:** can be a sign of dehydration or low intravascular volume

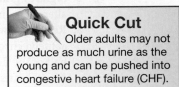

Quick Cut
Because water requirements vary. Fever, environmental temperature, and respiratory rate can increase insensible loss and increase maintenance requirements.

C. **Adjusting fluid rates and type for individual patients:** First, calculate the patient's maintenance rate, then adjust the amount up or down based on the need for resuscitation, or replacement of gastrointestinal (GI) losses, and the type based on type of losses (Table 1-2).

Quick Cut
Older adults may not produce as much urine as the young and can be pushed into congestive heart failure (CHF).

1. **Injury, illness, and surgery:** Can result in fluid losses due to blood loss, third spacing, insensible losses from diarrhea, fever, etc. Providing more than calculated maintenance fluid to replace losses (e.g., 1.5 or 2 × maintenance) is necessary, and rate adequacy can be judged from the above criteria.

2. **Hypervolemia and diuresis:** Patients who require diuresis already are overloaded with fluid, and intravenous (IV) fluids should be withheld; however, electrolyte or nutritional aspects of fluid administration may require water as a carrier for other substances during diuresis.

Table 1-2: Electrolyte Composition of Gastrointestinal Secretions

Organ	Volume/day	Na$^+$ (mEq/L)	K$^+$ (mEq/L)	Cl$^-$ (mEq/L)	HCO$_3^-$ (mEq/L)
Stomach	1–5 L	20–150	10–20	120–140	Nil
Duodenum	0.1–2 L	100–120	10–20	110	10–20
Ileum	1–3 L	80–140	5–10	60–90	30–50
Colon	0.1–2 L	100–120	10–30	90	30–50
Gallbladder	0.5–1 L	140	5	100	25
Pancreas	0.5–1 L	140	5	30 (higher when not stimulated)	115 (lower when not stimulated)

II. **Sodium:** Normally, people take 150–200 mEq of sodium daily, much of which is excreted in the urine.
   A. If the body needs to conserve sodium, it can reduce renal excretion to less than 1 mEq/day.
   B. Daily homeostasis is easily maintained with 1–2 mEq/kg/day.

III. **Potassium:** The normal daily intake of potassium is ~40–120 mEq/day, with about 10%–15% excreted in urine; an amount of 0.5–1 mEq/kg/day is appropriate to maintain homeostasis.

IV. **Maintenance IV:** Table 1-3 gives electrolyte concentrations of several IV fluids. Using the previous estimates for a 70-kg male, the weight formula for IV fluid would equal 110 mL/hr.
   A. Minimal sodium maintenance would require 70–140 mEq/day, and minimal potassium requirements would be 35–70 mEq/day.
   B. If 0.5% normal saline (NS) has 77 mEq/L sodium and 20 mEq/L potassium are added, then using 0.5% NS with 20 mEq/L potassium chloride at 110 mL/hr would equal about 2.6 L of fluid, 200 mEq of sodium, and 52 mEq of potassium . . . pretty close!

Water and Electrolyte Deficits and Excesses

I. **Water**
   A. **Hypovolemia**
      1. **Signs of acute volume loss:** include tachycardia, hypotension, and decreased urine output
      2. **Signs of gradual volume loss:** include loss of skin turgor, thirst, alterations in body temperature, and changes in mental status
      3. **Replacing water deficits:** Acute deficits should be replaced acutely; chronic deficits should be replaced more slowly, with half of the deficit replaced over the first 8 hours and the rest in 24–48 hours.
   B. **Hypervolemia:** well tolerated in healthy patients, who will just urinate the excess
      1. **Signs of acute hypervolemia:** acute shortness of breath, tachycardia
      2. **Signs of chronic hypervolemia:** peripheral edema, pulmonary edema

II. **Sodium:** close relationship to volume status
   A. **Hyponatremia (Na⁺ <130 mEq/L):** Figure 1-2
      1. **Causes**
         a. **Hyperosmolar:** hyperglycemia, mannitol infusion, or presence of other osmotically active particles that draw in water

Quick Cut
D5 ½ NS with 20 mEq/L potassium is a near-perfect maintenance fluid.

Quick Cut
Remember, based on a patient's specific need, maintenance fluids can be altered to optimize blood chemistry.

Quick Cut
In the case of hypernatremia with hypovolemia, do not allow the sodium concentration to drop more than 0.5–1 mEq/hr.

Quick Cut
Complications of acute CHF can arise in acutely hypervolemic patients with poor cardiac function.

Quick Cut
Diuresis may be needed in some chronically hypervolemic patients to reduce volume.

Quick Cut
For a hyponatremia workup, first check the serum osmolar value then, if needed, volume status.

Table 1-3: Electrolyte Concentration in Various Intravenous Fluids

Fluid	Na⁺ (mEq/L)	K⁺ (mEq/L)	Mg⁺⁺ (mEq/L)	Ca⁺⁺ (mEq/L)	Cl⁻ (mEq/L)	Lactate (mEq/L)	Osmolarity (mOsm/L)
Normal saline (0.9% NaCl)	154	0	0	0	154	0	308
½ normal saline (0.5% NaCl)	77	0	0	0	77	0	154
Hypertonic saline (3% saline)	513	0	0	0	513	0	1027
Lactated Ringer's	130	4	0	2.7	98	28	525
Plasmalyte*	140	5	3	0	98	0	294

*Plasmalyte also contains 27 mEq/L acetate and 23 mEq/L gluconate.

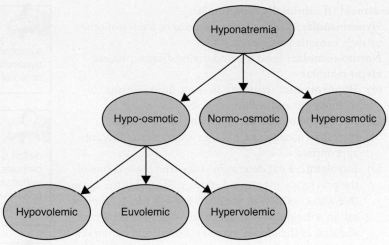

Figure 1-2: Hyponatremia.

b. **Normo-osmolar (pseudohyponatremia):**
   Hypertriglyceridemia, hyperlipidemia, and hyperproteinemia; large, minimally osmotic molecules *displace* water and interfere with the lab measurement of sodium.

c. **Hypo-osmolar**
   (1) **Hypovolemic:** renal losses, renal tubular acidosis, cerebral salt wasting, GI losses, "tea and toast syndrome," transcutaneous losses (burns, trauma)
   (2) **Hypervolemic:** The pathology is often related to low cardiac output (the kidneys see less blood flow, and free water is conserved) or hypoalbuminemic (e.g., cirrhosis) or other edematous states where salt (renin-angiotensin system) and free water (antidiuretic hormone [ADH]) cannot be excreted by the kidneys (e.g., renal failure, CHF, nephrotic syndrome).
   (3) **Euvolemic:** could be either of the states mentioned earlier, or (more frequently in the perioperative patient) **syndrome of inappropriate antidiuretic hormone (SIADH) secretion**, or others (e.g., glucocorticoid deficiency, hypothyroidism, water intoxication [psychogenic polydipsia])

2. **Symptoms**
   a. **Acute hyponatremia:** associated with acute cerebral edema, seizures, and coma
   b. **Chronic hyponatremia:** Well tolerated to Na^+ concentrations of 110 mEq/L; symptoms generally include confusion/decreased mental status, irritability, and decreased deep tendon reflexes.

3. **Diagnosis and categorization:** Clinical exam and lab determination of osmolar state are often enough for diagnosis, but, if in doubt (especially with hypo-osmolar hyponatremia), check urine osmolarity and sodium concentration.
   a. **Hypovolemic, hypo-osmolar hyponatremia:** urine Na^+ greater than 20 mEq/L = renal losses, less than 10 mEq/L = extrarenal losses
   b. **Hypervolemic, hypo-osmolar hyponatremia:** urine Na^+ greater than 20 mEq/L = renal failure; Na^+ less than 10 mEq/L = cirrhosis, heart failure
   c. **Euvolemic, hypo-osmolar hyponatremia:** urine osmolarity usually high; urine Na^+ usually greater than 20 mEq/L except in water intoxication

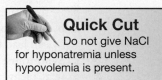
Quick Cut
Do not give NaCl for hyponatremia unless hypovolemia is present.

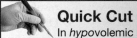
Quick Cut
In *hypo*volemic hypo-osmolar hyponatremia, total body sodium is also usually *low*, whereas in *hyper*volemic hypo-osmolar hyponatremla, total body sodium is usually *high*.

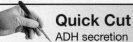
Quick Cut
ADH secretion can be stimulated by the stress response to trauma and surgery, causing free water retention and, in turn, euvolemic hypo-osmolar hyponatremia.

4. Treatment (if minimally symptomatic)
   a. Hyperosmolar: Correct hyperglycemia or source of other actively osmotic particles.
   b. Normo-osmolar: Treat the underlying disease process.
   c. Hypo-osmolar
      (1) Hypovolemic: Treat with isotonic fluid infusion to restore fluid and sodium deficits.
      (2) Hypervolemic: Treat underlying medical cause first, then usually salt and free water restrictions are appropriate.
      (3) Euvolemic: First determine if the true cause is one of the previously mentioned states; if SIADH is the cause, free water restriction usually is enough (do *not* replace salt in solution, which can paradoxically lower serum sodium, as the kidney excretes sodium and conserves water).

Quick Cut
With acutely symptomatic hypo-osmolar hyponatremia, give hypertonic or isotonic saline.

Quick Cut
If the sodium deficit is severe with hypo-osmolar, hypovolemic hyponatremia, *hypertonic* sodium replacement can be considered.

B. Hypernatremia (Na^+ >150 mEq/L)
   1. Categories
      a. Hypovolemia: Hypernatremia almost always represents a free water deficit; total body sodium may be low.
      b. Hypervolemia: Iatrogenic infusion of too much sodium can lead to hypervolemic hypernatremia, but this is rare.
   2. Symptoms: Can include those of volume depletion (e.g., tachycardia, hypotension) as well as other signs of dehydration (e.g., dry mucous membranes, decreased skin turgor); lethargy, confusion, and coma result from water shifts from the intracellular compartment in the central nervous system (CNS).
   3. Diagnosis/etiology (usually simple): high serum sodium with obvious free water losses; in surgical patients, fluid losses may be:
      a. Extrarenal: insensible losses due to fever, mechanical ventilation, burns, diarrhea, or measured losses from the GI tract
      b. Renal: excessive free water excretion
         (1) Osmotic diuresis from hyperglycemia or mannitol administration
         (2) High-output dilute urine from the polyuric phase of acute tubular necrosis (ATN)
   4. Treatment
      a. Hypovolemia: Need to replace volume; calculate free water deficit first:
         (1) Water deficit = 0.6 × body weight (kg) × (serum Na^+/140 − 1)
         (2) Replace half the deficit in the first 8 hours and the remainder in the next 16 hours.
         (3) If the hypovolemic state is severe (i.e., shock), initial resuscitation can be isotonic fluids; if the deficit is less severe, or once perfusion is adequate and the deficit reversed, switch to dextrose 5% in water (D5W) to complete the free water replacement.
      b. Hypervolemia
         (1) If the patient's total body water is increased, first decrease the amount of sodium administered.
         (2) If sodium intake (e.g., antibiotics, total parenteral nutrition [TPN]) cannot be decreased, free water can be infused to lower the serum sodium level, but this does not decrease the total body sodium or water content.
         (3) Diuretics can be used, but sodium can rise.
         (4) Also consider natriuresis

Quick Cut
Giving hypertonic sodium to patients with SIADH can make them worse. The patient will excrete the sodium via the kidneys and hold on to the water.

Quick Cut
Giving furosemide to hypernatremic patients can raise the sodium concentration, even in hypervolemic states. Use free water to equilibrate the sodium concentration prior to diuresis.

III. Potassium
   A. Hypokalemia (K^+ <3.5 mEq/L): *Severe* hypokalemia is defined as a serum potassium level of 3.0 mEq/L or less; in some patients (cardiac), a K^+ higher than 4.0 is desirable.
      1. Symptoms: Include ileus and weakness, and profound depletion results in cardiac dysrhythmias. Electrocardiogram (ECG) changes can become manifest below a K^+ of 3.0 mEq/L and include, in increasing order of severity, T-wave flattening or inversion, depressed ST segments, development

of U waves, prolonged QT interval, and finally ventricular tachycardia.

2. **Diagnosis/etiology (simple and based on blood chemistry):** rarely found in healthy humans with a normal diet and normal kidneys; causes fall in one of four categories:

   a. **Renal:** diuretics, vomiting (renal excretion of K^+ to preserve Na^+), renal tubular acidosis

   b. **Extrarenal:** diarrhea, burns

   c. **Intracellular shift:** insulin, alkalotic state

   d. **Medical disease:** hyperaldosteronism, Cushing syndrome

3. **Treatment**

   a. If symptoms are severe, administer potassium IV as needed to reduce symptoms.

   b. If symptoms are mild, infuse 20 mEq/hr maximum in the unmonitored patient and 40 mEq/hr in the monitored patient.

   c. Administration for more chronic conditions can be via the enteral route.

B. **Hyperkalemia ($K^+ \geq 6$ mEq/L)**

1. **Symptoms:** Rare but include diarrhea, cramping, nervousness, weakness, and flaccid paralysis; more often, cardiac dysrhythmias are manifest before other symptoms become severe, and ECG changes include **peaked T waves** and widened QRS and can eventually degenerate into ventricular fibrillation.

2. **Diagnosis/etiology (numerous):** among the more common are as follows:

   a. **Renal failure:** with inappropriate consumption and administration of K^+

   b. **Extracellular shift:** rhabdomyolysis, massive tissue necrosis, metabolic acidosis, hyperglycemia

   c. **Medical disease:** Addison disease, etc.

3. **Treatment**

   a. **Acutely symptomatic patient**

      (1) **IV calcium** stabilizes cardiac myocyte membranes and can prevent dysrhythmias (1 g Ca^{++} gluconate IV is a standard dose).

      (2) **Glucose/insulin** administration can be used to shift K^+ intracellularly acutely and quickly (1 ampule of D_{50} with 10 units of regular insulin is often enough).

      (3) **Bicarbonate** administration will also shift K^+ intracellularly.

   b. **To remove K^+ and to lower body stores permanently:**

      (1) Ion-exchange resin: used either by mouth or rectally and binds K^+ in the colon, facilitating excretion

      (2) Furosemide: only use if kidneys are able to excrete and closely monitor other electrolytes and fluid balance

      (3) Dialysis

IV. **Chloride**

A. **Hypochloremia ($Cl^- < 90$ mEq/L)**

1. **Symptoms:** usually associated with dehydration or hypokalemia due to vomiting or other GI loss

2. **Diagnosis/etiology**

   a. Stomach hydrochloric acid (HCl) is lost from vomiting, leading to low chloride and a buildup of bicarbonate, causing a **metabolic alkalosis.**

   b. It is often associated with **paradoxic aciduria.** Normally, the kidneys would excrete bicarbonate to reduce pH; however, as the dehydration worsens, the kidneys' drive to retain sodium predominates, and the kidney excretes both K^+ and H^+ to conserve sodium.

Quick Cut
More important than diagnosing hypokalemia is understanding the cause.

Quick Cut
Remember, serum K^+ concentration is not an indication of total body stores of potassium. If the serum K^+ is repleted but total body stores are low, serum K^+ will drop again quickly as K^+ shifts into cells.

Quick Cut
A general rule of thumb is that every 10 mEq of IV K^+ should raise serum concentration by 0.1 mEq/L.

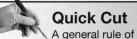

Quick Cut
Acutely, the goal is to stabilize the cardiac membrane and to lower serum potassium in the hypokalemic patient. Once the patient is stabilized, maneuvers to remove K^+ permanently from the body should be instituted.

3. **Treatment:** Replace the chloride and volume deficit with sodium chloride solutions and replace K^+ as needed.

B. **Hyperchloremia (Cl^- >110 mEq/L)**

1. **Cause:** The most common cause in surgical patients is the administration of large amounts of chloride in IV solutions (the chloride content in normal saline [154 mEq/L] is significantly higher than that in plasma [90–110 mEq/L]).

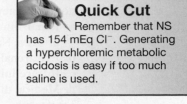

Quick Cut
Remember that NS has 154 mEq Cl^-. Generating a hyperchloremic metabolic acidosis is easy if too much saline is used.

2. **Diagnosis/etiology (easy—check the blood chemistry):** Excess chloride decreases the strong ion difference, thereby causing more water to dissociate and more H^+ ions to be present, leading to metabolic acidosis.

3. **Treatment:** Decrease the amount of chloride being infused; look for all sources (IV antibiotics) in addition to IV fluids (if isotonic saline needs to be administered for other reasons, consider sodium bicarbonate or sodium acetate to reduce chloride load [e.g., ½ NS with 1.5 amps $NaHCO_3^-$/L has 152 mEq/L Na^+, only 77 mEq/L chloride, and 75 mEq/L bicarbonate]).

V. Calcium

A. **Hypocalcemia (Ca^{++} <8 mg/dL)**

1. **Symptoms:** Include neuromuscular irritability with perioral and extremity numbness that may progress to carpopedal spasm and tetany; premature ventricular contractions can be reduced with treatment of hypocalcemia as prolongation of the QT interval is noted in these patients.

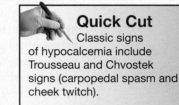

Quick Cut
Classic signs of hypocalcemia include Trousseau and Chvostek signs (carpopedal spasm and cheek twitch).

2. **Diagnosis/etiology (numerous)**

a. **Surgical patients:** Suppression of normal parathyroid function from the removal of adenomatous or hyperplastic glands is most common, followed by accidental damage of the parathyroids during thyroid surgery.

b. **Critically ill patients:** lactate, citrate from blood transfusions, and numerous medicines

c. **Other:** vitamin D deficiency, chronic renal failure, intestinal malabsorption, excess dietary or therapeutic (laxative) magnesium, mercury exposure, chelation therapy

3. **Treatment**

a. **Asymptomatic outpatients:** Can be supplemented orally—investigate possible medical causes (see previous discussion).

b. **Symptomatic patients:** Monitor and treat.

(1) If symptoms are mild, large doses of oral calcium are often adequate (especially in the postparathyroidectomy patient).

(2) Severely symptomatic patients should be repleted with IV calcium until symptoms resolve and an appropriate oral regimen is tolerated.

B. **Hypercalcemia (Ca^{++} ≥10.5 mg/dL)**

1. **Symptoms:** Fatigue, confusion, nausea, vomiting, diarrhea, dehydration, and anorexia are common; when related to hyperparathyroidism, renal calculi and ulcer disease are more common.

2. **Diagnosis/etiology (numerous)**

a. **Endocrine:** primary hyperparathyroidism (most common), thyrotoxicosis

b. **Malignancy:** most common (up to 20%–30% of cancer patients), often from osteolytic or parathyroid hormone–related protein (PTHrP)–secreting lesions

c. **Granulomatous disease:** sarcoidosis, tuberculosis

d. **Medications:** excess calcium ingestion, vitamin D toxicity, thiazide diuretics

e. **Other:** renal disease, milk alkali syndrome, familial hypocalciuric hypocalcemia

3. **Treatment**

a. **First-line therapy:** Aggressive isotonic resuscitation, leading to diuresis and calcium excretion; if unsuccessful, furosemide can be added.

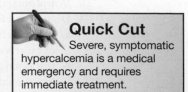

Quick Cut
Severe, symptomatic hypercalcemia is a medical emergency and requires immediate treatment.

b. **Medical therapy:** Medications to stop osteoclastic activity are the mainstream (i.e., bisphosphonates, calcitonin, and steroids are all used; plicacamycin is no longer available in the United States).

ACID–BASE DISTURBANCES

Regulatory Systems

I. **Carbon dioxide:** CO_2 production can exceed 15,000 mmol/day from metabolic processes (e.g., lung excretion). If Pco_2 increases, water dissociates and HCO_3^- and H^+ form based on the **Henderson-Hasselbalch equation**, thus decreasing pH. The reverse happens for lower Pco_2 concentrations. Either a loss of bicarbonate or a gain in protons can cause acidosis.

II. **Strong ions:** Ions that completely dissociate in water (e.g., Na^+, Cl^-, Ca^{++}, Mg^{++}, K^+). In a pure salt solution, ion concentrations are equal, and pH is neutral, whereas in plasma, cations outnumber anions. To maintain electrical neutrality, water dissociates, H^+ is excreted, and HCO_3^- concentration increases, creating a pH of 7.4, not 7.0.

III. **Weak acids:** Weak acids can exist as negatively charged molecules or accept H^+ and exist uncharged. These **buffering systems** include proteins and phosphates.

Quick Cut
The human body requires a very narrow pH range of 7.35–7.45 to function properly. Three main systems in the body maintain the pH within normal parameters: carbon dioxide, strong ions, and weak acids.

Quick Cut
The Henderson-Hasselbalch equation: $pH = pK \times \log [HCO_3^-/(0.03 \times Pco_2)]$.

Acidosis

The body's pH decreases when the Pco_2 increases, the concentration of HCO_3^- increases, the concentration of strong anions increases, or the concentration of weak acids increases. A pH less than 7.35 is considered pathologic, but patients can compensate from the following disorders of acid–base metabolism or have a mixed picture with a pH in the normal range.

Quick Cut
Acidosis is a pH-lowering process; *acidemia* is a low blood pH.

I. **Respiratory acidosis**

    A. Causes

        1. **Decreased ventilation** leads to increased CO_2 concentration. Any cause of depressed respirations can cause this pathology.

        2. **Increased CO_2 production.** Excess enteral or parenteral carbohydrate administration can increase the respiratory quotient and production of CO_2. Hospitalized patients may not be able to compensate.

    B. Treatment: The primary method for respiratory acidosis is to increase alveolar ventilation. In cases of drug overdose, this may be accomplished with appropriate reversing agents; however, most alveolar hypoventilation requires intubation with mechanical ventilation to clear CO_2 and return the pH to normal values.

II. **Metabolic acidosis** results either from HCO_3^- loss or accumulation of strong anions (measured or nonmeasured) or weak acids.

    A. Causes

        1. **Weak acid accumulation** (anion gap): Etiology includes loss of HCO_3^- to maintain electric neutrality.

            a. Acid accumulation can occur because of **renal failure** and the inability of the kidneys to clear acid by-products of metabolism.

            b. Lactic acidosis: A common cause is lactic acid, which results from inadequate tissue perfusion and anaerobic metabolism.

            c. Diabetic ketoacidosis: Acetoacetate and beta-hydroxybutyrate are weak acids.

            d. Toxins (polyethylene glycol, methanol): Methanol is metabolized to formaldehyde and then formic acid.

        2. **Strong anion accumulation:** normal anion gap

            a. Hyperchloremic acidosis: Excess chloride induces water to dissociate, H^+ to accumulate, and pH to drop.

        3. **Loss of bicarbonate:** normal anion gap

            a. Excess renal excretion of bicarbonate

            b. Diarrhea

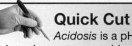

Quick Cut
To determine the etiology of metabolic acidosis, check the anion gap. If high, remember CUTE DIMPLES: cyanide, uremia, toluene, ethanol, diabetic ketoacidosis, isoniazid, methanol, propylene glycol, lactic acidosis, ethylene glycol, salicylates.

B. Treatment: The primary treatment for metabolic acidosis is correction of the underlying metabolic problem/disease and proper fluid and electrolyte management. Bicarbonate administration should *rarely* be used unless pH is dangerously low (<7.2) and the underlying defect is being corrected (exception: If the primary defect is excess loss of bicarbonate [diarrhea, renal tubular acidosis], bicarbonate therapy could be considered).

Alkalosis

I. **Respiratory alkalosis**
   A. **Causes**
      1. **Spontaneously breathing patient:** caused by alveolar ventilation increase and subsequent reduction in CO_2 levels (anxiety, pain, shock, sepsis, toxic substances [salicylate poisoning], or CNS dysfunction)
      2. **Mechanically ventilated patient:** Iatrogenic overventilation is common.

   > **Quick Cut**
   > Some processes (*think of pulmonary embolus!*) causing hypoxia or intrapulmonary shunts can lead to hypocarbia and alkalosis.

   B. **Treatment:** Includes decreasing minute ventilation and allowing CO_2 levels to return to normal. Most cases are self-limited, however, as patients cannot keep excessive ventilatory drive for extended periods.

II. **Metabolic alkalosis:** pH increases to higher than 7.45, and HCO_3^- is greater than 26 mEq/L.
   A. **Causes**
      1. Most common noniatrogenic cause of metabolic alkalosis is loss of gastric contents (HCl and large volumes of water are lost). To compensate for dehydration, the kidney excretes H^+ to conserve Na^+ (**paradoxical aciduria**). The concentration of strong anions is reduced, and water is less likely to dissociate, further decreasing H^+ and increasing pH.
      2. **Other causes**
         a. Drugs that limit renal excretion of HCO_3^- (e.g., steroids and diuretics)
         b. Overadministration of alkali (e.g., in ulcer therapy), acetate in TPN that is used to replace other anions, and citrate in transfused blood that is converted to CO_2 and water and then to HCO_3^- by the kidneys

   > **Quick Cut**
   > **Paradoxical aciduria:** The kidney exchanges H^+ for Na^+, so the urine may be acidic but the patient alkalotic.

   B. **Treatment:** The first step is to stop the loss of chloride and to replace the water and chloride with isotonic sodium chloride and potassium supplementation. For other causes, stopping the offending agent is usually sufficient.

Diagnosing Acid–base Disorders Based on the Blood Gas (Table 1-4)

Table 1-4: Acid–base Disorders

Disorder		Pco₂	HCO₃⁻	pH	Expected Compensation
Respiratory acidosis	Acute	↑	Normal	<7.35	1–4 mEq/L HCO₃⁻ for each 10 mm Hg Pco₂ rise
	Compensated	↑	↑	7.35–7.40	
Respiratory alkalosis	Acute	↓	Normal	>7.45	2–5 mEq/L HCO₃⁻ for each 10 mm Hg Pco₂ drop
	Compensated	↓	↓	7.40–7.45	
Metabolic acidosis	Acute	Normal	↓	<7.35	Expected Pco₂ = 1.5(HCO₃⁻) + 8
	Compensated	↓	↓	7.35–7.40	
Metabolic alkalosis	Acute	Normal	↑	>7.45	Expected Pco₂ = 0.7(HCO₃⁻) + 20
	Compensated	↑	↑	7.40–7.45	

COAGULATION

Hemostasis Mechanism Phases

I. **Primary hemostasis**

    A. **Platelet adherence:** The first step in controlling hemorrhage is platelet adherence to the injured vessel via glycoprotein (Gp) receptor Ib in conjunction with von Willebrand factor.

    B. **Platelet activation:** Activated platelets produce thromboxane A_2 and other vasoconstrictors, which reduce blood flow through the injured vessel. Gp IIb/IIIa is expressed, which promotes platelet–platelet adhesion (fibrinogen required) and **platelet plug** formation.

II. **Clot formation:** Tissue factor exposed due to vessel injury or in response to inflammation begins the **clotting cascade** (traditionally taught as having an intrinsic and extrinsic pathway; however, in vivo, both pathways act in concert).

    A. **Extrinsic pathway:** Tissue factor binds factor VII and activates it (VIIa). VIIa subsequently activates factor X. Xa then converts prothrombin to thrombin.

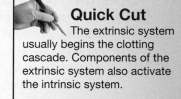

Quick Cut
The extrinsic system usually begins the clotting cascade. Components of the extrinsic system also activate the intrinsic system.

    B. **Intrinsic pathway:** In general, factor XIIa activates XI, then XIa activates IX. IX then converges with the extrinsic pathway by activating factor X. This pathway can be initiated either by exposure to a negatively charged surface (exposed collagen from a damaged vessel) or thrombin itself activates factor IX.

    C. **Both pathways converge at factor X:** Factor Xa then mediates conversion of prothrombin to thrombin with factor Va as a cofactor. Thrombin mediates fibrinogen conversion to fibrin. Finally, factor XIIIa mediates cross-linking of fibrin.

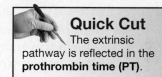

Quick Cut
The extrinsic pathway is reflected in the **prothrombin time (PT)**.

III. **Regulation and fibrinolysis:** The coagulation system is a *cascade*, meaning that each activated intermediate factor is able to activate many of the factors in subsequent steps. Thrombin itself acts as a positive feedback loop by activating factor IX. The fibrinolytic system acts to balance the coagulation cascade and to remove clots once healing has started.

    A. Tissue factor pathway inhibitor (TFPI) may inhibit TF–VIIa complexes.

        1. Protein C and protein S degrade factors V and VIII.

        2. Antithrombin III inhibits thrombin-Xa complexes.

        3. **Fibrinolysis:** Tissue-type plasminogen activator (t-PA) and urokinase-type plasminogen activator (uPA) mediate conversion of plasminogen to plasmin, which cleaves fibrin.

Coagulopathy

I. **History:** Lab studies should not be routinely ordered preoperatively in a patient with a negative history, whereas in a positive history, studies can be used to specify the diagnosis.

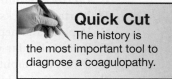

Quick Cut
The history is the most important tool to diagnose a coagulopathy.

    A. **Include any patient-perceived coagulopathy:** bruising, petechia, easy bleeding/nosebleeds, history of bleeding from other procedures (dental/surgical)

    B. **Family history**

    C. **Medical conditions/risk factors:** liver disease (cirrhosis), renal failure (uremia)

II. **Physical:** evidence of bruising or petechia

III. **Laboratory evaluation**

    A. **Platelet count:** normal is 150,000–400,000/mL blood

    B. **Bleeding time:** Measure of platelet function. Disorders of platelet function include uremia, drugs (aspirin, clopidogrel, Gp II B/III A inhibitors), von Willebrand disease, and low platelet count.

    C. **Prothrombin time:** PT measures the extrinsic cascade. Because factors II (thrombin), VII, and X are produced by the liver, PT represents a good measure of vitamin K–dependent coagulation factors and is therefore used to monitor warfarin therapy. The international normalized ratio (INR) is a normalization factor to equate lab values between labs.

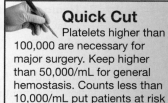

Quick Cut
Platelets higher than 100,000 are necessary for major surgery. Keep higher than 50,000/mL for general hemostasis. Counts less than 10,000/mL put patients at risk for spontaneous bleeding.

D. **Activated partial thromboplastin time (aPTT):** measures the intrinsic cascade and is useful for following patients on IV unfractionated heparin therapy

E. **Thrombin time:** Tests the conversion of fibrinogen to fibrin via thrombin; it is elevated when fibrinogen is depleted or nonfunctioning and in the presence of heparin.

F. **Thromboelastogram (TEG):** measures holistically clot formation and breakdown kinetics

G. **Activated clotting time (ACT):** rapidly determines effect of high-dose heparin; used in cardiac surgery

H. **Anti-factor Xa activity:** used to monitor low-molecular-weight heparin activity

> **Quick Cut**
> The TEG is rapidly becoming the standard of care test to identify bleeding disorders in trauma patients and in the intensive care unit (ICU).

Specific Hypocoagulopathic States

I. **First, ensure bleeding is not a surgical complication:** Do not necessarily blame postoperative bleeding on coagulopathy until surgical bleeding is ruled out.

II. **Liver disease:** In severe liver disease, hepatocytes cannot manufacture clotting factors. PT/INR is elevated. Treatment includes replacing factors with **fresh frozen plasma (FFP)**. Chronically, vitamin K can improve hepatic synthetic function.

III. **Renal disease:** Uremia causes platelet dysfunction. Treatment can be with DDAVP, which causes release of von Willebrand factor or FFP.

IV. **Disseminated intravascular coagulopathy (DIC):** Microvascular coagulation due to inflammation from sepsis, trauma, and other severe insults leads to a consumption and deficit of factors, leading to coagulopathy. The mainstay of treatment includes treating the underlying cause. Replacement of factors may exacerbate the condition; paradoxically, anticoagulant therapy may be beneficial.

V. **Consumption/dilution**
A. Due to severe trauma, sepsis, major surgery, and their attendant fluid resuscitation; treatment involves correcting the underlying cause and replacing factors with FFP.
B. Hypofibrinogen states need cryoprecipitate.
C. **Hypothermia and acidosis:** inhibit proper clotting mechanisms

VI. **Medically induced**
A. **Aspirin:** *permanently* binds cyclooxygenase (COX), preventing platelet aggregation
B. **Plavix:** blocks adenosine diphosphate (ADP)–mediated platelet aggregation
C. **Gp IIb/IIIA inhibitors:** inhibit platelet aggregation
D. **Warfarin:** blocks vitamin K–dependent liver synthesis of factors II, VII, IX, and X
E. **Heparin and heparinoids:** augment antithrombin-III function
F. **Low-molecular-weight heparin:** inhibits factor Xa
G. **Direct thrombin inhibitors:** argatroban, dabigatran
H. **Factor Xa inhibitors:** apixaban
I. **Fibrinolytics:** tissue plasminogen activator (tPA), urokinase, etc., mediate fibrinolysis

VII. **Hemophilia**
A. **Hemophilia A:** Congenital deficiency of factor VIII; treatment is factor replacement. FFP can be used in emergent situations.
B. **Hemophilia B:** Congenital deficiency of factor IX; treatment is factor replacement. FFP can be used in emergent situations.

VIII. **von Willebrand disease:** The most common congenital coagulopathy (1%–2% of adults) is deficiency of von Willebrand factor. Treatment is intranasal DDAVP in mild cases, IV DDAVP prior to surgical procedures, and cryoprecipitate or FFP in emergencies.

IX. **Others:** autoimmune diseases, cancer, snake venom

> **Quick Cut**
> Recombinant activated factor VII (rfVIIa) is approved for use in treating hemophiliacs who have developed antibodies to factors VIII and IX. Although not replacing the missing factors, supraphysiologic doses of rfVIIa cause a thrombin burst and clot to form, which has led to study of its efficacy to treat other coagulopathies, including warfarin therapy when quick reversal is needed (i.e., intracranial bleed) and in severe traumatic coagulopathy.

Specific Hypercoagulable States

I. **Surgical patients:** Surgery, trauma, and sepsis cause proinflammatory states that lead to a hypercoagulable state; therefore, surgical patients are at risk for **deep venous thrombosis (DVT).**

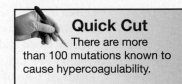

Quick Cut
Always assess your surgical patients for thromboembolic prophylaxis. Most hospitals have protocols now that must be followed.

    A. Major risk factors include major abdominal or pelvic surgery; orthopedic surgery, especially lower extremity; trauma, especially spine, pelvis, and lower extremity fractures; prolonged immobilization; cancer; smoking; obesity; central line placement; and others.

    B. Heparin 5,000 units subcutaneously every 8 hours or low-molecular-weight heparin subcutaneously daily or twice daily should be used; in patients who have contraindications to prophylaxis (intracranial bleed), inferior vena cava filters should be considered.

II. **Congenital risk factors:** Suspect if patients have multiple DVT or DVT without another known risk factor; treatment is usually anticoagulation.

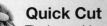

Quick Cut
There are more than 100 mutations known to cause hypercoagulability.

    A. **Protein S deficiency**
    B. **Protein C deficiency**
    C. **Factor V Leiden mutation**
    D. **Antithrombin III mutations**
    E. **Others**

PACKED RED BLOOD CELL TRANSFUSION THERAPY

Transfusion Risks

I. **Febrile reactions/allergic: most common immune reaction**

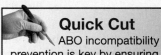

Quick Cut
The longer blood is stored, the worse it performs. Over time, cells lyse, and 2,3-diphosphoglycerate (2,3-DPG) levels fall, causing oxygen to bind more avidly.

    A. Usually related to either cytokines or donor leukocyte or other contaminants or a mild antibody response and is usually self-limited

    B. Can be prevented by leukodepletion and pretransfusion antipyretics

II. **Electrolyte disturbances**

    A. **Hyperkalemia:** Lysed cells can cause hyperkalemia.
    B. **Hypocalcemia:** Citrate in stored blood can bind calcium.

III. **Coagulopathy:** Packed red blood cells (pRBCs) do not contain clotting factors or platelet. Large-volume transfusion without these other products can cause a coagulopathy.

IV. **ABO incompatibility**

    A. **Etiology:** intravascular immune reaction, leading to clumping and lysis of red cells with mismatched blood

    B. **Signs and symptoms:** hemoglobinuria, fever, chills, coagulopathy, renal failure, and circulatory collapse

Quick Cut
ABO incompatibility prevention is key by ensuring correct patient identity and blood type to avoid consequent *preventable reactions*.

V. **Delayed hemolytic reaction:** usually takes 3–7 days to manifest

    A. **Signs and symptoms:** fever, malaise, hyperbilirubinemia, and decreasing hematocrit, usually related to minor antibody systems (e.g., Rh system)

    B. Usually but not always preventable with recipient antibody screening

    C. **Treatment:** hydration and supportive care

VI. **Disease transmission:** Many viruses are transmitted by blood, which was once a real risk. With modern screening methods (e.g., nucleic acid technology), the risk is theoretical and negligible.

    A. **HIV:** estimated to be 1:2,000,000
    B. **Hepatitis C:** estimated to be 1:2,000,000
    C. **Hepatitis B:** estimated to be 1:2,000,000

D. Others: Risks less known but have been described. Human t-lymphotropic virus (HTLV) 1 and 2, West Nile virus, Creutzfeldt-Jakob disease; overall risk of viral transmission may be as high as 1:50,000.

VII. Immunosuppression: Negative outcomes include the following:
  A. Morbidity: increased **infectious complications**, including ventilator-associated pneumonia
  B. Possible increases in **cancer recurrence** following potentially curative surgery
  C. Increased mortality: in ICU patients

Transfusion Indications

  I. Acute coronary disease: Standard trigger is 8 g/dL.

  II. Trauma patients: Exsanguinating patients (class III shock) should be given blood as resuscitation.
  A. Their Hgb measurement may still be high acutely, but they are losing blood and its attendant oxygen-carrying capacity.
  B. Blood/FFP ratios are being currently studied, but resuscitation with 1:1 ratio of blood/FFP with platelets every fourth round and minimal to no crystalloid.

  III. ICU patients: If needed, direct measurements of oxygen delivery and oxygen extraction can help to guide transfusion therapy to determine if extra oxygen-carrying capacity is needed.

  IV. General (non-ICU) patients: only transfuse if symptomatic (e.g., tachycardia, tachypnea, confusion, lethargy, and acidosis)

Transfusion Alternatives

  I. Elective surgery (if the time of blood loss is known)
  A. Autologous banked blood
  B. Epoetin alpha: can increase hct preoperatively to help avoid transfusion; useful in renal failure patients and those with chronic anemia
  C. Autotransfusion: recycle blood lost during surgery
  D. Acute normovolemic hemodilution
    1. Once a patient is anesthetized, blood can be removed, stored, and replaced with crystalloid or colloid to maintain euvolemia.
    2. Benefits
      a. Blood lost during surgery has a lower hct; therefore, fewer red cells are shed.
      b. Those that are shed can be replaced with fresh (not stored) autologous blood that was just removed.
  E. Directed donor: Risk of virus transmission is lower, but similar risks of immunomodulation and other reactions exist.
  F. Hemostatic agents: prevent blood loss in the first place
    1. FFP/cryoprecipitate: for patients with coagulopathy
    2. DDAVP: for platelet dysfunction, especially renal failure
    3. Tranexamic acid: inhibits serine proteases, including plasmin, and is therefore antifibrinolytic; increasingly used in trauma
    4. Lysine analogs: ϵ-aminocaproic acid
    5. Topical hemostatics: fibrin glue

  II. Acute unexpected blood loss
  A. Autotransfusion: may still be an option, if readily available
    1. Emergent aortic rupture
    2. Trauma laparotomy
    3. Hemothorax: Autotransfuse blood from the chest tube.
  B. Prevent further blood loss.

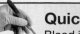

Quick Cut
Blood is an immunosuppressant associated with adverse outcomes in surgical patients. Only use when needed.

Quick Cut
Prior transfusion triggers of a hemoglobin (Hgb) of 10 g/dL or hematocrit (hct) of 30% were artificially set. *Transfusion decisions should be based on individual patient circumstances.* In general, it is safe to let the Hgb drop to 7 mg/dL and even lower in healthy, young individuals.

Quick Cut
Patients with *acute* coronary syndromes may need higher Hgb levels, but this is debatable.

Quick Cut
An Hgb transfusion trigger of 7 is as safe as 10 and reduces complications . . . even in those with a history of cardiac disease.

Quick Cut
Isotonic fluids can be used to support intravascular volume.

Quick Cut
Quick prevention of further blood loss is the best therapy for unexpected blood loss.

NUTRITION AND THE SURGICAL PATIENT

Energy Sources: Protein, Glucose, and Fat

I. **Protein**

  A. Requires conversion to glucose via hepatic gluconeogenesis to be used as a caloric fuel source

  B. Adequate intake is important for muscle mass maintenance and other protein-dependent, non–energy-producing processes.

II. **Glucose:** can be stored as glycogen and used as a short-term reservoir of energy

III. **Fat:** Majority of energy is stored as fat and to a lesser degree as protein (skeletal muscle).

Caloric and Protein Requirements

I. **Caloric requirements**

  A. **Basal metabolic rate (BMR):** amount of energy used by an unstressed, fasted individual at rest

  B. **Resting energy expenditure (REE):** amount of energy used by an unstressed, nonfasted individual at rest

  C. **Total energy expenditure (TEE):** actual amount of energy an individual uses

   1. TEE can increase significantly above REE by hypermetabolic conditions (e.g., surgery, trauma, sepsis, and burns).

   2. TEE can increased by voluntary work (e.g., exercise), whereas during starvation, the BMR decreases as the body adjusts to conserve body mass. Caloric requirements can be determined by indirect calorimetry or the **Fick equation**.

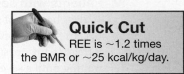

Quick Cut
REE is ~1.2 times the BMR or ~25 kcal/kg/day.

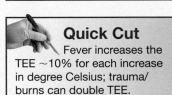

Quick Cut
Fever increases the TEE ~10% for each increase in degree Celsius; trauma/burns can double TEE.

II. **Protein Requirements**

  A. **Normal**

   1. Low because each protein molecule has a specific purpose and is therefore not generally available as an energy source

   2. Generally, daily protein requirements are only 0.8–1.0 g/kg/day, which is significantly less than the average American eats daily.

  B. **Starvation**

   1. The body makes every attempt to conserve protein. Because glycogen stores are metabolized within the first 24 hours of starvation, another source of glucose must be found for the tissues that cannot, or usually do not, use fats (i.e., brain cells, red and white blood cells). Proteins are broken down and converted to glucose in the liver by **gluconeogenesis** to supply the brain and blood cells with glucose.

   2. In unstressed starvation, protein catabolism can be prevented by exogenous administration of glucose. The brain adapts to use **ketones**, which are produced when fat is metabolized, and decreases the amount of protein that must be metabolized as a glucose source. After all of the available fat is metabolized, protein is degraded at a high rate until the total body protein stores are ~½ of baseline, at which time death occurs.

  C. **Severe illness**

   1. The body is not able to conserve energy and protein stores as it does during unstressed starvation.

   2. The **hormonal milieu** increases the BMR, decreases the ability to use fats and ketones, and thereby increases the dependence on glucose as an energy source. This glucose can come only from protein that is being degraded.

   3. As the degree of illness or injury increases, the **catabolic rate** increases accordingly, leading to a rapid breakdown of protein stores and multiorgan dysfunction if not checked. During the acute phase of severe illness or stressed starvation, protein catabolism is minimally affected by exogenous administration of glucose.

   4. **Primary treatment:** Eliminate the underlying cause of the stress response and provide enough calories and protein to replace metabolic and catabolic losses.

   5. As the illness begins to subside, the hormonal milieu changes, which leads to less retention of salt and water and a change from a catabolic protein environment to an **anabolic environment**. The nitrogen balance is positive, meaning that less nitrogen is lost than is administered to the patient. This balance represents protein that is being laid down and thus improvement of the patient's health.

Nutrition Status Evaluation

I. **Thin, cachectic patient:** Exhibits hollowed cheeks, no body fat, and very little muscle and is obviously in a poor nutritional state. Generally, patients who have acutely lost 10% of their body weight are considered malnourished and need nutritional support.

II. **Obese patient and well-developed patients:** may need as much nutritional support as the patient in a poor nutritional state, depending on the underlying disease process

III. **Previously well-nourished patient:** Generally able to endure a major operation and 5–10 days of starvation without an increase in morbidity or mortality. If the period of starvation extends beyond 10 days, nutritional support is necessary.

IV. **Patients with severe illness:** If unable to eat for more than 10 days because of surgery, consider early nutritional support. Because it takes several days to take effect, beginning such support if there is any question of nutritional deficit is more effective than waiting until a severe deficit occurs.

Therapy

I. **Goals:** The average hospitalized patient requires ~2,000 cal daily and ~60 g of protein.

   A. **Energy:** Determine caloric requirements to provide adequate energy substrates (i.e., carbohydrates, fats) and avoid excess calories in one of four ways.

      1. **Indirect calorimetry:** Measures amount of oxygen inhaled minus amount of oxygen exhaled to determine amount of oxygen consumed. Because oxygen consumption (VO_2) measured in mL O_2/min is directly correlated to kcal/day (1 mL O_2/min = ~7 kcal/day), measurement of the amount of oxygen consumed can determine daily caloric requirements.

      2. **Fick equation:** Amount of oxygen consumed, and therefore kcal required, is determined by multiplying the cardiac output by the arteriovenous oxygen content difference.

      3. **Harris-Benedict equations:** Daily caloric requirements are determined by calculating REE from gender-based equations using gender, height, weight, and age variable and then multiplying by an estimated stress factor.

      4. **Estimated REE (25 kcal/kg/day):** multiplied by an estimated stress factor

   B. **Protein:** Determine protein requirements in one of four ways.

      1. **Nitrogen balance:** The majority of catabolized protein is lost as urinary urea nitrogen, with ~2–4 g of nitrogen lost in stool. Protein grams divided by 6.25 equals nitrogen grams. Amount of nitrogen intake minus nitrogen output should be positive if adequate protein is given and the patient is not too catabolic.

      2. **Visceral protein measurement (e.g., albumin, transferrin, prealbumin)**

         a. Due to the long half-life of albumin, it should only be used to assess malnutrition in outpatient and elective surgery patients.

         b. Prealbumin has a shorter half-life and is more reflective of protein nutrition in hospitalized patients.

         c. A C-reactive protein (CRP) should be checked because elevated levels of inflammation (trauma/sepsis/burns) will alter visceral protein production away from prealbumin synthesis.

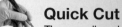

Quick Cut
The overall goal of nutritional support is to supply adequate energy in the form of calories and adequate protein for building proteins in the body.

Quick Cut
A ratio of 150 cal:1 g of protein is optimal. Mineral and trace elements are included in most formulas in adequate amounts to prevent deficiencies or toxicities.

Quick Cut
Fick equation: CO = $VO_2/(C_a - C_v)$, where CO = cardiac output, C_a = oxygen concentration of arterial blood, and C_v = oxygen concentration of mixed venous blood. $C_a - C_v$ is also known as the **arteriovenous oxygen difference**.

Quick Cut
Harris-Benedict gender-based equations:
Men: BMR = 88.362 + (13.397 × weight in kg) + (4.799 × height in cm) − (5.677 × age in years)

Women: BMR = 447.593 + (9.247 × weight in kg) + (3.098 × height in cm) − (4.330 × age in years)

Quick Cut
The protein requirement for most adults is ~0.8 g/kg/day (or 56 g for the hypothetical 70-kg patient). During severe illness with a high catabolic rate, this requirement may increase to 2 g/kg/day of protein or greater.

3. **Weight gain (poor method):** Because most patients needing nutritional support in the hospital are stressed, they tend to retain water and become edematous. Also, they will be catabolic and lose lean body weight despite the increase of their actual body weight from fluid gain.

4. **Observe the overall condition of the patient (best overall method):** Obtain nitrogen balances (maximum of twice weekly), follow visceral proteins (prealbumin/CRP twice weekly), and increase protein administration (although there is no theoretical limit to the maximum amount of protein that can be administered, protein in excess of the patient's needs will result in a rise in blood urea nitrogen [BUN]).

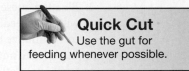

Quick Cut
When determining whether nutritional support is adequate for hospitalized patients, observing the patient's overall condition is better than monitoring weight gain alone.

II. **Enteral nutrition:** The preferred route to provide nutrition is enterally to maintain gut mucosal integrity and reduce complications. The gut is important in critically ill patients; if unused for even brief periods, the mucosa begins to atrophy and lose its barrier function, leading to bacterial translocation

Quick Cut
Use the gut for feeding whenever possible.

and worsening systemic inflammation. In addition to translocation, the atrophied mucosa is unable to digest food when food is ultimately presented, which leads to further delays in adequate nutrition.

A. **Formula compositions:** When possible, patients should be fed by mouth; however, with critical illness, aspiration risk, depressed mental status, or inability to take adequate calories or protein orally, administration of enteral feeding formulas is necessary. These formulas are designed to provide adequate nutrition and may be routine or ones that are highly specialized to serve the needs of unique patient populations.

1. **Standard formulas:** suitable for most patients
   a. Provide a balanced calorie/protein ratio with ~50%–65% of calories from carbohydrates, 10%–20% from proteins, and the rest from fats
   b. Caloric density is ~1.0–1.2 kcal/mL; they include the essential fats, minerals, and trace elements.

2. **Elemental formulas:** amino acid or small peptide–based for ease of digestion and lower residue in patients with short gut syndrome or distal enterocutaneous fistulas

3. **Calorie-dense formulas:** contain more calories per milliliter than standard formulas (typically 1.5–2.0 kcal/mL) for patients needing fluid restriction or very high caloric requirements

4. **Protein-dense formulas:** provide increased protein (20%–25% of calories) for patients with very high protein needs

5. **Fat-based formulas:** provide more calories from fats rather than glucose and attempt to reduce CO_2 production by altering the respiratory quotient for patients with compromised minute ventilation (e.g., severe chronic obstructive pulmonary disease [COPD] and acute respiratory distress syndrome [ARDS] patients)

6. **Immunomodulating formulas:** Provide glutamine and typically omega-3 fatty acids to enhance immunologic function; however, efficacy is mixed. Some recommend them for mechanically ventilated patients with systemic inflammatory response syndrome (SIRS) from sepsis, trauma, burns, acute lung injury (ALI), etc.

B. **Administration route**

1. Enteral nutrition formulas can be delivered by tubes placed into the GI tract directly (gastrostomy, feeding jejunostomy) or via the nose (nasogastric, nasoduodenal, or nasojejunal).

2. An abdominal radiograph to determine proper tube placement should be obtained prior to starting tube feedings on feeding tubes placed orally or nasally at the bedside.

3. Postpyloric placement (jejunostomy, nasoduodenal, nasojejunal) is associated with earlier tolerance but is more difficult, leading to potential delays in initiation of enteral nutrition.

4. Early initiation of enteral nutrition (<48 hours) is associated with fewer complications and should be used even in the immediate postoperative period following abdominal surgery or trauma.

C. **Administration rate:** Enteral nutrition should be started as continuous infusion.
  1. A reasonable starting point is full strength at 20 mL/hr and increased by 20 mL/hr every 6–12 hours until the goal rate is obtained or excessive residuals are noted.
  2. The goal rate is determined by the patient's caloric needs and the caloric density of the formula.
  3. Gastric residual volumes of tube feedings should be checked every 4 hours for excessive residual volumes (>500 mL), even if feedings are postpyloric.
    a. If residual volumes are high, the infusion should be stopped and then resumed after 4 hours.
    b. If residuals continue to be high, the cause (ileus, obstruction) should be sought.
D. **Complications**
  1. Gastric content aspiration is the most common complication of enteral nutrition but can be reduced by monitoring residual volumes and maintaining the head of the bed up 30 degrees.
  2. Bloating, mesenteric ischemia (rare), and diarrhea may occur with tube feedings, but adjustments in composition and rate can minimize these issues.
  3. Inadequate nutritional supplementation caused by frequent feeding cessation is not uncommon unless concerted efforts are made to avoid it.

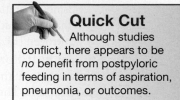

Quick Cut
Although studies conflict, there appears to be *no* benefit from postpyloric feeding in terms of aspiration, pneumonia, or outcomes.

III. **Parenteral (IV) nutrition:** TPN allows the provision of adequate nutrition when the GI tract is usable due to malabsorption, obstruction, fistulas, or anatomic changes. Combined enteral and parenteral administration is sometimes beneficial.
A. **Formula composition:** TPN solutions should contain components of nutritional requirements because other sources may not be available.
  1. **Carbohydrates:** Predominantly as glucose solution; provide ~50% of total calories and cause TPN to have a high osmolality. Partial (or peripheral) parenteral nutrition (PPN) contains lower concentration of glucose and is not significantly hyperosmolar.
  2. **Amino acid solution:** provide ~10% of total calories and importantly providing essential amino acids for metabolism, especially in hypercatabolic patients
  3. **Fats:** administered either continuously or intermittently as lipid emulsion and are necessary to avoid essential fatty acid deficiency
    a. Lipid emulsions also provide the most calories in the smallest volume (fat has the highest caloric density) and produce less CO_2 (lowest respiratory quotient), which may be important in patients with volume restrictions or compromised ventilation.
    b. Administration of lipid emulsions can lead to hypertriglyceridemia; levels should be routinely monitored.
  4. **Electrolytes:** include the monovalent cations, sodium and potassium; the divalent cations, calcium and magnesium; and the anions, chloride and acetate (converted to bicarbonate in the liver), which can be adjusted as needed
  5. **Vitamins and trace elements:** Must be provided to avoid acquired deficiencies; specifically, the exogenous administration of B vitamins, vitamin E/selenium (lipid peroxidation and free radical scavenging), zinc (wound healing, immunity), and chromium (insulin sensitivity) should be considered in patients receiving TPN.
  6. **Medications:** May be incorporated into TPN; parenteral stress ulcer prophylaxis medications and insulin are the most frequently added.
B. **Administration route:** usually via a percutaneously placed venous line with the tip located in the vena cava
C. **Administration rate:** TPN is typically provided continuously at a rate that provides adequate calories to meet the patient's needs and depends on caloric density and degree of hypermetabolism.
  1. Commonly, patients are started at half the goal rate for 12 hours before advancing to the full rate to avoid severe hyperglycemia.
  2. Some advocate decreasing the TPN rate by half for 6–12 hours prior to stopping to avoid hypoglycemia.
  3. Cycling to allow patients to be disconnected for periods of time during the day can be accomplished but should only be prescribed by experienced personnel and on selected patients.

Quick Cut
The high osmolality of TPN causes phlebitis and sclerosis if infused into a peripheral vein (less hyperosmolar PPN can be delivered via a peripheral vein but typically does not meet caloric needs).

D. Complications

1. Include those related to line placement (hemothorax, pneumothorax); infections (line sepsis, pneumonia, acalculous cholecystitis); hyperglycemia (associated with increased infection risk and death); hepatic dysfunction; and abnormalities in electrolytes, vitamins, fatty acids, and trace elements

2. TPN is associated with higher morbidity and mortality than enteral nutrition usually due to infectious and hepatic complications. In patients unable to receive adequate enteral nutrition, this increased risk is unavoidable.

THE INTENSIVE CARE UNIT

Specialized Intensive Care Unit Care and Monitoring

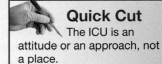

Quick Cut
The ICU is an attitude or an approach, not a place.

I. **Intensive patient care:** The acuity of a patient's condition may require close nursing and physician observation and management, which can only be provided in an ICU setting, where one nurse cares for only one or two patients at a time and physicians are present at all times.

II. **Management specific to the ICU:** provides critically ill patients with specific care and monitoring not typically available in other hospital units

A. **Airway control (endotracheal intubation):** placement of an artificial airway to prevent airway obstruction or to provide mechanical ventilation

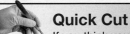

Quick Cut
If you think you might have to intubate a patient . . . *do it*! It is easier to extubate an intubated patient than to resuscitate from respiratory arrest.

1. **Placement:** Artificial airways can be placed translaryngeally, either orotracheal or nasotracheal, or directly into the trachea by an incision in the lower anterior neck (**tracheostomy**).

2. **Cricothyroidotomy:** perform when intubation is required emergently and cannot be performed translaryngeally

3. **Assessment for intubation:** The decision to intubate a patient by whichever route is a critical decision with serious consequences if performed too late. Assess early and repeat frequently based on patient acuity; it is not simple but should include at least the following:

   a. **Respiratory rate (RR):** most simple to assess
      (1) The normal RR is 12–16 breaths per minute (bpm).
      (2) If a patient's RR is greater than 40 bpm, intubate.
      (3) If a patient is breathing 30–40 bpm, initiate therapy to get RR less than 30 bpm, or the patient will tire and go into respiratory failure (most humans cannot sustain RRs of >30 bpm for very long without fatigue).
      (4) Low RRs are almost always caused by a neurologic disorder (e.g., alcohol, drugs, head injury), which will determine if intubation is needed.

   b. **Respiratory effort:** represents the **work of breathing**
      (1) Patients exerting a significant effort (i.e., using accessory respiratory muscles, having difficulty speaking in full sentences, forcibly exhaling, or uncomfortably inhaling) typically need intubation.
      (2) If left to progress without intervention, these patients become overly tired with progressive hypoventilation and potential respiratory arrest.

   c. **Hypoxia:** can be an indication for intubation but also manageable by noninvasive increased oxygen concentrations. Intubation facilitates both increased **fraction of inspired oxygen** (Fio2) and airway pressure provision to reduce intrapulmonary shunt and improve oxygenation.

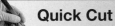

Quick Cut
Patients with acute arterial oxygen saturations less than 92% typically need supplemental oxygen or intubation to improve their oxygenation status.

   d. **Impending airway obstruction:** indication for intubation to prevent complete obstruction and loss of the airway
      (1) Anatomic (e.g., from trauma, tumors, edema, or vocal cord abnormalities) and functional changes (e.g., from depressed neurologic status from head trauma, drugs, anesthesia, or stroke) can interfere with airway patency.

(2) With concern for impending airway obstruction, intubate early for controlled passage of the endotracheal tube.

B. **Ventilator support:** Most common reason to be admitted to an ICU. Once the decision has been made to intubate, next decide how to manage the ventilator patient. Ventilator support should address **ventilation** and **oxygenation.** Mode of ventilation (see the following discussion) will alter how these are achieved; however, more commonly, mode influences patient tolerance of mechanical ventilation.

1. **Ventilation:** determines CO_2 elimination and depends on alveolar minute ventilation

    a. **Alveolar minute ventilation:** total minute ventilation − dead space ventilation

    b. **Total minute ventilation:** product of RR × tidal volume, expressed as L/min. To decrease P_{CO_2}, also adjust RR and tidal volume with increases in minute ventilation.

2. **Oxygenation (or P_{O_2}):** determined by the partial pressure of alveolar oxygen and the intrapulmonary shunt

    a. Increasing F_{IO_2} will increase alveolar oxygen, whereas increasing mean airway pressure (e.g., by increasing **positive end-expiratory pressure [PEEP]**) will decrease shunt and increase P_{O_2}.

3. **Mode of ventilation:** Determines how the ventilator will provide a mechanical breath to the patient and is based on pressure or volume. (Many other modes exist than are discussed here, but these will suffice in most patients.)

    a. **Synchronized intermittent mandatory ventilation (SIMV):** provides a preset rate and tidal volume

    (1) Spontaneous breathing by the patient provides additional minute ventilation (tidal volume × rate) dependent on the patient's work of breathing capability.

    (2) The work of breathing is shared between the machine's minute ventilation and the patient's spontaneous minute ventilation.

    (3) Usual mode of ventilation when weaning a patient: By turning down the ventilator rate, the patient assumes more work of breathing until the ventilator is no longer needed.

    (4) Pressure support (see the following discussion) can be added to facilitate spontaneous breaths.

    b. **Assist or volume control (AC/VC):** provides a preset rate and tidal volume, and all additional patient breaths are fully assisted by the ventilator to the preset tidal volume

    (1) Minute ventilation becomes the result of the preset tidal volume × (the preset ventilator's + patient's rates).

    (2) This allows the patient to receive full ventilatory support without expending extra energy on the work of breathing.

    c. **Pressure support (PS):** Rather than providing a preset volume or rate, this mode pressurizes the ventilator circuit to a preset level when the patient initiates a breath and maintains that level until the patient stops inhaling. The patient is able to initiate and terminate the respiratory cycle in this mode.

    (1) Inspired tidal volume: determined by the amount of PS and the patient's intrinsic work of breathing capacity

    (2) Increasing PS reduces the work of breathing for the same tidal volume or allows a larger tidal volume for the same amount of work.

    (3) PS facilitates weaning from the ventilator.

    (4) Usual starting point: 5–10 mm Hg above the baseline pressure (continuous positive airway pressure [CPAP]/PEEP) and can be used alone or in combination with SIMV

    d. **CPAP and PEEP:** These modes are similar in that both result in the ventilator circuit being pressurized to a specified level above atmospheric at all times, during inspiration and expiration.

    (1) This primary means of increasing oxygenation increases mean airway pressure and the number of inflated alveoli, which increases lung surface area available for gas exchange and decreases intrapulmonary shunt.

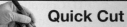

Quick Cut
Except for occasional cases of chronically ventilated patients, all patients requiring mechanical ventilation will be managed in an ICU.

Quick Cut
For any patient receiving ventilatory support, ventilator-associated lung injury is an inherent risk to mechanical ventilation.

Quick Cut
Increase mean airway pressure (increase PEEP, switch modes) for improvements in oxygenation. Change minute ventilation for improvements in ventilation.

(2) Usually, CPAP/PEEP of 5 mm Hg above atmospheric pressure is used and is increased as necessary to improve oxygenation.

(3) Because these modes increase intrathoracic pressure at higher levels, they can decrease venous return to the heart and therefore CO.

(4) PEEP is used with SIMV and AC, whereas CPAP is used with PS.

4. Rate: After mode, the next parameter to set is rate (normal, ~10–12 bpm).

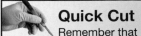

Quick Cut
Remember that if the patient is severely acidotic, he or she may have been compensating with the respiratory system and may require a much higher RR.

   a. Higher rates may be necessary to decrease the Pco_2 if higher minute ventilation or lower tidal volumes are required.

   b. No rate is needed for PS.

5. Tidal volume: Normal tidal volume is 5 mL/kg, but ventilated patients are usually set at 6–8 mL/kg.

   a. Higher volumes are needed to overcome dead space and to ensure alveolar filling.

   b. With decreasing lung compliance (e.g., with ARDS), smaller tidal volumes of 4–6 mL/kg have been shown to reduce mortality.

   c. Adjust volume as the patient's condition requires.

   d. Occasionally, permissive hypercapnia is beneficial to avoid barotrauma.

6. Routine ventilator support starting point: The ventilator settings described previously allow management of most ventilatory problems. Depending on the patient's condition, other modes are available to ventilate patients, but these suffice for routine ventilatory management.

   a. Mode: SIMV; however, if no work of breathing is desired, use the AC mode.

   b. Rate: 10–12 bpm

   c. Tidal volume: 6–8 mL/kg (4–6 mL/kg if the patient has ALI or ARDS)

   d. PS: 5–10 mm Hg (not used in AC/VC)

   e. PEEP/CPAP: 5–10 mm Hg

   f. Fio_2: 0.4

   g. Modify settings for the patient's condition: higher Fio_2 and/or higher PEEP if the patient is hypoxic, lower PEEP if hypotensive, faster rate if acidotic, etc.

7. Extubation: Ventilator weaning is the progressive transfer of the work of breathing from the ventilator to the stable patient.

Quick Cut
Patients with a significant acidosis with or without compensation should not be extubated without careful consideration of the underlying cause.

   a. Muscle atrophy: Ventilator patients are usually in a catabolic state, thus breaking down muscle protein for fuel. Because patients on complete ventilator support do no work of breathing, their respiratory muscles rapidly atrophy.

   b. Stable patient: Adjust the amount of ventilatory support to allow the patient to do some work of breathing to keep the respiratory muscles intact. As the patient's condition improves, the RR delivered by the ventilator is decreased until the patient adequately assumes the work of breathing.

   c. Spontaneous breathing trial (SBT): This daily test has been shown to shorten mechanical ventilation duration. The patient who passes the SBT with adequate parameters (described below), is awake enough to control airway, and has acceptable acid–base balance may be ready for extubation. The SBT can be a low amount of CPAP and pressure support (5 mm Hg for each) or more classically (and more predictive of successful extubation) be a flow-by oxygen trial off the ventilator.

     (1) Rapid shallow breathing index (RR bpm ÷ by tidal volume in L) less than 100 (some use a lower number, for example, 60 or 80, for PS trials)

     (2) Vital capacity: greater than 15–20 mm Hg

     (3) Negative inspiratory force greater than 20 cm H_2O

     (4) Arterial blood gases: The patient must have acceptable blood gases as well as spirometry values.

       (a) Oxygen saturation should be higher than 90% due to the limitations of providing high oxygen concentrations via face mask.

       (b) Pco_2 should be 35–45 mm Hg with pH of 7.35–7.45.

C. **Hemodynamic and other invasive monitoring:** Mainstays in modern ICUs are the arterial line for blood pressure; the pulmonary artery catheter for COs, pulmonary artery wedge pressures, and mixed venous oxygen saturation; and the intracranial catheter for intracranial pressure (ICP) monitoring. However, pulmonary artery catheters are now used much less, with noninvasive technologies such CO measurement based on arterial line tracings and cardiac performance based on echocardiography.

> **Quick Cut**
> Monitoring with invasive techniques such as arterial lines, pulmonary artery catheters, and ICP take place only in the ICU.

1. **Arterial catheter:** Usually placed in one of the accessible radial arteries. If a radial artery cannot be cannulated, other sites are femoral, axillary, and brachial arteries.

   a. The arterial line provides continuous blood pressure monitoring and is a simple, nonpainful source for blood sampling.

   b. Three pressure measurements obtained: systolic, diastolic, and mean.

      (1) **Systolic:** highest cardiac cycle pressure recorded

      (2) **Diastolic:** lowest cardiac cycle pressure recorded

      (3) **Mean:** Measured by integrating the area under the curve of the cardiac pressure wave. The mean pressure can be indirectly determined as $(BP_{systolic} - 2 \times BP_{diastolic})/3$ and represents the pressure available to perfuse the organs.

2. **Pulmonary artery (Swan-Ganz) catheter:** Flow-directed catheter inserted into a subclavian or jugular vein with an inflatable balloon on its tip to float through the heart and into the pulmonary artery. It has an opening (port) in the tip distal to the balloon, another opening in its side at a position that rests in the vena cava or right atrium, and a **thermistor** (a temperature-measuring device) near the distal port (Fig. 1-3). Extra ports may infuse medications.

   a. **Pulmonary capillary wedge pressure (PCWP)/occlusion pressure (PCOP):** When the catheter is in position in a distal pulmonary artery, the balloon is inflated and occludes antegrade blood flow, thereby allowing the distal port to measure retrograde pressure from the left atrium, an indirect measure of left ventricular preload. By assessing ventricular preload, alterations in fluid therapy can be made to maximize CO based on the **Starling curve.**

   > **Quick Cut**
   > Swan-Ganz catheters are only used in special circumstances, but knowledge of them helps in understanding non-invasive measurement of cardiovascular physiology.

   b. **Thermodilution methodology:** The catheter is able to determine CO by accurately measuring changes in blood temperature (thermodilution) after introduction of a known thermal challenge.

   c. **Mixed venous oxygen saturation (SvO$_2$):** can be assessed by either aspirating blood from the distal port or by using oximetry located on the distal tip

      (1) SvO$_2$ provides a means to determine if the amount of oxygen being pumped by the heart (*oxygen delivery*) is adequate for the amount of oxygen the body needs (*oxygen consumption*).

   > **Quick Cut**
   > SvO$_2$ is one of the best measures readily available to determine if shock is present.

      (2) Normal SvO$_2$: ~70%; if oxygen consumption is elevated or oxygen delivery is decreased, saturation will be less than 70%.

      (3) If the SvO$_2$ is persistently low (60% or less), oxygen delivery is insufficient, and organ dysfunction will occur.

      (4) Using similar technology, a less invasive but not as accurate method for determining SvO$_2$ can be obtained from the end of a central venous catheter.

   d. **Systemic vascular resistance (SVR)/pulmonary vascular resistance (PVR):** By knowing the CO, the mean arterial pressure (MAP), and the central venous pressure (CVP), SVR and PVR can be calculated (MPAP, mean pulmonary artery pressure; 80, a conversion factor).

   > **Quick Cut**
   > The basic information that can be gathered from the pulmonary artery catheter includes left atrial and left ventricle preload pressures, CO, SvO$_2$, SVR, and PVR.

      (1) $SVR = [(MAP - CVP)/CO] \times 80$; normal: 800–1,200 dynes.second/cm^5

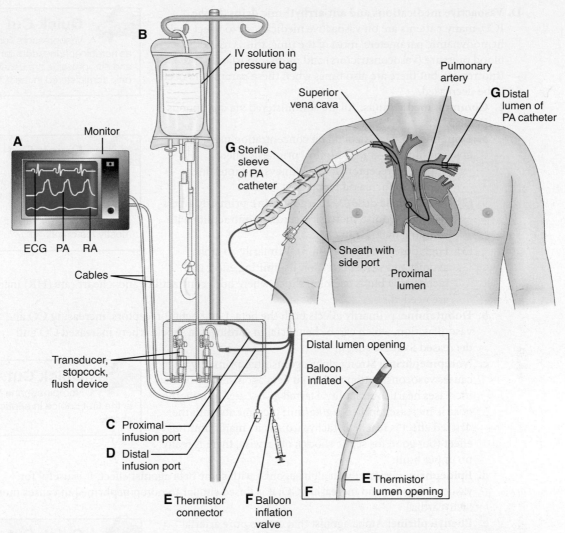

Figure 1-3: Pulmonary artery (*PA*) catheter and pressure monitoring systems. (*A*) Bedside monitor that connects with cables to (*B*) the pressure monitoring systems (includes IV solution in a pressure bag, IV tubing, and two transducers with stopcocks and flush devices). This system connects to (*C*) the proximal infusion port that opens in the right atria and is used to infuse fluids or medications and monitor central venous pressures and (*D*) the distal infusion port. This port opens in the PA and is used to monitor PA pressures. (*E*) The thermistor connector is attached to the bedside cardiac monitor to obtain CO. (*F*) An air-filled syringe is attached to the balloon inflation valve during catheter insertion and measurement of PA wedge pressure. (*G*) PA catheter positioned in the pulmonary artery. Note the sterile sleeve over the PA catheter. The PA catheter is threaded through the sheath until it reaches the desired position in the PA. The side port on the sheath is used to infuse medications or fluids. ECG, electrocardiogram; RA, right atrium. (From Farrell M, Dempsey J. *Smeltzer and Bare's Textbook of Medical-Surgical Nursing*, 2nd ed. Philadelphia: Lippincott Williams & Wilkins; 2010.)

            (2) $PVR = [(MPAP - PCWP)/CO] \times 80$; normal: 20–120 dynes $\times$ second/cm^5

            (3) Low SVR indicates systemic inflammation or other distributive shock states (e.g., sepsis).

            (4) High SVR indicates other shock states with inadequate CO.

    e. Other: Additional data can be gleaned, which is beyond this book's scope. As noted, nearly all of it can now be obtained noninvasively.

        (1) Pulmonary artery pressures: can be estimated by echocardiography

        (2) CO/SVR: can be measured with a simple A-line tracing and the appropriate hardware and software

D. Vasoactive medications and antiarrhythmic drips: In the
ICU, many patients are on vasoactive medications to affect their
hemodynamic parameters; most of the time, this is to increase
blood pressure (vasoconstrictors) and more importantly CO
(inotropes), but there are also times when these parameters need
to be decreased.

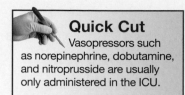

Quick Cut
Vasopressors such
as norepinephrine, dobutamine,
and nitroprusside are usually
only administered in the ICU.

1. **Common medications:** All are administered via continuous
   IV drip.
   a. **Dopamine:** Effects depend on concentration used.
      (1) Low dose (1–3 μg/kg/min): primarily affects
          dopamine receptors in the kidneys and intestine,
          leading to increased blood flow
      (2) Intermediate dose (3–10 μg/kg/min): primarily a beta-
          receptor agonist, increasing cardiac contractility with
          resulting increase in CO
      (3) High dose (>10 μg/kg/min): Primarily an alpha
          agonist and vasoconstrictor. Its limiting effect is
          tachycardia but is useful in shock where both contractility and a heart rate (HR) increase
          are needed.

Quick Cut
Renal dose
dopamine is sometimes used
in certain patient populations
(cardiac surgery), but its
use as a natriuretic agent is
mostly historical.

   b. **Dobutamine:** primarily affects both the beta-1 and beta-2 receptors, increasing CO and
      vasodilatation, which can be beneficial in cardiogenic shock, where increased CO and
      decreased SVR are sought
   c. **Norepinephrine:** Strong alpha agonist that primarily
      causes vasoconstriction with mild beta agonist activity that
      increases heart contractility. Started at 1–2 μg/kg/min, the
      dose is increased in 1–2-μg/kg/min increments until the
      desired effect is reached. Tachycardia is its major limiting
      effect (but good for septic shock); otherwise, there is really
      no upper limit.

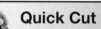

Quick Cut
Norepinephrine
is the first choice in septic
shock.

   d. **Epinephrine:** Primarily an alpha agonist with some beta agonist effect. It is useful for
      vasoconstriction and increasing CO; it is dosed similar to norepinephrine but causes more
      tachycardia.
   e. **Phenylephrine:** Alpha agonist that causes pure arterial
      constriction but is not very potent. Drips are usually begun
      at ~50 μg/min and increased in increments of 50 μg/min
      until a total dose of 300 μg/min is reached, when a more
      potent vasoconstrictor is needed.

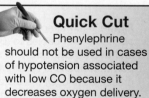

Quick Cut
Phenylephrine
should not be used in cases
of hypotension associated
with low CO because it
decreases oxygen delivery.

2. **Common vasodilators:** Occasionally, patients have
   hypertension and need their blood pressure lowered or
   their SVR will be excessively high and need vasodilation. In
   cardiogenic shock, lowering the afterload by decreasing SVR
   will increase CO and get the patient out of shock.
   a. **Nitroprusside:** Primarily an arterial vasodilator. The
      initial dose is 0.3 μg/kg/min, with a maximum dose of
      3 μg/kg/min. It can result in reflex tachycardia, and one of
      its metabolites is cyanide.

Quick Cut
Nitroprusside used
in large doses for a prolonged
period can cause cyanide
poisoning and acidosis.

   b. **Nitroglycerin:** primarily a venodilator and a coronary
      artery dilator that decreases venous preload to decrease diastolic wall tension and to allow
      better heart contraction if it has been overstretched
      (1) Also allows better diastolic blood flow to the heart itself and may increase CO
      (2) Primarily used in cases of coronary ischemia
      (3) Dosing starts at 5 μg/min and increases in 5–20-μg/min increments until the desired
          effect is obtained.
   c. **Labetalol:** acts a mixed alpha- and beta-blocker in IV form
   d. **Esmolol:** pure beta-blocker
   e. **Nicardipine:** potent calcium channel blocker

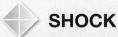

SHOCK

Definition

Shock is the clinical syndrome resulting from inadequate tissue perfusion to maintain normal cellular metabolism. Essentially, it is inadequate oxygen delivery to meet oxygen demand.

I. **Oxygen delivery equation:** $DO_2 = [1.39 \times Hgb \text{ (grams)} \times Sao_2 + (0.003 \times Pao_2)] \times CO$.

   A. Pao_2 contributes very little to oxygen delivery.

   B. $Hgb \times Sao_2$ represents the blood's oxygen-carrying capacity.

   C. CO is determined by $HR \times$ stroke volume (SV), and SV is determined by cardiac preload, contractility, and afterload.

   D. With inadequate oxygen delivery: "fix" **Hgb, Sao₂, HR, preload, contractility,** and **afterload**.

II. **Types of shock:** Shock can result from poor oxygen delivery or (in rare cases) from increased demand; Table 1-5 summarizes types of shock based on analysis of the patient's hemodynamic profile.

   A. **Hypovolemic shock:** Most common type of shock, and hemorrhage is the most common reason for hypovolemia. Loss of plasma volume (e.g., with major burns, third spacing, or GI losses) can also result in hypovolemia. Decreased **preload** decreases CO and oxygen delivery to cells. Loss of red cell volume reduces **Hgb** levels.

      1. **Clinical presentation and mortality:** Depend on the magnitude and duration of shock. Increased lactate production occurs as normal aerobic cellular metabolism progresses to less energy efficient anaerobic metabolism (fewer adenosine triphosphate [ATP] produced), resulting in cellular damage and death.

      2. **Treatment (preload restoration):** blood and plasma volume

         a. Aggressive volume administration is needed, preferably through two large-bore IV catheters.

         b. Stop ongoing blood loss and transfuse blood as needed.

         c. Consider central venous access for monitoring and high-flow fluid administration.

   B. **Cardiogenic shock:** caused by myocardial ischemia, CHF, and valvular diseases

      1. Blood volume remains normal or increased, but loss of **contractility** or other impediments to forward flow results in decreased perfusion.

      2. **Treatment:** Restore pump function either by increasing **contractility** or decreasing **afterload** so the weak pump has an easier time generating flow. Nitroglycerine can help reverse cardiac ischemia if blood pressure will tolerate it.

   C. **Neurogenic shock:** caused by vasovagal response, cervicothoracic spinal cord injury, or spinal anesthesia

      1. Loss of sympathetic tone leading to peripheral vasodilatation can result in poor perfusion.

      2. **Treatment:** First increase **preload**, then increase **afterload** with phenylephrine or norepinephrine if unresponsive.

   D. **Septic shock:** Toxins released by microbes result in profound hyperinflammatory physiologic derangements, including third spacing of fluids (decreased **preload**), cardiac dysfunction (poor **contractility**), and reduction in SVR (decreased **afterload**).

      1. Septic shock results in progressive maldistributive hypoperfusion: CO may be decreased, normal, or increased, depending on the degree of hypovolemia and the severity of the inflammatory insult. The hyperinflammatory response is characterized by increased cellular metabolism and

Quick Cut
The six variables to adjust to improve oxygen delivery are Hgb, Sao₂, HR, preload, contractility, and afterload.

Quick Cut
Reversing shock as early as possible is critical for reducing organ failure and complications in the ICU.

Quick Cut
Although hypotension occurs with hypovolemia, the important concept is loss of perfusion, not decreased pressure.

Quick Cut
Bleeding hypovolemic shock patients should get blood.

Quick Cut
Resuscitate hemorrhage by transfusing pRBCs and FFP in a 1:1 ratio with platelets for every 4 units . . . minimize crystalloid.

Quick Cut
Restoring pump function in cardiogenic shock may reduce blood pressure, but blood pressure is not the goal . . . perfusion is!

Table 1-5: Types of Shock Based on Hemodynamic Profile Analysis

Type of Shock	Heart Rate	Blood Pressure Changes	Left Heart Filling Pressures (CVP/PAOP)	Systemic Vascular Resistance	Cardiac Output/ Index	Mixed Venous Oxygen Saturation (SvO$_2$)
Hypovolemic	Elevated	First: none Second: narrow pulse pressure/ elevated diastolic Third: systolic hypotension	Low	High	Low	Low
Cardiogenic	Usually increased	Usually decreased	High*	High	Low	Low
Neurogenic	Normal or decreased	Decreased	Low	Low	Decreased (loss of cardiac compensation)	Low
Obstructive	Usually increased but could be decreased	Decreased	Usually high*	High	Low	Low
Septic: Early:	Elevated	Usually low	Normal or low	Low	Low, normal, or high	Normal or high
After fluid resuscitation (late):	Elevated or normal	Normal or low	Elevated	Low	Normal or High	Often high

*Right ventricular failure can lead to increased central venous pressure (CVP), but decreased capillary wedge pressure, pulmonary embolus, and tension pneumothorax can also lead to high CVP but low or normal pulmonary artery occlusion pressure (PAOP) pressures. In tamponade, all filling pressures are elevated.

oxygen demand. Cellular hypoperfusion and anaerobic metabolism are associated with organ dysfunction and death.

2. **Treatment:** includes antibiotics, controlling the infection source, and reversing shock
   a. First use fluids to increase CVP to 8–12 (**preload**).
   b. Follow lactate/SvO$_2$ levels.
      (1) If they are deranged, transfuse blood to an **Hgb** of 10.
      (2) Use norepinephrine to maintain MAP higher than 65 mm Hg as **afterload** may be low.
      (3) If lactate/SvO$_2$ is still deranged, add dobutamine to increase CO (**contractility**).
E. **Obstructive shock:** The hallmark is CO with elevated CVP resulting in tissue hypoperfusion from a physical obstruction (e.g., tension pneumothorax, cardiac tamponade, massive pulmonary embolism, venous air embolism, and severe cardiac valvular stenosis).
1. **Treatment:** fluid resuscitation (**preload**) followed by prompt resolution of the obstruction, often through procedural means
   a. **Tension pneumothorax:** An injured lung develops a one-way valve that allows air into but not out of the pleural space.
      (1) Trapped air creates an increase in pleural pressure, displacing the heart and mediastinal structures (e.g., vena cava, aorta) and compressing them to the contralateral side with decreased venous return to the heart.
      (2) A chest tube placed on the affected side relieves the problem.
   b. **Cardiac tamponade:** Blood or fluid accumulates around the heart in the pericardium.
      (1) The resulting increased pressure in the pericardial sac impairs venous return into the right atrium, decreasing CO.
      (2) **Treatment**: Drain the pericardium to allow venous return to increase and CO to normalize.

    c. Pulmonary embolism: Blocks blood flow through the pulmonary artery, resulting in decreased CO and hypoxia. Treatment ranges from anticoagulation through operative pulmonary thrombectomy.

    d. Abdominal compartment syndrome is increased pressure in the abdomen that compresses the IVC and decreases preload.

    e. Mechanical ventilation with excessive PEEP (positive end-expiratory pressure) may increase intrathoracic pressure and lead to obstructive shock.

F. Miscellaneous shock: often distributive (reduced **afterload**) in nature (e.g., anaphylaxis, adrenal insufficiency)

    1. Cyanide toxicity impairs oxygen usage directly.

    2. In some patients (e.g., Jehovah's Witnesses, who do not accept blood transfusions for religious reasons), the **Hgb** level is so low that it causes shock and poor oxygen delivery.

    3. Severe hypoxia from respiratory failure or ALI/ARDS can also lead to shock (**oxygen saturation**).

Chapter 2

Essentials of General Surgery

Natasha Hansraj and Douglas J. Turner

WOUNDS

Skin
I. **Characteristics:** Skin is the largest organ of the body and comprises three layers.
   A. **Epidermis:** composed of stratified squamous epithelial cells aiding in protection
   B. **Dermis:** connective tissue with papillary digitation into the epidermis composed of collagen fibers, hair follicles, capillaries, and sweat glands
   C. **Hypodermis (subcutaneous tissue):** deepest layer; loose, fat-containing vascular tissue

II. **Fascia:** connective tissue able to withstand tension

Wound Healing
I. **Healing:** comprises three stages
   A. **Inflammatory (days 1–10):** influx of polymorphonuclear leukocytes and macrophages, cytokine release, and epithelialization
   B. **Proliferative (days 2–21):** Fibroblasts appear, producing collagen and granulation tissue; neovascularization occurs to overcome ischemia.
   C. **Remodeling (3 weeks–1 year):** Collagen fibers remodel to increase strength but collagen amount remains the same. Type 1 collagen is predominant in wounds after 3 weeks.

II. **Strength of tissue:** Tissue strength grows with healing and is therefore stronger with longer times from the initial wound. At 20 days, strength is 20% of normal; 40 days, 40% of normal; and at 1 year, it is 70% of normal.

Wound Classification
I. **Clean:** uninfected operative site without crossing a mucosal barrier

II. **Clean contaminated:** Respiratory, gastrointestinal (GI), or genitourinary (GU) tract is entered in controlled conditions (e.g., appendix or biliary surgery).

III. **Contaminated:** open accidental wounds or gross GI spillage

IV. **Dirty:** old wounds with devitalized tissue, purulence, or perforated viscus

Quick Cut
Wound classification is important because it predicts the risk of infectious complications in the postoperative wound.

Wound Repair
I. **Purpose:** to restore injured tissue to its normal function and integrity

II. **Types**
   A. **Primary intention:** All layers are sutured; used for clean cases causing minimal scarring (Fig. 2-1).
      1. **Advantage:** most cosmetic
      2. **Disadvantage:** Bacterial colonization can lead to wound infection and breakdown.

Quick Cut
The most important factor in healing is collagen deposition providing tensile strength.

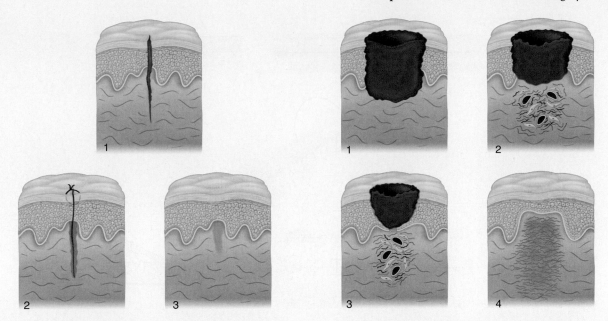

A Healing by primary intention (wounds with approximated edges) **B** Healing by secondary intention (wounds with separated edges)
Figure 2-1: Wound healing by primary and secondary intention. (Image modified from Rubin E, Farber JL. *Pathology*, 4th ed. Philadelphia: Lippincott Williams & Wilkins; 2005, with permission.)

    B. **Secondary intention:** Fascia is closed, leaving subcutaneous and skin layers open to heal spontaneously; used for contaminated wounds (see Fig. 2-1).
      1. **Mechanism:** Healing results from re-epithelialization from wound edges and sweat glands along with granulation tissue. Myofibroblasts aid in wound contracture.
      2. **Advantage:** minimal risk of infection
      3. **Disadvantage:** requires dressing changes and leads to broad scars
    C. **Delayed primary intention:** Wounds are initially left open for repeated debridement. Once healthy granulation tissue is present without signs of infection, wound defect is closed by sutures or flaps.

Wound Closure

    I. **Stitch:** Sutures can be interrupted or continuous.
      A. **Interrupted closure:** series of sutures tied individually after passage through both sides of the wound
        1. **Advantage:** allows better alignment, especially in wounds with irregular edges
        2. **Disadvantage:** requires longer time for closure
      B. **Continuous closure (running stitch):** Stitches are placed one after the other with the same suture and tied only at the end.
        1. **Advantage:** faster; provides equal tension from bite to bite
        2. **Disadvantage:** can strangulate tissue and carries the risk of complete unraveling of entire closure with suture fracture
    II. **Approach:** Sutures can be sewn in a simple or complex manner (Fig. 2-2).
      A. **Simple suture:** equidistant bites taken through the skin and subcutaneous tissue from one side to the other
      B. **Vertical mattress suture:** Needle is placed in the skin in a far–far, reverse direction, near–near fashion.
      C. **Horizontal mattress suture:** Parallel bites are taken in a far–far, move along incision and reverse the direction, far–far fashion.

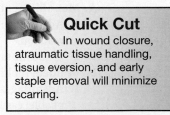

Quick Cut
In wound closure, atraumatic tissue handling, tissue eversion, and early staple removal will minimize scarring.

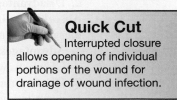

Quick Cut
Interrupted closure allows opening of individual portions of the wound for drainage of wound infection.

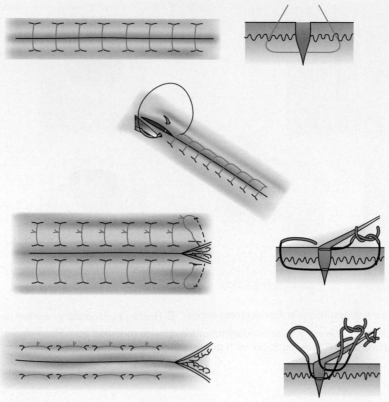

Figure 2-2: Suture techniques include interrupted, continuous, and mattress suturing.

Suture Characteristics

I. **Suture size:** Diameter of the suture. As the number of 0s increases, diameter decreases (i.e., 5-0 [00000] is smaller than 4-0 [0000]).

II. **Suture material:** divided into monofilament versus braided, absorbable versus nonabsorbable (Table 2-1)

A. **Monofilament:** made of a single strand
   1. **Advantage:** Less drag through tissue causes less tissue reaction.
   2. **Disadvantage:** easily breaks; needs more knots to secure

B. **Braided:** multifilament
   1. **Advantages:** greater shear strength; softer, more flexible, pliable; easily passes through tissue; and needs fewer knots
   2. **Disadvantage:** can tear fragile tissue and be a nidus for infection

C. **Absorbable suture:** degrades over time because it is made of collagen, which is enzymatically digested, or synthetic polymers, which hydrolyze causing less tissue reaction (Fig. 2-3)
   1. **Advantages:** Decreased risk of infection because they are nonpermanent. Ideal for biliary and GU tracts, where foreign body would be a nidus for stone formation and infection.
   2. **Disadvantage:** Patients with impaired healing or infection increase rate of suture degradation. Therefore, if the suture loses strength before the wound heals, dehiscence can result.

D. **Nonabsorbable suture:** permanent foreign body that is encapsulated by fibroblasts (see Fig. 2-3)
   1. **Uses:** used in heart valves, hernias, and vascular anastomosis. This suture is preferred when healing may be slow or requires long-term reinforcement (hernia repair) or when the consequences of suture failure are high (blood vessels and heart valves).
   2. **Disadvantage:** nidus for infection

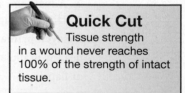

Quick Cut
Tissue strength in a wound never reaches 100% of the strength of intact tissue.

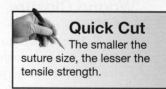

Quick Cut
The smaller the suture size, the lesser the tensile strength.

Table 2-1: Types of Suture Materials

Sutures	Material	Monofilament vs. Braided	Half-life	Natural vs. Synthetic	Comments and Typical Uses
Absorbable sutures					
Gut (catgut)	Collagen from intestine—beef serosa or sheep submucosa	Monofilament	7–10 days	Natural	Originally from cats; packaged in alcohol, must be kept wet; rarely used
Chromic gut (chromic catgut)	Chromate-tanned gut	Monofilament	2 weeks	Natural	Ties well; packaged in alcohol, must be kept wet; less used than in years past
Polyglactin-910 polyglycolic acid	Synthetic polymer	Braided	2–3 weeks	Synthetic	**Bowel, subcutaneous** tissue, fascia
Polydioxanone polyglyconate	Synthetic polymer	Monofilament	4 weeks	Synthetic	Fascia, bowel, biliary, and **urinary tract**
Poliglecaprone 25	Synthetic polymer	Monofilament	1–2 weeks	Synthetic	Subcuticular skin closure
Permanent sutures					
Silk	Silk-organic protein, fibroin	Braided	~20 years	Natural	Best handling, hemostasis
Polyester	Polyester	Braided	Permanent	Synthetic	Heart valves, fascia; known for potential for harboring infection
Polypropylene	Polypropylene	Monofilament	Permanent	Synthetic	Cardiovascular, hernias, fascia
Nylon	Nylon	1. Monofilament 2. Braided	Permanent	Synthetic	1. Skin 2. Looks and handles like silk
Cotton, linen	Plant derived	Braided	Permanent	Natural	Obsolete due to extent of resulting tissue reaction
Stainless steel	316L stainless	Monofilament	Permanent, can fracture after years	Synthetic	Sternum, hernias; difficult to handle, sharp ends
ePTFE*	ePTFE	Porous monofilament	Permanent	Synthetic	Cardiovascular, hernias; has properties of both braided and monofilament
Staples	1. Skin-steel 2. Stapling devices—titanium	Monofilament	Permanent	Synthetic	Skin staples: faster than sutured closures. Stapling devices: used for bowel anastomoses; vascular closures, bronchial closures

*ePTFE, expanded polytetrafluoroethylene.

◆ SURGICAL TUBES AND DRAINS

Drains

I. Types

    A. **Closed drains:** Drain connects to the body cavity in closed system.

        1. **Gravity drains (e.g., Foley):** Tubes are attached to a reservoir at a lower height.

        2. **Underwater seal drainage system (e.g., chest tubes):** prevents air and fluid from re-entering the body

        3. **Suction drain (e.g., Jackson-Pratt):** Apply suction to evacuate larger volumes of fluid and remove dead space.

Quick Cut
Tubes and drains allow exit of excess or abnormal body fluids, but may clog. In this case, low drain output may not represent adequate drainage.

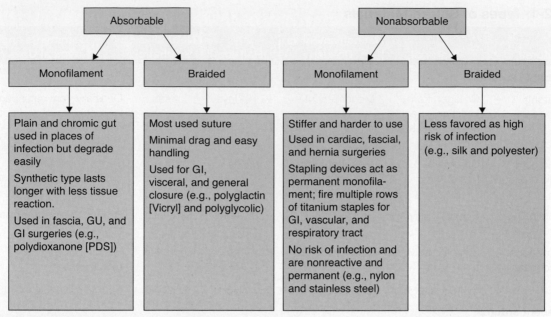

Figure 2-3: Major suture types by category.

B. **Open drains (e.g., Penrose):** Open at both ends to allow pus to drain.

C. **Sump drains (e.g., nasogastric [NG] tubes):** double-lumen catheters allowing air and irrigation fluid to enter through one lumen while suction is applied to the other lumen

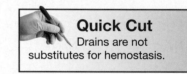

Quick Cut
Drains are not substitutes for hemostasis.

II. **Complications:** Drains should be removed once their purpose has been met to minimize complications.

A. **Colonization:** Microorganisms increase the risk of infection.

B. **Corrosion:** Rigid drains can corrode into nearby organs and vessels.

C. **Necrosis:** Excessive suction can lead to necrosis.

D. **Retraction:** Drains can retract into the body or can be sutured in place internally.

GI Tubes

I. **Gastrostomy tubes:** Inserted in the stomach through the skin for feeding purposes or prolonged gastric decompression. The epithelialized tract forms after several weeks in place, then closes in 6–24 hours once the tube is removed.

II. **Sengstaken-Blakemore/Minnesota tubes:** NG tubes with inflatable esophageal and gastric balloons to tamponade esophageal variceal bleed

III. **NG tubes:** can be used for relieving partial small bowel obstruction

IV. **Jejunostomy tubes:** provide nutrition to those unable to tolerate gastric feeds

V. **Rectal tubes:** large-caliber tubes inserted through the anus into the rectum for decompression

Catheters

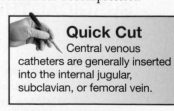

Quick Cut
Central venous catheters are generally inserted into the internal jugular, subclavian, or femoral vein.

I. **Central venous catheters:** single-, double-, or triple-lumen tubes placed with their tips in the superior vena cava

A. **Purpose:** Administer fluids, pressors, parental nutrition, or hemodialysis.

B. **Complications:** infection leading to bacteremia or pneumothorax

1. **Central line–associated bloodstream infections:** ~40,000 occur in the United States per year.

2. **Minocycline or rifampin:** Central venous catheters coated with either of these agents have been demonstrated to lower bloodstream infections without contributing to antibiotic resistance.

II. **Peripherally inserted central catheters (PICCs):** placed through the antecubital vein into a central vein

III. **Port:** similar to a central venous catheter with access under the skin; commonly used for chemotherapy

IV. **Cuffed central venous catheters (e.g., Hickman):** Tunnelled catheters used for long-term access for hemodialysis, chemotherapy, and parental nutrition. The Dacron cuff permits ingrowth of granulation tissue to secure the line and act as a mechanical barrier to infection.

V. **Peritoneal dialysis catheters:** inserted into the peritoneal cavity for peritoneal dialysis

HERNIAS

Overview

I. **Definition:** Abnormal protrusion of contents through a defect into a separate body cavity. Most commonly, hernias are present on the abdominal wall.

II. **Incidence and etiology:** In both men and women, 70% of hernias occur in the inguinal region.
   A. **Congenital defects:** include indirect inguinal hernia
   B. **Loss of tissue strength and elasticity:** from aging or repetitive stress, as in hiatal hernia
   C. **Trauma (especially operative trauma):** Normal tissue strength is altered surgically and can lead to the development of hernia.
   D. **Increased intra-abdominal pressure:** contributes to hernia symptoms; may result from the following:
      1. **Heavy lifting**
      2. **Coughing, asthma, and chronic obstructive pulmonary disease (COPD)**
      3. **Bladder outlet obstruction (e.g., benign prostatic hypertrophy)**
      4. **Prior pregnancy**
      5. **Ascites and abdominal distention**
      6. **Obesity**

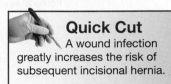

Quick Cut
A wound infection greatly increases the risk of subsequent incisional hernia.

III. **Descriptive terms**
   A. **Reducible:** Hernia contents can be pushed back into their normal position.
   B. **Incarcerated:** Hernia contents cannot be reduced.
   C. **Obstructing:** Hernia contains bowel that is kinked and obstructs the GI tract.
   D. **Strangulated:** Tissue contained in the hernia is ischemic and will necrose due to blood supply compromise.
   E. **Sliding:** Wall of the hernia sac is partly formed by a retroperitoneal structure, such as the colon or the bladder, rather than being formed completely by peritoneum.
   F. **Richter hernia:** Only one side of the bowel wall is trapped in the hernia (typically, the antimesenteric side). The incarcerated portion of bowel can necrose and perforate in the absence of obstructive symptoms.

Quick Cut
A Richter hernia can perforate without signs and symptoms of obstruction.

IV. **Complications:** Hernias should be repaired electively to alleviate symptoms and to prevent the development of major complications.
   A. **Intestinal obstruction**
   B. **Intestinal strangulation with bowel perforation**

Inguinal Hernia

I. **Anatomy of the inguinal region:** Figures 2-4 and 2-5
   A. **Internal inguinal ring:** opening in the transversalis fascia lateral to the inferior epigastric vessels
   B. **External inguinal ring:** opening in the external oblique aponeurosis
   C. **Inguinal canal:** communication between the internal and external rings
      1. **Anterior wall:** formed by the external oblique aponeurosis
      2. **Inferior wall:** formed by the inguinal ligament (**Poupart ligament**)
      3. **Roof (superior wall):** made up of fibers of the internal oblique and transversus abdominis muscles, forming the **conjoint tendon**
      4. **Posterior wall (floor):** formed by the transversalis fascia
         a. **Hesselbach triangle:** located within floor
         b. **Triangle constituents:** formed laterally by the inferior epigastric artery, inferiorly by the inguinal ligament, and superomedially by the lateral border of the rectus sheath

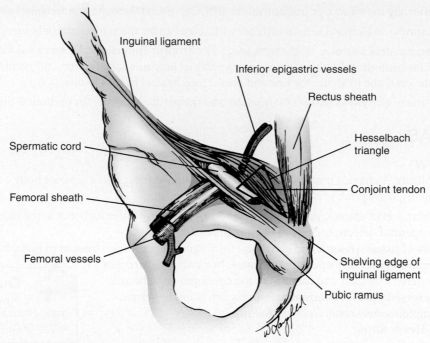

Figure 2-4: Inguinal anatomy.

5. **Round ligament:** traverses the inguinal canal in women
6. **Spermatic cord structures:** Pass through both rings in the inguinal canal and into the scrotum in men. Structures include the following:
   a. **Arteries:** testicular and cremasteric
   b. **Veins:** pampiniform plexus
   c. **Vas deferens**
   d. **Processus vaginalis:** evagination of peritoneum that accompanies testicle descent through the abdominal wall

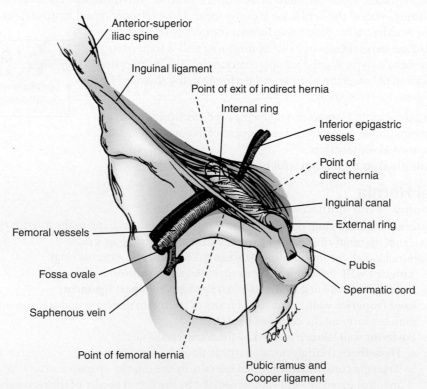

Figure 2-5: Sites of inguinofemoral hernias.

e. **Nerves:** Ilioinguinal and genital branch of the genitofemoral nerves are within the inguinal canal but are external to the cremasteric fascia.

> **Quick Cut**
> A patent processus vaginalis is a congenital indirect inguinal hernia.

II. **Types**
A. **Indirect inguinal hernias:** passes from the peritoneal cavity through the **internal inguinal ring** (i.e., lateral to the epigastric vessels)
   1. **Spermatic cord hydrocele:** may occur if the processus vaginalis is incompletely obliterated
   2. **Incidence:** Indirect inguinal hernias are the most common type of hernia and are 5× more common than direct hernias.
      a. **Gender:** 10× more common in men than in women. At least 5% of men develop an inguinal hernia.
      b. **Age:** may occur from infancy to old age but generally occur by the fifth decade of life
   3. **Pediatric inguinal hernia:** Almost always indirect and has a high risk of incarceration. It is more common on the right (75%).
B. **Direct inguinal hernias:** occurs through the floor of the inguinal canal (i.e., through **Hesselbach triangle**; see Fig. 2-4) because of an acquired weakness in the tissue

> **Quick Cut**
> The inferior epigastric vessels are the anatomic landmarks that distinguish indirect from direct inguinal hernias.

   1. **Site:** Direct hernias occur medial to the epigastric vessels and are direct protrusions of abdominal structures into the floor of the canal posterior to the spermatic cord. It is not contained in the cord as is an indirect hernia.
   2. **Sac:** broadly based defect; much less often associated with strangulation than an indirect inguinal hernia
   3. **Cause:** increases in occurrence with age and is related to physical activity
C. **Recurrent inguinal hernia:** Usually recurs as a direct hernia. Most commonly, the defect occurs in the most medial aspect of the repair of the floor of the inguinal canal.
D. **Pantaloon hernias:** combinations of direct and indirect hernias in which the hernia sac passes both medially and laterally to the epigastric vessels
E. **Femoral hernias:** occurs along the femoral sheath in the **femoral canal** (see Figs. 2-4 and 2-5)
   1. **Site:** Hernia contents protrude posterior to the inguinal ligament, anterior to the pubic ramus periosteum (i.e., **Cooper ligament**), and medial to the femoral vein. The hernia traverses the femoral canal and may also turn cephalad once it has exited the foramen ovale and can cross anteriorly to the inguinal ligament.
   2. **Sac:** Narrow neck; 30%–40% of femoral hernias become incarcerated or strangulated.
   3. **Cause:** more common in women than in men and are associated with female gender, prior pregnancy, and prior inguinal hernia repair

III. **Diagnosis:** based on history and physical examination
A. **History:** May include the appearance of a lump in the groin. The mass may be intermittently present and may be painful. Its appearance is often associated with activity.
B. **Physical examination:** Done with the patient in both supine and standing positions; mass may be visible, and its size and visibility may depend on the patient's position. The mass may be tender or may be reducible with gentle pressure.
C. **Differential diagnosis:** includes hydrocele, varix (especially if thrombosed), lymphadenopathy, lipoma of the spermatic cord, undescended testicle, abscess, or tumor

IV. **Repair:** Surgery is the only curative procedure for inguinal hernias. Most patients develop symptoms, so routine repair is recommended for even minimally symptomatic patients.
A. **Indirect inguinal hernia:** Repair involves returning hernia contents into the peritoneal cavity.
   1. **Division and/or ligation of the base of the hernia sac at the level of the peritoneal cavity:** Sac is **always anteromedial** to the cord at the level of the internal ring.
   2. **In adults:** To prevent recurrence, the internal inguinal ring must be tightened in addition to repair of any defect of the floor of the inguinal canal.
B. **Direct inguinal hernia:** Repair is based on reinforcement of the inguinal canal floor after invaginating the hernia sac.
C. **Femoral hernia:** Repair involves approaching the femoral sheath through the floor of the inguinal canal. The space is usually closed by apposing the posterior reflection of the inguinal ligament to Cooper ligament (**Cooper ligament repair**).

D. **Inguinal canal floor:** Repair can be done with many techniques. Two classic techniques used less commonly now are described first, and then two newer techniques are described.

1. **Bassini repair:** Transversalis fascia and conjoint tendon above are sutured to the reflection of the inguinal ligament (i.e., the shelving edge of Poupart ligament) below.

   a. **In men:** Spermatic cord is returned to its normal anatomic location between the reinforced inguinal canal floor and the external oblique aponeurosis.

   b. **In women:** Round ligament may be ligated and the internal ring closed.

2. **Cooper ligament repair (McVay method):** similar to the Bassini repair except that the transversalis fascia and conjoint tendon are sutured to Cooper ligament

   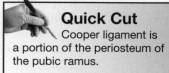

   Quick Cut
   Cooper ligament is a portion of the periosteum of the pubic ramus.

   a. **Relaxing incision:** Because Cooper ligament is more posterior than the inguinal ligament and subjects the repair to increased tension, this counterincision is often made superiorly and allows the conjoint tendon to be sutured to Cooper ligament with less tension.

   b. **Disadvantage:** Tension is the problem with this technique, causing both postoperative pain and early and late recurrences.

3. **Shouldice repair:** Uses the transversalis fascia, which is divided longitudinally and imbricated upon itself in two layers. The internal oblique muscle and conjoint tendon are then sutured to the reflection of the inguinal ligament in two layers.

4. **Prosthetic mesh repairs (Lichtenstein repairs):** have supplanted other techniques

   a. **Procedure:** involves repairing the inguinal floor by using mesh to close the space, suturing it (as in a Bassini repair) to the transversalis fascia and conjoint tendon above and to the reflection of the inguinal ligament below

   b. **Open and laparoscopic techniques:** Used to place polypropylene mesh to reinforce the weakened transversalis fascia. Open techniques also place mesh into the defect.

   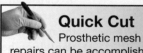

   Quick Cut
   Prosthetic mesh repairs can be accomplished by an open or a laparoscopic approach.

   1. **Indirect hernias:** Cone-shaped polypropylene mesh may be placed adjacent to (anteromedial to) the spermatic cord.

   2. **Direct hernias:** Cone-shaped mesh is used to "plug" the transversalis fascia defect.

V. **Recurrence rates:** Vary depending on the type of hernia; generally, inguinal hernias recur in less than 10% of cases. This figure is usually higher for hernias at other sites.

VI. **Special situations**

A. **Strangulation or necrosis of the incarcerated bowel:** If the bowel returns to the peritoneal cavity spontaneously before visual examination, the abdomen is usually opened to resect any necrotic bowel.

B. **Recurrent hernias or hernias with large defects:** may require the insertion of prosthetic material such as polypropylene mesh to repair the abdominal wall defect adequately

C. **Pediatrics:** Simple high ligation of the hernia sac is used for hernias in this age group. No floor repair is needed.

D. **Truss:** device that exerts external compression over the hernia defect; used only when surgery cannot be safely performed or when the patient refuses surgery

Abdominal Wall Hernias

I. **Umbilical hernias:** occur through the defect where the umbilical structures passed through the abdominal wall

A. **Incidence:** Occur 10× more often in women than in men. The defect is common in children but usually closes by age 2 years, and less than 5% persist into later childhood and adult life.

Quick Cut
In adults, umbilical hernias are often associated with increased intra-abdominal pressure as with ascites or pregnancy.

B. **Repair:** with small umbilical hernias, consists of a simple transverse repair of the fascial defect

II. **Epigastric hernias (epiploceles):** result from a defect in the linea alba above the umbilicus

A. **Incidence:** Occur more commonly in men (3:1 ratio); 20% are multiple at the time of repair.

B. **Repair (simple suturing):** associated with a recurrence rate as high as 10%

III. **Ventral hernias:** occur in the abdominal wall in areas other than the inguinal region
  A. **Incisional hernia:** most common type of ventral hernia; results from poor wound healing in a previous surgical incision and occurs in up to 20% of abdominal incisions
    1. **Common causes:** include wound infection, advanced age, obesity, general debilitation or malnutrition, improper surgical technique, or a postoperative increase in abdominal pressure (ascites or pulmonary complications)
    2. **Repair:** Performed after the patient has recovered from the prior surgical trauma. Requires definition of the adequate fascial edges surrounding the defect, closure with nonabsorbable sutures, and use of prosthetic mesh (polypropylene or ePTFE) when the defect is too large to be closed primarily.
  B. **Spigelian hernias:** protrude through the abdominal wall along the semilunar line (the lateral edge of the rectus muscle) at the semicircular line of Douglas (below the umbilicus)
  C. **Obturator hernias:** occur in the pelvis through the obturator foramen and can cause pain along the obturator nerve (midanterior thigh), referred to as **Howship-Romberg sign**
  D. **Lumbar hernias:** occur on the flank and are seen in the superior (Grynfeltt) and inferior (Petit) triangles
  E. **Perineal hernias:** occur in the pelvic floor usually after surgical procedures such as an abdominoperineal resection
  F. **Peristomal hernias:** develop adjacent to an intestinal ostomy

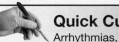

Quick Cut
Spigelian hernias are lateral epigastric hernias that may be difficult to diagnose.

POSTOPERATIVE COMPLICATIONS

Postoperative Fever

I. **"5 W's":** useful mnemonic for common causes of postoperative fever
  A. **Wind:** Pulmonary complications occur on postoperative days 1–3, usually as a result of incisional pain, shallow breathing, and depressed cough from narcotics.

Quick Cut
Remember the 5 "W's" for postoperative fever.

    1. **Atelectasis:** Due to peripheral collapse of alveoli. Treated with pulmonary toilet (i.e., deep breathing, early ambulation, and incentive spirometer) to recruit most of the alveoli. More severe cases may need bronchoscopy to remove a mucus plug.
    2. **Pneumonia:** presents as fever, cough, leukocytosis, and pulmonary infiltrate on chest x-ray
  B. **Water:** Urinary tract infections occur on postoperative days 3–5 due to urinary catheterization; aided by early postoperative removal of catheters.
  C. **Wound infections:** Usually cause fever postoperative days 3–7. More virulent forms (streptococcal or *Clostridium* infections) cause necrotizing infection earlier.
  D. **Walk:** Deep venous thrombosis (DVT) usually occurs in the lower extremities and can cause fever at any postoperative point. Immobilization and hypercoagulable state associated with surgery can increase the risk of thrombosis. Complications of DVT can include pulmonary emboli with associated tachycardia, tachypnea, and hypoxemia.
  E. **Wonder drugs:** Any drug can cause "drug fever," especially antibiotics, which are often used empirically.

II. **Others:** Less common causes include anastomotic leak after bowel surgery, sinusitis, pancreatitis, pseudomembranous colitis, postpericardiotomy syndrome (5–7 days postoperatively), and perirectal abscess.

Myocardial Infarction (MI)

I. **Perioperative MI:** often non–ST-segment elevation MI (NSTEMI)

II. **Symptoms:** presents as shortness of breath, chest pain, or arrhythmias

III. **Treatment:** Mortality from perioperative MI is 30%; therefore, suspicion requires electrocardiography (ECG), troponins, telemetry, and early management.

Quick Cut
Arrhythmias, especially atrial fibrillation, are common after surgery due to changes in electrolytes or volume status.

Fluid Status

I. **Hypovolemia:** common early after surgery due to third-space fluid sequestration

II. **Symptoms:** presents as tachycardia, hypotension, and oliguria

III. **Treatment:** hydration

IV. **Overhydration:** On postoperative days 3–4, the body begins to mobilize this fluid intravascularly with high renal output, causing congestive heart failure, tachyarrhythmias, or pulmonary congestion with impaired oxygenation requiring further diuresis.

SURGICAL INFECTIONS

Surgical Site Infection

I. **Definition:** infection present in any location along the surgical tract

II. **Common organisms:** *Staphylococcus aureus* most common infection overall
   A. *Escherichia coli*: most common gram-negative rod
   B. *Bacteroides fragilis*: most common anaerobe

III. **Features:** fever on postoperative days 5–8 with local tenderness, cellulitis, drainage, and wound dehiscence

IV. **Treatment:** Superficial infections need incision and drainage; deeper wound infections or necrosis need operative debridement and antibiotics.

V. **Prophylactic antibiotics:** Given preoperatively to combat bacterial contamination of tissue during operative period. Follow these general rules.

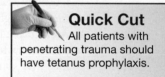

Quick Cut
Prophylactic antibiotics are best given shortly before incision in the operating room.

   A. **Significant risk for postoperative infection exists.**
   B. **Discontinue after surgery (usually before 1 day).**
   C. **Antibiotics effective against the pathogens most likely present.**
   D. **Benefits should outweigh risks of allergy or superinfection.**

Tetanus Injection

I. **Active immunization:** Tetanus toxoid injections provide protective titers in 30 days; given in infancy with boosters every 10 years.

II. **Prophylaxis:** any person with penetrating injury

Quick Cut
All patients with penetrating trauma should have tetanus prophylaxis.

   A. **Unknown tetanus status:** must receive tetanus immunization
   B. **If more than 5 years since last immunization:** must receive a booster
   C. **Contaminated wounds without immunization:** require *both* tetanus toxoid and passive immunity with tetanus immune globulin (protective for 1 month)

III. **Devitalized tissue:** must be debrided

IV. **Antibiotics:** High doses of penicillin are administered prophylactically with extensive necrosis or suspected *Clostridium tetani* infection.

Abscesses

I. **Cutaneous abscess**
   A. **Furuncle (boil):** cutaneous staphylococcal abscess associated with acne and skin disorders
   B. **Carbuncle:** spreads through the dermis into subcutaneous tissues; common with diabetes
   C. **Hidradenitis suppurativa:** Infections of the apocrine sweat glands in the groin and axilla that occur as chronic recurrent abscesses and are often caused by staphylococci. Treatment includes drainage, antibiotics, and excision of the involved area containing multiple abscesses or sinus tracts.

II. **Intra-abdominal abscesses:** Most common sites are the subphrenic and subhepatic spaces, pelvis, and periappendiceal and pericolonic areas.
   A. **External:** caused by penetrating trauma or surgical procedure
   B. **Internal:** caused by a perforated viscus (e.g., appendix) or bacterial seeding (e.g., tubo-ovarian abscess)
   C. **Clinical features:** fever, pain, leukocytosis, tachycardia, and sepsis
   D. **Diagnosis:** Needs high clinical suspicion. Computed tomography (CT) or ultrasound can confirm diagnosis.
   E. **Treatment:** Mainstay is drainage.
      1. **Unilocular abscess:** can be drained percutaneously
      2. **Multilocular abscess:** Complex or necrotic debris may require surgical drainage.

Cellulitis

I. **Definition:** inflammation of the dermal and subcutaneous tissue due to nonsuppurative bacterial invasion

II. **Clinical features:** Produces erythema, edema, and tenderness. May invade the lymphatics, causing red tender streaks (lymphangitis).

III. **Treatment:** antibiotics, usually penicillin because *Streptococcus* is usually the causative organism

Necrotizing Fasciitis

I. **Definition:** Infection introduced through a puncture wound or surgical incision that has a rapidly progressive measurable mortality rate. Pathologically, it invades through fascial planes, causing vascular thrombosis and tissue necrosis.

II. **Clinical features:** Patient becomes toxic with fever and tachycardia.
A. **Overlying skin:** may appear normal or may have hemorrhagic bullae with edema and crepitus
B. **Discharge:** foul smelling if present
C. **Tests:** Plain x-ray or CT scan reveals air in the soft tissue.

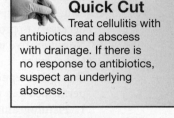

Quick Cut
Treat cellulitis with antibiotics and abscess with drainage. If there is no response to antibiotics, suspect an underlying abscess.

III. **Cause:** multiple organisms; microaerophilic beta-hemolytic streptococci, staphylococci, or aerobes and anaerobes

IV. **Treatment:** aggressive surgical debridement of all devitalized tissue and high-dose antibiotics

Clostridium Myositis and Gas Gangrene

I. *Clostridium perfringens:* causative agent; anaerobic, gram-positive bacilli secreting alpha-lecithinase toxin

II. **Wound characteristics:** The following make wounds susceptible to this infection:
A. **Extensive necrosis:** creates a redox potential for the anaerobe
B. **Impaired blood flow to the area:** as in vascular thrombosis
C. **Gross contamination**
D. **Immunocompromise:** as in diabetes or patients on steroid therapy

III. **Clinical features:** can occur as early as 6 hours after injury
A. **Presentation:** severe pain (out of proportion to exam), weakened pulse, diaphoresis, tenderness to touch, and crepitus
B. **Tests:** Falling hematocrit and rising bilirubin from hemolysis. Gram-positive bacilli with spores without white blood cells in drainage and air in soft tissue on x-ray.

III. **Treatment:** Extensive debridement of tissue; delay is usually catastrophic.

GASTROINTESTINAL FISTULA

I. **Definition:** Abnormal communication between two or more hollow organs or between a hollow organ and the body surface. Named according to the sites they connect (e.g., enterocutaneous fistula connects the small bowel and skin).

II. **Causes**
A. **Congenital:** as in tracheoesophageal fistula
B. **Operative:** as in anastomotic breakdown
C. **Inflammation:** as in Crohn disease
D. **Malignancy:** in which tumor destroys tissue (e.g., sigmoid cancer invades into the bladder)
E. **Radiation**

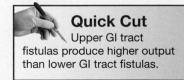

Quick Cut
To remember causes for nonhealing fistulae, use the mnemonic FRIENDS: **F**oreign body, **R**adiation, **I**nflammation, **E**pithelialization, **N**eoplasm, **D**istal obstruction, and **S**epsis/infection.

III. **Evaluation and management:** Determine cause (e.g., diverticulitis or cancer) and volume of drainage (low output has higher rate of closure) and examine to determine location.
A. **Fluid and electrolyte disturbances:** Correct electrolyte losses.
1. **Stomach:** Output is rich in H^+ and Cl^-, causing hypokalemic metabolic alkalosis; replace with D5 ½ normal saline with K^+.

Quick Cut
Upper GI tract fistulas produce higher output than lower GI tract fistulas.

2. **Pancreatic/biliary:** High bicarbonate content; can cause dehydration and metabolic acidosis. Replace with lactated Ringer with HCO_3^-.

3. **Small intestine:** Drainage is rich in K^+ and bicarbonate; replace with lactated Ringer with HCO_3^-.

4. **Large intestines:** Higher potassium loss. Replace with lactated Ringer with K^+.

B. **Infection/sepsis:** Organ leak contaminates sterile spaces, causing abscess/peritonitis.

1. **CT/magnetic resonance imaging (MRI):** can determine undrained abscesses associated with the fistula if persistent fever

2. **Healing:** requires appropriate antibiotic and drainage

C. **Malnutrition:** High caloric needs during infection and either loss of nutrition or poor absorption require early advent of total parental nutrition (TPN).

D. **Inhibit organ secretion:** Use H_2 blockers for the stomach and octreotide with the pancreas.

E. **Skin care:** Output can cause skin excoriation; drains, collection bags, or surgical diversion are necessary to protect the skin.

F. **Nonoperative management:** Bowel rest, TPN, and minimizing drainage can allow fistula to heal in 1–2 months.

G. **Operative repair:** If nonhealing, then operative repair can be performed in a nonseptic, well-nourished patient.

> **Quick Cut**
> GI fistulas may result from trauma or surgery, inflammation, malignancy, or radiation. The main complications from these fistulas are infectious and nutritional.

1. **Fistulogram:** First, determine anatomy and exclude distal obstruction with contrast by mouth, rectum, or into the fistula.

2. **Resection:** With current management, the fistula tract and affected bowel are resected with anastomosis to restore bowel continuity.

3. **Mortality:** Current management has lowered the mortality rate to 5%–15%.

H. **Sepsis prevention:** Enteric and colonic fistulas are complications after trauma, surgery, diverticulitis, cancer, inflammatory bowel disease, and radiation warranting a mortality rate of 6%–33% mostly due to sepsis. Initial management depends on hydration, nutritional support, and octreotide to decrease output and drainage of abscesses, with repair of 25%–75% of fistulas at 3 months.

Chapter 3

Medical Risk Factors in Surgical Patients

Susan B. Kesmodel, Natalia Kubicki, and Mayur Narayan

GENERAL ASPECTS FOR EVALUATION AND MANAGEMENT OF THE SURGICAL PATIENT

Assessment of Medical Comorbidities and Risk Factors

I. **Preoperative evaluation:** first step in ensuring successful surgical outcomes
   A. **Short-term risk:** perioperative period including intraoperative and up to 48 hours postoperative
   B. **Long-term risk:** up to 30 days postoperative

> **Quick Cut**
> In most cases when patients are undergoing elective, noncardiac procedures, minimal preoperative testing is necessary.

II. **Comprehensive history and physical exam:** to identify existing medical problems and other risk factors that may impact surgical outcomes
   A. **Medical history:** Focus on underlying medical conditions, prior difficulties with anesthesia, and the following:
      1. **Medications:** current prescriptions, over-the-counter, alternative medications and supplements, and allergies to medications
      2. **Physiologic parameters:** including volume and nutritional status, and presence of infection
      3. **Substance abuse:** history of tobacco, excessive alcohol use, and drug use
      4. **Familial disorders:** bleeding disorders or problems with anesthesia
   B. **Physical exam:** include evaluation of the following:
      1. **Cardiac function:** heart rate, irregular heart rhythm, heart murmur, lower extremity (LE) edema, jugular venous distention
      2. **Pulmonary function:** accessory muscle use, cyanosis, chest wall deformity, abnormalities on auscultation
      3. **Volume status/renal function:** blood pressure (BP), skin turgor, mucous membrane moistness, presence of dialysis access, edema
      4. **Hepatic function:** jaundice, ascites, hepatomegaly, muscle wasting, spider angiomata, telangiectasias
      5. **Nutritional status:** body mass index, temporal wasting
      6. **Coagulation disorders:** petechiae, ecchymoses, thromboses

Preoperative Testing

I. **Recommendations for preoperative testing:** Ultimately it is the surgeon who must decide on the extent of testing based on the preoperative assessment of the patient and the expected risks of the surgery. Guidelines are listed in Table 3-1.

A. **Elective surgery:** Routine preoperative testing should be performed selectively in these patients based on history; although elderly patients have a higher incidence of abnormal laboratory values, routine testing based on age alone may not impact outcome.

B. **Emergency surgery:** Goal of testing is to identify pre-existing medical conditions and acute organ dysfunction that may impact surgical outcome so that these problems can be monitored during the perioperative period. Most patients will have laboratory and noninvasive testing that includes a complete blood count (CBC), comprehensive medical panel, coagulation profile, electrocardiogram (ECG), and chest x-ray.

C. **Type of surgery:** Also influences extent of preoperative testing; patients undergoing more complicated surgical procedures, where greater fluid shifts and blood loss are expected, will require a more comprehensive assessment. Severity of surgical procedures stratified by the risk of cardiac complications is shown in Table 3-2.

> **Quick Cut**
> Routine preoperative testing for elective surgery is not associated with a decrease in surgical complications. Only American Society of Anesthesiologists (ASA) classification and type of surgical procedure were independent predictors of postoperative complications.

> **Quick Cut**
> Operative morbidity and mortality is increased in patients undergoing emergency surgery. If time permits, electrolyte abnormalities, hypovolemia, acid–base disorders, and coagulopathy should be corrected preoperatively.

Table 3-1: General Guidelines for Preoperative Testing in the Surgical Patient

Complete blood count	• History of chronic kidney disease, liver disease, cardiovascular disease, hematologic disorders, and malignancy • History of anemia or bleeding disorders • Patients undergoing cardiovascular surgery or other high-risk surgical procedures • Patients undergoing intermediate-risk surgical procedures with comorbid conditions • History of malignancy • Pregnant patients • Extremes of age
Basic metabolic panel (electrolytes, creatinine, glucose)	• History of chronic kidney disease, liver disease, endocrine disorders, and diabetes • Use of medications associated with electrolyte abnormalities • Patients undergoing cardiovascular or other high-risk surgery • Patients undergoing intermediate or high-risk surgical procedures with comorbid conditions
Coagulation parameters	• History of chronic kidney disease, liver disease, cardiovascular disease, and pulmonary disease • History of a bleeding disorder • Patients taking anticoagulants • Patients undergoing high-risk surgical procedures
Liver function tests	• History of liver disease • History of malignancy
Electrocardiogram	• Patients with a history of cardiovascular disease or risk factors for cardiovascular disease who are undergoing intermediate or high-risk surgical procedures • Patients with no risk factors undergoing high-risk surgery
Chest radiograph	• History of chronic obstructive pulmonary disease, asthma, or cardiac disease • Recent upper respiratory infection • Abnormal history and physical examination findings • Patients undergoing cardiovascular or thoracic surgery • Patient age older than 50 years undergoing upper abdominal surgery • Consider for patients who are smokers
Urinalysis	• New urinary symptoms • Urologic procedures • Implantation of foreign material

Table 3-2: Stratification of Noncardiac Surgical Procedures by Cardiac Risk

Low risk (<1%)	Breast and other soft tissue, dental, endocrine, eye, gynecologic, minor orthopedic or urologic, plastic surgery
Intermediate risk (1%–5%)	Intraperitoneal, intrathoracic, carotid and endovascular aneurysm repair, head and neck, neurologic, major orthopedic
High risk (>5%)	Aortic and other major vascular procedures

II. **ASA classification:** ASA physical status classification used to assess the degree of systemic illness in patients prior to surgery is shown in Table 3-3.

III. **Infection control:** Surgical site infections are one of the most common postoperative complications; however, use of antibiotics in the perioperative setting has been shown to decrease their incidence.
   A. **Dosing:** One preoperative dose is sufficient for most cases and should be dosed within 60 minutes of the surgical procedure except for vancomycin, which should be dosed 60–120 minutes prior to surgery.
   B. **Choice:** should target the most likely pathogens based on the surgical site
   C. **Duration:** Prolonged duration of antibiotic use is discouraged.
   D. **Redosing:** should be based on the half-life of the drug, duration of the surgical procedure, and degree of blood loss

IV. **Venous thromboembolism (VTE):** one of the most common complications following surgery
   A. **Risk factors:** include advanced age; prolonged immobility; malignancy; history of VTE; fractures of the pelvis, hip, or LE; type of surgery; major trauma; obesity; stroke; and myocardial infarction (MI)
   B. **Preoperative prophylaxis:** Guidelines are based on severity of the surgery and patient comorbidities (Table 3-4).
      1. **High-risk patients:** Low-dose unfractionated heparin (LDUH) or low-molecular-weight heparin (LMWH) should be started preoperatively; otherwise, initiate as early in the postoperative period as possible.
         a. **Graduated compression stockings (GCS) and intermittent pneumatic compression (ICP):** start preoperatively to decrease venous stasis, improve blood flow velocity, and increase fibrolytic activity
         b. **Postoperative:** Early ambulation in this period is essential.
         c. **High-risk orthopedic procedures:** Consider extending prophylaxis for 30 days after surgery.

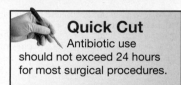

Quick Cut
Increasing ASA score correlates with postoperative morbidity and mortality as well as a longer duration of surgery, increased intraoperative blood loss, longer requirement for postoperative ventilatory support, and longer hospital admission.

Quick Cut
Antibiotic use should not exceed 24 hours for most surgical procedures.

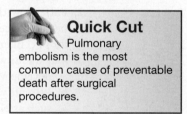

Quick Cut
Pulmonary embolism is the most common cause of preventable death after surgical procedures.

Table 3-3: American Society of Anesthesiologists Physical Status Classification

Class	Description
I	Healthy patient
II	Mild systemic disease with no functional limitation
III	Severe systemic disease with definite functional limitation
IV	Severe systemic disease that is a constant threat to life
V	Moribund patient unlikely to survive 24 hours with or without operation

Table 3-4: Guidelines for Venous Thromboembolism Prevention in Patients Undergoing Surgery

Level of Risk	Prevention Strategy
Low risk	
Minor surgery in patients younger than age 40 years with no risk factors	Early mobilization
Moderate risk	
Minor surgery with risk factors Surgery in patients age 40–60 years with no risk factors	LDUH every 12 hours, LMWH ≤3,400 units daily, GCS, or IPC
High risk	
Surgery in patients older than age 60 years Surgery in patients age 40–60 years with risk factors	LDUH every 8 hours, LMWH >3,400 units daily, or IPC
Highest risk	
Surgery in patients with multiple risk factors Hip or knee arthroplasty or hip fracture Major trauma or spinal cord injury	LMWH >3,400 units daily, fondaparinux, oral vitamin K antagonists, or GCS/IPC and LDUH/LMWH

LDUH, low-dose unfractionated heparin; LMWH, low-molecular-weight heparin; GCS, graduated compression stockings; IPC, intermittent pneumatic compression.
Adapted from Guyatt GH, Akl EA, Crowther M, et al; American College of Chest Physicians Antithrombotic Therapy and Prevention of Thrombosis Panel. Antithrombotic therapy and prevention of thrombosis: American College of Chest Physicians evidence-based clinical practice guidelines. *Chest.* 2012;141(2)(Suppl):7S–47S.

2. **Patients with recent VTE events:** If anticoagulation must be discontinued for an extended period, placement of an inferior vena cava (IVC) filter should be considered; major indications for IVC filter placement include the following:
   a. Patients who are refractory to medical anticoagulation and develop VTE while on medical therapy
   b. Patients who develop complications of anticoagulation such as bleeding and thrombocytopenia
   c. Contraindication to anticoagulation such as recent traumatic brain injury or recent major abdominal hemorrhage
   d. Free-floating thrombus in the ileofemoral region at increased risk of dislodging and leading to VTE

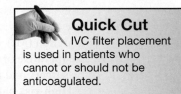

Quick Cut
IVC filter placement is used in patients who cannot or should not be anticoagulated.

EVALUATION OF THE SURGICAL PATIENT WITH CARDIAC DISEASE

General Aspects
I. **Risk assessment:** Extensive research has focused on preoperative assessment of cardiac risk and prevention of postoperative complications. Postoperative MI is associated with hospital mortality rates of 15%–25%.

Quick Cut
Perioperative cardiac mortality remains the leading cause of death after anesthesia and surgery.

II. **Primary goal:** Identify comorbid conditions that may adversely impact operative outcomes and attempt to optimize or correct these conditions preoperatively.

Assessment of Cardiac Disease and Risk Factors for Cardiac Disease
I. **Past medical history:** should focus on history of cardiac disease, cardiac interventions, and other medical conditions that are risk factors for the development of cardiovascular disease
   A. **Presence of comorbid conditions:** Diabetes mellitus (DM), pulmonary disease, and chronic kidney disease (CKD) may increase the risk of perioperative cardiac complications.
   B. **Other:** Obtain complete list of current medications and assess functional status.

II. **Physical examination:** Assess body habitus, jugular venous distention, LE edema, cyanosis, surgical scars, and presence of indwelling pacemakers or automatic implantable cardioverter-defibrillators (AICDs).
   A. **Vital signs:** including BP in both arms
   B. **Auscultation of heart sounds:** Evaluate for rhythm, murmurs, or other signs of cardiac dysfunction.
   C. **Peripheral pulses:** Presence of peripheral vascular disease (PVD) may indicate coronary artery disease (CAD) even in the asymptomatic patient.

III. **Cardiac history**
   A. **Hypertension (HTN):** Mild (stage 1) or moderate (stage 2; systolic blood pressure [SBP] <180 mm Hg and diastolic blood pressure [DBP] <110 mm Hg) is not an independent risk factor, but stage 3 (SBP ≥180 mm Hg and DBP ≥110 mm Hg) is a risk factor for the development of cardiac complications.

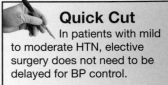

Quick Cut
In patients with mild to moderate HTN, elective surgery does not need to be delayed for BP control.

   B. **Angina:** Table 3-5 shows the Canadian Cardiovascular Society angina classification system based on the degree of symptoms with physical activity; patients with class III or class IV angina have an increased risk of cardiac complications during surgery.
   C. **Valvular heart disease:** Critical aortic stenosis is associated with increased risk of perioperative cardiac complications; these patients cannot increase cardiac output because of outflow obstruction.
      1. **Aortic or mitral regurgitation:** Operative risk is related to the status of left ventricular function.
      2. **Prosthetic heart valves:** Patients are at risk for valve thrombosis and thromboembolic complications.
   D. **Congestive heart failure (CHF):** increases risk of pulmonary edema
   E. **Pacemakers and AICDs:** may be affected intraoperatively by electrocautery devices

IV. **ECG indications:** chest pain, history of CAD, CHF, DM, HTN, PVD, morbid obesity, valvular heart disease, and exercise intolerance
   A. **Exclusions:** ECG is not routinely needed in minimal-risk procedures and in patients aged younger than 65 years.
   B. **Timing:** ECG within 1 year is adequate for most patients and most surgical procedures; however, in patients with CAD, an ECG should be obtained within 30 days or following the last episode of cardiovascular symptoms if within 1 year.
   C. **Abnormal findings:** evidence of prior MI, bundle branch block (BBB), bifascicular block, atrioventricular (AV) block, prolonged QT, right ventricular hypertrophy, arrhythmia

Preoperative Risk Assessment Stratification Tools

I. **American College of Cardiology/American Heart Association:** Patients undergoing noncardiac procedures are stratified into three groups based on risk of developing cardiac complications: low risk (<1%), intermediate risk (1%–5%), and high risk (5%).

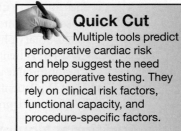

Quick Cut
Multiple tools predict perioperative cardiac risk and help suggest the need for preoperative testing. They rely on clinical risk factors, functional capacity, and procedure-specific factors.

II. **Goldman Risk Index (Original Cardiac Risk Index):** identified perioperative fatal and nonfatal cardiac events; divides patients into four risk classes based on points obtained from history, physical exam, preoperative testing, and type of operation (Table 3-6)

Table 3-5: Canadian Cardiovascular Society Classification of Angina

Class	Description
0	Asymptomatic
I	Angina only during strenuous or prolonged physical activity
II	Slight limitation, angina only during vigorous physical activity
III	Moderate limitation, symptoms with activities of daily living
IV	Severe limitation, inability to perform activity without angina or angina at rest

Table 3-6: Goldman Risk Index

Risk Factor	Points
Active heart failure: preoperative third heart sound or jugular venous distention	11
Myocardial infarction in the past 6 months	10
≥5 premature ventricular complexes/min before surgery	7
Rhythm other than sinus	7
Age older than 70 years	5
Emergency surgery	4
Significant aortic stenosis	3
Intraperitoneal, intrathoracic, or aortic surgery	3
Markers of poor general medical condition (e.g., renal dysfunction, liver disease, lung disease, electrolyte imbalance)	3

From Goldman L, Caldera DL, Nussbaum SR, et al. Multifactorial index of cardiac risk in noncardiac surgical procedures. *New Engl J Med*. 1977; 297(16):845–850.

III. **Revised Cardiac Risk Index (modified from the Original Cardiac Risk Index):** assigns predictors of cardiac complications from history and type of surgery
   A. **History:** ischemic heart disease, CHF, cerebrovascular disease (stroke or transient ischemic attack), diabetes requiring insulin use, or CKD (creatinine >2 mg/dL)
   B. **Type of surgery:** suprainguinal vascular, intraperitoneal, or intrathoracic
   C. **Risk for cardiac death, nonfatal MI, and nonfatal cardiac arrest:** based on number of predictors
      1. **0 predictor:** 0.4%
      2. **1 predictor:** 0.9%
      3. **2 predictors:** 6.6%
      4. **Greater than 3 predictors:** greater than 11%

IV. **New York Heart Association (NYHA):** functional classification
   A. **Class I:** Patients with cardiac disease without physical activity limitations; ordinary physical activity does not cause undue fatigue, palpitations, or dyspnea.
   B. **Class II:** Patients with cardiac disease that slightly limits physical activity but who are comfortable at rest; ordinary physical activity results in fatigue, palpitations, or dyspnea.
   C. **Class III:** Patients with cardiac disease resulting in marked limitation of physical activity but who are comfortable at rest; less than ordinary activity causes fatigue, palpitations, or dyspnea.
   D. **Class IV:** Patients with cardiac disease who cannot do any physical activity without discomfort; symptoms are present even at rest or with minimal exertion.

Additional Noninvasive and Invasive Cardiac Testing

I. **Echocardiogram:** may be considered in patients with prior abnormal ECG findings, known history of CAD or CHF, dyspnea with unknown cause, and to evaluate left ventricular function

II. **Noninvasive myocardial perfusion assessment:** indicated for patients with a functional capacity less than 4 metabolic equivalents of exercise (METs) or unknown capacity (e.g., unable to climb a flight of stairs) and for patients with moderate functional capacity undergoing high-risk surgery

III. **Exercise stress testing:** measures functional capacity to identify the presence of cardiac arrhythmias or myocardial ischemia and estimates perioperative cardiac risk and long-term prognosis

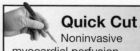

Quick Cut
Noninvasive myocardial perfusion assessment is *not* recommended for patients undergoing intermediate-risk surgical operations with no clinical risk factors or for patients undergoing low-risk surgical procedures.

IV. **Noninvasive stress testing:** includes radionuclide myocardial imaging, stress echocardiography, and dobutamine echocardiography

A. **Perioperative cardiac risk:** directly related to extent of jeopardized myocardium identified

B. **Patients with unstable myocardial ischemia:** Perform coronary angiography or stabilize with aggressive medical treatment rather than stress testing.

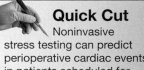

Quick Cut
Noninvasive stress testing can predict perioperative cardiac events in patients scheduled for noncardiac surgery who are unable to exercise.

Perioperative Management and Approaches to Risk Reduction

I. **Modifiable risk factors:** For elective surgical procedures, health and lifestyle modifications should be implemented preoperatively.

A. **Health management:** Control BP, cholesterol, and DM and use antiplatelet agents or anticoagulation.

B. **Lifestyle modification:** aerobic exercise greater than 150 minutes per week, smoking cessation, weight loss, and diet modification

II. **Perioperative beta-blocker therapy:** Beta-blockers are effective in preventing severe BP fluctuations and can reduce the number and duration of perioperative coronary ischemic episodes.

A. **Indications:** patients who are already on beta-blockers, particularly those with history of arrhythmia or MI and patients undergoing intermediate-risk surgery with clinical risk factors for ischemic heart disease

B. **Initiation:** If beta-blockers are indicated, they should be started at least 2 weeks before elective surgery.

C. **Titration:** should be titrated to a heart rate of 60–80 beats per minute in the absence of hypotension and should be tapered off slowly to minimize risk of withdrawal

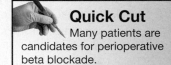

Quick Cut
Many patients are candidates for perioperative beta blockade.

III. **Perioperative alpha-adrenergic agonists:** used as anesthetic adjuvants and analgesics

A. **Primary effect:** sympatholytic, reducing peripheral norepinephrine release

B. **Advantages:** reduce requirement for intravenous (IV) or inhaled anesthetics and has been shown to decrease MI and perioperative mortality rates in patients undergoing vascular surgery

C. **Clonidine:** selective agonist for alpha$_2$-adrenoreceptors

1. **Oral antihypertensive effects:** result from central and peripheral attenuation of sympathetic outflow

2. **Withdrawal:** May precipitate hypertensive crises; labetalol can be used to treat clonidine withdrawal.

Quick Cut
Traditionally, α-adrenergic agonists were used only as anti-hypertensives. Now, their use is increasing for sedative, anxiolytic and analgesic effects."

D. **Dexmedetomidine:** highly selective alpha$_2$-receptor agonist available as an IV solution

1. **Usual dosing:** infusion of 0.3–0.7 μg/kg/hr

2. **Effects:** shown to increase sedation, analgesia, and amnesia; decreases heart rate, cardiac output, and circulating catecholamines; minimizes need for narcotics when used perioperatively in patients with obstructive sleep apnea (OSA)

IV. **Coronary artery revascularization:** should be performed in patients with stable angina who have significant left main coronary artery stenosis or three-vessel disease

A. **Other indications:** recommended for patients with high-risk unstable angina, non–ST-segment elevation MI, and acute ST elevation

B. **Elective noncardiac surgery:** not recommended within 4 weeks of coronary revascularization

C. **Elective noncardiac surgery:** not recommended within 4–6 weeks of bare-metal coronary stent implantation or within 12 months of drug-eluting coronary stent implantation

D. **Elective procedures with significant risk of perioperative bleeding:** should be deferred until patients have completed an

Quick Cut
Routine prophylactic coronary revascularization is not recommended for patients with stable CAD before noncardiac surgery.

appropriate course of thienopyridine therapy (ticlopidine or clopidogrel)
1. **For patients treated with drug-eluting stents:** Aspirin should be continued if possible.
2. **Antiplatelet therapy:** should resume as soon as possible in the postoperative period to prevent late stent thrombosis

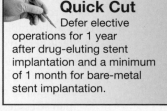

Quick Cut
Defer elective operations for 1 year after drug-eluting stent implantation and a minimum of 1 month for bare-metal stent implantation.

V. **Maintenance of normothermia:** Body temperature 36.6°C ± 0.5°C is recommended for most procedures except during periods in which mild hypothermia is intended to provide organ protection.

VI. **3-Hydroxy-3-methylglutaryl-coenzyme A (HMG-CoA) reductase inhibitors:** should be started for patients who have known vascular disease, elevated low-density lipoprotein cholesterol, or ischemia
   A. **Should be continued:** for patients undergoing noncardiac surgery and for those who are already taking statins
   B. **Other indications:** Statin use may also be considered for patients undergoing vascular and intermediate-risk surgical operations.

Invasive Hemodynamic Monitoring

I. **Arterial line:** Allows for continuous direct BP monitoring and frequent arterial blood gas (ABG) sampling; consider in critically ill patients and in patients in whom large volume shifts or blood loss is expected.

II. **Pulmonary artery catheter (Swan-Ganz):** consider in patients at risk for major hemodynamic disturbances or in elderly patients with known cardiac history
   A. **Precautions:** Patient disease, surgical procedure, and practice setting should be weighed prior to insertion.
   B. **Data interpretation:** Lack of experience in interpreting pulmonary artery catheter data may cause more harm than benefit.

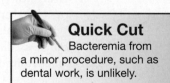

Quick Cut
Pulmonary artery catheters are not recommended for routine use.

III. **Transesophageal echocardiography (TEE):** consider in critically ill patients to help determine the cause of an acute or persistent hemodynamic abnormality
   A. **Advantages:** superior to transthoracic echocardiography (TTE) in providing structural and functional detail
   B. **Disadvantages:** invasive procedure that requires intubation

Bacterial Endocarditis Prophylaxis

I. **In general:** no longer recommended based solely on the risk of acquiring infective endocarditis (IE)

II. **Indications:** Cardiac conditions associated with high adverse outcomes from IE include prosthetic cardiac valve, previous IE, congenital heart disease, and cardiac transplant recipients who develop cardiac valvulopathy.

III. **Regimen:** Amoxicillin PO or ampicillin, cefazolin, or ceftriaxone IV; if allergic to penicillin, use clindamycin or azithromycin.

Quick Cut
Bacteremia from a minor procedure, such as dental work, is unlikely.

Quick Cut
Antibiotic prophylaxis solely to prevent IE is not recommended for genitourinary or gastrointestinal tract procedures.

Postoperative Complications

I. **MI:** Most perioperative MIs occur during the first 3–5 days when patients shift extracellular fluid intravascularly in a process known as *autodiuresis*.
   A. **Signs and symptoms:** Postoperative MIs may be associated with new-onset CHF, arrhythmias, or changes in mental status rather than chest pain.
   B. **Emergency surgery:** places patients at a higher risk for perioperative cardiac events than elective surgery

Quick Cut
Patients with a history of an MI, pathologic Q waves on preoperative ECG, or an MI within the past 30 days are at major risk for MI.

II. **Arrhythmias:** Majority of surgery patients exhibit abnormalities in heart rate or rhythm; however, only ~5% of these are clinically significant.

III. **Pulmonary edema:** may occur in patients with a history of CHF due to volume overload and HTN

IV. **Thromboembolic events:** May occur in patients with prosthetic heart valves in whom anticoagulation has been discontinued; anticoagulation should be restarted as soon as possible.

Quick Cut
The hospital mortality rate of patients who have a postoperative MI after noncardiac surgery is 20%.

Quick Cut
Postoperative arrhythmias may be caused by metabolic abnormalities, ischemia, and hypoxia, and these problems should be identified and corrected.

EVALUATION OF THE SURGICAL PATIENT WITH LUNG DISEASE

Pulmonary Function Assessment

I. **General aspects:** Patients with chronic lung disease are more susceptible to postoperative pulmonary complications that may include atelectasis, pneumonia, exacerbation of chronic lung disease, and respiratory failure requiring mechanical ventilation. Because these complications are associated with longer hospital stays and increased morbidity and mortality, identifying pulmonary risk factors preoperatively allows appropriate testing and risk modification may be undertaken prior to surgery.

II. **History and physical examination:** should alert the physician that pulmonary disease exists
   A. **Patient history:** Age older than 50 years has been identified as an independent risk factor for postoperative pulmonary complications.
   B. **Review of systems:** chronic cough, excessive sputum production, wheezing, exercise intolerance, and dyspnea
   C. **Social history:** tobacco use
   D. **Medical history:** chronic obstructive pulmonary disease (COPD), obesity, OSA, pulmonary HTN, asthma, emphysema, prior lung surgery, neuromuscular disorders, CHF, and recurrent bronchitis or pneumonia
   E. **Physical examination:** scoliosis; chest wall abnormalities; abnormalities on auscultation including wheezing, rales, and rhonchi; prolonged expiration; cyanosis; finger clubbing; jugular venous distention; and scars from prior surgery

III. **Preoperative studies:** Laboratory and imaging evaluation should be obtained only in select patients at higher risk for postoperative pulmonary complications.
   A. **Chest radiograph:** Routine preoperative chest x-rays are not necessary in all patients.
   B. **ABGs:** Assess the adequacy of ventilation and oxygenation.
   C. **ASA risk classification:** Greater than class II confers a more than four-fold increased risk of postoperative pulmonary complications.
   D. **Pulmonary function tests (PFTs):** In the absence of a history significant for COPD or asthma, routine preoperative spirometry has not been shown to predict postoperative pulmonary complications in extrathoracic surgery.
   E. **Preoperative spirometry and ABGs:** may be considered in patients with findings that suggest pulmonary disease such as planned thoracic procedures, productive cough and dyspnea, greater than 20/pack/year history of cigarette smoking, abnormal chest radiograph findings, and morbid obesity
   F. **Patients undergoing thoracic surgical procedures:** Specific criteria have been established for the minimum pulmonary function necessary to tolerate pulmonary resection.

Quick Cut
Chest x-rays should be performed in patients with known cardiopulmonary disease or in patients older than age 50 years who are undergoing upper abdominal, thoracic, or aortic aneurysm surgery.

Quick Cut
No single PFT is an absolute contraindication to surgery.

Quick Cut
Failure of PFTs to improve after bronchodilator therapy may be an indication of high pulmonary risk.

Preoperative Risk Modification

I. **Cease cigarette smoking:** should be stopped at least 6–8 weeks before elective surgery in order to significantly reduce postoperative complications

II. **COPD:** Antibiotics should be administered prior to surgery in patients with acute bronchitis, productive cough, or purulent sputum production. Elective surgery should be delayed until after treatment and symptoms have resolved.

III. **Asthma:** Patients should be managed preoperatively with antibiotics, bronchodilators, beta$_2$ agonists, and steroids.

IV. **Obesity:** Obese patients have a restrictive respiratory pattern that leads to an increased incidence of postoperative atelectasis.

> **Quick Cut**
> The importance of ambulation and incentive spirometry use should be reviewed with patients preoperatively.

Operative Considerations

I. **Anesthesia:** General anesthesia may cause a small but significant drop in functional residual capacity for up to 2 weeks postoperatively.

A. **Neuromuscular blockade:** Impairs ciliary and diaphragmatic function; to minimize residual blockade following surgery, avoid use of long-acting agents.

B. **Endotracheal intubation and inhalation anesthetics:** may exacerbate bronchospasm

C. **Mechanical ventilation:** leads to an increased risk of pneumothorax in susceptible patients due to barotraumas

D. **Neuraxial blockade (spinal or epidural anesthesia):** results in a lower rate of pulmonary complications when compared to general anesthesia

II. **Operative factors:** influence the risk of pulmonary complications

A. **Surgical location:** Thoracotomy and upper abdominal surgeries are associated with the greatest risk of postoperative pulmonary complications.

B. **Minimally invasive surgery:** May reduce postoperative pulmonary complications due to improvement in postoperative lung volumes and a decrease in postoperative pain. Intraoperative CO_2 retention may occur due to insufflation.

> **Quick Cut**
> Higher abdominal incisions have an increased risk of pulmonary complications relative to lower abdominal incisions.

C. **Type of incision:** Horizontal incisions have a lower incidence of respiratory complications including hypoxemia and atelectasis when compared to vertical incisions.

D. **Length of surgery:** Surgery lasting more than 3 hours and emergency surgery are associated with increased pulmonary complications.

Perioperative Management

I. **Lung expansion:** Lung expansion techniques reduce postoperative pulmonary complications; these include incentive spirometry, cough, deep breathing, continuous positive airway pressure (CPAP), postural drainage, chest physiotherapy, and intermittent positive pressure breathing.

> **Quick Cut**
> The maximal reduction in pulmonary complications is achieved when patient teaching on interventions is started preoperatively.

II. **Extubation:** Following the completion of surgery; adequate ventilation and oxygenation must be maintained, the airway must remain patent, and aspiration must be prevented with suctioning and head turning.

A. **Protocol-based weaning of mechanical ventilation:** decreases ventilator time and reduces the incidence of ventilator-associated pneumonia

B. **Reintubation:** can be prevented with aggressive management including bronchodilator therapy, frequent suctioning, and noninvasive ventilation with CPAP or bilevel positive airway pressure (BiPAP)

III. **Adequate pain control:** helps to minimize pulmonary complications by improving patient comfort

A. **Medication:** Avoid excessive narcotic or benzodiazepine use to minimize oversedation and respiratory depression.

B. **Epidural anesthesia:** can provide excellent postoperative pain control and may reduce pulmonary complications

> **Quick Cut**
> Adequate pain control allows for earlier ambulation and improves the ability of patients to cough and perform deep breathing exercises.

Pulmonary Complications

I. **Atelectasis:** most common postoperative pulmonary complication

   A. **Hypoxemia with atelectasis:** usually begins on the second postoperative day

   B. **Early hypoxemia:** may signal hypoventilation from residual anesthesia, airway edema, or obstruction

II. **Pneumonia:** typically occurs within 5 days of surgery

   A. **Cause:** frequently caused by gram-negative bacteria and *Staphylococcus aureus*

   B. **Treatment:** includes collection of respiratory cultures and initiation of antibiotics

III. **Other significant complications:** include bronchospasm (which can be treated with short-acting inhaled beta$_2$ agonists), pulmonary edema, pneumothorax, pulmonary embolism, adult respiratory distress syndrome, and aspiration

> **Quick Cut**
> Postoperative pulmonary complications are almost as common as postoperative cardiac complications, and they can lead to increased hospital lengths of stay and increased mortality after surgery.

EVALUATION OF THE SURGICAL PATIENT WITH RENAL DISEASE

Renal Function Assessment

I. **History:** should focus on medical conditions that are risk factors for the development of kidney disease such as a known history of CKD, prior episodes of acute kidney injury (AKI), any surgical procedures on the kidney and urinary tract, and nephrotoxic medications

   A. **Underlying systemic diseases:** include diffuse atherosclerosis, DM, HTN, autoimmune diseases, and collagen vascular disease

   B. **Medications:** Thorough review is important to identify any nephrotoxic medications that have the potential to contribute to AKI.

   C. **Other:** Prior history of bleeding problems; determine if the patient is dialysis dependent.

II. **Physical examination:** should focus on the following:

   A. **Signs of volume overload:** pulmonary rales, jugular venous distension, and peripheral edema

   B. **Signs of cardiovascular disease:** cardiac murmurs, diminished peripheral pulses, jugular venous distension, or peripheral edema

   C. **Evidence of coagulopathy:** including petechiae and ecchymoses

   D. **Central nervous system changes:** including lethargy and altered mental status

   E. **Pericardial or pleural rubs and decreased basilar breath sounds:** may indicate pleural effusions

III. **Laboratory testing and diagnostic studies:** should include the following:

   A. **Basic metabolic panel:** Assess for electrolyte abnormalities and blood urea nitrogen (BUN) and creatinine levels.

   B. **CBC:** to evaluate for anemia; iron studies if anemia is present

   C. **Bleeding time**

   D. **Calculations:** Creatinine clearance and glomerular filtration rate (GFR) to determine renal function may be performed using the Crockcroft-Gault formula and the Modification of Diet in Renal Disease (MDRD) Study Equation.

     1. **Crockcroft-Gault formula:**

$$\frac{(140 - \text{age}) \times \text{lean body weight [kg]}}{\text{Cr [mg/dL]} \times 72}$$

     2. **For women:**

$$\frac{(140 - \text{age}) \times \text{lean body weight [kg]} \times .85}{\text{Cr [mg/dL]} \times 72}$$

> **Quick Cut**
> Patients with CKD commonly need surgery: Access for dialysis is nearly universal, as well as general surgical problems.

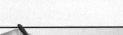

> **Quick Cut**
> Cardiovascular disease is the most common cause of mortality in patients with CKD.

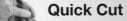

> **Quick Cut**
> Standard formulas estimate the degree of renal function and allow appropriate dosing of medications.

Table 3-7: National Kidney Foundation Classification of Chronic Kidney Disease

Stage	Description	GFR (mL/min per 1.73 m²)
1	Kidney damage with normal or increased GFR	≥90
2	Kidney damage with mild decreased GFR	60–89
3	Moderately decreased GFR	30–59
4	Severely decreased GFR	15–29
5	Kidney failure	<15 (or dialysis)

GFR, glomerular filtration rate.

     3. **MDRD Study Equation:** GFR, in mL/min per 1.73m² = 186.3 × SCr (exp[−1.154]) × age (exp[−0.203]) × (0.742 if female) × (1.21 if black)

  E. Other: Drug levels should be measured, chest radiograph should be obtained to assess volume status, and ECG should be obtained and compared to prior ECGs.

IV. Classification of CKD: defined as either kidney damage or decreased kidney function for at least 3 months (Table 3-7)

  A. Proteinuria: principal indicator of kidney damage

  B. GFR: single best measure of kidney function

  C. Level of kidney function: determines stage of CKD regardless of underlying diagnosis

Preoperative Management

I. Fluid and electrolyte homeostasis: altered in patients with renal disease and results in HTN and the following:

  A. Sodium and water retention: can exacerbate CHF and peripheral edema

  B. Hyperkalemia: Attempts should be made to normalize K⁺ levels.

    1. Treatment: Sodium bicarbonate, insulin and glucose in combination, and beta agonists may be given to temporarily shift K^+ intracellularly.

    2. Exchange resins: Sodium polystyrene sulfonate (Kayexalate) may be given orally or by enema.

    3. Dialysis: may also be used

  C. Metabolic acidosis: may be corrected by either bicarbonate administration or with dialysis

  D. Hypocalcemia: due to decreased active vitamin D formation

  E. Hyperphosphatemia: caused by secondary hyperparathyroidism

II. Hematologic functions: altered

  A. Anemia: Occurs as a result of decreased erythropoietin production; erythropoietin may be given preoperatively if the surgery is elective.

  B. Coagulation defects are expected to occur as a result of altered platelet adhesion and aggregation in uremic patients.

III. Cardiac and other vascular abnormalities: more common and include atherosclerosis, pericarditis, and pericardial effusions

IV. Nutritional status: impaired due to decreased body stores of nitrogen and protein, which may lead to poor wound healing

V. Dialysis: Routine hemodialysis should be performed to prevent volume overload, metabolic acidosis, and hyperkalemia.

  A. Peritoneal dialysis exchanges: Should occur up until the time of surgery; the peritoneal dialysate should be drained immediately prior to surgery.

  B. Temporary hemodialysis: may be used after abdominal surgery

> **Quick Cut**
> Hemodialysis should be performed within 24 hours of elective surgery.

Operative Variables

I. Anesthesia: Renal failure affects the metabolism of different anesthetic drugs due to changes in renal excretion and protein binding.

  A. Inhalational agents: Decrease GFR and urinary excretion of sodium. Fluoride ion accumulation with the use of some agents can lead to renal toxicity.

B. **Muscle relaxants:** Succinylcholine administration leads to increases in serum K^+, and atracurium undergoes enzymatic degradation in plasma and can be safely used in patients with renal insufficiency.

C. **Benzodiazepines:** Highly protein-bound agents; renal failure causes decreased protein binding and increased accumulation of the active form, which leads to prolonged sedation.

D. **Morphine:** Should be used cautiously due to its prolonged sedative effects. Propoxyphene and meperidine should be avoided in patients with renal failure due to accumulation of neurotoxic metabolites.

> **Quick Cut**
> Narcotics may have prolonged effects in patients with renal dysfunction, making fentanyl the narcotic of choice.

II. **Vascular access**

A. **Arteriovenous fistulas and grafts:** Special care must be taken to protect the access site of dialysis patients.

1. **Position:** Arm should be positioned to avoid prolonged pressure and possible thrombosis.

2. **Blood draws and BP monitoring:** should be performed on the opposite limb

3. **Evaluation:** Graft should be evaluated preoperatively and postoperatively to ensure patency.

B. **Central line placement:** Central venous access should be placed on the opposite side of existing vascular access for dialysis.

> **Quick Cut**
> Central line placement in the subclavian vein should be avoided to prevent subclavian stenosis that may affect the ability to create future vascular access fistulas and grafts.

III. **Anemia and blood loss:** Severe anemia should be corrected; blood transfusion should be avoided if possible to prevent antibody formation and hyperkalemia.

IV. **Hypotension:** should be avoided to prevent decreased renal perfusion and acute tubular necrosis (ATN)

V. **Antibiotics:** must be dosed appropriately for renal function

Postoperative Complications

I. **General aspects:** Postoperative complications are common in patients with CKD, most commonly hyperkalemia, AKI, infection, hemodynamic instability, bleeding, arrhythmias, anemia, and loss of vascular access.

II. **Hyperkalemia:** Can be managed by shifting K^+ intracellularly or by eliminating K^+ from the body. If ECG changes (e.g., peaked T waves, P wave loss, widened QRS) occur, IV calcium should be given to protect against ventricular fibrillation and cardiac arrest.

> **Quick Cut**
> Surgical mortality in patients with end-stage renal disease ranges from 1% to 4%; however, the risk increases five-fold for emergency surgical procedures.

III. **Coagulopathy:** can be managed with desmopressin (DDAVP), conjugated estrogens, and cryoprecipitate

IV. **AKI:** more common in patients with CKD

A. **Risk factors:** include increasing age, depressed cardiac function, existing kidney disease, HTN, PVD, DM, emergency surgery, and cardiovascular procedures

B. **Management:** should focus on avoiding nephrotoxins, correcting electrolyte abnormalities and acid–base disorders, and maintaining renal perfusion through euvolemia

> **Quick Cut**
> The most common cause of AKI is ATN.

EVALUATION OF THE SURGICAL PATIENT WITH LIVER DISEASE

Hepatic Function Assessment

I. **Thorough history and physical examination:** will help to provide information regarding possible liver disease

A. **History:** should focus on any prior episodes of liver dysfunction, upper gastrointestinal bleeding, hereditary liver disorders, exposure to infections agents (e.g., blood transfusions, tattoos), prior adverse reactions to inhalational anesthetics, and other risk factors (e.g., alcohol abuse, drug abuse)

> **Quick Cut**
> The severity of liver dysfunction and the nature of the surgical procedure correlate with operative risk.

> **Quick Cut**
> Hepatic insufficiency increases the risk of complications and death in the postoperative period.

    B. Physical examination: should include an assessment of the following:
1. **Clinically evident features of liver dysfunction:** jaundice, ascites, peripheral edema, muscle wasting, testicular atrophy, palmar erythema, spider angiomas, gynecomastia, hepatosplenomegaly, and liver nodularity
2. **Signs of portal HTN:** including caput medusa (dilated periumbilical vessels) or splenomegaly
3. **Evidence of hepatic encephalopathy:** including asterixis and changes in mental status

II. Laboratory testing and diagnostic studies: Routine assessment of liver function in surgical patients is only necessary if there is clinical suspicion for underlying liver disease.

> **Quick Cut**
> Laboratory studies may be normal despite the presence of significant liver disease.

    A. Useful tests: include aspartate aminotransferase (AST), alanine aminotransferase (ALT), bilirubin (total, direct, and indirect), alkaline phosphatase, albumin, and prothrombin time

    B. Platelet count: may be abnormal in patients with portal HTN

    C. Hepatitis serologies: should be sent in patients where exposure to these viral agents is suspected

III. Liver biopsy: may be performed preoperatively to assess degree of cirrhosis

Operative Risk Assessment and Stratification

I. Underlying liver disease: includes the following:

    A. Acute hepatitis: Increases surgical morbidity and mortality. Surgery should only be performed in patients with acute hepatitis if it is emergent.

    B. Chronic hepatitis: Also increases operative morbidity and mortality; however, elective procedures may be performed in patients whose liver function is well compensated.

    C. Cirrhosis: Operative outcomes are influenced by the degree of hepatic dysfunction and the type of surgical procedure.

    D. Obstructive jaundice: In patients with distal biliary obstruction who are not undergoing liver resection, biliary drainage does not seem to decrease significantly perioperative morbidity. For proximal biliary obstruction where liver resection will be performed as part of the surgical procedure, preoperative biliary drainage may be more important.

II. Severity of underlying liver disease: The Child-Turcotte-Pugh score and the Model for End-Stage Liver Disease (MELD) score are two classification systems that can be used to assess degree of hepatic dysfunction.

    A. Child-Turcotte-Pugh classification system: Calculated from the patient's serum bilirubin, albumin level, prothrombin time, degree of ascites and encephalopathy. Operative mortality for elective surgical procedures is ~10% in Child class A, 30% in Child class B, and greater than 50% in Child class C patients.

> **Quick Cut**
> MELD has replaced Child's classification in clinical practice. The MELD score may also be predictive: For every 1-point increase in the MELD score, there is a 1% increase in operative mortality.

    B. MELD score: Linear regression model calculated from a patient's bilirubin level, creatinine, and international normalized ratio (INR) is most commonly used to stratify patients for liver transplantation. Operative mortality in patients with a MELD score less than 8 is ~5% but may increase to greater than 50% in patients with a MELD score greater than 20.

III. Type of surgical procedure: Morbidity and mortality in patients with hepatic dysfunction is greatest for open abdominal and cardiac procedures; emergency surgery is also associated with increased morbidity and mortality.

Anesthetic Considerations

I. General aspects: Decreased hepatic perfusion at baseline increases the susceptibility of the liver to hypoxemia and hypoperfusion intraoperatively. Hepatic dysfunction may also alter drug metabolism and prolong the effects of medications.

II. Inhalation anesthetics: reduce splanchnic perfusion and hepatic blood flow to some extent

    A. Isoflurane: associated with minimal hepatic metabolism and does not impair hepatic blood flow and is therefore the inhalational anesthetic of choice in patients with liver dysfunction

    B. Halogenated inhalational agents: should be avoided in patients with a history of hepatotoxicity after inhalational anesthesia

III. Muscle relaxants: Neuromuscular blockade may be prolonged after administration of nondepolarizing muscle relaxants. Atracurium and cisatracurium are recommended as they undergo peripheral enzymatic degradation and are not metabolized in the liver.

IV. Narcotics and benzodiazepines: Drug action can be prolonged in patients with hepatic dysfunction due to altered metabolism.

    A. Narcotics metabolized in the liver: Morphine, hydrocodone, and oxycodone should be avoided. Fentanyl may be used because its metabolism is not affected by hepatic dysfunction.

    B. Benzodiazepine metabolism: Midazolam and diazepam are affected by hepatic dysfunction. The clearance rate of oxazepam and temazepam are not affected because they are not metabolized in the liver.

Perioperative Management

I. Fluid and electrolyte balance: Perioperative hypotension should be avoided to prevent worsening hepatic function.

    A. Ascites: can be managed with diuretics, fluid and sodium restriction, and paracentesis

    B. Hypomagnesemia: common in patients with chronic liver disease and should be corrected

    C. Lactate metabolism impairment: may result in significant acid–base disturbances that may require fluid resuscitation or dialysis

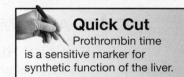

Quick Cut
Perioperative care should focus on correcting physiologic abnormalities and providing supportive care as organ dysfunction develops.

II. Coagulopathy

    A. Prothrombin time: May be elevated secondary to vitamin K deficiency (lack of factors II, VII, IX, and X) or failure of synthetic function. Treatment may be instituted with vitamin K or fresh frozen plasma.

    B. Thrombocytopenia: may be present in patients with portal HTN and splenomegaly and can be treated with platelet transfusion as needed

Quick Cut
Prothrombin time is a sensitive marker for synthetic function of the liver.

III. Hepatic dysfunction: Worsening hepatic function is the most common postoperative problem in patients with liver disease and may manifest as worsening hepatic encephalopathy, jaundice, ascites, coagulopathy, and hypoglycemia.

    A. Encephalopathy: May be treated with protein restriction and the use of lactulose. Narcotics and sedatives that precipitate hepatic encephalopathy should be avoided.

    B. Jaundice: Correctable causes such as biliary obstruction should be identified and managed.

    C. Ascites: can be managed with diuretics, sodium and water restriction, and paracentesis

    D. Coagulopathy: can be treated with vitamin K, fresh frozen plasma, cryoprecipitate, desmopressin acetate, and platelet transfusion

    E. Hypoglycemia: may occur in patients with worsening liver failure and should be treated with glucose infusion

Chapter 4

Life-Threatening Disorders: Acute Abdominal Surgical Emergencies

Laura S. Buchanan and Jose J. Diaz

ACUTE ABDOMEN

Definition and History

I. **Acute surgical abdomen:** acute onset of severe abdominal pain and usually merits emergent or urgent surgical evaluation

II. **Pain characteristics:** can give clues to pathology (Fig. 4-1)
   A. **Gradual, midabdominal, nonspecific progressive pain:** suggests visceral irritation from a worsening process
   B. **Severe, sudden onset of pain:** suggests perforation and may be localized or diffuse
   C. **Gradual pain that has sudden severe component:** can suggest perforation of previous pathology such as appendicitis
   D. **Crampy, intermittent pain:** suggests bowel obstruction

III. **Diet and bowel changes**
   A. **Anorexia, nausea, and vomiting:** commonly accompany an acute intra-abdominal inflammatory process
   B. **Changes in bowel habits:** nonspecific in most conditions
      1. **Bloody diarrhea:** suggests ischemia or infection, as in ischemic colitis, *Salmonella*, or intussusception
      2. **Absence of bowel movement or flatus:** significant in obstruction

IV. **Systemic signs**
   A. **Chills and fever:** nonspecific but raise concern for sepsis secondary to abdominal pathology
      1. **Uncomplicated appendicitis/diverticulitis:** typically associated with low-grade fever
      2. **Perforation:** usually has fever greater than 38°C
   B. **Unplanned weight loss:** raises concern for undiagnosed malignancy
   C. **Abdominal distension:** concern for possible pathologic bowel distension or an intra-abdominal mass
   D. **Rigid abdomen:** common in cases of gastrointestinal (GI) tract perforation

Quick Cut
Many surgical consults address time-sensitive and life-threatening disease, often requiring rapid evaluation, resuscitation, and definitive management.

Quick Cut
Emergent means immediate; *urgent* refers to minimal delay.

Quick Cut
Childhood intussusception may produce a characteristic bloody diarrhea classically referred to as "currant jelly" stools.

Quick Cut
A rigid abdomen is synonymous with diffuse peritonitis and almost always indicates the need for emergent surgery.

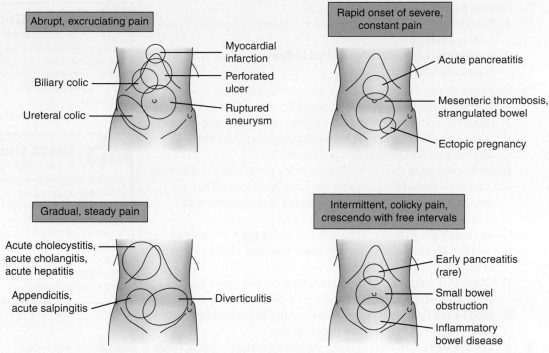

Figure 4-1: Acute abdomen. (From Doherty GM, Boey JH. The acute abdomen. In: Way LW, Doherty GM, eds. *Current Surgical Diagnosis and Treatment*, 11th ed. New York: McGraw-Hill; 2003:506, with permission.)

V. Pertinent medical history

A. **Previous abdominal surgery:** predisposes to adhesive disease with potential obstruction

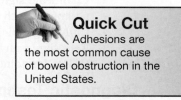

Quick Cut
Adhesions are the most common cause of bowel obstruction in the United States.

    1. Malignancy history may be elicited in this portion of questioning.

    2. Previous episodes of similar symptoms may have undergone medical evaluation and records can be obtained.

B. **Previous illness in other systems:** may be causal or associated with the current episode

    1. **Urinary tract infection (UTI) and obstruction:** can present as with acute abdominal pain

    2. **The reproductive system (especially in women):** can mimic acute abdominal pathology with ovarian cyst rupture, endometriosis, and *mittelschmerz* (pain with ovulation).

    3. **Atrial fibrillation:** suggests an embolic process causing intestinal ischemia

    4. **Diabetes mellitus:** Associated with infection; sudden poor glucose control can indicate sepsis.

Physical Exam

I. **Systemic signs:** Can include fever, tachypnea, hypotension, and dysrhythmias, all of which contribute to severity of illness and indicate that the patient may need resuscitation. Observation can reveal jaundice, dehydration, and mental status changes.

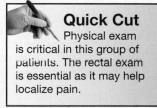

Quick Cut
Physical exam is critical in this group of patients. The rectal exam is essential as it may help localize pain.

II. **Abdominal exam:** includes observation, auscultation, and palpation

A. **Observation:** may reveal obvious hernias, local erythema, distension, or asymmetry

B. **Auscultation:** Abscess of bowel sounds suggests peritoneal inflammation, whereas increased, frequent, or high-pitched sounds can indicate obstruction.

C. **Palpation:** should be done so as to minimize distress to the patient by beginning away from the point of maximal pain

D. **Peritoneal signs:** Indicate visceral irritation and include rebound pain, involuntary guarding, and pain with slight motion of the bed. These patients will be lying still, usually flat.

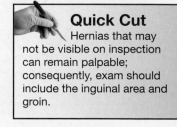

Quick Cut
Hernias that may not be visible on inspection can remain palpable; consequently, exam should include the inguinal area and groin.

III. **Rectal exam:** can localize tenderness
  A. **Presence of blood:** raises concern for ischemia, malignancy, or hemorrhoids
  B. **Prostatitis (can cause generalized abdominal pain):** may be diagnosed with rectal exam

IV. **Specific signs:** Specific findings include the following:
  A. **Murphy sign:** Pain in the right upper quadrant (RUQ) with inspiration while the examiner palpates under the right costal margin as seen in acute cholecystitis; the patient will cease inspiratory effort during this maneuver.
  B. **McBurney sign:** Pain at McBurney point (one third the distance from the anterior iliac spine to the umbilicus) typically after migration from the periumbilical region is characteristic of appendicitis (Fig. 4-2).
  C. **Rovsing sign:** Pain (or rebound pain) in the right lower quadrant (RLQ) with palpation of the left lower quadrant (LLQ) is typical in appendicitis.
  D. **Obturator sign:** Pain with internal rotation of a flexed leg is associated with appendicitis and pelvic abscess.
  E. **Psoas sign:** Pain with hip extension or hip flexion against pressure is seen in retrocecal appendicitis.
  F. **Markle sign:** Pain with shaking the bed or patient's foot is a sign of generalized peritoneal inflammation.
  G. **Charcot triad:** Fever, jaundice, and RUQ pain occurs in cholangitis.
  H. **Reynold pentad:** Fever, jaundice, RUQ pain, mental status change, and shock/sepsis indicates a severe form of cholangitis.
  I. **Chandelier sign:** Pain with manual palpation of the cervix during bimanual exam is due to pelvic peritonitis, such as PID or abscess.
  J. **Cullen sign:** Bluish ecchymosis in the periumbilical region is caused by retroperitoneal hemorrhage.
  K. **Kehr sign:** pain in the left shoulder, referred from irritation pathology in the left upper quadrant (LUQ), including splenic rupture or subdiaphragmatic abscess

Diagnostic Testing

I. **Laboratory evaluation**
  A. **Complete blood count (CBC) with differential:** Can reveal anemia and dehydration and suggest infection. A normal or low white count can be seen in the setting of infection in immunosuppressed patients including elderly and diabetic patients.
  B. **Serum electrolytes:** can detect chemical abnormalities typically secondary to the abdominal process including acute renal injury, acidosis, and alkalosis
  C. **Elevated lactate levels:** Can indicate underresuscitation, ischemia, or necrotic tissue. It is also elevated in liver failure.

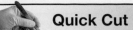
Quick Cut
A digital rectal exam is an essential part of the examination of patient presenting with abdominal or perineal pain—it is not optional.

Quick Cut
In men, testicular torsion requires emergent intervention and can present with sudden lower abdominal pain. Pelvic exam in women can suggest intrauterine pregnancy, ectopic pregnancy, pelvic inflammatory disease (PID), and ovarian mass.

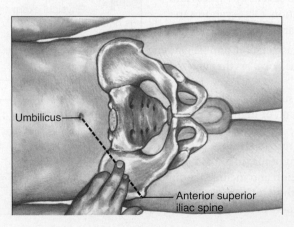

Umbilicus

Anterior superior iliac spine

Figure 4-2: McBurney point. (Lippincott Nursing Advisor. Philadelphia: Lippincott Williams & Wilkins; 2009.) Retrieved from http://clineguide.ovid.com/gateway?resourcenursingadvisor&docid=cc978-1-58255-511-9)

D. **Urine analysis:** can rule in or out a UTI or kidney stone

E. **Amylase and lipase:** Can suggest pancreatitis. Amylase is less specific and can be elevated with other intestinal pathology.

F. **Coagulation studies:** essential for all patients suspected of needing operative intervention

G. **Beta-human chorionic gonadotropin:** indicated for all women of childbearing potential

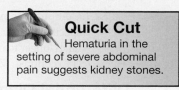

Quick Cut
Hematuria in the setting of severe abdominal pain suggests kidney stones.

II. **Imaging:** Determined by the patient presentation, but all patients with acute abdomen should have an upright chest x-ray, abdominal flat plate, and flat and upright abdominal x-rays or a lateral decubitus view.

A. **Findings**

1. **Free air:** air typically seen under the diaphragm (Fig. 4-3)

a. **Perforations:** present in 80% of proximal perforations (gastroduodenal) but only 25% of distal perforations (colonic)

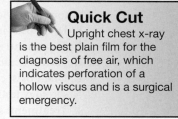

Quick Cut
Upright chest x-ray is the best plain film for the diagnosis of free air, which indicates perforation of a hollow viscus and is a surgical emergency.

b. **Abdominal manipulation:** less common causes such as peritoneal dialysis or recent laparoscopic surgery

2. **Pneumatosis intestinalis:** appears as small bubble-like air collections within the intestinal wall; may indicate ischemia or contained perforation

3. **Pneumobilia:** appears as air tracking within the liver and is caused by connections between the biliary and intestinal system, cholangitis, gallstone ileus, or recent endoscopic retrograde cholangiopancreatography (ERCP)

4. **Portal venous gas:** seen with necrotic tissue in the drainage bed of the portal system, typically the small intestine, appendix, or colon

5. **Sentinel loop air (in adults):** abnormal; can be due to obstruction, or it can indicate pathology in a nearby organ

B. **Abdominal ultrasound:** imaging test of choice for cholecystitis

1. **Findings**

a. **Gallbladder wall thickening and pericholecystic fluid**

b. **Shadows from gallstones:** may also be evident

2. **In pregnancy:** often used for evaluation of potential appendicitis

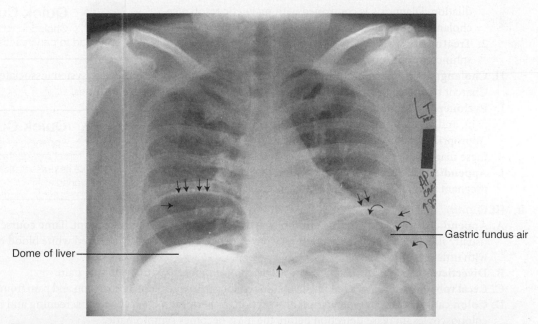

Dome of liver

Gastric fundus air

Figure 4-3: Free air. The straight arrows at the top left represent the diaphragm. The horizontal arrow at left points to the free air. On the right, the uppermost arrows show the diaphragm, and the curved arrows illustrate the outline of the stomach. The lone central arrow signifies the gastroesophageal junction. (Smith W. *Radiology 101*, 4th ed. Philadelphia: Lippincott Williams & Wilkins; 2013.)

C. **Computed tomography (CT) of the abdomen/pelvis:** Gives more specific information than any other single study; however, it often takes longer to obtain and ideally requires oral (PO) and intravenous (IV) contrast, which may be contraindicated in an acutely ill patient.

> **Quick Cut**
> CT scans are useful but should never replace a detailed history and physical examination.

Differential Diagnosis

I. **RUQ pain**

A. **Cholecystitis:** Pain is typically worse with fatty foods, often with history of previous episodes of similar pain and cholelithiasis.

> **Quick Cut**
> When establishing a differential diagnosis for abdominal pain, consider location first.

   1. **Diagnosis:** improved with RUQ ultrasound
   2. **Treatment:** antibiotics and cholecystectomy

B. **Hepatitis:** acutely can present with RUQ pain and tenderness
   1. **Diagnosis:** confirmed with liver function tests (LFTs) and serology testing
   2. **Treatment:** supportive and nonsurgical

C. **Peptic ulcer disease:** includes gastric and duodenal ulcer disease and is associated *Helicobacter pylori* infection
   1. **Presentation:** pain, bleeding, obstruction, or perforation
   2. **Treatment:** includes antimicrobials as well as proton pump inhibitors (PPIs)

D. **Pancreatitis:** Pain can result in patients sitting, leaning forward to achieve pain relief.
   1. **Diagnosis:** Serum amylase and lipase are elevated. CT scanning with IV contrast is necessary to determine if necrosis is present.
   2. **Treatment:** Patients require aggressive fluid resuscitation and monitoring.

> **Quick Cut**
> Acute pancreatitis is most commonly caused by alcohol intake or gallstones.

E. **Liver mass:** Typically causes pain only if stretching the hepatic capsule. Biliary obstruction from a mass is characteristically painless jaundice.

F. **Gastritis:** Can present with acute abdominal pain. More serious causes of pain must be eliminated and supportive care offered.

G. **Choledocholithiasis:** caused by gallstones lodging in the common bile duct and usually associated with some element of biliary obstruction
   1. **Diagnosis:** Elevated bilirubin and transaminases are suspicious when imaging reveals direct evidence of choledocholithiasis or common bile duct dilation. Diagnosis is confirmed with magnetic resonance cholangiopancreatography (MRCP) or ERCP.
   2. **Treatment:** ERCP is also potentially therapeutic with sphincterotomy and stone extraction.

> **Quick Cut**
> Choledocholithiasis can lead to pancreatitis.

H. **Cholangitis:** Infection of the biliary system ascending into the intrahepatic system associated with Charcot triad and Reynold pentad; 95% of cases are associated with gallstones.

I. **Pyelonephritis and nephrolithiasis:** Typically present with flank pain, and nephrolithiasis typically has associated hematuria. Appropriate history and laboratory evaluation should lead to these diagnoses.

J. **Appendicitis:** Pain may have an atypical location, especially in pregnant women with displacement caused by an enlarged uterus.

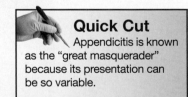

> **Quick Cut**
> Appendicitis is known as the "great masquerader" because its presentation can be so variable.

II. **RLQ pain**

A. **Appendicitis:** Typically starts periumbilical with radiation to McBurney point. Time course is usually short hours to a day. Patient may have normal or only slightly elevated white blood cell count with little or no fever.

B. **Diverticulitis:** Typically a left side or pelvic pain can present with right-side pain.

C. **Cecal volvulus:** torsion of a redundant cecum resulting in a closed loop obstruction and pain from ischemia

D. **Colon cancer:** Can present as pain, obstruction, or perforation. Fecal occult screening and routine colonoscopies increase detection before the mass becomes symptomatic.

E. **Meckel diverticulum:** Occurs in 2% of population, only 2% of which are symptomatic, and most occur within 2 ft of the ileocecal valve.

F. **Renal system:** Other conditions include UTI, nephrolithiasis, and pyelolithiasis.

G. **Reproductive system:** gynecologic pain, prostatitis, and testicular torsion

III. **LUQ pain**
   A. **Peptic ulcer disease**
   B. **Gastritis**
   C. **Splenic rupture or inflammation**
   D. **Hiatal hernia**
   E. **Boerhaave syndrome**
   F. **Mallory-Weiss tear**

IV. **LLQ pain**
   A. **Diverticulitis:** can present with uncomplicated inflammation, contained abscess, free perforation, or bleeding
   B. **Sigmoid volvulus:** results from torsion of the sigmoid colon
   C. **Colon cancer**
   D. **UTI, nephrolithiasis, pyelonephritis**
   E. **Gynecologic, prostatitis, testicular torsion**

V. **Medical conditions masquerading as a surgical abdomen**
   A. **Pneumonia**
   B. **Myocardial infarction**
   C. **Pericarditis**
   D. **Malignancy**
   E. **Diabetic ketoacidosis**
   F. **Acute hepatitis**
   G. **Rare causes:** include acute polyserositis, rheumatic fever, porphyria, sickle cell crisis, and lead intoxication

OBSTRUCTION

History

I. **Symptoms:** Include nausea, vomiting, crampy abdominal pain, and decreased or absence of flatus and stool (all of which, in the absence of pain, suggest ileus). History of similar episodes or slow progression of symptoms suggests a chronic etiology.

II. **Previous surgical history:** Extremely important because obstruction with previous abdominal surgery is usually adhesive disease and can potentially improve with non-operative management. However, in the absence of previous surgery, the source of obstruction may be malignancy, perforation, or volvulus and requires intervention.

> **Quick Cut**
> Most SBO due to adhesions can be resolved with nasogastric decompression and supportive care.

Physical Exam

I. **Abdominal exam:** Significant for distension. Emesis character including nonbilious, bilious, and feculent can suggest location of obstruction.

II. **Incarcerated hernias:** Detailed exam should look for hernias, including inguinal and femoral.

Diagnostic Studies

I. **Laboratory analysis:** important because patients often present not only with dehydration but also with significant electrolyte and acid–base abnormality

II. **Abdominal x-ray:** may reveal air in a nonanatomic location with a hernia
   A. **Cecal and sigmoid volvulus:** have characteristic distended colon loops visible on plain film
   B. **Small bowel obstruction (SBO):** Normal abdominal x-ray shows air in the gastric and colon area, but distended, air-filled loops of small bowel are consistent with SBO (Fig. 4-4). Multiple air-fluid levels on plain radiographs also indicate obstruction.

Differential Diagnosis

I. **Mechanical obstruction:** due to physical blockage of the intestine by internal or external mass, stricture, or intestinal twisting and can occur in the small or large intestine
   A. **Terminology**
      1. **Acute obstruction:** can occur over hours and rapidly progress
      2. **Chronic obstruction:** develops over weeks to months and is characterized by malnutrition and chronic illness

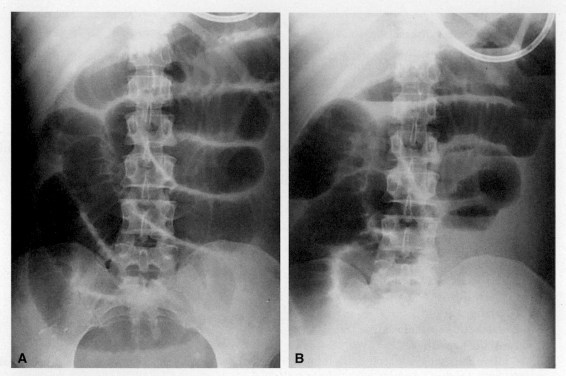

Figure 4-4: A,B: Small bowel obstruction. Part A is a supine film, and Part B is an upright x-ray. Note the air-fluid levels visible in Part B. (From Yamada T, Alpers DH, Laine L, et al. *Textbook of Gastroenterology*, 4th ed. Philadelphia: Lippincott Williams & Wilkins; 2003.)

3. **Strangulating obstruction:** Occurs when the blood supply to the affected segment of bowel is compromised, leading to gangrene and perforation. Signs of strangulation include continuous pain, fever, tachycardia, peritoneal signs, acidosis and leukocytosis, and indicate progressive ischemia.

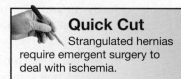
Quick Cut
Strangulated hernias require emergent surgery to deal with ischemia.

4. **Incarceration:** Refers to a hernia that cannot be reduced; an incarcerated hernia may also be strangulated.
5. **Closed loop obstruction:** Both limbs of a segment of bowel are obstructed.
    b. **Distention:** As the more proximal bowel distends, symptoms of obstruction develop.
    c. **Closed loop:** more prone to perforation because it cannot decompress

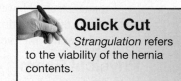
Quick Cut
Strangulation refers to the viability of the hernia contents.

6. **Partial obstructions:** Allow small or intermittent amounts of matter through; these may respond well to conservative management.
    a. **Clinically:** Patients may pass small amounts of gas or stool.
    b. **Radiographically:** Gas or contrast will be seen passing into the colon.
7. **Intussusception:** Occurs when the bowel folds within its own lumen (think of a sock removed hastily and folded into itself). May occur spontaneously in pediatric patients, but in adults, the lead point is suspicious for tumor.

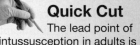
Quick Cut
The lead point of intussusception in adults is presumed to be a tumor and must be investigated.

8. **Perforating obstruction:** occurs when the proximal bowel overdistends, resulting in perforation
B. **Location:** can partially be indicated by exam findings
    1. **Gastric outlet obstruction:** Results in early satiety and nonbilious emesis. This is typically a chronic onset.
    2. **Small intestinal obstruction:** will result in bilious or feculent emesis

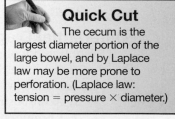
Quick Cut
The cecum is the largest diameter portion of the large bowel, and by Laplace law may be more prone to perforation. (Laplace law: tension = pressure × diameter.)

3. **Large intestinal obstruction:** may not result in emesis until late in its course after the entire proximal small bowel has dilated

C. **Causes**

1. **Adhesions resulting from previous surgery:** Most common cause; partial adhesive obstructions are first managed conservatively.

2. **Malignancy:** Without history of prior surgery, a mass is the most common diagnosis; treatment requires removal or bypass and tumor-specific treatment.

3. **Hernias:** common source of obstruction caused by migration of an intestinal segment through the hernia defect

   a. **Internal hernias:** occur when a bowel segment migrates through an internal opening within the abdominal cavity

   b. **Treatment:** reduction of hernia contents and hernia repair

4. **Less common causes:** include congenital lesions (webs, malrotation), inflammatory lesions (Crohn disease, diverticulitis), foreign bodies, radiation, and trauma

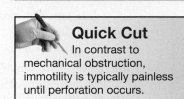

Quick Cut
Mechanical obstructions can be extraluminal (adhesion, hernias) or intraluminal (mass, bezoar).

II. **Functional obstruction:** inability to move intestinal contents typically due to impaired motility

A. **Ileus (paralytic or adynamic):** diffuse intestinal lack of motility

1. **Causes:** occurs after surgery, peritoneal irritation, and electrolyte abnormality

2. **Treatment:** includes fluid and nutritional support as well as electrolyte replacement

B. **Colonic pseudo-obstruction (Ogilvie syndrome):** impaired motility of the colon commonly seen after back or hip surgery

Quick Cut
In contrast to mechanical obstruction, immotility is typically painless until perforation occurs.

HEMORRHAGE

Terminology

I. **GI bleeding:** Common emergent surgical consult. In all patients, priority is placed on resuscitation and, when necessary, transfusion. Upper GI bleed is defined as bleeding proximal to the ligament of Treitz; lower GI bleed includes all other GI locations.

II. **Hematemesis:** Emesis of blood that is bright red or the color of coffee grounds. It is due to bleeding proximal to the ligament of Treitz.

Quick Cut
With all hemorrhagic sources, initial treatment includes control of hemorrhage, resuscitation, and reversal of coagulopathy.

III. **Hematochezia:** passage of bright red blood from the rectum and can be due to bleeding from an upper or lower source

IV. **Melena:** passage of black stools due to blood in the GI system and also can occur with upper or lower GI hemorrhage

V. **Currant jelly stool:** mixture of blood and mucus typically described in children with intussusception

Evaluation

I. **Localization:** First step in evaluation; upper GI hemorrhage may present as hematochezia, melena, or even bright red blood per rectum.

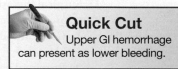

Quick Cut
Upper GI hemorrhage can present as lower bleeding.

A. **Nasogastric (NG) and gastric lavage:** Evaluates for gastric and duodenal sources. NG lavage must contain bile to be negative. If there is no bile in the NG lavage, then a duodenal bleed may still be missed.

B. **Endoscopy:** Can visualize the stomach, duodenum, and colon. Therapeutic interventions can offer treatment as well.

C. **Radiographic imaging:** Includes tagged red cell scan and angiography; these are more useful in lower GI bleeding.

D. **Capsule endoscopy or push enteroscopy:** can visualize the small intestine in stable patients with resolved or intermittent bleeds

II. Differential

A. Upper GI bleed: Most common causes are peptic ulcers, esophagogastric varices, vascular malformations, and Mallory-Weiss tears.

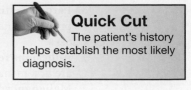

Quick Cut
The patient's history helps establish the most likely diagnosis.

1. **History of ulcer disease or nonsteroidal anti-inflammatory drug use:** bleeding peptic ulcer
2. **History of gastroesophageal reflux disease (GERD):** esophagitis
3. **History of heavy alcohol use:** bleeding varices or gastritis
4. **Recent retching:** Mallory-Weiss tear
5. **Weight loss:** upper GI malignancy

B. Lower GI bleed: Includes all other sources of GI bleeding including jejunum, ileum, colon, and rectum, whereas upper GI bleeding can present with only lower bleeding. Blood is cathartic and passes quickly through the intestine. Upper sources of bleeding must be evaluated and ruled out.

1. **Common causes:** Lower bleeding is most commonly diverticular hemorrhage and bleeding vascular malformations.
2. **Less common causes:** include malignancy, polyps, hemorrhoids, fissures, ischemic colitis, Meckel diverticulum (most common source in pediatrics), infectious colitis, and inflammatory bowel disease (IBD)

III. Treatment: requires resuscitation, localization of bleeding source, cessation of immediate hemorrhage, and prevention of future episodes

A. Initial approach: Because patients with GI bleed may present in hemorrhagic shock, the initial approach must include assessment of ABCs (airway, breathing, circulation), establishment of two large-bore IV lines, and administration of appropriate fluids/blood, depending on illness severity.

B. Localization: determined by history, physical, and diagnostic testing

1. **Rectal exam:** Every exam for bleeding must include a rectal exam.
2. **NG tube for lavage and aspiration:** can diagnose an upper GI source but does not rule out an upper GI source if negative
3. **Esophagogastroduodenoscopy (EGD):** can both localize and treat or rule out upper GI sources of hemorrhage
4. **Tagged red blood cell scan:** identifies active bleeding by gross location (LUQ) but will not give specifics of anatomic location

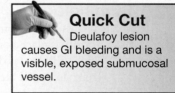

Quick Cut
Dieulafoy lesion causes GI bleeding and is a visible, exposed submucosal vessel.

   a. Detect bleeds of 0.5 mL/min but requires a delay of up to several hours while the study is being performed
   b. Because the tagged cells remain in circulation, if the study is negative, and the patient rebleeds, the test can be repeated within 24 hours.
5. **Angiography:** can identify the vessel with bleeding and potentially embolize to provide treatment; can detect bleeding at a rate of 0.5–1.0 mL/min
6. **Colonoscopy:** can be difficult in an unprepped colon full of blood but if successful can also be therapeutic with clips, epinephrine injections, and cauterization

C. Nonsurgical treatment: includes endoscopy, angiography, and embolization

1. **Vasopressin infusion:** will not stop bleeding but may temporize to give time for treatment
2. **Ulcer treatment:** includes PPI drip and treatment for *H. pylori*

D. Surgical therapy: indicated for persistent hemorrhagic shock (fails resuscitation) and recurrent bleeding despite maximal therapy

Quick Cut
Only 10% of upper GI bleeds require surgical intervention.

1. **Gastroduodenostomy:** performed if no lesion has been identified
2. **Proximal gastrectomy:** performed if no source is seen
3. **Subtotal colectomy:** performed if lower GI bleeding has not been localized before operative intervention, but this procedure his high mortality and can be complicated by rebleeding if the source is not included in the resected colon

Study Questions for Part I

Directions: *Each of the numbered items in this section is followed by several possible answers. Select the ONE lettered answer that is BEST in each case.*

1. A healthy adult presents for a pre-employment physical. What will be the largest component of his or her body by mass?

   A. Protein
   B. Water
   C. Calcium
   D. Sodium
   E. Potassium

2. An 80-year-old man with a history of ischemic cardiomyopathy is hypotensive and oliguric after major abdominal surgery. Initial fluid resuscitation produces only transient improvements. He is transferred to the intensive care unit for further management. A pulmonary artery catheter could be used to measure all of the following *except*:

   A. Left atrial filling pressure
   B. Cardiac output
   C. Ejection fraction
   D. Mixed venous oxygen saturation
   E. Systemic vascular resistance

3. A 25-year-old man is injured in the arm with a knife. What is the first mechanism responsible for hemostasis?

   A. Extrinsic clotting system
   B. Vessel constriction
   C. Intrinsic clotting system
   D. Platelet activation
   E. Fibrinolytic system

4. A 27-year-old woman is experiencing perioral and extremity numbness the morning after a neck operation. What is the cause of her symptoms?

   A. Hypokalemia
   B. Hypercalcemia
   C. Hypocalcemia
   D. Hypochloremia
   E. Hyperkalemia

5. A 55-year-old woman undergoes laparotomy for small bowel obstruction. During lysis of adhesions, an enterotomy is made in the obstructed, but viable, bowel, and a large amount of fecal-looking bowel contents are spilled into the abdomen. The incision would now be considered what kind of wound?

   A. Clean contaminated
   B. Secondary
   C. Infected
   D. Contaminated
   E. Clean

6. A critically ill 55-year-old man is in septic shock in the intensive care unit after removal of a nonviable small bowel. What is the most reliable measurement of arterial blood pressure?

   A. Arterial line diastolic
   B. Noninvasive systolic
   C. Arterial line mean
   D. Arterial line systolic
   E. Noninvasive mean

7. Delayed primary closure would be the most appropriate wound closure technique for which of the following procedures?

   A. Removal of perforated appendix
   B. Repair of wound dehiscence 1 week after elective left colectomy
   C. Emergency drainage of a diverticular abscess with sigmoid resection and end colostomy
   D. Vagotomy and pyloroplasty for bleeding duodenal ulcer
   E. Repair of an incisional hernia 12 weeks after an elective left colectomy complicated by a wound infection and a resultant incisional hernia

8. A 55-year-old man with insulin-dependent diabetes presents to the emergency department with acute abdominal pain. His heart rate is 130 beats per minute, his blood pressure is 90/60 mm Hg, and his oral temperature is 101.8°F. His respiratory rate is 28 breaths per minute (bpm). The abdominal examination demonstrates diffuse peritonitis. What should be the first step in the evaluation and management of this patient?

   A. Volume resuscitation
   B. Abdominal radiograph
   C. IV antibiotics
   D. CT scan
   E. Immediate laparotomy

9. A 57-year-old man underwent a laparoscopic splenectomy for idiopathic thrombocytopenic purpura (ITP). He subsequently develops a persistent output of 100 mL daily of amylase-rich fluid from a drain placed at the time of surgery. All of the following would be expected to prevent spontaneous resolution of this problem *except*:

   A. Octreotide administration
   B. Pancreatic duct stricture
   C. Infection
   D. Nonabsorbable suture in distal pancreatic duct
   E. Epithelialization of the tract

10. For appropriate procedures, antibiotic prophylaxis for bacterial endocarditis should be administered in patients with a history of which of the following?

    A. Mitral valve prolapse without regurgitation
    B. Automatic implantable cardiac defibrillator placement
    C. Aortic valve replacement
    D. Coronary artery bypass graft
    E. Surgically repaired ventricular septal defect

11. Which of the following procedures would be expected to have the greatest impact on postoperative pulmonary function?

    A. Low anterior resection
    B. Femoropopliteal bypass
    C. Subtotal gastrectomy
    D. Open cholecystectomy
    E. Total abdominal hysterectomy

12. Which of the following is a criterion for emergent preoperative dialysis?

A. Potassium (K^+) 5.0, without arrhythmia
B. Arterial pH 7.30, anion gap 8
C. Pericardial friction rub
D. Blood urea nitrogen 105
E. Creatinine 5.5

13. Preoperative coagulation studies should be obtained on which of the following patients?

A. A 35-year-old woman on aspirin, prior to varicose vein surgery
B. A 65-year-old diabetic man, prior to inguinal hernia repair
C. A 70-year-old jaundiced woman, prior to choledochojejunostomy
D. A 45-year-old woman prior to bilateral prophylactic mastectomy with transverse rectus abdominis myocutaneous flap reconstructions
E. A 50-year-old man with stable angina, prior to coronary artery bypass

Directions: *The group of items in this section consists of lettered options followed by a set of numbered items. For each item, select the lettered option(s) that is(are) most closely associated with it. Each lettered option may be selected once, more than once, or not at all.*

Questions 14–17

Match the clinical situation with the appropriate type of drain.

14. Nasogastric decompression

15. Spontaneous pneumothorax

16. Diffuse peritonitis from perforated duodenal ulcer

17. Splenectomy for ruptured spleen

A. Jackson-Pratt closed drain

B. No drain

C. Underwater seal drain

D. Sump drain

18. A 50-year-old woman with chronic obstructive pulmonary disease is hospitalized with small bowel obstruction. On the evening of her second day, she is acutely anxious and is breathing at a rate of 24 bpm. After pain medications and reassurance, her oxygen saturations are 92% on 2 L of oxygen, and her tachypnea increases to 30 beats per minute. On exam, she has labored breathing but no other acute findings. What is the best course of action?

A. Increase oxygen by nasal cannula to 3 L
B. Elective intubation
C. Diuresis with furosemide
D. Additional narcotics to suppress breathing rate
E. Computerized tomography of abdomen to assess bowel obstruction

19. A 24-year-old man presents with a traumatic wound to the left extremity. It had been injured in a fall 4 days previously. At home, the patient noted increased redness, pain, and swelling, with the discharge of some foul-smelling pus. In the emergency department, he has a temperature of 102°F, heart rate of 132 beats per minute, and systolic blood pressure of 85 mm Hg. The leg is tensely distended, extremely tender, and there is some purulent drainage around a region of necrotic skin. The most appropriate treatment for this patient is:

A. Oral antibiotics
B. IV isotonic fluids
C. Phenylephrine
D. Low-dose dopamine
E. Intubation and drainage of the abscess

20. A 30-year-old man presents with a mass in his right groin. It is not tender and is a bulge that is more prominent on standing and with exercise. On examination, you find a 3-cm protrusion into the right scrotum that completely resolves with gentle pressure. The most appropriate management is:

    A. Broad-spectrum antibiotics
    B. Tumor markers, including alpha-fetoprotein
    C. Elective surgical repair
    D. Observation only
    E. CT scan of the abdomen and pelvis

21. A 52-year-old woman undergoes uneventful partial colectomy for a large polyp of the sigmoid colon. During the procedure, placement of a Foley catheter demonstrates good urine output. Four days later, she develops a fever. Which of the following is the LEAST likely cause of her fever?

    A. Pneumonia
    B. Wound infection
    C. UTI
    D. Perirectal abscess
    E. Deep venous thrombosis (DVT)

22. A 30-year-old man presents for elective repair of a right-sided inguinal hernia. He has no significant medical history, and his physical examination is positive only for the presence of a reducible right-sided hernia. The operative plan is an open inguinal hernia repair with mesh. The most appropriate preoperative workup for this patient is:

    A. Chest x-ray, electrocardiogram (ECG)
    B. CBC, basic metabolic panel (BMP)
    C. Urinalysis
    D. Noninvasive stress test
    E. Coagulation profile only

23. A 60-year-old woman has diabetes and end-stage renal disease on hemodialysis. She undergoes emergency surgery for perforated peptic ulcer, which is uneventful. On postoperative day 2, she has chest pain and an ECG, which shows peaked T waves. The best initial maneuver is:

    A. IV calcium
    B. IV insulin
    C. Oral potassium
    D. Oral calcium
    E. IV morphine

24. A 40-year-old woman presents with acute abdominal pain. She describes the pain as high in the epigastrium, perhaps moving a little to the right side. The pain comes with meals and has been present on and off over the past 6 months. After lunch today, the patient developed severe pain, low-grade fever, and nausea. Her vital signs show no fever, heart rate of 85 beats per minute, and normal blood pressure. On exam, she is markedly tender under the right costal margin and cannot take a full breath during that part of the examination. The best initial test for this patient is:

    A. Abdominal CT scan
    B. RUQ ultrasound
    C. Abdominal magnetic resonance enterography (MRE)
    D. EGD
    E. Liver–spleen scanning

25. An 18-year-old man presents with 12 hours of abdominal pain. It was originally periumbilical then migrated to his right side. Over the past 2 hours, he has developed some nausea but has not had any emesis. On examination, he has pain on the right side when palpating the left side. The name for this sign is:

    A. McBurney sign
    B. Obturator sign
    C. Psoas sign
    D. Markle sign
    E. Rovsing sign

26. A 15-year-old boy is admitted with a history and physical findings consistent with appendicitis. Which finding is most likely to be positive?

    A. Pelvic crepitus
    B. Iliopsoas sign
    C. Murphy sign
    D. Flank ecchymosis
    E. Periumbilical ecchymosis

27. A 50-year-old man is admitted with massive bright red rectal bleeding. He recently had a barium enema that demonstrated no diverticular or space-occupying lesion. Nasogastric suction reveals no blood but does produce yellow bile. The patient continues to bleed. What is the next diagnostic step?

    A. Repeat barium enema
    B. Colonoscopy
    C. Upper GI series
    D. Mesenteric angiography
    E. Small bowel follow-through with barium

28. A 15-year-old boy awakens with sudden onset of RLQ and scrotal tenderness accompanied by nausea and vomiting. Which of the following is the most appropriate diagnosis and represents a surgical emergency?

    A. Acute prostatitis
    B. Acute epididymitis
    C. Torsion of the testicle
    D. Acute appendicitis
    E. Gastroenteritis

29. Massive bleeding from the lower GI tract is occurring in a 55-year-old man who is otherwise healthy. After continued bleeding equivalent to one unit of blood, what should be the initial management?

    A. Emergency laparotomy and total colectomy and ileoproctostomy
    B. Emergency laparotomy and colostomy with operative endoscopy
    C. Arteriography to identify the bleeding site after anoscopy and sigmoidoscopy have ruled out a distal site
    D. Infusion of vitamin K and fresh frozen plasma
    E. Colonic irrigation with iced saline solution

Questions 30–31

A 45-year-old man is seen in the emergency department after vomiting bright red blood. He has no previous symptoms. He drinks one alcoholic beverage a day.

30. What is the most reliable method for locating the lesion responsible for the bleeding?

    A. Upper GI series
    B. Exploratory laparotomy
    C. Upper endoscopy
    D. Arteriography
    E. Radionuclide scanning

31. After several hours in the hospital, he begins to have recurrent bleeding. He is transferred to a critical care bed and is persistently hypotensive despite transfusion of 9 units of packed red blood cells. Which is the most appropriate next step in management of this patient?

    A. Upper endoscopy with attempt at cauterization of bleeding
    B. Transport to the interventional radiology unit to identify and embolize bleeding source
    C. Placement of a Blakemore tube to temporarily tamponade bleeding and to allow for stabilization of blood pressure
    D. Laparotomy to control bleeding
    E. Infusion of vasopressin and additional units of blood

32. A 45-year-old woman who has had a hysterectomy presents to the emergency department with abdominal pain and vomiting. A mechanical small bowel obstruction is seen on the abdominal radiograph. What is the most likely cause for this obstruction?

    A. Carcinoma of the colon
    B. Small bowel cancer
    C. Adhesions
    D. Incarcerated inguinal hernia
    E. Diverticulitis

33. A 25-year-old man is admitted with a history of sudden onset of severe midepigastric abdominal pain. Upright chest radiograph reveals free intraperitoneal air. What is the therapy for this patient?

    A. Upper endoscopy
    B. Barium swallow
    C. Gastrografin swallow
    D. Observation
    E. Laparotomy

Answers and Explanations

1. **The answer is B** (Chapter 1, Fluid and Electrolytes, Normal Body Composition, I A). The normal adult human body is made up of 50%–70% water. The water is contained in three primary compartments of the body: intracellular, extracellular, and intravascular. On average, two thirds of the body is made of water; in the hypothetical 70-kg man, this is 46 L. Of this 46 L, two thirds is intracellular (30 L), and one third is extracellular (16 L). Of the extracellular portion, three fourths is interstitial (12 L), and one fourth is intravascular (4 L). This approximation gives a good starting point when beginning to estimate fluid resuscitation, replacement, and maintenance.

2. **The answer is C** (Chapter 1, The Intensive Care Unit, Specialized Intensive Care Unit Care and Monitoring, II C 2). A pulmonary artery catheter can be useful in distinguishing cardiac dysfunction from other causes of shock in certain patients. It will allow the treating physician to measure left atrial filling pressure from the port in the tip via back pressure through the lungs. Cardiac output is measured via thermal dilution. Mixed venous oxygen saturation can be measured by drawing a sample from the catheter. Systemic vascular resistance can be calculated from the cardiac output, mean arterial pressure, and central venous pressure.

3. **The answer is B** (Chapter 1, Coagulation, Hemostasis Mechanism Phases, I A). The first mechanism activated when there is damage to a vessel is constriction, which is an effort to stop blood flow. This is followed by platelet activation, which produces a platelet plug. The intrinsic and extrinsic pathways are then activated to form a fibrin clot. The fibrinolytic system is the body's mechanism to dissolve established clots.

4. **The answer is C** (Chapter 1, Fluid and Electrolytes, Water and Electrolyte Deficits and Excesses, V A 1). Hypocalcemia can induce neuromuscular irritability, including perioral and extremity numbness. This can progress to carpopedal spasm and tetany. The most common cause of hypocalcemia is parathyroid surgery to treat hypercalcemia, resulting in rebound hypocalcemia.

5. **The answer is D** (Chapter 2, Wounds, Wound Classification, I–IV). The wound described is a contaminated wound due to the gross spill of contaminated material. A clean wound is one made through normal, antiseptically prepared skin and encounters no infected or colonized areas. A clean-contaminated wound is similar to a clean wound except that a contaminated or potentially contaminated area (e.g., bowel, bronchus, urinary tract), which has been prepared to the best of one's ability and presents minimal contamination, has been opened. An infected wound is one that already has an established infection present. Secondary is a type of wound closure and not a classification of a wound.

6. **The answer is C** (Chapter 1, The Intensive Care Unit, Specialized Intensive Care Unit Care and Monitoring, II C 1). The arterial line mean pressure is the most accurate and is the most physiologically useful measurement of blood pressure. It may be very accurate but often has limited clinical usefulness and must be used cautiously. Noninvasive blood pressures are not very accurate in critically ill patients. Noninvasive blood pressure measurements are notoriously high in hypotensive patients and low in hypertensive patients.

7. **The answer is A** (Chapter 2, Wounds, Wound Repair, II C). Delayed primary intention is appropriate for contaminated wounds, such as a ruptured appendix without abscess formation. Wound dehiscences are closed with retention sutures that include all layers, including the skin, because the fascial strength has been compromised. Infected wounds are packed open to heal by secondary intention, as with drainage of a diverticular abscess. Clean and clean-contaminated wounds can be closed primarily, as with incisional hernia repair (clean) and vagotomy/pyloroplasty (clean contaminated).

8. **The answer is A** (Chapter 1, Shock, Definition, II D). Intra-abdominal sepsis in a diabetic patient may be complicated by the development of ketoacidosis and dehydration. The patient presents with a condition that will likely require emergent surgical intervention. Initial management should be directed at restoration of the patient's circulating blood volume and optimization of his physiologic status prior to possible laparotomy. The serum glucose, electrolytes, and pH should be determined and abnormalities corrected. Measurement of hourly urine output will allow assessment of the adequacy of resuscitation. Abdominal radiographs should be obtained to look for free intraperitoneal air, and broad-spectrum IV antibiotics should be administered, but fluid resuscitation takes top priority. A CT scan may not be indicated in the patient who, on physical examination and history, clearly has peritonitis.

9. **The answer is A** (Chapter 2, Gastrointestinal Fistula, III D). Enterocutaneous fistulas typically respond to conservative management and spontaneously close when conditions are favorable. Octreotide has been shown to decrease pancreatic fistula output and clearly does not inhibit resolution. Distal obstruction (pancreatic duct stricture), infection, foreign body (nonabsorbable suture), and epithelialization all inhibit resolution.

10. **The answer is C** (Chapter 3, Evaluation of the Surgical Patient with Cardiac Disease, Bacterial Endocarditis Prophylaxis, II). In 1997, the American Heart Association updated guidelines to clarify recommendations for antibiotic prophylaxis for the prevention of bacterial endocarditis. In general, appropriate prophylaxis should be given to patients with underlying structural cardiac defects (e.g., prosthetic cardiac valves, significant valvular disease, hypertrophic cardiomyopathy, complex congenital heart disease, surgically constructed systemic-pulmonary shunts) who undergo procedures leading to bacteremia with organisms likely to cause endocarditis (e.g., major dental work or invasive procedures of the respiratory, GI, or genitourinary tracts).

11. **The answer is C** (Chapter 3, Evaluation of the Surgical Patient with Lung Disease, Operative Considerations, II A). Major upper abdominal surgery performed via a vertical midline incision would be expected to have the greatest impact on postoperative pulmonary function. Other operative factors would include thoracotomy, residual intraperitoneal sepsis, age older than 59 years, prolonged preoperative hospitalization, colorectal or gastroduodenal surgery, procedure longer than 3.5 hours, and higher body mass index. Lower abdominal and extremity surgery are associated with fewer pulmonary complications when compared with thoracic and upper abdominal surgery.

12. **The answer is C** (Chapter 3, Evaluation of the Surgical Patient with Renal Disease, Preoperative Management, V). Indications for emergent dialysis include life-threatening hyperkalemia, severe metabolic acidosis secondary to retained organic acids, uremic pericarditis, and volume overload. The serum creatinine and blood urea nitrogen levels reflect the underlying renal dysfunction but will not necessarily mandate emergent preoperative dialysis.

13. **The answer is C** (Chapter 3, Table 3-1). Preoperative evaluation with routine coagulation studies is neither cost-effective nor routinely indicated. Patients with a history of postsurgical bleeding or ongoing acute hemorrhage, patients on oral anticoagulation, patients with liver disease or hepatobiliary obstruction, malnourished patients, and patients unable to give an adequate history should have prothrombin time, partial thromboplastin time, and platelet counts checked preoperatively.

14–17. **The answers are 14-D, 15-C, 16-B, and 17-A** (Chapter 2, Surgical Tubes and Drains, Drains, I C). Sump drains are needed to adequately decompress the stomach. When the pleural space requires drainage, a chest tube is placed and connected to an underwater seal so that air and fluid cannot reflux into the chest. This is needed because of the negative intrathoracic pressure generated with each inspiration. Diffuse peritonitis cannot be drained, as the peritoneal contents quickly "wall off" foreign bodies such as drains; discrete intraperitoneal collections can be drained. Splenectomy jeopardizes the pancreatic tail, which is in close proximity to the splenic hilum. When the area is obscured, as with the hematoma accompanying splenic rupture, the integrity of the pancreas cannot be assured, and the potential pancreatic fluid leak is drained with a closed-suction drain such as a Jackson-Pratt drain.

18. **The answer is B** (Chapter 1, The Intensive Care Unit, Specialized Intensive Care Unit Care and Monitoring, II). The patient is clearly showing signs of increased work of breathing and is hyperventilating at an unsustainable rate. It would be reasonable to give anxiolytics or to order a chest radiograph to assess this patient. Increasing the oxygen by nasal cannula may result in marginal improvement in saturation but will not address any underlying condition. Diuresis is appropriate for fluid overload. Narcotics will suppress breathing rate but only at significant doses and run the risk of hypoventilation. CT scan of the abdomen will not be diagnostic and may remove the patient from an appropriately monitored setting.

19. **The answer is E** (Chapter 1, Shock, Definition, II D). The patient is showing signs of septic shock. The primary treatment is source control (drainage of the leg abscess), systemic antibiotics, and supportive care (intubation and fluid resuscitation). Oral antibiotics alone would be insufficient to treat this critically ill patient. Although IV fluids would help support the patient, they do not address the infection. Phenylephrine is useful for neurogenic shock, and low-dose dopamine support is not necessary in this instance.

20. **The answer is C** (Chapter 2, Hernias, Inguinal Hernia, IV). The patient presents with signs and symptoms of an inguinal hernia. The presence of a hernia is an indication for surgical repair. Antibiotics may be indicated in cases of infection, but the patient has no signs of lymphadenopathy. Tumor markers are useful in the workup of testicular masses suspicious for malignancy. In general, imaging is not needed prior to undertaking hernia repair.

21. **The answer is D** (Chapter 2, Postoperative Complications, Postoperative Fever, I). The 5 W's provide common causes of fever: wound, wind (pneumonia), water (UTI), walking (DVT), and "wonder drugs" (typically antibiotics). Other infections may cause fever, but in the immediate postoperative setting, a new abscess remote from the operative site is unlikely.

22. **The answer is C** (Chapter 3, General Aspects for Evaluation and Management of the Surgical Patient, Preoperative Testing, I, and Table 3-1). The patient does not require preoperative cardiac testing given his age, lack of symptoms, and low–cardiac risk surgery. CBC and BMP are reserved for cases in which there is a clinical suspicion of disease or higher risk surgery. Coagulation parameters are necessary in those on anticoagulation or those with a history of bleeding. Urinalysis is indicated in those patients where a foreign body implant is planned, in this case, mesh.

23. **The answer is A** (Chapter 3, Evaluation of the Surgical Patient with Renal Disease, Preoperative Management, I B). The patient is showing signs and symptoms of hyperkalemia. The ultimate treatment is elimination of potassium, best accomplished through dialysis. For immediate cardiac protection, IV calcium stabilizes cardiac myocytes and prevents ventricular fibrillation. IV insulin helps shift potassium intracellularly and is useful as part of the treatment. IV morphine helps with myocardial infarction.

24. **The answer is B** (Chapter 4, Acute Abdomen, Diagnostic Testing, II B). The patient has signs and symptoms consistent with acute cholecystitis and demonstrates a positive Murphy sign. The initial test of choice is an RUQ ultrasound, which may demonstrate a thickened gallbladder wall, pericholecystic fluid, ductal dilatation, or gallstones. Abdominal CT scan is reasonable for patients with abdominal pain but is neither sensitive nor specific for biliary pathology. MRE is a reasonable test for small bowel disease, such as Crohn disease. EGD may evaluate gastric pathology such as ulcer, but the clinical situation does not fit this patient. In acute cholecystitis, hepatic iminodiacetic acid (HIDA) scanning is reasonable but after an ultrasound is performed.

25. **The answer is E** (Chapter 4, Acute Abdomen, Physical Exam, IV C). The patient presents with a classic history for appendicitis. All of the listed signs may be present in acute appendicitis. Rovsing sign is pain on the right when palpating the left side, as the peritoneum is distended internally to touch the inflamed appendix. McBurney sign is pain at McBurney point in the RLQ. Obturator sign is pain on internal rotation of the leg. Psoas may reflect retrocecal appendicitis, pain on extension of the leg. Markle sign represents diffuse peritonitis, with pain on shaking the bed.

26. The answer is B (Chapter 4, Acute Abdomen, Physical Exam, IV E). The iliopsoas sign is pain in the lower abdomen and psoas region that is elicited when the thigh is flexed against resistance. It suggests an inflammatory process, such as appendicitis. Crepitus suggests a rapidly spreading gas-forming infection. Murphy sign is elicited by palpating the RUQ during inspiration and suggests acute cholecystitis. Flank and periumbilical ecchymoses suggest retroperitoneal hemorrhage.

27. The answer is D (Chapter 4, Hemorrhage, Evaluation, III B). The most likely cause of massive lower GI bleeding in the absence of diverticula is an angiodysplastic lesion of the colon, particularly the right colon. An upper GI series and small bowel studies should be done only after an exhaustive colonic workup has failed to demonstrate the source of bleeding. Colonoscopy in the face of massive bleeding is unreliable and difficult and carries the risk of colonic perforation. In addition, it will not usually demonstrate an angiodysplastic lesion. A repeat barium enema is also unlikely to help. The most helpful study in this patient would be selective mesenteric angiography.

28. The answer is C (Chapter 4, Acute Abdomen, Physical Exam, IV). The history described would be more typical for either testicular torsion or acute epididymitis, of which only torsion represents a surgical emergency. Torsion of the testicle is likely the result of an abnormal attachment of the tunica vaginalis around the cord that allows the testis to twist (bell-clapper deformity). Compromise of the blood supply causes exquisite pain and produces gangrene and atrophy of the testis unless the torsion is treated immediately. Torsion is usually seen in young males, most often occurring spontaneously and even during sleep. It is associated with an onset of severe pain and is accompanied by nausea, vomiting, and abdominal pain. Acute prostatitis may present with vague abdominal pain. A more typical presentation for appendicitis would be pain preceded by nausea or anorexia. This presentation is not typical for gastroenteritis (which is not a surgical emergency).

29. The answer is C (Chapter 4, Hemorrhage, Evaluation, III B 6). Arteriography is most often used as the initial evaluation step for continued bleeding after anorectal bleeding sources have been eliminated by endoscopy. Arteriography allows identification of diverticular bleeding as well as an angiodysplastic lesion of the right colon. Surgery is generally not indicated until 4–6 units of blood have been shed. Coagulation products are of no use unless the patient has abnormal clotting studies. Saline lavage of the colon is not a routine procedure.

30–31. The answers are 30-C (Chapter 4, Hemorrhage, Evaluation, III B 3) **and 31-D** (Chapter 4, Hemorrhage, Evaluation, III D). Upper endoscopy is the most reliable method for precisely locating the site of upper GI bleeding. Endoscopy can almost always be used unless bleeding is massive. Patients who are unstable or have blood losses requiring more than 6 units of blood within a 24-hour period require surgical intervention. Unstable patients should not typically be transported to interventional radiology. A Blakemore tube is only useful for bleeding esophageal varices. This patient, who does not have a history indicative of cirrhosis, is unlikely to have bleeding from varices.

32. The answer is C (Chapter 4, Obstruction, Differential Diagnosis, I C 1). Obstructing adhesive bands after abdominal surgery are the most common cause of intestinal obstruction. They may be diffuse or solitary. A partial small bowel obstruction often responds to conservative management with nasogastric decompression and hydration. Complete small bowel obstruction typically requires operative intervention.

33. The answer is E (Chapter 4, Acute Abdomen, Diagnostic Testing, II A 1). Free air within the peritoneal cavity signals perforation of a hollow viscus. It is present in about 80% of gastroduodenal perforations. Because free peritoneal air is rarely secondary to other causes, additional studies in this patient would not be necessary before laparotomy.

Thoracic Disorders

Chapter Cuts and Caveats

Part II

CHAPTER 5

Principles of Thoracic Surgery:

◆ Symptoms of malignancy or a radiologic abnormality suspicious for a neoplasm (e.g., coin lesion on a screening chest x-ray, symptoms of dyspnea, or enlarged lymph nodes on physical exam) necessitate aggressive diagnosis because a delay can result in significant growth or metastasis and increase mortality.

◆ Small cell carcinoma is considered a systemic disease that begins in the lung and metastasizes early. It is rarely amenable to surgical resection, and chemotherapy is the primary treatment.

◆ Non–small cell carcinoma begins as a more local disease that spreads to local and regional lymph nodes before becoming systemic, making surgical resection more likely to be curative.

◆ Mesothelioma usually presents in a late stage with low cure rates, but early stages can be cured with extrapleural pneumonectomy.

◆ Spontaneous pneumothorax occurs in young asthenic adults due to a rupture of apical blebs. First episodes are treated with chest tube, but recurrent or bilateral episodes undergo thoracoscopic excision of the blebs and pleural abrasion.

◆ Empyema is treated with (1) antibiotics, (2) pus evacuation, and (3) re-expansion of the lung.

◆ With mediastinal masses, the location accurately formulates the differential diagnosis and focuses the clinical evaluation: Anterior location suggests lymphoma, thyroid, teratoma/germ cell tumors, or thymoma (which can present with myasthenia gravis, be diagnosed with antiacetylcholine receptor antibodies, and be cured with resection); middle suggests lymphoma, sarcoid, metastatic lung cancer, and cysts; and posterior suggests neurogenic tumors.

CHAPTER 6

Heart:

◆ Many new technologies and minimally invasive interventions are being used to treat coronary artery and valvular disease. Initial treatment of coronary artery disease should consist of lifestyle changes. More aggressive interventions should be used based on the symptoms, extent of disease, and the risk/benefit ratio for the intervention.

◆ Cardiac catheterization is the basis for determining coronary artery anatomy as well as many endoluminal interventions.

◆ Patients with left main coronary artery disease have a reduced survival, making it a primary indication for coronary artery revascularization.

◆ The internal mammary artery graft, which has a 90% or better patency rate at 10 years, has superior patency over other grafts.

◆ Mechanical valves have a long lifetime but require long-term anticoagulation to prevent thromboembolic events. Biologic prosthesis valves have a shorter lifetime but no need for anticoagulation.

◆ Acute pericardial tamponade may occur with as little as 100 mL of fluid and can be relieved by pericardiocentesis. Traumatic tamponade usually requires surgical exploration.

Chapter 5

Principles of Thoracic Surgery

Jinny Ha and Whitney Burrows

GENERAL PRINCIPLES OF THORACIC SURGERY

Thoracic Cavity Anatomy

I. **Chest wall:** Formed by the sternum, ribs, vertebral column, intercostal muscles, intercostal vessels, and nerves (Fig. 5-1). Its inferior border is the diaphragm; it is lined internally by the parietal pleura.

II. **Mediastinum:** anatomic region between the pleural cavities for the length of the thorax (Fig. 5-2)

> **Quick Cut**
> The intercostal bundle runs on the undersurface of the ribs.

A. **Anterior compartment:** extends from the undersurface of the sternum to the pericardium and contains the thymus gland, lymph nodes, ascending and transverse aorta, and great veins

B. **Visceral compartment:** extends from the pericardium to the anterior longitudinal spinal ligament and contains the pericardium, heart, trachea, hilar structures of the lung, esophagus, phrenic nerves, and lymph nodes

C. **Paravertebral sulci:** potential spaces that contain the sympathetic chains, intercostal nerves, and descending thoracic aorta

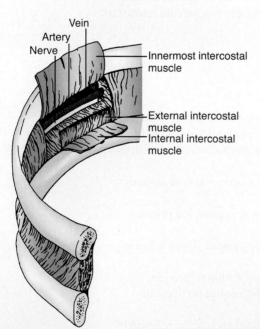

Figure 5-1: Chest wall. (Adapted from Way L. Thoracic wall, pleura, lung, and mediastinum. In: Way LW, ed. *Current Surgical Diagnosis and Treatment*, 10th ed. Stamford, CT: Appleton & Lange; 1983:319.)

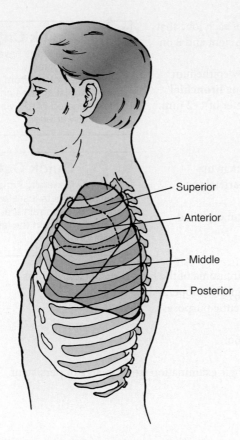

Figure 5-2: Anatomic compartments of the mediastinum.

- Superior
- Anterior
- Middle
- Posterior

III. Lungs and tracheobronchial tree

A. **Right lung:** has three lobes—the upper, middle, and lower—separated by two **fissures** (Fig. 5-3)

B. **Left lung:** has two lobes—the upper and the lower

1. **Lingula:** portion of the upper lobe

2. **Single oblique fissure:** separates lobes

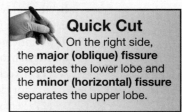

Quick Cut
On the right side, the **major (oblique) fissure** separates the lower lobe and the **minor (horizontal) fissure** separates the upper lobe.

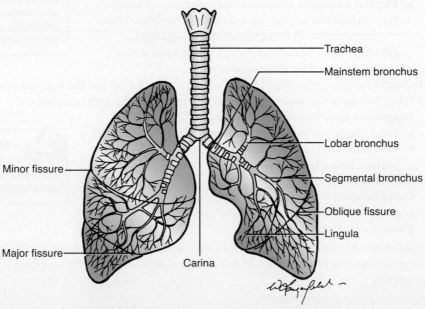

- Trachea
- Mainstem bronchus
- Lobar bronchus
- Segmental bronchus
- Oblique fissure
- Lingula
- Minor fissure
- Major fissure
- Carina

Figure 5-3: Lungs and tracheobronchial tree. (Courtesy of Thomas C. King and Craig R. Smith. Columbia Presbyterian Hospital, New York.)

C. **Bronchopulmonary segments:** Intact sections of each lobe that have a separate blood supply; there are 10 on the right and 8 on the left.

D. **Tracheobronchial tree:** Formed from respiratory epithelium with reinforcing cartilaginous rings; the branching **bronchial tubes** are progressively smaller, down to a diameter of 1–2 mm.

E. **Blood supply:** dual
   1. **Pulmonary artery:** Blood is **unoxygenated**.
   2. **Bronchial artery:** Blood is **oxygenated**.

F. **Lymphatic vessels:** present throughout the parenchyma
   1. **Lymphatic flow in the pleural space:** from parietal to visceral pleura
   2. **Lymphatic drainage within the mediastinum:** cephalad

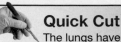

Quick Cut
The lungs have a dual blood supply: oxygenated blood from the bronchial arteries and unoxygenated blood via the pulmonary arteries.

Quick Cut
Generally, lymphatic drainage affects ipsilateral nodes, but contralateral flow often occurs from the left lower lobe.

General Thoracic Procedures

I. **Endoscopy**

A. **Laryngoscopy:** Occasionally important when carcinoma of the lung is suspected. Tumor involvement of the recurrent laryngeal nerves signifies inoperability.

B. **Bronchoscopy:** useful for diagnostic and therapeutic purposes
   1. **Diagnostic uses:** include the following:
      a. To confirm a lung or tracheobronchial tumor
      b. To identify the source of hemoptysis
      c. To obtain specimens for culture and cytologic examination from an area of persistent pulmonary atelectasis or pneumonitis
      d. To obtain tissue biopsy
   2. **Therapeutic uses:** include the following:
      a. To remove a foreign body
      b. To remove retained secretions (e.g., from aspiration of gastric contents)
      c. To drain lung infections, such as abscesses
   3. **Types:** include the following:
      a. **Rigid bronchoscopy:** allows visualization of the trachea and main bronchi to the individual lobes
         (1) Excellent for biopsies of endobronchial lesions and for clearing of thick secretions
         (2) Performance of rigid bronchoscopy under local anesthesia requires considerable skill.
      b. **Flexible fiberoptic bronchoscopy:** used more frequently
         (1) Particularly helpful for visualizing lobar bronchi and biopsy in small bronchopulmonary segments
         (2) Although rigid bronchoscopy is preferred, it may also be used for clearing secretions.

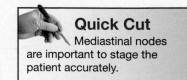

Quick Cut
Flexible bronchoscopy is especially useful when the patient is intubated, as it preserves the airway during the procedure.

C. **Mediastinoscopy:** Lighted hollow instrument is inserted behind the sternum at the tracheal notch and directed along the anterior surface of the trachea in the pretracheal space.
   1. **Diagnostic uses:** include the following:
      a. Direct biopsy of paratracheal and subcarinal lymph nodes
      b. Useful for diagnosing sarcoidosis, lymphoma, and various fungal infections
   2. **Mortality rate:** less than 0.1%
   3. **Complications:** include hemorrhage, pneumothorax, and injury to the recurrent laryngeal nerves, although the incidence is extremely low

Quick Cut
Mediastinal nodes are important to stage the patient accurately.

III. **Scalene node biopsy:** performed before the use of computed tomography (CT)/positron emission tomography (PET) scans and fine-needle aspiration (FNA) for lung cancer; used if FNA is nondiagnostic

IV. **Diagnostic pleural procedures**

A. **Thoracentesis:** Pleural effusions are examined for organisms in suspected infections and cytologically in suspected malignancies. Positive cytologic findings prove a tumor to be inoperable.

B. **Pleural biopsy:** Either percutaneous or open pleural biopsy yields a positive diagnosis in 60%–80% of patients with tuberculosis or cancer when a pleural effusion or pleural-based mass is present.

V. **Lung biopsy**

A. **Diagnostic uses:** Percutaneous lung biopsy may be used for either a localized peripheral lesion or a diffuse parenchymal process.

B. **Types:** include the following:

1. **CT-directed FNA biopsy:** may obtain tissue for tumor diagnosis, but sampling errors do exist

a. **Other uses:** may also be useful for infections and inflammatory processes

b. **Complications:** pneumothorax and hemorrhage

2. **Open lung biopsy:** necessary if needle biopsy fails at diagnosis

VI. **Thoracic exposure:** provided by various **thoracic incisions**, including the following:

A. **Median sternotomy:** exposes heart, pericardium, and structures in the anterior mediastinum (Fig. 5-4)

B. **Posterolateral thoracotomy:** exposes lung, esophagus, and posterior mediastinum (Fig. 5-5)

C. **Axillary thoracotomy:** for limited exposure of the upper thorax during procedures such as first-rib resection, upper lobe biopsy, or sympathectomy

D. **Anterolateral thoracotomy:** for rapid exposure in cases of unstable cardiovascular status that cannot tolerate a lateral incision; also allows for excellent airway control (Fig. 5-6)

E. **Anterior parasternal mediastinotomy (Chamberlain procedure, left side):** 2- to 3-cm parasternal incision allows mediastinoscope into the mediastinum or, more commonly, direct visualization and biopsy of mediastinal lymph nodes (para-aortic [level 6] and aortopulmonary window [level 5]).

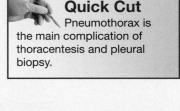

Quick Cut
Pneumothorax is the main complication of thoracentesis and pleural biopsy.

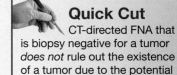

Quick Cut
CT-directed FNA that is biopsy negative for a tumor *does not* rule out the existence of a tumor due to the potential for sampling error.

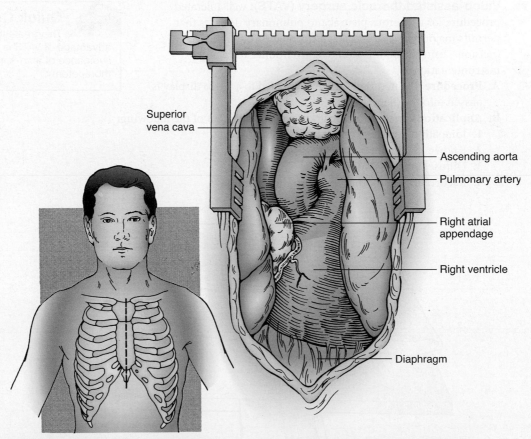

Figure 5-4: Median sternotomy. (Adapted from Kirklin JW, Barratt-Boyes BG. Hypothermia, circulatory arrest, and cardiopulmonary bypass. In: Kirklin JW, Barratt-Boyes BG, eds *Cardiac Surgery*. New York: Wiley; 1986:62.)

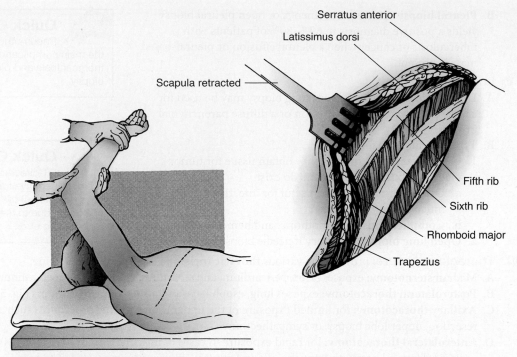

Serratus anterior
Latissimus dorsi
Scapula retracted
Fifth rib
Sixth rib
Rhomboid major
Trapezius

Figure 5-5: Posterolateral thoracotomy. (Adapted from Bryant LR, Morgan CV Jr. Chest wall, pleura, lung, mediastinum. In: Schwartz SI, Shires GT, Spencer FC, eds. *Principles of Surgery*, 5th ed. New York: McGraw-Hill; 1989:634.)

VII. Video-assisted thoracic surgery (VATS): well-tolerated procedure for numerous pleural and pulmonary diseases that permits major procedures to be performed through minor incisions, using a combination of conventional and unique instrumentation

A. Procedure: Lighted rigid scope connected to a video display is passed into the pleural space.

B. Applications: include the diagnosis or management of the following:
1. Idiopathic exudative pleural effusion
2. Known malignant pleural effusion
3. Diffuse interstitial lung disease
4. Recurrent pneumothorax or persistent air leak

Quick Cut
The greatest advantage of VATS is the avoidance of a rib-spreading thoracotomy.

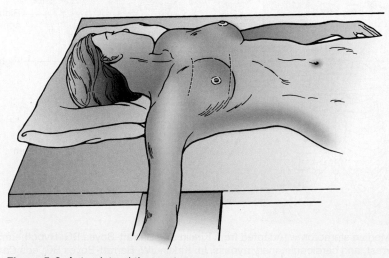

Figure 5-6: Anterolateral thoracotomy.

5. Indeterminate peripheral solitary pulmonary nodules
6. Mediastinal cyst
7. Anatomic lobectomy (in experienced hands only)

CHEST WALL DISORDERS

Chest Wall Deformities

I. **Pectus excavatum (funnel chest):** Depression of the sternum is the most common chest wall deformity.
   A. **Symptoms:** usually asymptomatic but it may cause some cardiopulmonary symptoms
   B. **Surgery:** may be performed for moderate to severe deformities between age 8 years to prior to end of adolescence

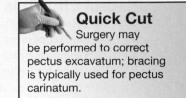

Quick Cut
Surgery may be performed to correct pectus excavatum; bracing is typically used for pectus carinatum.

   1. **Modified Ravitch:** open
   2. **Nuss procedure:** closed or minimally invasive approach that involves inserting a metal bar through lateral incisions to raise the sternum

II. **Pectus carinatum (pigeon breast):** Protrusion deformity of the anterior sternum, rarely causing symptoms. Bracing is an option, with surgery performed for cosmetic reasons.

III. **Poland syndrome:** unilateral absence of costal cartilages, pectoralis muscle, and breast. Surgery is indicated for protection of the underlying thoracic structures and for cosmesis.

IV. **Thoracic outlet syndrome (TOS)**
   A. **Clinical presentation:** Can manifest into three different forms (neurogenic, arterial, and venous) but symptomatology can overlap

Quick Cut
TOS is caused by compression of the neurovascular bundle—the brachial plexus and subclavian artery and vein.

   1. **Neurogenic:** combination of motor and sensory symptoms from compression of the brachial plexus. Patients can have upper extremity (UE) weakness or pain affecting the neck, shoulder, and arm.
   2. **Arterial:** Symptoms are related to compression of the subclavian artery, which can include pain, pallor, paresthesia, and UE coolness.
   3. **Venous:** presents with unilateral swelling of UE with associated cyanosis or rubor due to compression or thrombosis of subclavian vein
   B. **Diagnosis:** Clinical; based on a detailed history and physical examination. Cervical spine films to rule out disk disease and chest x-ray to evaluate for bony abnormalities (i.e., cervical rib) should be performed.

Quick Cut
Surgery for TOS may involve first-rib resection, anterior scalenectomy, or brachial plexus neurolysis.

   C. **Treatment:** initially conservative, using a focused physical therapy program for 4–6 weeks

Chest Wall Tumors

I. **Benign tumors**
   A. **Chondroma:** Most common benign tumor of the chest wall; it occurs at the costochondral junction.
   B. **Fibrous dysplasia of the rib:** Occurs posteriorly or on the lateral portion of the rib. It is not painful, and it grows slowly.
   C. **Osteochondroma:** occurs on any portion of the rib

II. **Malignant tumors:** include fibrosarcoma, chondrosarcoma, osteogenic sarcoma, myeloma, and Ewing sarcoma

III. **Treatment:** involves wide excision and reconstruction using autologous grafts, prosthetic grafts, or both

PLEURAL AND PLEURAL SPACE DISORDERS

Spontaneous Pneumothorax

I. **Epidemiology:** usually occurs in tall, thin males ages 10–30 years. Other risk factors include smoking, chronic obstructive pulmonary disease (COPD), family history, Marfan syndrome, homocystinuria, and thoracic endometriosis.

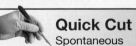

Quick Cut
Spontaneous pneumothorax occurs when a **subpleural bleb** ruptures into the pleural space and allows secondary lung collapse.

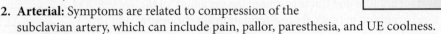

II. **Symptoms:** include pleuritic chest pain and dyspnea

III. **Diagnosis:** made by physical examination and chest radiograph

IV. **Treatment:** chest tube drainage of the pleural space
   A. **Indications for surgery:** include recurrent pneumothorax (ipsilateral), persistent air leak for 3–5 days, incomplete lung expansion, hemopneumothorax
   B. **Procedure:** stapling of apical blebs and pleural abrasion

> **Quick Cut**
> Surgery is generally reserved for pneumothorax that does not resolve with chest tube drainage.

Pleural Effusions

I. **Transudative effusions:** result from systemic disorders that cause an increased hydrostatic pressure (congestive heart failure [CHF]) or states associated with decreased oncotic pressure (hypoalbuminemia) allowing the accumulation of *protein-poor* plasma filtrate in the pleural space. Treatment is directed toward the underlying process; thoracentesis provides diagnosis and symptomatic relief.

II. **Exudative effusions:** result from the local pleural pathology, which increases the permeability of the pleura, allowing accumulation of a *protein-rich* plasma filtrate within the pleural space. Treatment usually requires chest tube drainage and/or pleurodesis.

> **Quick Cut**
> Transudative effusions are systemic and protein poor; exudative effusions are local and protein rich.

Pleural Empyema

I. **Pathophysiology:** evolves in three stages
   A. **Exudative phase:** Onset to 7 days; fluid is initially produced.
   B. **Fibrinopurulent phase:** Days 7–21; deposits of fibrin on the pleura form loculations, and the fluid is turbid or purulent.
   C. **Chronic or organized phase:** More than 21 days; fibrin and pleura fuse and thicken around the periphery of the fluid, resulting in frank abscess formation and/or pleural rind or peel.

> **Quick Cut**
> Pus in the pleural space usually accumulates secondary to pulmonary infection.

II. **Diagnosis:** Made by thoracentesis in a patient with pleural effusion, leukocytosis, and fever; the aspirated pleural fluid is sent for biochemistry studies, and if on gross examination the fluid is very cloudy or smells foul, an empyema is likely to be present.

> **Quick Cut**
> Stages of empyema: I, exudative phase; II, fibrinopurulent phase; and III, chronic or organized phase.

III. **Treatment:** Recent use of image-guided catheters followed by pleural lytic therapy using tissue plasminogen activator has demonstrated impressive results in successfully draining empyemas.
   A. **Early empyemas:** may be treated with aspiration and hhantibiotics
   B. **Established empyemas:** Usually have thicker fluid and need continuous closed drainage. Loculated empyemas may require surgical drainage via VATS or open thoracotomy.
   C. **Chronic empyemas:** If unresponsive to chest tube drainage, may require open drainage via localized rib resection, especially for debilitated patients.

> **Quick Cut**
> Positive pleural cultures, low pH (<7.1), low glucose (<50 mg/dL), and high lactate dehydrogenase content (>1,000 IU/dL) are consistent with empyema.

> **Quick Cut**
> Decortication and evacuation of empyema should be performed for lung re-expansion in chronic empyema.

Pleural Tumors and Mesothelioma

I. **Overview:** Majority of pleural lesions are metastases from other primary malignancy.

II. **Localized benign mesotheliomas:** Are *not related* to asbestos exposure; these lesions are treated by wide local excision.

III. **Malignant mesothelioma:** *Related* to prior asbestos exposure and presents with a pleural effusion. It has a poor prognosis; the role of surgery is primarily for diagnosis and palliation.

> **Quick Cut**
> Primary tumors of the pleura are rare.

PULMONARY INFECTIONS

Lung Abscess

I. **Etiology:** Aspiration of oropharyngeal contents is the most common cause. It occurs in the dependent segments of the lung; these infections are most often mixed flora, but anaerobic organisms may predominate.

II. **Treatment:** Intravenous antibiotics are the mainstay for lung abscesses.
   A. **Image-guided percutaneous drainage:** often effective for large abscesses
   B. **Indications for surgery:** include failure of the abscess to resolve with antibiotic therapy, hemorrhage, inability to rule out cavitating carcinoma, giant abscess (>4–6 cm in diameter), or rupture into pleural space resulting in a pyopneumothorax

> **Quick Cut**
> Symptoms of lung abscess are similar to those associated with pneumonia. Radiographs will demonstrate a cavitary lesion with an air-fluid level.

SOLITARY PULMONARY NODULES (COIN LESIONS)

Overview

I. **Presentation:** well-circumscribed lesions usually less than 3 cm in diameter that are completely surrounded by normal lung parenchyma

II. **Initial assessment:** should always start with a thorough history and physical with focus on smoking history, history of cancer, hemoptysis, and age

> **Quick Cut**
> Solitary pulmonary nodules have a broad differential, including congenital, inflammatory, neoplastic, and vascular etiologies.

Imaging

I. **Thin-section CT:** important for characterizing a pulmonary nodule
   A. **Margins:** Irregular, lobulated, or spiculated edges are suggestive of malignancy.
   B. **Calcifications:** Typically associated with benign lesions; different patterns of calcification can be seen in granulomatous disease and hamartomas.
   C. **Growth:** Comparison with previous imaging is important. Size stability more than 2 years is highly associated with benign lesions.

II. **PET scan:** has sensitivity of 95% and lower specificity of 80%
   A. **False negatives:** can occur for bronchoalveolar carcinomas, carcinoids, and tumor less than 1 cm in diameter
   B. **False positives:** can occur in the setting of recent infection or granulomatous diseases

>
> **Quick Cut**
> **Corona radiata sign**, which is the spiculated appearance of a lesion from fine linear strands extending outward, is highly suspicious of a malignancy.

Invasive Diagnostic Techniques

I. **Bronchoscopy:** with endobronchial biopsy and/or brushings can be useful for centrally located lesions

II. **Transthoracic FNA:** Can be used for peripherally located lesions. Possible complications include hemorrhage and pneumothorax.

III. **Excisional biopsy:** allows for definitive pathologic diagnosis

BRONCHOGENIC CARCINOMA

Overview

I. **Epidemiology:** Bronchogenic carcinoma is the leading cause of cancer death among men and women in the United States.
   A. **Locally advanced or metastatic disease:** 75% of patient presentations
   B. **Age:** Middle-aged and elderly; 90% of cases occur between ages 40 and 80 years.

II. **Risk factors:** 90% of all lung carcinomas are *related to smoking*; occupational and environmental carcinogens include asbestos, tar, radon, soot, nickel, arsenic, and chromium.

> **Quick Cut**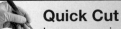
> Lung cancer is the leading cause of cancer death and has a 5-year survival rate of 15%.

Pathology

I. **Histologic distribution:** Most common lung neoplasm is a metastatic lesion from another primary malignancy (secondary lung cancer). Lung cancers are classified into two major types.

    A. **Small cell lung carcinomas:** 20% of primary lung cancers

    B. **Non–small cell lung carcinomas:** 80% of primary lung cancers

> **Quick Cut**
> The most common lung neoplasm is a metastatic deposit from another primary malignancy.

II. **Non–small cell lung carcinomas**

    A. **Adenocarcinoma:** Now the most common lung carcinoma; lesions are typically located in the periphery and arise from bronchioles and terminal alveolar units.

    B. **Noninvasive adenocarcinoma:** formerly called *bronchoalveolar carcinoma*; variant of adenocarcinoma

        1. **Forms (three):** solitary nodule, multinodular form, and a diffuse/pneumonic form

        2. Overrepresented in nonsmokers

    C. **Squamous cell carcinoma:** second most common subtype

        1. **Location:** Most occur centrally in the lung fields and arise from the respiratory mucosa of lobar and segmental bronchi.

        2. **Tumor characteristics:** Bulky and is associated with obstruction; it undergoes central necrosis and cavitation.

III. **Small cell anaplastic (oat cell) carcinoma:** highly malignant; represents <15%–25% of all malignant lung tumors

    A. **Histology:** reveals clusters, nests, or sheets of small, round, oval, or spindle-shaped cells with dark nuclei and a scanty cytoplasm

        1. **Electron microscopy:** reveals neurosecretory cytoplasmic granules

        2. **Classification:** neuroendocrine tumors of the amine precursor uptake and decarboxylation (APUD) system

    B. **Staging classifications:** early metastasis by lymphatic and vascular routes

        1. **Limited disease:** localized to one hemithorax with ipsilateral regional node involvement

        2. **Extensive disease:** metastasis outside the hemithorax

    C. **Treatment:** Involves a combination of chemotherapy and radiotherapy. Surgery may be indicated in those with early lesions.

    D. **Prognosis:** overall quite poor

> **Quick Cut**
> Treatment for non-small cell lung cancer is primarily surgical. Treatment for small cell carcinoma is chemotherapy and radiation.

IV. **Other rare tumors:** Undifferentiated large cell carcinoma, bronchial adenoma, papilloma, and sarcomas are rare.

Clinical Presentation

I. **Pulmonary symptoms:** may include unrelenting cough, dyspnea, chest pain, hemoptysis, wheezing, and pneumonic symptoms

II. **Extrapulmonary symptoms**

    A. **Metastatic extrapulmonary manifestations:** include weight loss, malaise, headache, nausea and vomiting related to brain metastases, and bone pain

> **Quick Cut**
> A chronic, unrelenting cough is the most common symptom of lung cancer.

    B. **Nonmetastatic extrapulmonary manifestations (paraneoplastic syndromes):** secondary to hormonelike substances that are elaborated by the tumor and include Cushing syndrome, hypercalcemia, myasthenic neuropathies, hypertrophic osteoarthropathies, and gynecomastia

III. **Pancoast tumor:** invades the superior sulcus involving the thoracic outlet and results in shoulder pain from invasion of muscle, radicular arm pain from invasion of C8 and T1 nerve roots, and **Horner syndrome**

> **Quick Cut**
> Horner syndrome is ptosis, miosis, enophthalmos, and anhidrosis.

Diagnosis and Staging

I. **Abnormal chest radiograph:** Most common finding; more likely to represent carcinoma in patients age 40 years and older. The tumor may present as a nodule, an infiltrate, or as atelectasis.

II. **CT scan:** reveals the extent of the tumor and the possibility of mediastinal lymph node metastasis

III. **PET scan:** routinely used to assess the primary tumor and the mediastinal lymph nodes and to screen for metastatic disease

IV. **Bronchoscopy:** assesses for bronchial involvement and resectability in **central** lesions, and tissue is obtained for cytologic examination

V. **Mediastinoscopy or mediastinotomy:** obtains mediastinal lymph nodes for pathologic examination and aids in staging

VI. **Percutaneous needle biopsy:** may be used for peripheral lesions to obtain tissue for cytologic examination

VII. **Staging:** fundamental for the evaluation of treatment protocols and based on information obtained during the preoperative evaluation, findings at mediastinoscopy, thoracotomy, and pathologic findings of the surgical specimens. Definitions of tumor size (T), lymph node metastasis (N), and distant metastasis (M) comprise the **TNM classification of carcinoma of the lung** by the revised International Clinical Staging System (Table 5-1).

Table 5-1: Tumor-Node-Metastasis Classification of Lung Cancer

T (primary tumors)
TX: Tumor is proved by the presence of malignant cells in bronchopulmonary secretions but is not visualized on a radiograph or by bronchoscopy or any tumor that cannot be assessed, such as one in a retreatment staging.
T0: No evidence of primary tumor
TIS: Carcinoma in situ

T1: Tumor that is ≤3 cm in greatest dimension, surrounded by lung or visceral pleura and with no evidence of invasion proximal to a lobar bronchus at bronchoscopy
   T1a: Tumor <2 cm in size
   T1b: Tumor 2–3 cm in size

T2: Tumor >3 cm but <7 cm in greatest dimension or a tumor of any size that either invades the visceral pleura or has associated atelectasis or obstructive pneumonitis that extends to the hilar region that involves less than an entire lung; at bronchoscopy, the proximal extent of demonstrable tumor must be within a lobar bronchus or at least 2 cm distal to the carina.
   T2a: Tumor >3 but <5 cm in size
   T2b: Tumor >5 cm but <7 cm in size

T3: Tumor >7 cm in size or one that directly invades into the chest wall (including superior sulcus tumors), diaphragm, mediastinal pleura, parietal pericardium, or phrenic nerve or a tumor in the main bronchus <2 cm from the carina without involving the carina; also, any associated atelectasis or obstructive pneumonitis involving the entire lung or a separate nodule in the same lobe
T4: Tumor of any size with invasion of the mediastinum or involving the heart, great vessels, trachea, esophagus, vertebral body, or carina; in addition, satellite tumor nodules that occur within a different ipsilateral lobe
N (nodal involvement)
N0: No demonstrable metastasis to regional lymph nodes
N1: Metastasis to lymph nodes in the peribronchial or the ipsilateral hilar region, or both, including direct extension
N2: Metastasis to ipsilateral mediastinal lymph nodes and subcarinal lymph nodes
N3: Metastasis to contralateral mediastinal lymph nodes, contralateral hilar lymph nodes, ipsilateral or contralateral scalene, or supraclavicular lymph nodes
M (distant metastasis)
M0: No (known) distant metastasis

M1:
   M1a: Separate tumor in a contralateral lobe; tumor with pleural nodules or malignant pleural effusions
   M1b: Distant metastasis

Treatment

I. **Surgical treatment**
   A. **Pulmonary resection:** Such as lobectomy, extended lobectomy, or pneumonectomy, is the mainstay of curative therapy for early-stage bronchogenic carcinoma. A regional lymphadenectomy is routinely performed primarily for prognostic (staging) purposes rather than therapeutic intent.
      1. **Lobectomy:** used in disease localized to one lobe
      2. **Extended resections and pneumonectomy:** used when the tumor involves a fissure or centrally located tumors
      3. **Wedge resections or bronchial segmentectomy:** may be used in localized disease in high-risk patients
   B. **Contraindications for thoracotomy:** 50% of all patients with lung carcinomas are not candidates for thoracotomy.
      1. **N2 disease:** extensive ipsilateral mediastinal lymph node involvement, particularly high paratracheal and subcarinal
      2. **N3 disease:** any contralateral mediastinal lymph node involvement
      3. **Other:** distant metastases, malignant pleural effusion, superior vena cava syndrome, recurrent laryngeal nerve involvement, phrenic nerve paralysis, or poor pulmonary function (relative contraindication)

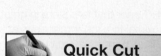

> **Quick Cut**
> A "popcorn" appearance on x-ray suggests **hamartoma**, an overgrowth of cartilage that is the most common benign lung lesion.

II. **Adjuvant therapy:** Further treatment using radiotherapy, chemotherapy, or both is indicated for some advanced-stage tumors.
   A. **Postoperative adjuvant chemotherapy:** now indicated in all resected non–small cell lung cancer patients **stage Ib** and higher, demonstrating a small but statistically significant survival benefit
   B. **Preoperative chemotherapy and radiation therapy:** can be given to select patients with IIIa (N2) disease to sterilize their mediastinal node disease

BRONCHIAL ADENOMAS

Overview

I. **Characteristics:** Carcinoid tumors, which comprise 80%–90% of bronchial adenomas, occur mainly in the proximal bronchi (20% mainstem bronchi, 60% lobar or segmental bronchi, and 20% peripheral parenchyma).
   A. **Carcinoid tumors:** arise from basal bronchial stem cells, which, in the process of malignant transformation, differentiate in the direction of **neuroendocrine** tissue
   B. **Growth:** They grow slowly and protrude endobronchially, often causing some degree of bronchial obstruction.
   C. **Peptide production:** can produce many different types, most commonly serotonin, which can, but very rarely does, lead to carcinoid syndrome if released into systemic circulation

> **Quick Cut**
> The term **adenoma** is a misnomer because all of these lesions are all **malignant neoplasms** that arise from the tracheobronchial tree.

II. **Signs and symptoms:** Cough, recurrent infection, hemoptysis, pain, and wheezing. Patient may report a long history of recurrent pneumonia or asthma.
III. **Diagnosis:** Chest x-ray may reveal a mass with or without associated atelectasis or pneumonia. CT better describes the local extent or the presence of distant metastasis. A tissue sample via bronchoscopy or FNA can be performed.
IV. **Treatment:** surgical excision
   A. **Lobectomy:** Most commonly performed procedure; rarely does it require a pneumonectomy.
   B. **Octreotide:** can be used for patients with unresectable disease with symptoms of carcinoid syndrome
V. **Prognosis:** should be greater than 85% 5-year survival for typical carcinoid tumors, decreasing to less than 50%–70% for the atypical variant

Adenoid Cystic Carcinoma (Cylindroma)

I. **Characteristics:** comprises <10% of bronchial adenomas
   A. **Location: occurs more centrally** in the lower trachea/carina area and in the orifices of the mainstem bronchi
   B. **Metastases:** tends to occur late, but about one third of patients present with metastases

II. **Treatment:** En bloc excision of the tumor, including peribronchial tissue and regional lymph nodes. **Radiation therapy** should be considered in all inoperable patients and in those with residual tumor after resection.

III. **Prognosis:** less favorable than in the case of a carcinoid tumor

Mucoepidermoid Carcinoma

I. **Characteristics:** account for less than 1% of bronchial adenomas

    A. Location: Distribution in the tracheobronchial tree is similar to that with carcinoid tumors.

    B. Most are low grade.

II. **Treatment:** Principles that are outlined for carcinoid tumors apply to low-grade mucoepidermoid carcinoma. High-grade variants should be approached and managed like other bronchial carcinomas.

METASTATIC TUMOR

Treatment

I. **Treatment:** Most metastatic tumors to the lung are not resected. In highly selected cases, surgery is indicated.

II. **Single or multiple metastatic tumors:** can be removed from the lung as part of the treatment protocol

>
> **Quick Cut**
> Metastatic tumors are common to the lung, which may be the only site of metastases from a nonpulmonary primary tumor.

III. **Complete resectability:** Associated with longer survival than unresectable disease. Long-term survival more than 5 years can be 20%–30% of all patients with completely resected pulmonary metastases.

TRACHEAL DISORDERS

Anatomy

I. **Structure:** Trachea is <11 cm from the cricoid to the carina and 1.8–2.3 cm in diameter.

    A. Cartilage: Encircled by 18–22 cartilaginous rings. The **cricoid cartilage** is the only complete tracheal ring; the remaining rings have a membranous portion posteriorly.

    B. Mobility: Vertical; when the neck is extended, 50% of the trachea is in the neck; when the neck is flexed, the entire trachea is behind the sternum.

II. **Blood supply:** Segmental and shared with the esophagus; blood is supplied by the inferior thyroid, subclavian, superior intercostal, internal mammary, and the innominate arteries and the bronchial circulation.

Tracheal Neoplasms

I. **Types**

    A. Primary neoplasms: rare

        1. Squamous cell carcinomas: Most common variant of these rare tumors. They may be exophytic, may cause superficial ulceration, or may be multiple.

        2. Adenoid carcinoma: grows slowly

        3. Other: include carcinosarcomas, pseudosarcomas, mucoepidermoid carcinomas, squamous papillomas, chondromas, and chondrosarcomas

    B. Secondary tumors: usually from the lung, esophagus, or thyroid gland

II. **Diagnosis:** Bronchoscopy provides diagnosis.

    A. Radiographic studies: include chest x-ray, CT scan, tracheal tomogram, and fluoroscopy for laryngeal evaluation

    B. Pulmonary function testing: mandatory if carinal or pulmonary resection is contemplated

III. **Treatment:** Tracheal resection; up to 50% may be removed.

    A. Resection: Adequate mobilization can usually be obtained by flexing the patient's neck, although laryngeal or hilar release techniques are sometimes necessary. An **end-to-end anastomosis** is performed.

    B. Incisions

        1. Cervical incision: used for resection of the upper half of the trachea

        2. Posterolateral thoracotomy: used for the lower portion of the trachea

        3. Combined cervical incision and median sternotomy: can expose entire trachea

IV. **Prognosis:** similar to that for resectable carcinoma of the lung

MEDIASTINAL LESIONS

Anterior Compartment Lesions

I. **Thymomas:** Thymic tumors are among the most common tumors of the anterosuperior mediastinum in the adult.

Quick Cut
Fifty percent of patients with thymomas have associated myasthenia gravis.

 A. **Incidence:** Thymomas are most common in the fifth and sixth decades of life; males and females are equally affected.

 B. **Diagnosis:** Most patients are asymptomatic, and the tumor is discovered incidentally on a routine chest radiograph.

  1. **Symptoms:** when present, relate to invasion by malignant thymomas and consist of chest pain, dyspnea, or superior vena cava syndrome

Quick Cut
Thymic tumors that are not associated with myasthenia gravis require exploration and total removal of the tumor.

  2. **Chest x-ray:** Lateral view is helpful because small tumors may be obscured by the great vessels in posteroanterior chest radiographs.

 C. **Surgical treatment:** Most are removed through a sternal-splitting median sternotomy.

II. **Teratomas**

 A. **Incidence:** Occur most frequently in adolescents; 80% are benign.

 B. **Etiology:** Originate from the branchial cleft pouch in association with the thymus gland. Ectodermal, endodermal, and mesodermal elements are present.

 C. **Diagnosis:** Radiographically may appear as smooth-walled cystic lesions or as lobulated solid lesions. Calcification is often present.

 D. **Treatment:** surgical excision

III. **Lymphomas:** Symptoms include cough, chest pain, fever, and weight loss.

Quick Cut
Fifty percent of patients with lymphoma have mediastinal lymph node involvement.

 A. **Diagnosis:** chest radiograph and lymph node biopsy, using either mediastinoscopy or anterior mediastinotomy

 B. **Treatment:** nonsurgical

IV. **Germ cell tumors:** Rare; occur with an incidence of less than 1% of all mediastinal tumors. They metastasize to pleural lymph nodes, the liver, bone, and the retroperitoneum.

 A. **Histologic types:** seminoma, embryonal cell carcinoma, teratocarcinoma, choriocarcinoma, and endodermal sinus tumor

 B. **Symptoms:** chest pain, cough, and hoarseness caused by invasion of the vagus nerves

 C. **Diagnosis:** combination of radiographs and serum tumor markers (**beta-human chorionic gonadotropin** and **alpha-fetoprotein**)

 D. **Treatment**

  1. **Seminomas:** complete surgical resection followed by postoperative radiotherapy

  2. **Nonseminomas:** combination chemotherapy

 E. **Adjuvant therapy:** Seminomas are very radiosensitive, and the other cell types may benefit from chemotherapeutic agents.

Visceral Compartment Lesions

I. **Pericardial cysts:** Usually asymptomatic and are seen on a chest radiograph. Surgery is usually done as a diagnostic procedure.

Quick Cut
Visceral compartment lesions are usually cystic, most commonly pericardial cysts or bronchogenic cysts.

II. **Bronchogenic cysts:** Generally arise posterior to the carina and may cause pulmonary compression, which can be life-threatening, particularly in infancy. The usual treatment is surgical excision.

III. **Ascending aortic aneurysms:** included as middle mediastinal masses due to the location of the great vessels in this compartment

THORACIC TRAUMA

Immediate Life-Threatening Injuries

Quick Cut
Fewer than 25% of patients with chest injuries require surgical intervention.

I. **Airway obstruction:** Quickly leads to hypoxia, hypercapnia, acidosis, and cardiac arrest. The highest priority is rapid evaluation and securing the upper airway by clearing out secretions, blood, or foreign bodies; endotracheal intubation; or cricothyroidotomy.

II. **Tension pneumothorax:** implies that the pleural air collection is under positive pressure, significant enough to cause a marked mediastinal shift away from the affected side and cardiopulmonary collapse

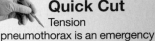

> **Quick Cut**
> Tension pneumothorax is an emergency that requires immediate needle decompression and presents with hypotension.

   A. **Causes:** Check-valve mechanism allows air to escape from the lung into the pleural space, which cannot be vented and can cause *sudden death*.

   B. **Clinical presentation:** Collapsed lung results in chest pain, shortness of breath, and decreased or absent breath sounds on the affected side. Hypotension results from mediastinal shift, which compresses the vena cava and obstructs venous return to the heart.

   C. **Treatment:** Thorax must be decompressed by an intercostal tube with underwater seal and suction.

III. **Open pneumothorax:** Open wound in the chest wall has exposed the pleural space to the atmosphere.

   A. **Clinical presentation:** Open wound allows air movement through the defect during spontaneous respiration, causing ineffective alveolar ventilation.

   B. **Treatment:** Involves covering the wound and inserting a thoracostomy tube. Later, debridement and closure of the wound may be necessary.

IV. **Massive hemothorax:** occurs with the rapid accumulation of blood in the pleural space, which causes both compromised ventilation as well as hypovolemic shock

> **Quick Cut**
> Surgery is indicated if a chest tube placed for hemorrhage has an initial output of more than 1 L or drainage of more than 200 mL/hr over 4 hours.

   A. **Treatment:** entails securing intravenous access and beginning volume resuscitation and placement of a thoracostomy tube

   B. **Complications**

   1. **Fibrothorax:** If the hemothorax is inadequately drained, this may develop and requires decortication.

   2. **Hemorrhage:** indication for surgical exploration

V. **Cardiac tamponade:** occurs with the rapid accumulation of blood in the pericardial sac, which causes compression of the cardiac chambers and decreased diastolic filling resulting in decreased cardiac output

   A. **Clinical presentation:** hypotension, tachycardia, and jugular venous distention with muffled heart sounds

   B. **Treatment:** prompt pericardial decompression either by pericardiocentesis (if in extremis) or surgical pericardiotomy

VI. **Flail chest:** Blunt chest trauma, causing extensive anterior and posterior rib fractures or sternocostal disconnection, results in paradoxical chest wall movement.

> **Quick Cut**
> Flail chest is defined as at least two fractures in two or more ribs, which produces a free floating segment of chest wall.

   A. **Clinical presentation:** Paradoxical chest wall movement interferes with the mechanics of respiration and can cause acute alveolar hypoventilation. Morbidity is related to underlying lung injury.

   B. **Treatment:** Adequate pain control (intercostal blocks or epidural narcotics) and aggressive pulmonary toilet. Mechanical ventilation may be required in severe cases.

Potentially Life-Threatening Injuries

I. **Tracheobronchial disruption:** usually occurs within 2 cm of the carina

   A. **Diagnosis:** made by bronchoscopy; suspected with the following:

   1. Collapsed lung fails to expand, following placement of a thoracostomy tube.

   2. Massive air leak persists.

   3. Massive progressive subcutaneous emphysema is present.

   B. **Treatment:** primary repair

II. **Aortic disruption:** Results from a deceleration injury in which the mobile ascending aorta and arch move forward, whereas the descending thoracic aorta remains fixed in position by the mediastinal pleura and intercostal vessels. This movement causes a tear at the aortic isthmus, just distal to the takeoff of the left subclavian artery.

  A. **Clinical presentation:** Usually results in fracture of the intima and media with the adventitia remaining mainly intact. However, complete disruption of all layers can occur with the hematoma contained only by the intact mediastinal pleura.
  B. **Chest radiograph findings:** widened mediastinum, indistinct aortic knob, depressed left mainstem bronchus, apical cap, deviation of trachea to the right, and left pleural effusion
  C. **Diagnosis:** confirmed by an aortogram or CT angiography
  D. **Treatment:** Involves strict blood pressure control with short-acting antihypertensives and open repair with interposition graft. Some centers treat with placement of endovascular stents.

III. **Diaphragmatic disruption:** results from blunt trauma to the chest and abdomen, producing a radial tear in the diaphragm, beginning at the esophageal hiatus
  A. **Diagnosis:** Chest radiograph shows evidence of the stomach or colon in the chest.
  B. **Treatment:** Immediate placement of a nasogastric tube (if not already in place) will prevent acute gastric dilatation, which can produce severe, life-threatening respiratory distress.
    1. **Next step:** urgent transabdominal repair with simultaneous treatment of any intra-abdominal injuries
    2. **Transthoracic repair:** If rupture is not diagnosed until 7–10 days later, this is recommended to free any adhesions to the lung that might exist.

IV. **Esophageal disruption:** usually results from penetrating rather than blunt trauma
  A. **Clinical presentation:** causes rapidly progressive mediastinitis
  B. **Treatment:** wide mediastinal drainage and primary closure with tissue reinforcement (pleura, intercostal muscle, or stomach)

V. **Cardiac contusion:** results from direct sternal impact; ranges in severity from clinically silent to cardiac rupture
  A. **Functional complications:** arrhythmias, myocardial rupture, ventricular septal rupture, left ventricular failure, and coronary artery rupture or thrombosis
  B. **Diagnosis:** electrocardiography, cardiac enzymes, and echocardiogram
  C. **Treatment:** cardiac and hemodynamic monitoring, appropriate pharmacologic control of arrhythmias, and inotropic support if cardiogenic shock develops

VI. **Pulmonary contusion:** most common injury associated with thoracic trauma
  A. **Causes:** Blunt trauma produces capillary disruption with subsequent intra-alveolar hemorrhage, edema, and small airway obstruction.
  B. **Diagnosis:** chest radiograph, arterial blood gas, and clinical symptoms of respiratory distress
  C. **Treatment:** fluid restriction, supplemental oxygen, vigorous chest physiotherapy, adequate analgesia (epidural narcotics), and prompt chest tube drainage of any associated pleural space complication

Chapter 6

Heart

A. Claire Watkins, D. Bruce Panasuk, William R. Alex,
Richard N. Edie, and James S. Gammie

ACQUIRED HEART DISEASE

Overview

I. **Epidemiology**
   A. **Heart disease:** leading cause of death (38%) in North America
   B. **Myocardial infarction (MI):** 3 million annually in the United States; mortality rate of 10%–15%

II. **Signs and symptoms**
   A. **Dyspnea:** caused by pulmonary congestion, resulting from increased left atrial pressure
   B. **Peripheral edema:** result of significant right-sided congestive heart failure (CHF)
   C. **Chest pain:** caused by angina pectoris, MI, pericarditis, aortic dissection, pulmonary infarction, pulmonary embolism (PE), or aortic stenosis
   D. **Palpitations:** cardiac arrhythmia; often indicates ischemia
   E. **Hemoptysis:** associated with mitral stenosis, pulmonary hypertension, and pulmonary infarction
   F. **Syncope:** result of mitral stenosis, aortic stenosis, heart block, or arrhythmia
   G. **Fatigue:** result of decreased cardiac output (CO)

III. **Physical examination:** should include the following:
   A. **Blood pressure:** measured in both arms and legs
   B. **Peripheral pulses**
      1. **Pulsus parvus et tardus:** may be seen with aortic stenosis
      2. **Aortic insufficiency:** causes wide pulse pressure with a "water-hammer pulse" (short, intense peripheral pulses)
   C. **Neck vein distention:** correlates with internal jugular vein filling; may be caused by cardiac tamponade, tricuspid regurgitation, or right heart failure
   D. **Heart**
      1. **Inspection and palpation:** of the precordium
         a. **Normal point of maximum impulse (PMI):** felt at the midclavicular line, fifth intercostal space
         b. **Left ventricular hypertrophy:** PMI is increased and displaced laterally.
         c. **Right ventricular hypertrophy:** parasternal heave
      2. **Auscultation:** quality of heart tones, type of rhythm, murmurs, rales, and gallops

IV. **Preoperative management:** Obtain baseline chest radiograph and electrocardiogram (ECG).
   A. **Echocardiography:** defines ventricular function and ejection fraction (EF) and assesses for valvular disease

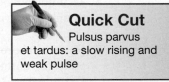

Quick Cut
Pulsus parvus et tardus: a slow rising and weak pulse

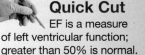

Quick Cut
EF is a measure of left ventricular function; greater than 50% is normal. EF(%) = stroke volume (SV) × 100 end diastolic volume (EDV).

B. Cardiac catheterization: Right heart catheterization is used to determine pulmonary artery pressure (PAP), CO, pulmonary capillary wedge pressure (PCWP), and the presence of left-to-right shunts ("step up"). Left heart catheterization includes coronary artery angiography and ventriculography (to determine EF).

C. Pulmonary function studies: patients with known pulmonary disease

> **Quick Cut**
> Cardiac catheterization is the gold standard for defining coronary artery anatomy and disease.

V. Cardiac arrest

   A. Causes: include anoxia/hypoxemia, ischemia/coronary thrombosis/MI, and electrolyte disturbances (i.e., myocardial depressants, such as anesthetic agents, antiarrhythmic drugs, or digitalis; conduction disturbances, and vagotonic maneuvers)

   B. Immediate cardiopulmonary resuscitation (CPR): ABCs

     1. Airway: endotracheal intubation; surgical airway if airway obstruction

     2. Breathing: ventilatory and oxygen support with an Ambu bag or a ventilator

     3. Circulation

       a. Cardiac massage: Closed chest cardiac compressions. With cardiac tamponade, acute massive hemothorax, or an unstable sternum, open chest massage is usually required.

       b. Electrical defibrillation: if cardiac arrest is from ventricular fibrillation

       c. Drug therapy: Commonly used agents include the following:

         (1) Epinephrine: inotrope, chronotrope, vasopressor

         (2) Calcium: optimizes inotropic effects

         (3) Sodium bicarbonate: to treat associated acidosis

         (4) Vasopressor agents: to support blood pressure

         (5) Atropine: to reverse bradycardia

       d. Blood volume: replace if necessary

> **Quick Cut**
> Anoxic brain injury results after 3–4 minutes of cardiac arrest. CPR can maintain cerebral perfusion.

> **Quick Cut**
> Acidosis and hypocalcemia *suppress* the myocardium, thereby impairing ventricular function. Hyperkalemia and hypomagnesemia *excite* the myocardium and are arrhythmogenic.

VI. Extracorporeal circulation (cardiopulmonary bypass): provides the surgeon with a motionless heart and a bloodless field while simultaneously perfusing the different organ systems with oxygenated blood (Fig. 6-1)

   A. Technique: Blood is drained from the venous system, passed through an oxygenator and a heat exchanger, and pumped back anteriorly.

   B. Myocardial protection: Hypothermia and **cardioplegia** are protective during the ischemia induced by the procedure.

     1. Widespread total body inflammatory response: initiates humoral amplification systems, including the coagulation cascade, fibrinolytic system, complement activation, and the kallikrein-kinin system.

     2. Vasoactive substance release: epinephrine, norepinephrine, histamine, and bradykinin

     3. Sodium and free water retention: causes diffuse edema

> **Quick Cut**
> In the OR, the high potassium concentration in cardioplegic solutions allows arrest of the heart and minimization of myocardial energy consumption.

VII. Prosthetic valves (Fig. 6-2): can be tissue or mechanical materials

   A. Tissue valves: Porcine aortic valves or bovine pericardial tissue do not require long-term anticoagulation but have limited durability and may fail gradually over time. Aortic tissue valves can be expected to last 10–20 years, and mitral tissue valves last 10–15 years.

   B. Mechanical valves: require lifetime anticoagulation therapy to prevent thrombosis/embolism but typically last for life

   C. Risks: Stroke risk of 1%–2% per year. Both tissue and mechanical valves have a similar risk of prosthetic valve endocarditis.

>
> **Quick Cut**
> Major complications of cardiopulmonary bypass include stroke and other embolic events, vascular injury or aneurysm, air embolism, hemolysis, and platelet dysfunction.

>
> **Quick Cut**
> The risk of stroke is higher for mitral valves than aortic valves.

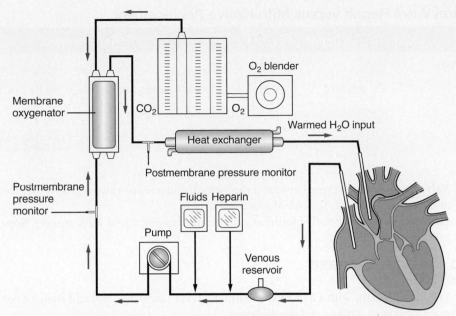

Figure 6-1: Extracorporeal membrane oxygenation (ECMO) setup.

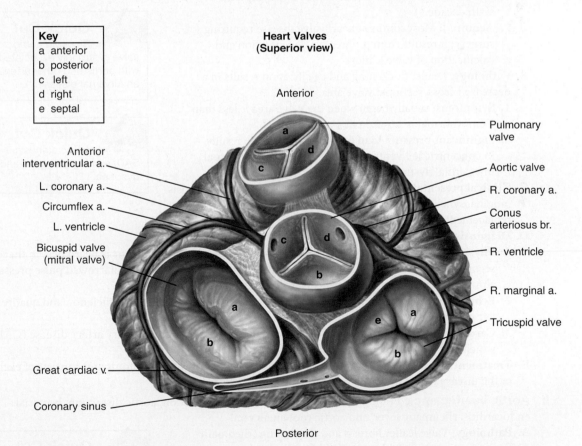

Key	
a	anterior
b	posterior
c	left
d	right
e	septal

Heart Valves (Superior view)

Figure 6-2: Heart valves. (Asset provided by Anatomical Chart Co.)

Table 6-1: Mitral Valve Repair versus Mitral Valve Replacement

	Repair	Replacement
Operative mortality	1%	6%
Anticoagulation	Not required	Mandatory for 3 months for tissue, life for mechanical
Reoperation	<10% at 20 years	10–15 years for tissue
Stroke risk	0.04%/year	1%–2%/year

    D. Valve selection: Choosing between a mechanical and a tissue valve depends on the risk of long-term anticoagulation versus the risk of reoperation.

    E. Heart valve repair: Possible for most patients undergoing mitral valve surgery. Repair is superior to replacement (Table 6-1).

Aortic Valvular Disease

I. Aortic stenosis

    A. Etiology: Patients with a history of **rheumatic fever** rarely have isolated stenosis but usually have a mixed lesion of stenosis and insufficiency.

        1. Congenital: Bicuspid aortic valves occur in 1%–2% of the population. These usually develop calcific changes by the fourth decade and symptoms by the sixth decade.

        2. Acquired: Most common heart valve disease requiring surgery; it results from progressive degeneration and calcification of valve leaflets.

>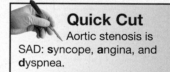
> **Quick Cut**
> Bicuspid aortic valve is strongly associated with aortic and other arterial aneurysmal disease.

    B. Pathology: Leaflet thickening and calcification results in a decreased cross-sectional valve area.

        1. Symptoms: usually begin when the valve area is less than 1 cm^2 (normal is 2.5–3.5 cm^2)

        2. Significant pressure load on the left ventricle: results in concentric left ventricular hypertrophy and eventual myocardial dysfunction

> **Quick Cut**
> Aortic stenosis is SAD: **s**yncope, **a**ngina, and **d**yspnea.

    C. Clinical presentation: Patients with symptomatic aortic stenosis (angina, syncope, arrhythmia, and dyspnea) require aortic valve replacement due to the likelihood of sudden death.

    D. Diagnosis

        1. Physical examination: Classic systolic crescendo–decrescendo murmur is heard best in the second right intercostal space but may radiate to the carotid arteries. A narrowed pulse pressure along with pulsus parvus et tardus is frequently found.

        2. Echocardiography: estimates the degree of stenosis, any associated insufficiency, and quality of left ventricular function

        3. Cardiac catheterization: identifies the presence of concomitant coronary artery disease (CAD), which is present in 50% of surgical patients

    E. Treatment: Surgical correction is recommended for patients with symptoms and consists of excision of the diseased valve and replacement with a prosthetic valve.

II. Aortic insufficiency: Etiologies include myxomatous degeneration, aortic dissection, bacterial endocarditis, rheumatic fever, and aortic root aneurysm.

    A. Pathology: Valve leaflet fibrosis and shortening (rheumatic fever), aortic annulus dilatation (Marfan syndrome or aortic aneurysm), or myxomatous leaflet degeneration imposes a significant **volume load** on the left ventricle leading to left ventricular dilatation.

> **Quick Cut**
> Uncorrected aortic annulus dilation may lead to left ventricular failure with pulmonary congestion.

    B. Clinical presentation: Early symptoms include palpitations secondary to ventricular arrhythmias and dyspnea on exertion; later, severe CHF is seen, and death results from progressive cardiac failure.

C. **Diagnosis**
 1. **Physical examination**
  a. **Murmur:** Characteristic diastolic murmur is heard along the left sternal border and radiates to the axilla.
  b. **Pulse pressure:** Often increased; water-hammer pulses are characteristic.
 2. **Echocardiography:** used to quantitate the degree of insufficiency and to assess left ventricular ejection performance
 3. **Cardiac catheterization:** used to determine the presence of associated CAD
E. **Treatment:** Aortic valve replacement surgery to avoid decompensation is recommended for patients with severe insufficiency and any one of the following symptoms: left ventricular systolic dysfunction (EF <50%), severe left ventricular dilation (end-systolic dimension >55 mm, end-diastolic dimension >75 mm), undergoing another cardiac surgery, and acute onset.

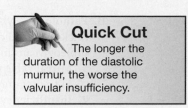

Quick Cut
The longer the duration of the diastolic murmur, the worse the valvular insufficiency.

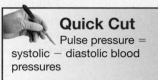

Quick Cut
Pulse pressure = systolic − diastolic blood pressures

Mitral Valve Disease

I. **Mitral stenosis:** Although only 50% of patients report a history of rheumatic fever, this condition is thought to be the cause of almost all mitral stenosis.
 A. **Pathology:** Interval between rheumatic fever and the manifestation of mitral stenosis is 10–25 years.
  1. **Underlying pathologic changes:** fusion of the commissures and leaflet thickening with or without shortening of the chordae tendineae
  2. **Cross-sectional area of the mitral valve:** normal = 4–6 cm^2; mild stenosis = 2–2.5 cm^2; moderate = 1.5–2 cm^2; and severe = 1–1.5 cm^2
  3. **Pathophysiologic changes:** increased left atrial pressure, pulmonary hypertension, atrial fibrillation, decreased CO, and increased pulmonary vascular resistance
 B. **Clinical presentation:** Dyspnea is the most significant symptom, indicating pulmonary congestion and increased left atrial pressure.
  1. **Other manifestations:** paroxysmal nocturnal dyspnea and orthopnea, chronic cough and hemoptysis, pulmonary edema, systemic arterial embolization (usually from a left atrial thrombus), and atrial fibrillation
  2. **Long-standing pulmonary hypertension:** may result in right ventricular failure and secondary tricuspid regurgitation
 C. **Diagnosis**
  1. **Physical examination:** Typical patient is thin and cachectic; auscultation reveals the **classic triad** of an apical diastolic rumble, an opening snap, and a loud first heart sound.
  2. **Chest x-ray:** typically shows a prominent pulmonary vasculature in the upper lung fields
  3. **ECG:** may be normal or may show P-wave abnormalities, signs of right ventricular hypertrophy, and right axis deviation
  4. **Echocardiography:** used to determine the morphology of the valve and the severity of the stenosis
  5. **Cardiac catheterization:** used to calculate the mitral valve cross-sectional area, the mitral valve end-diastolic pressure gradient, PAP, and any associated valvular or coronary artery disease
 D. **Treatment:** Surgery is recommended for all patients with symptomatic stenosis. The choice of operative approach depends on the extent of these changes.
  1. **Commissurotomy:** Opening of the fused commissures can be accomplished under direct vision during surgical mitral valve repair or percutaneously by balloon mitral valvuloplasty.
  2. **Mitral valve replacement:** required for severe disease of the chordae tendineae and papillary muscles
II. **Mitral insufficiency**
 A. **Etiology:** degenerative mitral valve disease
  1. **Ventricular dilation:** also called *functional mitral regurgitation*, alters valvular geometry; occurs with ischemic or idiopathic cardiomyopathy
  2. **Other:** infective endocarditis and rheumatic fever

Quick Cut
Think of mitral stenosis in a thin patient with dyspnea, opening snap, and a diastolic rumble.

Quick Cut
In selected patients, balloon valvuloplasty and open commissurotomy have equivalent results.

B. **Pathology:** Myxomatous degeneration is the most common cause and is characterized by leaflet thickening and chordal elongation. Structural alterations of collagen and abnormal accumulation of proteoglycans in the leaflet tissue are also seen.
   1. **Mitral valve prolapse:** present in 2%–3% of the population, but most do not develop significant mitral regurgitation and do not require surgery
   2. **Insufficiency secondary to rheumatic fever:** Pathogenesis is similar to that in mitral stenosis.
   3. **Pathophysiologic changes:** increased left atrial pressure during systole, late-appearing pulmonary vascular changes (e.g., increased pulmonary vascular resistance), and increased left ventricular stroke volume (SV)
C. **Clinical presentation:** Many years may elapse between the first evidence of insufficiency and symptom development.
   1. **Symptoms:** dyspnea on exertion, fatigue, and palpitations
   2. **Atrial fibrillation:** Distention of the left atrium causes elevated left atrial pressure.
D. **Diagnosis**
   1. **Physical examination:** reveals a holosystolic blowing murmur at the apex that radiates to the axilla, accompanied by an accentuated apical impulse
   2. **Echocardiography:** can accurately quantitate the degree of mitral regurgitation and can demonstrate underlying anatomic abnormalities of the valve (e.g., leaflet prolapse, ruptured chordae tendineae, annular dilation, leaflet restriction, annular calcification, presence of vegetations, etc.), degree of left atrial enlargement, extent of left ventricular dysfunction, and the presence of associated tricuspid regurgitation
   3. **Cardiac catheterization:** determines presence of CAD
E. **Treatment:** Only patients with severe regurgitation should be considered for surgery. Careful echocardiographic assessment of the degree of regurgitation should be performed.
   1. **Surgical indications:** severe regurgitation in addition to the following (however, growing evidence demonstrates that asymptomatic patients with severe mitral regurgitation enjoy improved long-term survival with early operation):
      a. **Symptoms:** New York Heart Association (NYHA) class II or above (Table 6-2)
      b. **Evidence of left ventricular dysfunction:** EF less than 60%, ventricular dilation (end-systolic dimension >40 mm), and development of atrial fibrillation or significant pulmonary hypertension
   2. **Mitral valve repair:** performed when possible either by quadrangular resection of the posterior leaflet or insertion of an annuloplasty ring (cloth-covered ring that stabilizes and sometimes decreases the size of the mitral valve annulus)

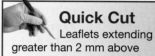
Quick Cut
Of patients undergoing cardiac surgery, 12% have atrial fibrillation; 25% develop postoperative atrial fibrillation.

Quick Cut
Leaflets extending greater than 2 mm above the mitral valve annulus is echocardiographic evidence of prolapse.

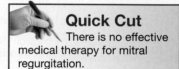
Quick Cut
There is no effective medical therapy for mitral regurgitation.

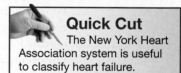
Quick Cut
The New York Heart Association system is useful to classify heart failure.

Tricuspid Valve, Pulmonic Valve, and Multiple Valvular Diseases

I. Tricuspid stenosis and insufficiency
A. **Etiology**
   1. **Organic tricuspid stenosis:** always caused by rheumatic fever, most commonly associated with mitral valve disease

Table 6-2: New York Heart Association Functional Classification of Heart Failure

Class I	No symptoms
Class II	Mild symptoms during ordinary activity
Class III	Significant symptoms during any activity
Class IV	Symptoms even while at rest

(Symptoms are typically angina and dyspnea.)

2. **Functional tricuspid insufficiency:** result of right ventricular dilatation secondary to pulmonary hypertension and right ventricular failure, most commonly from mitral valve disease
3. **Tricuspid insufficiency:** sometimes seen in carcinoid syndrome, lupus, or secondary to blunt trauma or to bacterial endocarditis (intravenous [IV] drug abuse)

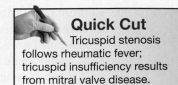

Quick Cut
Tricuspid stenosis follows rheumatic fever; tricuspid insufficiency results from mitral valve disease.

B. **Pathology**
 1. **Stenosis secondary to rheumatic fever:** Pathogenesis is similar to that in mitral valve disease.
 2. **Elevation of right atrial pressure secondary to stenosis:** leads to peripheral edema, jugular venous distention, hepatomegaly, and ascites

C. **Clinical presentation**
 1. **Isolated tricuspid insufficiency:** usually well tolerated
 2. **Right-sided heart failure:** When this occurs, symptoms (e.g., edema, hepatomegaly, and ascites) develop.

D. **Diagnosis**
 1. **Physical examination:** Prominent jugular venous pulse may be observed.
    a. **Tricuspid insufficiency:** Produces a systolic murmur at the lower end of the sternum; the liver may be pulsatile.
    b. **Tricuspid stenosis:** produces a diastolic murmur in the same region
 2. **Chest x-ray:** enlargement of the right side of the heart
 3. **Echocardiography:** estimates the amount of tricuspid valve pathology and should include an evaluation of any associated aortic or mitral valve lesions and right heart function
 4. **Cardiac catheterization:** most accurate guide to diagnosing tricuspid disease

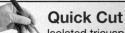

Quick Cut
Isolated tricuspid disease, especially tricuspid insufficiency, may be well tolerated without surgical intervention.

E. **Treatment:** In mild to moderate insufficiency associated with mitral valve disease, opinion varies concerning the need for surgery.
 1. **Extensive insufficiency associated with mitral valve disease:** Consensus is that either valve repair (usually with an annuloplasty ring) or (rarely) valve replacement is appropriate.
 2. **Significant stenosis:** commissurotomy or valve replacement

II. **Pulmonic valve disease**
 A. **Pathology:** Acquired lesions are uncommon; carcinoid syndrome may produce pulmonic stenosis.
 B. **Treatment:** surgical repair or valve replacement when warranted by the degree of dysfunction

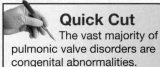

Quick Cut
The vast majority of pulmonic valve disorders are congenital abnormalities.

III. **Multiple valvular disease**
 A. **Pathology:** Multiple valves may be involved in rheumatic fever.
 B. **Treatment:** involves repair or replacement of all valves with significant dysfunction

Quick Cut
Patients with multi-valvular disease have signs and symptoms dictated by the most severely affected valve.

Coronary Artery Disease

I. **Etiology and epidemiology:** most common cause of death in the United States; four times more prevalent in men than in women, although the incidence in women is rapidly increasing
 A. **Atherosclerosis:** Predominant pathogenetic mechanism; uncommon causes include vasculitis, radiation injury, and trauma.
 B. **Risk factors:** Those identified by epidemiologic studies include hypertension (risk minimized when blood pressure <140/90 mm Hg), smoking, hypercholesterolemia (risk minimized when cholesterol <200 mg/dL, low-density lipoprotein <100 mg/dL, and high-density lipoprotein >40 mg/dL), family history of heart disease, diabetes, and obesity.

Quick Cut
CAD accounts for 500,000 deaths per year.

II. **Pathophysiologic effects:** Ischemic disease of the myocardium causes decreased ventricular compliance and cardiac contractility and myocardial necrosis; ventricular dysfunction following ischemia occurs secondary to irreversible myocardial necrosis.
 A. **Hibernating myocardium:** dysfunctional muscle that improves with revascularization
 B. **Stunned myocardium:** temporary dysfunction following revascularization

III. Clinical presentation: CAD may take one of the following forms:

    A. Angina pectoris: Typically presents as substernal chest pain lasting 5–10 minutes. Precipitated by emotional stress, exertion, or cold weather and is relieved by rest.

        1. Stable angina: unchanged for a prolonged period

        2. Unstable angina: shows a change from a previously stable pattern or new-onset angina

        3. Other: angina at rest and postinfarction angina

    B. MI: ischemic ECG changes and troponin elevation

    C. Other: CHF or sudden death

IV. Diagnosis: Angina pectoris due to CAD is most often made from the patient's history.

> **Quick Cut**
> A 75% stenosis in coronary artery cross-sectional area is the point at which a lesion significantly impedes coronary blood flow.

    A. Cardiac catheterization: Diagnostic gold standard for CAD. Location and size of coronary lesions can be both diagnosed and treated. Left ventricular function may be assessed by the ventriculogram and hemodynamic measurements.

    B. ECG: Normal in up to 75% of patients when they are at rest without pain. ST-segment changes and T-wave changes may be seen, and evidence of a previous infarction may be apparent.

    C. Exercise stress testing: evaluates inducible ischemia, ventricular dysfunction, and associated ECG changes

    D. Radio thallium scan of the heart: delineates ischemic and infarcted areas of myocardium

V. Treatment

    A. Medical treatment: Management of CAD is initiated with medical therapy in patients with stable angina and with no evidence of CHF.

> **Quick Cut**
> Medical management of CAD focuses on control of risk factors.

        1. Drugs: aspirin, beta-blockers, statins, aldosterone blockade, and antihypertensives

        2. Additional therapy: low-fat diet, smoking cessation, and a graded exercise program

    B. Catheter-based coronary interventions

        1. Balloon angioplasty: Balloon dilation to relieve the obstruction. Stenosis often recurs.

        2. Coronary stenting: Metal stent is placed in the lesion to keep it from closing over time ("restenosis"). Stent may be "bare metal" or may be coated with a drug (e.g., sirolimus) that elutes over time to prevent restenosis.

    C. Coronary artery bypass surgery (CABG): construction of bypass grafts to downstream segments of the affected coronary arteries to re-establish normal blood flow to the myocardium

> **Quick Cut**
> CABG 10-year patency rates: internal mammary artery more than 90%, saphenous vein ~50%.

        1. Common grafts (Fig. 6-3): left internal mammary artery to left anterior descending (LAD) coronary artery, reversed saphenous vein grafts constructed from the ascending aorta to the target vessel, and radial artery or right internal mammary artery grafts

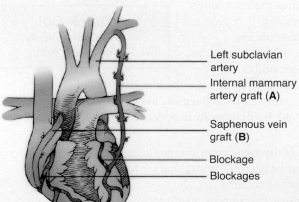

Left subclavian artery

Internal mammary artery graft (**A**)

Saphenous vein graft (**B**)

Blockage

Blockages

Figure 6-3: Coronary artery bypass surgery. (From Rosdahl CB, Kowalski MT. *Textbook of Basic Nursing*, 10th ed. Philadelphia: Lippincott Williams & Wilkins; 2011.)

2. **Indications:** left main disease greater than 50% stenosis, proximal LAD or circumflex disease greater than 70% stenosis, triple-vessel disease (especially with EF <50%), proximal LAD with other vessel disease, angina refractory to medical management, or failed percutaneous coronary intervention

3. **Increased survival:** with left main disease and triple-vessel disease with decreased ventricular function or with diabetes

4. **Prognosis:** Overall mortality is 2%–3%; risk is increased in patients with renal failure, urgency of operation, pulmonary disease, peripheral vascular disease, and history of stroke or diabetes.

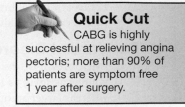

Quick Cut
CABG is highly successful at relieving angina pectoris; more than 90% of patients are symptom free 1 year after surgery.

VI. **Surgical treatment of MI complications:** Mechanical complications of MI are increasingly rare with early revascularization.

A. **Ventricular aneurysms:** Myocardium remodels following infarction and can thin or become aneurysmal.

1. **Indications for repair:** CHF, ventricular arrhythmias, or (rarely) systemic thromboembolization

2. **Coronary revascularization:** may also be warranted at the same time

B. **Ruptured ventricle:** Rare; the untreated mortality rate is 100%.

C. **Rupture of the interventricular septum (postinfarct ventricular septal defect [VSD]):** carries mortality rate of 50% without immediate operation

D. **Papillary muscle dysfunction or rupture:** Posterior papillary muscle is usually involved.

1. **Treatment:** mitral valve replacement or repair

2. **Long-term survival:** depends on the extent of myocardial damage

Quick Cut
Placement of an intra-aortic balloon pump can help maintain patients with infarct-related VSD or papillary muscle rupture until surgery.

Cardiac Tumors

I. **Benign tumors:** Myxomas are the single most common benign cardiac tumors. Most are located in the left atrium. Others include rhabdomyosarcomas (most common in childhood), papillary elastofibromas, and lipomas as well as either pedunculated or sessile myxomas (50% of benign cardiac tumors), 75% of which are located in left atrium

II. **Malignant tumors:** Overall, account for 20%–25% of all primary cardiac tumors. Sarcomas and angiosarcomas are the most common.

III. **Metastatic tumors:** occur more frequently than primary cardiac tumors (benign or malignant)

A. **Autopsy studies:** show cardiac involvement by metastatic disease in ~10% of cancer deaths

B. **Types:** Renal cell carcinoma, neuroblastoma, melanoma, lymphoma, and leukemia are the tumors that most often metastasize to the heart.

Quick Cut
Malignant tumors originating from the heart carry a very poor prognosis.

IV. **Clinical presentation:** Myxomas typically result in embolization. Additional presentations include CHF, pericardial effusion and tamponade, and arrhythmia.

V. **Treatment:** surgical excision

Cardiac Trauma

I. **Penetrating injury (through the anterior chest wall):** most likely to injure the right ventricle

A. **Bleeding into the pericardium:** common

B. **Pericardial tamponade:** may result; manifested by distended neck veins, hypotension, pulsus paradoxus, and distant heart sounds

Quick Cut
Pericardial effusions (blood) can be visualized on subxiphoid windows of a focused assessment with sonography for trauma exam.

II. **Blunt trauma:** usually more extensive than is appreciated

A. **Diagnosis:** History of a significant blow to the chest, with or without fractured ribs or sternum, should create a high index of suspicion of a cardiac contusion or infarction.

1. **Serial ECGs and cardiac enzyme studies:** should be obtained

2. **Echocardiography:** helps determine myocardial injury

3. **New murmurs:** should be investigated with imaging

4. **Monitoring:** similar to a patient with MI because of similar myocardial injury

B. **Treatment:** Blunt trauma may cause rupture of a tricuspid, mitral, or aortic valve, requiring treatment by valve replacement or repair.

Pericardial Disorders

I. **Pericardial effusion:** Pericardium responds to noxious stimuli by increasing fluid production; volume as small as 100 mL may produce symptomatic tamponade if the fluid accumulates rapidly, whereas larger amounts may be tolerated if the fluid accumulates slowly.

   A. **Treatment:** pericardiocentesis or by tube pericardiostomy via a subxiphoid approach

   B. **Chronic effusions (e.g., those that occur with malignant involvement of the pericardium):** may require pericardiectomy via left thoracotomy or sternotomy

II. **Pericarditis**

   A. **Acute pericarditis**

   1. **Causes:** staphylococcal or streptococcal infection (acute pyogenic pericarditis is uncommon and is usually associated with a systemic illness), viral infection, uremia, traumatic hemopericardium, malignant disease, and connective tissue disorders

   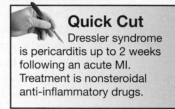

   Quick Cut
   Dressler syndrome is pericarditis up to 2 weeks following an acute MI. Treatment is nonsteroidal anti-inflammatory drugs.

   2. **Treatment:** Manage the underlying cause. Open pericardial drainage may be required. Most cases resolve without serious sequelae.

   B. **Chronic pericarditis:** Etiology is often impossible to establish. It may go unnoticed until it results in the chronic constrictive form, causing chronic tamponade.

   C. **Chronic constrictive pericarditis:** presents with dyspnea on exertion, easy fatigability, marked jugular venous distention, ascites, hepatomegaly, and peripheral edema

   1. **Diagnosis:** Pericardium may become calcified, which is evident on chest x-ray. Cardiac catheterization may be needed to confirm.

   Quick Cut
   ECG changes seen in pericarditis include ST elevations in all leads, not one distribution.

   2. **Treatment:** Once the diagnosis has been established in the symptomatic patient, pericardiectomy should be undertaken with or without cardiopulmonary bypass.

CONGENITAL HEART DISEASE

Overview

I. **Incidence:** <3 in 1,000 births

II. **Etiology:** often unknown

   A. **Rubella (occurring in the first trimester of pregnancy):** known to cause patent ductus arteriosus (PDA)

   B. **Down syndrome:** associated with endocardial cushion defects

III. **Types in decreasing order:** VSD, transposition of the great vessels, tetralogy of Fallot, hypoplastic left heart syndrome, atrial septal defect (ASD), PDA, coarctation of the aorta, and endocardial cushion defects

IV. **Common presentations:** easy fatigability and decreased exercise tolerance, poor feeding habits and poor weight gain, frequent pulmonary infections, and signs of cyanosis (indicating a right-to-left shunt)

V. **Physical examination:** Abnormalities in growth and development should be identified.

   A. **Cyanosis and clubbing of the fingers:** may be noted

   B. **Heart examination:** should proceed in the same manner as in the adult

   1. **Systolic murmurs:** frequently found in infants and small children and may not be clinically significant, but a gallop rhythm is of great clinical importance

   2. **CHF in children:** frequently manifested by hepatic enlargement

VI. **Diagnosis:** Echocardiogram and often catheterization are required.

Patent Ductus Arteriosus

I. **Pathophysiology:** Hypoxia and prostaglandins E_1 (PGE_1) and E_2 (PGE_2) act to keep the ductus open in utero. In the normal-term infant, blood circulation through the pulmonary vascular bed results in elevated oxygen levels and prostaglandin breakdown, which results in closure of the ductus within days.

II. **Clinical presentation**
   A. **Common complaints:** dyspnea, fatigue, and palpitations, signifying CHF and/or pulmonary hypertension
   B. **May be seen in combination with other defects:** VSD and coarctation of the aorta

III. **Diagnosis** based primarily on the physical findings and echocardiogram
   A. **Physical examination:** Classic continuous "machinery-like" murmur may be absent until age 1 year.
      1. **Pulses:** widened pulse pressure and bounding peripheral pulses
      2. **Cyanosis:** right-to-left shunt from pulmonary vascular disease

IV. **Treatment**
   A. **Surgical management:** ligation of the ductus, reserved for premature infants with severe pulmonary dysfunction, infants who suffer from CHF within the first year of life, and asymptomatic children with a patent ductus that persists until age 2–3 years
   B. **Indomethacin:** This prostaglandin inhibitor can achieve closure in premature infants with symptomatic simple PDA.

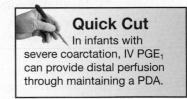

Quick Cut
Most preterm infants weighing less than 1.5 kg will have a PDA.

Coarctation of the Aorta

I. **Overview:** severe narrowing, located adjacent to the ductus arteriosus that may be fatal in the first few months of life
   A. **Associated intracardiac defects:** Up to 60% of patients have PDA, VSD, and bicuspid aortic valve.
   B. **Incidence:** twice as common in males

II. **Clinical presentation:** often asymptomatic for varying periods of time
   A. **CHF:** shortly after birth
   B. **Other:** Headaches, epistaxis, lower extremity (LE) weakness, and dizziness may be seen in the symptomatic child.

III. **Diagnosis**
   A. **Physical findings:** upper extremity (UE) hypertension, absent or diminished LE pulses, and a systolic murmur
   B. **Chest x-ray:** may reveal "rib notching" in older children, representing collateral pathways via intercostal arteries
   C. **Echocardiography:** suggests the degree of flow limitation and other associated anomalies
   D. **Cardiac catheterization:** usually recommended to define location and any associated cardiac defects

IV. **Treatment:** surgical correction for symptomatic patients or asymptomatic children ages 5–6 years
   A. **Operative procedures:** resection and end-to-end anastomosis, prosthetic patch graft, and subclavian arterial flap (in which the distal subclavian artery is transected and a proximal-based subclavian artery flap is used to enlarge the aorta at the level of the coarctation)
   B. **Complications:** residual hypertension, spinal cord injury due to ischemia during surgery, postoperative mesenteric vasculitis related to hypertension, and postoperative aneurysm at the site of the operative repair

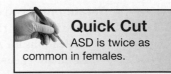

Quick Cut
In infants with severe coarctation, IV PGE$_1$ can provide distal perfusion through maintaining a PDA.

Atrial Septal Defects

I. **Classification**
   A. **Ostium secundum defect:** most common ASD, found in the midportion of the atrial septum
   B. **Sinus venosus defect:** located high up on the atrial septum, often associated with anomalies of pulmonary venous drainage
   C. **Ostium primum defects:** components of atrioventricular septal defects, located on the atrial side of the mitral and tricuspid valves

II. **Pathophysiology:** Atrial pressures are equal on both sides of a large ASD (Fig. 6-4).
   A. **Direction of shunt:** Because atrial emptying occurs during ventricular diastole, direction of shunt at the atrial level is

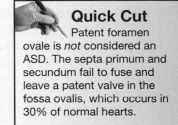

Quick Cut
ASD is twice as common in females.

Quick Cut
Patent foramen ovale is *not* considered an ASD. The septa primum and secundum fail to fuse and leave a patent valve in the fossa ovalis, which occurs in 30% of normal hearts.

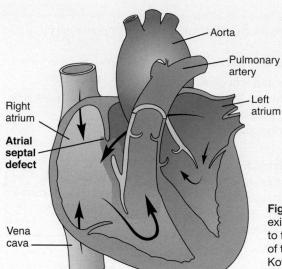

Aorta

Pulmonary artery

Left atrium

Right atrium

Atrial septal defect

Vena cava

Figure 6-4: Atrial septal defect. In an ASD, an abnormal communication exists between the atria, allowing blood to be shunted from the left atrium to the right atrium through the atrial septum. This hole is usually the area of the foramen ovale, which normally closes at birth. (From Rosdahl CB, Kowalski MT. *Textbook of Basic Nursing*, 10th ed. Philadelphia: Lippincott Williams & Wilkins; 2011.)

determined by the relative compliances of the ventricles. Because the right ventricle is more compliant, the flow is left to right across an ASD.

B. **Increased pulmonary blood flow:** Causes mild growth retardation, and **pulmonary vascular obstructive disease** may develop, which results in the right ventricle becoming less compliant than the left, with blood flow shunting right to left across the ASD.

III. **Clinical presentation**
A. **Infancy and early childhood:** mild dyspnea and easy fatigability
B. **Children:** reduced exercise tolerance and recurrent respiratory infections
C. **Adults:** atrial fibrillation and CHF
D. **Other:** Patients may present with neurologic symptoms (cerebrovascular accident or transient ischemic attack) or Eisenmenger syndrome.

> **Quick Cut**
> Eisenmenger syndrome is a sequence of events: 1, congenital left to right shunt (from septal defect or PDA); 2, subsequent pulmonary hypertension; 3, this increased pressure reverses the shunt; and 4, cyanotic symptoms develop.

IV. **Diagnosis**
A. **Physical examination:** systolic murmur in the left second or third intercostal space and a fixed, split, second heart sound
B. **Chest x-ray:** moderate enlargement of the right ventricle and prominence of the pulmonary vasculature
C. **ECG:** right ventricular hypertrophy
D. **Echocardiography:** defines the ASD and notes the direction of shunting
E. **Cardiac catheterization:** Determines the "step-up" in oxygen saturation in the right atrium. The amount of left-to-right shunt may be calculated.

V. **Treatment:** Based on the size of the left-to-right shunt; some (<6 mm) may close spontaneously. Surgery carries a mortality risk of less than 1%; ideal timing is age 4–5 years, before the child goes to school.
A. **Indications for ASD closure:** Pulmonary blood flow is more than 1.5 times greater than the systemic blood flow, neurologic events, heart failure, arrhythmia, or right ventricular volume overload.
B. **Approach:** Closure may be attempted percutaneously in the catheterization laboratory.

Ventricular Septal Defects
I. **Classification:** Figure 6-5.
A. **Membranous defect:** most common ventricular, 70%–80%
B. **Muscular defects:** may be single or multiple (10%–15%)
C. **Inlet defect:** atrioventricular canal type, endocardial cushion defect, 5% of isolated defects
D. **Outlet defects:** 5%–10% (also called *supracristal* or *conoseptal defects*)

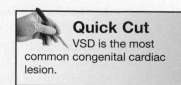

> **Quick Cut**
> VSD is the most common congenital cardiac lesion.

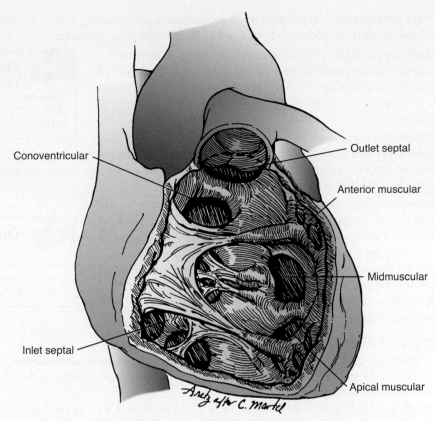

Figure 6-5: Location of congenital septal defects. (Reprinted with permission from Kaiser LR, Kron IL, Spray TL. *Mastery of Cardiothoracic Surgery*. Philadelphia: Lippincott-Raven; 1998:688.)

II. **Pathophysiology:** Ventricular pressures can be equal on either side of a large VSD (Fig. 6-6).

A. **Direction of shunt:** Determined by the relative resistances of the pulmonary and systemic circuits. Because the pulmonary vascular resistance is lower than the systemic vascular resistance, flow is left to right across a VSD.

B. **Increased pulmonary blood flow:** Left-to-right shunting leads to pulmonary hypertension, decreased right ventricular compliance, and Eisenmenger syndrome (irreversible pulmonary vascular obstructive disease).

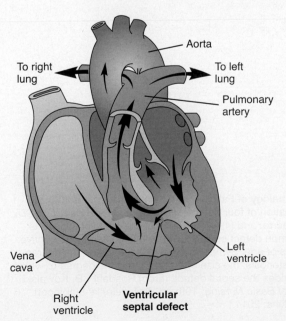

Figure 6-6: Ventricular septal defects. In a VSD, a hole is in the wall of the septum that separates the left and right ventricles. Normally, deoxygenated blood flows through the superior vena cava and inferior vena cava into the right atrium, right ventricle, and pulmonary artery. In a VSD, some oxygen-rich blood from the left ventricle flows through the defect and recirculates through the lungs. (From Rosdahl CB, Kowalski MT. *Textbook of Basic Nursing,* 10th ed. Philadelphia: Lippincott Williams & Wilkins; 2011.)

C. **Other adverse effects of pulmonary overcirculation:** poor feeding, failure to thrive, frequent respiratory tract infections, and increased pulmonary vascular resistance

III. **Clinical presentation:** Children with large defects usually have dyspnea on exertion, easy fatigability, and an increased incidence of pulmonary infections. Severe cardiac failure may be seen in infants but is less common in children.

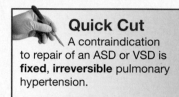

Quick Cut
Fifty percent of VSDs are associated with PDA, aortic coarctation, or tetralogy of Fallot.

IV. **Diagnosis**
   A. **Physical examination:** harsh pansystolic murmur
   B. **Chest x-ray and ECG:** show evidence of biventricular hypertrophy if large
   C. **Cardiac catheterization:** determines the severity of the left-to-right shunt, pulmonary vascular resistance, and the location

V. **Treatment:** surgical closure
   A. **Indications:** symptomatic or outlet or inlet VSDs; asymptomatic children with significant shunts who have not had spontaneous closure by age 2 years, PAP 0.5 times greater than systemic blood pressure, or pulmonary blood flow greater than 1.5 times systemic blood flow

Quick Cut
A contraindication to repair of an ASD or VSD is **fixed, irreversible** pulmonary hypertension.

   B. **Operative mortality risk (<5%):** related to the degree of preoperative pulmonary vascular disease

Tetralogy of Fallot

I. **Pathophysiology:** One of the most common **cyanotic congenital heart disorders**; consists of obstruction of the right ventricular outflow tract, a large anterior VSD, right ventricular hypertrophy, and an overriding aorta (Fig. 6-7).
   A. **Pentalogy of Fallot:** with the addition of an ASD (which is of little physiologic significance)
   B. **Direction of shunt:** Because resistance to right ventricular outflow exceeds the systemic vascular resistance, the shunt is right to left, resulting in desaturation of the blood and cyanosis.

II. **Clinical presentation:** **Cyanosis** and **dyspnea on exertion** are routinely seen. Children soon learn that by **squatting**, they can temporarily alleviate these symptoms. These are 'Tet spells.'
   A. **Squatting:** increases the systemic vascular resistance, which decreases the magnitude of right-to-left shunt and causes an increase in pulmonary blood flow

Tetralogy of Fallot

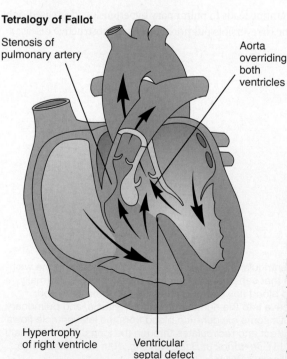

Stenosis of pulmonary artery

Aorta overriding both ventricles

Hypertrophy of right ventricle

Ventricular septal defect

Figure 6-7: Tetralogy of Fallot. Tetralogy of Fallot is characterized by the combination of four defects: (1) pulmonary stenosis, (2) VSD, (3) overriding aorta, and (4) hypertrophy of the right ventricle. It is the most common defect causing cyanosis in children who survive beyond 2 years of age. Symptom severity depends on the degree of pulmonary stenosis, the size of the VSD, and the degree to which the aorta overrides the septal defect. (From Rosdahl CB, Kowalski MT. *Textbook of Basic Nursing*, 10th ed. Philadelphia: Lippincott Williams & Wilkins; 2011.)

B. **Cyanosis:** Seen at birth in 30% of the cases, by the first year in 30%, and later in childhood in the remainder. Polycythemia and clubbing accompany it.

C. **Exercise tolerance:** limited because of the inability to increase pulmonary blood flow

III. **Diagnosis**

A. **Physical examination:** Reveals clubbing of the digits and cyanosis. A harsh systolic murmur of pulmonary stenosis is often heard.

B. **Cardiac catheterization:** determines the level of pulmonic outflow obstruction and the size of the pulmonary arteries

IV. **Treatment:** Total correction is undertaken after age 4–6 months.

A. **Surgery:** Risk depends on patient's age and the degree of cyanosis; prior to correction, sufficient hydration and avoidance of upper respiratory infections are imperative.

B. **Palliative options prior to repair for high-risk, symptomatic patients:** balloon pulmonary valvuloplasty and systemic-to-pulmonary (Blalock-Taussig) shunt

> **Quick Cut**
> Tet spells: episodes of severe cyanosis incited by dehydration, crying, or straining that may be relieved by squatting.

Transposition of the Great Arteries

I. **Pathophysiology:** occurs when the aorta arises from the morphologic right ventricle and the pulmonary artery arises from the morphologic left ventricle, resulting in two independent parallel circuits

II. **Survival:** depends on communication between the right and left sides of the heart through an ASD, VSD, or PDA

III. **Diagnosis:** echocardiogram and cardiac catheterization (in the setting of additional intracardiac or extracardiac anomalies or inadequate shunting)

IV. **Treatment**

A. **Balloon atrial septostomy:** performed to facilitate mixing of blood with inadequate shunting; followed by definitive surgical correction

B. **Arterial switch:** division of the great arteries with transfer of the coronaries and proper anastomoses of the aorta to the left and pulmonary artery to the right ventricles

Study Questions for Part II

Directions: *Each of the numbered items in this section is followed by several possible answers. Select the ONE lettered answer that is BEST in each case.*

1. A 19-year-old man is brought to the emergency room. He has no significant medical history, but he does smoke one pack of cigarettes per day. He is complaining of dyspnea and has a blood pressure of 150/70 mm Hg. Breath sounds are diminished on the left. What is the best initial treatment for this patient?

    A. Chest tube drainage
    B. Supplemental oxygen only
    C. Needle decompression of the left chest
    D. Computed tomography (CT) scan of the thorax
    E. Emergent surgical exploration

2. In the same patient, which of the following is an indication for surgery?

    A. Family history of recurrent spontaneous pneumothorax
    B. Persistent air leak after 3 days of chest tube drainage
    C. Identification of an apical bleb on chest CT
    D. Evidence of life-threatening respiratory compromise on initial presentation
    E. History of one prior episode successfully treated with conservative management on the contralateral side

3. A patient is brought to the emergency department with a stab wound to the right chest in the fourth intercostal space in the midaxillary line. The patient is hypotensive, complains of shortness of breath, and is found to have absent breath sounds on the right side of the chest. Which step should come next in the management of this patient?

    A. Chest radiograph
    B. Chest tube insertion
    C. Needle thoracentesis
    D. Local wound exploration
    E. Pericardiocentesis

Questions 4–5

A chest radiograph of a 55-year-old man involved in a high-speed motor vehicle accident shows a widened mediastinum and pneumomediastinum. EKG shows sinus tachycardia with frequent premature ventricular contractions.

4. All of the following maneuvers are appropriate at this time *except*:

    A. Aortogram
    B. Bronchoscopy
    C. Continuous cardiac monitoring
    D. Left thoracotomy
    E. Endotracheal intubation

5. Expected physiologic changes due to blunt chest trauma include all but which of the following?

    A. Elevated P_{CO_2}
    B. Increased compliance
    C. Elevated alveolar–arterial (A-a) gradient
    D. Decreased ventricular contractions
    E. Elevated shunt fractions

Questions 6–7

A 70-year-old patient on antibiotic therapy for necrotizing bacterial pneumonia is found to have a large pleural effusion.

6. In addition to continued antibiotics, what should be the next step in management of this patient?

   A. Sputum culture and sensitivity
   B. Chest tube insertion
   C. Thoracentesis
   D. Thoracotomy and decortication
   E. Rib resection and open drainage

7. A sample of pleural fluid is cloudy and thick, with a pH of 7.2. What should be the next therapeutic step?

   A. Video-assisted thoracoscopic surgery with talc pleurodesis
   B. Chest tube drainage
   C. Repeat thoracentesis
   D. Thoracotomy and decortication
   E. Rib resection drainage

8. A routine chest radiograph for a 55-year-old man with a 50 pack-year smoking history shows a peripherally located 1.5-cm noncalcified lesion of the upper lobe of the left lung. No evidence of this lesion appeared on a chest radiograph 5 years earlier. What should be the next step in this patient's management?

   A. Observation with serial chest radiographs
   B. Thoracotomy
   C. Bronchoscopy
   D. Biopsy
   E. Sputum cytology

9. A 35-year-old man is involved in a high-speed motor vehicle collision. He arrives in the emergency room in respiratory distress. Radiographs taken during the initial evaluation reveal an air-fluid level in the left chest. Management includes all of the following *except*:

   A. Establishment of a secure airway
   B. Immediate placement of a nasogastric tube
   C. Urgent thoracotomy to repair the injury
   D. Placement of adequate peripheral vascular access
   E. Urgent laparotomy to repair injury

10. Which of the following forms of congenital heart disease is most common?

   A. Transposition of the great vessels
   B. Tetralogy of Fallot
   C. ASD
   D. PDA
   E. VSD

11. A 32-year-old man is referred for a 1-cm lesion of the right upper lobe of the lung. The lesion appears calcified. Previous chest radiograph taken 1 year prior demonstrates the lesion to be present at the same size. Further workup and treatment would include which of the following?

   A. CT scan–guided biopsy
   B. Radiation therapy
   C. Surgical excision
   D. Antibiotics
   E. Observation with repeat chest x-ray

12. A 57-year-old male patient with a 60 pack-year smoking history is referred for a 1.5-cm solitary mass in the right upper lobe. CT scan demonstrates no evidence of lymph node involvement. What should further workup or treatment include?

    A. Radiation therapy
    B. Open lung biopsy
    C. Chemotherapy
    D. Right upper lobectomy
    E. Repeat chest x-ray in 6 months

13. A 22-year-old female is referred for evaluation of a 2-cm middle mediastinal mass discovered on routine chest radiograph. What is the most likely diagnosis?

    A. Bronchogenic cyst
    B. Lymphoma
    C. Neurogenic tumor
    D. Thymoma
    E. Adenocarcinoma

14. A 78-year-old previously healthy man is admitted to the emergency department complaining of angina, dyspnea, and near syncope. ECG is normal, and a loud systolic murmur is heard in the second right interspace with radiation to the carotids. What is the most likely diagnosis in this patient?

    A. MI
    B. Pericarditis
    C. Mitral regurgitation
    D. Aortic stenosis
    E. Aortic insufficiency

15. Which of the following is not a risk factor for CAD?

    A. Hypertension
    B. Smoking
    C. Diabetes
    D. Renal failure
    E. Hypercholesterolemia

16. A 72-year-old female patient is admitted with unstable angina. Cardiac catheterization reveals severe triple-vessel CAD. The optimal treatment of this patient would include which of the following?

    A. Coronary artery bypass surgery
    B. Observation
    C. Medical management (nitrates, beta-blockers)
    D. Coronary angioplasty
    E. Tissue plasminogen activator

17. A 72-year-old male patient with a history of syncope and dyspnea presents for evaluation for peripheral vascular surgery. Physical examination reveals a systolic crescendo–decrescendo murmur that radiates to the carotid arteries. As he is symptomatic, his diseased valve would typically have an area of less than which of the following?

    A. 1 cm^2
    B. 1.5 cm^2
    C. 2 cm^2
    D. 3 cm^2
    E. 4 cm^2

18. A 29-year-old man is evaluated for a cerebral vascular accident. Physical examination reveals a systolic ejection murmur at the left second interspace and a fixed split second heart sound. What is the most likely diagnosis?

    A. VSD
    B. ASD
    C. Mitral stenosis
    D. Aortic insufficiency
    E. Ventricular aneurysm

19. A 40-year-old man is in a major motor vehicle collision with ejection from the driver's seat. On arrival, his blood pressure is 70/40 mm Hg, with a pulse of 125 beats per minute. He has a chest tube inserted which releases 1,500 mL of blood and no change in vital signs. The most appropriate approach to this patient is:

    A. Median sternotomy
    B. CT scan with IV contrast
    C. Left posterolateral thoracotomy
    D. Right posterolateral thoracotomy
    E. Anterolateral thoracotomy

20. A 46-year-old post office worker presents with complaints of numbness and occasional pain in the left arm. Exam reveals a normal pulse and no edema of the left arm, but symptoms seem to be worse when the patient stretches her arm above her head. The best initial test is:

    A. Chest x-ray
    B. Serum potassium
    C. Angiography
    D. CT scan of the left shoulder
    E. Pulmonary function tests (PFTs)

21. A 70-year-old female with a history of 50 pack-years of cigarette smoking presents with a chronic cough. Physical exam reveals coarse breath sounds bilaterally, and chest x-ray suggests low lung volumes with a 2-cm spiculated lesion in the periphery of the left lower lobe. Biopsy suggests adenocarcinoma, and a metastatic workup is negative. The most appropriate treatment is:

    A. Chemotherapy
    B. Radiation therapy
    C. Left lower lobectomy
    D. Left pneumonectomy
    E. Wedge excision

22. A 54-year-old female presents with 6 months of mild shortness of breath, lower extremity edema, and occasional heart palpitations. ECG reveals normal sinus rhythm. Echocardiogram shows moderate to severe mitral regurgitation, EF of 50%, and moderately dilated left atrium. Cardiac catheterization reveals normal coronary arteries. What is the best therapeutic option for this patient?

    A. Diuresis and repeat echocardiogram in 6 months
    B. Mitral valve replacement
    C. Anticoagulation and Holter monitor
    D. Mitral valve repair

23. A 65-year-old male suffers an ST-elevation MI and is treated with a drug-eluting stent in the mid LAD artery, aspirin, clopidogrel, simvastatin, and metoprolol. He remains hemodynamically stable and initially recovers cardiac function with an EF of 45% on hospital day 3. However on hospital day 5, he is short of breath and edematous with mild hypotension and a new harsh holosystolic murmur. Which of the following will not be helpful in his continued management?

A. Intra-aortic balloon pump
B. Echocardiogram
C. Surgical repair
D. Volume resuscitation
E. Transfer to an intensive care unit

Answers and Explanations

1. **The answer is A** (Chapter 5, Pleural and Pleural Space Disorders, Spontaneous Pneumothorax). The patient has signs and symptoms of spontaneous pneumothorax. After a confirmatory x-ray, treatment with a chest tube is the best initial treatment. Needle decompression is indicated in cases of tension pneumothorax. Additional imaging, such as with CT, is not initially indicated but may be required if there is no resolution. Supplemental oxygen may help with pneumothorax resorption but is not sufficient to allow complete resolution.

2. **The answer is E** (Chapter 5, Pleural and Pleural Space Disorders, Spontaneous Pneumothorax, IV A). Indications for definitive surgical management of spontaneous pneumothorax include recurrence (ipsilateral or contralateral), persistent air leak greater than 3–5 days, incomplete expansion of the lung, and hemopneumothorax.

3. **The answer is C** (Chapter 5, Thoracic Trauma, Immediate Life-Threatening Injuries, II C). The patient has signs and symptoms consistent with a tension pneumothorax. This life-threatening situation should be treated immediately by needle thoracentesis. A chest tube insertion should follow this maneuver. A chest radiograph is not necessary to confirm the diagnosis and will only delay treatment. Local wound exploration has no role in the management of stab wounds of the chest. Pericardiocentesis is the choice when evidence indicates pericardial tamponade.

4–5. **The answers are 4-D** (Chapter 5, Thoracic Trauma, Potentially Life-Threatening Injuries, II D) **and 5-B** (Chapter 5, Thoracic Trauma, Immediate Life-Threatening Injuries, VI). Causes for the chest radiograph and ECG findings are multiple and include aortic rupture, cardiac tamponade, tracheobronchial disruption, hypoxia, and cardiac contusion. A more precise diagnosis would be mandatory before undertaking thoracotomy because operative strategy would depend on which injury is present.

   Blunt thoracic trauma with or without flail chest results in chest wall muscle damage and pain, with resultant splinting and loss of chest wall elasticity. Intra-alveolar hemorrhage and interstitial edema reduce pulmonary parenchymal elasticity. Therefore, both lung and chest wall compliance decrease. PCO_2, A-a gradient, and shunt fractions would probably be elevated, and ventricular contractions would probably be decreased.

6–7. **The answers are 6-C** (Chapter 5, Pleural and Pleural Space Disorders, Pleural Effusions, II) **and 7-B** (Chapter 5, Pleural and Pleural Space Disorders, Pleural Empyema, III B). The patient developing a pleural effusion in the setting of an underlying pneumonia requires thoracentesis for diagnosis. The character of the fluid described is consistent with that present in an empyema. Initial treatment of an empyema should involve closed chest tube drainage. Thoracotomy and decortication or rib resection may be required when the empyema is not adequately drained by the chest tube or is otherwise not amenable to closed drainage. Video-assisted thoracoscopic surgery pleurodesis is not standard treatment for an empyema.

8. **The answer is D** (Chapter 5, Solitary Pulmonary Nodules [Coin Lesions], Invasive Diagnostic Techniques). The patient has a solitary pulmonary nodule. He is older than age 40 years, and the characteristics do not favor a benign lesion, such as concentric calcification. In addition, the lesion was not present on the chest radiograph 5 years earlier. Diagnosis is mandatory for determining whether the lesion is malignant. This can be done by needle biopsy or thoracoscopic biopsy.

9. **The answer is C** (Chapter 5, Thoracic Trauma, Potentially Life-Threatening Injuries, III). This patient is presenting with a diaphragmatic disruption, as evidenced by the identification of the stomach in the chest. Treatment involves standard resuscitation principles, (airway, breathing, circulation), placement of a nasogastric tube to prevent acute gastric dilatation (which can produce severe, life-threatening respiratory distress), and urgent transabdominal repair of the diaphragmatic defect. If diagnosis is delayed by 7–10 days, transthoracic repair is preferred to facilitate the freeing of any adhesions to the lung.

10. The answer is E (Chapter 6, Congenital Heart Disease, Overview, II). The most common forms of congenital heart disease are, in decreasing order, VSD, transposition of the great vessels, tetralogy of Fallot, hypoplastic left heart syndrome, ASD, and PDA.

11. The answer is E (Chapter 5, Solitary Pulmonary Nodules [Coin Lesions], Imaging, I C). Isolated lung nodules less than 1.0 cm are known as coin lesions. Workup should include a detailed history, noting any use of tobacco products or previous malignancy. Any prior chest radiographs should be obtained. A calcified lesion that has not enlarged over a 2-year period suggests a benign process. In this patient, observation with follow-up x-ray is indicated. Any change in the lesion is an indication for biopsy.

12. The answer is D (Chapter 5, Bronchogenic Carcinoma, Treatment, I A). The appropriate treatment is surgical lobectomy. Observation with repeat chest x-ray is not warranted with a smoking history.

This patient is in clinical stage I, based on tumor size and nodal status. There is no clear benefit in biopsying the lesion. Chemotherapy and radiation may be indicated in certain stage IIIa lesions or in locally advanced disease.

13. The answer is A (Chapter 5, Mediastinal Lesions, Visceral Compartment Lesions, II). The most common middle mediastinal mass is a bronchogenic cyst. Lymphoma, thymoma, and germ cell tumors are commonly located in the anterior mediastinum. Middle mediastinal lesions include bronchogenic and pericardial cysts. Metastatic adenocarcinoma may involve the pleural surfaces; however, lesions are often small and multiple.

14. The answer is D (Chapter 6, Acquired Heart Disease, Aortic Valvular Disease, I D). Angina, syncope, and dyspnea are the classic symptoms of aortic stenosis. Physical examination generally reveals a systolic ejection murmur in the second right intercostal space. An ECG and serial cardiac enzymes should be obtained to rule out cardiac ischemia. The murmur of aortic insufficiency is diastolic with a clinical picture of heart failure.

15. The answer is D (Chapter 6, Acquired Heart Disease, Coronary Artery Disease, I B). Risk factors for CAD are the same as those for vascular disease in general—smoking, diabetes, obesity, hypertension, and hypercholesterolemia. Although renal failure is often associated with CAD, this is because of the frequent association with other risk factors, such as hypertension and diabetes.

16. The answer is A (Chapter 6, Acquired Heart Disease, Coronary Artery Disease, V C 2). This patient has severe triple-vessel coronary disease. Studies have shown a significant survival advantage for patients in this category who are treated with surgical revascularization rather than with medical management or angioplasty. Additional benefit may be realized in patients with compromised ventricular function.

17. The answer is A (Chapter 6, Acquired Heart Disease, Aortic Valvular Disease, I B 1). This patient has aortic stenosis. Symptoms usually begin when the valve area is less than 1 cm^2.

18. The answer is B (Chapter 6, Congenital Heart Disease, Atrial Septal Defects, III D). Echocardiogram searching for thrombus or septal defect should be obtained in a younger patient who suffers from a cerebral vascular accident. A second interspace murmur and fixed splitting of the second heart sound are classic findings in ASD. Anticoagulation for 4–6 weeks with elective repair of the ASD is the indicated treatment.

19. The answer is E (Chapter 5, Thoracic Trauma, Immediate Life-Threatening Injuries, IV B). Anterolateral thoracotomy is the procedure of choice. The patient meets criteria for operative intervention as the initial chest tube output exceeds 1 L. The best initial incision in the hemodynamically unstable patient is anterolateral thoracotomy.

20. The answer is A (Chapter 5, Chest Wall Disorders, Chest Wall Deformities, IV A 1). The patient has signs and symptoms consistent with neurogenic thoracic outlet syndrome. There may be a cervical rib causing compression of the brachial plexus. Chest x-ray is the initial diagnostic study, followed by a course of physical therapy to alleviate the compression. The patient's symptoms are unlikely to be caused by an electrolyte disturbance. Angiography is not indicated given the normal pulse exam. Shoulder films may rule out fracture, but CT would be indicated for questions of ligamentous injury. PFTs are useful for lung pathology only.

21. **The answer is C** (Chapter 5, Bronchogenic Carcinoma, Treatment, I A 1). The best definitive management of a lung cancer is excision, and formal lobectomy is the procedure of choice. Wedge excision is used in cases of patients that are too high risk to tolerate anatomic resection, and pneumonectomy is reserved for those patients with more diffuse disease in one lung. Chemotherapy and radiation have a role in advanced disease palliation.

22. **The answer is D** (Chapter 6, Acquired Heart Disease, Mitral Valve Disease, II E 2). This patient meets American Heart Association/American College of Cardiology criteria for surgical correction of mitral regurgitation given her symptoms, depressed EF and likely atrial fibrillations. In the setting of mitral regurgitation, an EF below 60% represents decreased function. Mitral valve repair is preferred to replacement when possible. Although treating volume overload and atrial fibrillation will be important aspects in the medical management of mitral insufficiency, surgical correction is indicated and outcomes are improved with earlier intervention.

23. **The answer is D** (Chapter 6, Acquired Heart Disease, Coronary Artery Disease, VI C). This patient is presenting with a postinfarction VSD. Most immediately, an echocardiogram will be necessary to determine the location and size of the VSD. Given his mild hypotension, an intra-aortic balloon pump will help support hemodynamics until repair can be done. Catheter-based repairs are not likely to be helpful, as friable, injured myocardium surrounding the VSD does not offer suitable attachment point for any percutaneous devices. The diagnosis of a postinfarct VSD mandates surgical repair, which should be done within 24 hours to optimize survival. Volume resuscitation in the setting of impending cardiogenic shock will only serve to advance the disease state.

Part III

Vascular Disorders
Chapter Cuts and Caveats

CHAPTER 7

Arterial Disease:

◆ An untreated TIA is associated with a 40% chance of a second TIA or stroke within 2 years. CEA, if done for more than 70% stenosis, lowers the 2-year major stroke rate to 9%, whereas medical treatment with antiplatelet therapy has a 26% rate.

◆ The CEA perioperative risk of a major stroke is 1%–3% and is dependent on the surgeon.

◆ Acute arterial embolism often is secondary to cardiac thrombi, such as with atrial fibrillation, acute MI, and valvular disease.

◆ Occlusive disease of the distal aorta and iliac and femoral arteries (inflow disease) may produce claudication, rest pain, or tissue loss. When it is limb threatening, it should be evaluated and revascularized. Inflow disease should generally be revascularized before outflow disease.

◆ Claudication is reversible ischemia of the leg and is managed by lifestyle modification, including a supervised exercise program; smoking cessation; control of diabetes, hyperlipidemia, and hypertension; and antiplatelet therapy. Revascularization is reserved for patients in whom the claudication interferes with an active lifestyle.

◆ The hallmarks of ischemia are the 6 P's: pain, pulselessness, paralysis, pallor, paresthesias, and poikilothermia.

◆ Rest pain is constant pain, usually across the forefoot, and indicates severe ischemia. Tissue loss is imminent, and urgent evaluation and revascularization is appropriate.

◆ There are three important facets to a vascular bypass patency: (1) inflow: if blood flow into the bypass is not strong, the bypass will thrombose; (2) the conduit: if the conduit has a technical problem, such as a twist, kink, narrowing, or anything else that impedes flow, the bypass will thrombose; and (3) outflow: if the vessels distal to the bypass are obstructed for any reason, the bypass will thrombose.

◆ Revascularization longer than 6 hours after acute ischemia may result in a severely impaired limb or even require amputation.

◆ Compartment syndrome may occur following revascularization and is caused by increased tissue pressure (20–40 mm Hg) obstructing capillary blood flow to the tissues (because the compartment pressure does not reach arterial pressure, the patient will not present with the signs of arterial occlusion and may have a normal distal pulse).

◆ Both open and endovascular repairs of the aorta have excellent long-term durability. Endoleaks are leaks in the space between an endograft and the native vessel, and most should be repaired.

◆ Elective repair of AAA at least 5.5 cm in men and 5 cm in women in greatest diameter is appropriate if the patient is likely to tolerate the procedure and has a life expectancy of more than 2 years.

◆ More than 95% of AAAs arise infrarenally.

- The presence of AAA and new-onset abdominal pain should be urgently evaluated for leak or rupture and repaired if present: ~50% of ruptured AAAs result in death prior to treatment. Repaired ruptured AAAs have a high incidence for postoperative complications, especially MI and acute renal failure.
- Descending thoracic aortic dissection is usually treated with medical therapy to control hypertension.
- Surgical or endovascular repair is reserved for leaks, rupture, or occlusion of aortic branches.
- Proximal dissection is a surgical emergency due to risk of coronary occlusion, aortic regurgitation, and tamponade.

CHAPTER 8

Venous and Lymphatic Disease:

- Surgery is a proinflammatory state, and all surgical patients are at increased risk of lower extremity DVT. Many patients may have no symptoms or physical findings.
- Initial DVT treatment is anticoagulation with heparin followed by warfarin.
- Risk factors for DVT are summarized in the Virchow triad: stasis, hypercoagulable states, and endothelial injury.
- Proven lower extremity DVT prophylaxis includes intermittent pneumatic compression devices and low-dose anticoagulation.
- IVC filters may prevent lower extremity DVTs from becoming a PE in special situations: those who fail anticoagulation or those who cannot tolerate anticoagulation (such as hemorrhagic stroke or trauma).
- Upper extremity DVT: usually refers to thrombosis of the axillary or subclavian vein.
    - Secondary UEDVT is increasing in incidence due to increased use of upper extremity catheters. Pulmonary embolus may occur in up to 1/3rd of patients, and post-thrombotic syndrome of the arm is common; thus anticoagulation with heparin followed by warfarin is appropriate in most cases.
    - Primary UEDVT (Paget-Schroetter Syndrome) is rare and typically related to extreme arm exercise in sports (effort thrombosis) or thoracic outlet syndrome. It may be amenable to urgent catheter directed thrombolytic therapy aimed at preventing post-thrombotic syndrome, followed by investigation for etiology.
- PE is diagnosed with CT pulmonary angiogram. PE patients are best treated with systemic anticoagulation.

Chapter 7

Arterial Disease

Garima Dosi and Robert S. Crawford

GENERAL PRINCIPLES

Pathophysiology
Atherosclerosis

I. **Characteristics:** starts as a fatty streak and can progress to complex plaques, characterized by intimal ulceration or intraplaque hemorrhage

II. **Clinical manifestations:** Can be distal from embolization or local from stenosis causing partial blockage and diminished distal flow or occlusion and complete luminal blockage. Also determined by the acuity of the lesion and presence of collateral circulation.

III. **Risk factors:** diabetes mellitus (DM), tobacco use, hypertension (HTN), and hyperlipidemia

LOWER EXTREMITY ARTERIAL OCCLUSIVE DISEASE

Classification

I. **Based on lesion location:** Figure 7-2 shows the lower extremity (LE) arterial tree.

A. **Suprainguinal aortoiliac occlusive disease (AIOD):** involves the aorta and iliacs up to the level of inguinal ligament

B. **Infrainguinal disease:** arteries distal to inguinal ligament (femoral, popliteal, and tibial systems), including femoropopliteal disease and infrageniculate tibial disease

II. **Based on symptomatology:** includes noncritical and critical limb ischemia

A. **Intermittent claudication:** Symptoms are reproducible; rest brings relief. This is *not* a limb-threatening condition.

1. **Inciting event:** walking or exercise
2. **Primary symptom:** pain in affected muscle groups (calf)
3. **Risk of major limb amputation:** ~1% per year

B. **Neurogenic claudication:** Patient presents with history of back pain. Pain radiates down the leg, with associated paresthesia, and can occur with standing.

Quick Cut
Vascular surgeons encounter a wide variety of clinical manifestations of arterial disease; Figure 7-1 demonstrates that the lesions have some common pathophysiologic features.

Quick Cut
Atherosclerosis is the most common cause of arterial occlusive disease and can affect any vascular bed in the body.

Quick Cut
In acute arterial occlusion, collateral circulation does not have time to develop, resulting in acute ischemia and tissue loss.

Quick Cut
Fewer than 5% of patients with intermittent claudication progress to critical limb ischemia.

Quick Cut
Vasculogenic claudication requires ambulation; neurogenic claudication may occur while standing or at rest.

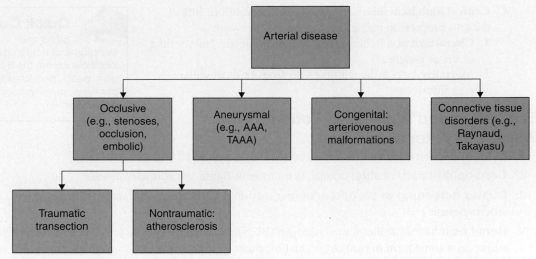

Figure 7-1: The spectrum of arterial disease. *AAA*, abdominal aortic aneurysm; *TAAA*, thoracoabdominal aortic aneurysm.

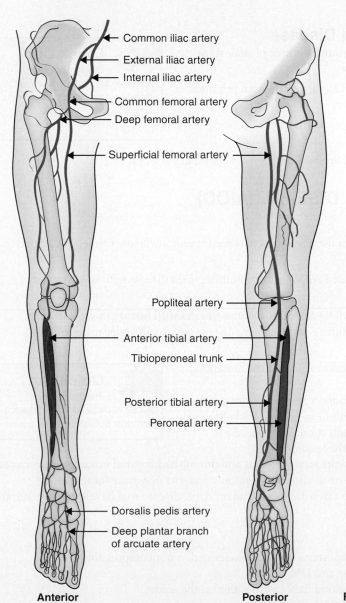

Figure 7-2: The arterial tree of the lower extremity.

C. **Critical limb ischemia:** Limb-threatening condition; 30% of patients progress to major amputation within a year.
   1. **Characteristics:** ischemic rest pain or tissue loss (nonhealing ulcers or gangrene)
   2. **Mortality:** ~25% die within 1 year from cardiovascular complications.

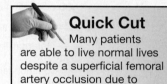

Quick Cut
Signs and symptoms of acute arterial insufficiency are the 6 P's: **p**ain, **p**allor, **p**aresthesia, **p**aralysis, **p**ulselessness, and **p**oikilothermia.

Evaluation and Workup of Patients with Peripheral Arterial Disease

I. **Evaluation:** starts with a detailed history and thorough physical exam

II. **Cardiopulmonary status:** critical, as many have significant coronary disease

III. **Duplex screening of carotid arteries:** may demonstrate concomitant cerebrovascular atherosclerosis

IV. **Renal assessment:** Blood urea nitrogen (BUN) and creatinine levels are required, as most patients will require some form of contrast evaluation either by digital subtraction angiography (DSA) or computed tomography angiography (CTA).

V. **Atherosclerotic risk factors:** Initiate best medical management of DM, HTN, hyperlipidemia, and smoking cessation.

Natural History of Untreated Disease

I. **Collateral circulation:** develops around the area of stenosis or occlusion to provide distal blood flow

II. **Superficial artery occlusion:** Collateral vessels from profunda femoris reconstitute the popliteal artery.

III. **Geniculate collaterals:** develop around the knee to provide collateral blood flow

IV. **In AIOD:** Collaterals arise from iliac, lumbar, and internal mammary arteries.

Quick Cut
Many patients are able to live normal lives despite a superficial femoral artery occlusion due to collateral flow.

AORTOILIAC OCCLUSIVE DISEASE (AIOD)

General Aspects

I. **Anatomic location:** Atherosclerosis usually begins in the infrarenal aorta; over time, this can extend and may result in total occlusion.

II. **Extent:** Patients can either have isolated AIOD or have multisegment disease with involvement of infrainguinal vasculature.

III. **Risk factors:** Those with isolated AIOD are usually young females with history of smoking and hypercholesterolemia; patients with diffuse multisegment disease are usually older male with DM and HTN.

IV. **Clinical presentation:** Blue toe syndrome can be the presenting symptom in AIOD.
   A. **Intermittent claudication:** Distribution is in the buttock and thigh and suspected in patients with near-normal ankle-brachial index (ABI) who complain of claudication. Exercise ABI is helpful in uncovering the level of the lesion.
   B. **Leriche syndrome:** buttock claudication, impotence, and diminished femoral pulses; seen in males
   C. **Blue toe syndrome:** Produced by small cholesterol emboli; patients may have focal areas of ischemia in the feet. More common in patients with aneurysmal disease that have extensive mural thrombus.

Quick Cut
The hallmark of AIOD is diminished or absent femoral pulses.

Diagnostic Investigations

I. **ABI:** correlates with patient's functional status and can be elevated in noncompressible medial calcinosis as in end-stage renal disease and DM
   A. **Procedure:** Blood pressure is measured in both arms, then at the ankle.
   B. **Calculation:** Divide systolic ankle pressure by highest of the two brachial pressures (Table 7-1).

Table 7-1: Standardized Classification of Disease Based on Ankle-Brachial Index

1.13–1.0	Normal
0.9–1.0	Minimal arterial disease; asymptomatic
0.5–.09	Claudication, mild to moderate disease
<0.5	Rest pain; severe disease

An ABI of approximately 1 is normal. Higher values indicate calcified vessels, and lower values indicate the presence of arterial disease.

II. **Noninvasive vascular lab studies:** involves measurement of segmental pressure and waveform analysis at each arterial segment (thigh, calf, ankle, and toes) and duplex evaluation of the lower limb arteries
   A. **Segmental pressure and pulse volume recording (PVR):** will demonstrate differences in pulse pressure
   B. **Timing:** Segmental pressure measurements may be performed after graded exercise treadmill test.

III. **CTA:** most common test for localizing lesions but with limitations of radiation exposure and possible renal insufficiency from intravenous (IV) contrast

Quick Cut A difference of 20 mm Hg between segments is diagnostic of a functionally significant lesion.

IV. **Magnetic resonance angiography (MRA):** has same advantages as CTA but more expensive
   A. **Gadolinium contrast:** carries the risk of nephrogenic systemic fibrosis in patients with renal insufficiency
   B. **Other limitations:** False negatives can occur in patients with previous endovascular interventions.

V. **DSA:** still considered the gold standard; commonly performed during a planned intervention

Treatment

I. **Medical therapy:** First line of therapy for all patients with claudication; best management of their atherosclerotic risk factors and smoking cessation should be instituted in all patients as well as antiplatelet therapy with aspirin.
   A. **HMG-CoA reductase inhibitors:** recommended even in patients with acceptable lipid profiles due to the additional cardiovascular protective effects
   B. **Cilostazol:** Phosphodiesterase-3 inhibitor that causes vasodilation through smooth muscle cell relaxation and inhibition of platelet aggregation. Contraindicated in congestive heart failure (CHF).

Quick Cut Cilostazol is the only drug that has shown some improvement in absolute walking distance in patients with intermittent claudication.

II. **Graded exercise program:** Very effective at encouraging development of collaterals and alleviating symptoms. Ambulation should be an early part of any treatment algorithm for claudication.

III. **Operative intervention:** Indications include lifestyle-limiting claudication, ischemic rest pain, or evidence of tissue loss.
   A. **Angioplasty/stent:** performed via transfemoral or brachial approach
      1. **Advantages:** Distal aorta and iliacs can be treated with balloon angioplasty and stent placement; 5-year patency rate is excellent.
      2. **Site-related complications:** bleeding or hematoma, pseudoaneurysm; arteriovenous fistula, iliac artery dissection, thrombus formation, and distal embolization

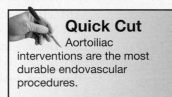

Quick Cut Aortoiliac interventions are the most durable endovascular procedures.

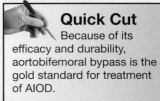

Quick Cut Because of its efficacy and durability, aortobifemoral bypass is the gold standard for treatment of AIOD.

   B. **Open procedures:** may include direct reconstruction or extra-anatomic approaches if the patient has severe comorbidities or infection
      1. **Aortobifemoral bypass:** Five-year patency of this procedure is 90% and 75% at 10 years. Procedure is as follows:
         a. **Step 1:** midline laparotomy and aortic exposure
         b. **Step 2:** Proximal anastomosis is performed between the graft (Dacron or polytetrafluoroethylene [PTFE]) and aorta in end-to-end or end-to-side fashion.

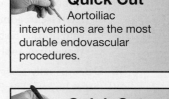

c. **Step 3:** Limbs of the bifurcated prosthetic graft are tunneled retroperitoneally and anastomosed to femoral arteries.

2. **Femoral-femoral bypass:** Performed for unilateral iliac disease; the contralateral femoral artery serves as arterial inflow.

a. **Procedure:** Prosthetic graft is tunneled either subcutaneously or in space of Retzius and anastomosed to femoral arteries.

b. **Patency:** 5-year rate of 75%

3. **Axillobifemoral bypass:** Performed in patients with AIOD who are high-risk candidates for open aortic revascularization; axillary artery serves as the arterial inflow. Five-year patency rate of 60%–85%.

FEMOROPOPLITEAL OCCLUSIVE DISEASE

General Aspects

I. **Anatomic extent and location:** Occlusive disease is most frequently seen in the superficial femoral artery (SFA).

II. **Disease severity:** ranges from flow-limiting stenosis to complete occlusion in the superficial femoral and popliteal arteries

III. **Risk factors:** Atherosclerosis is the most important risk factor; other causes include popliteal entrapment, dissection, embolization, or aneurysmal degeneration.

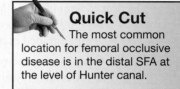

Quick Cut
The most common location for femoral occlusive disease is in the distal SFA at the level of Hunter canal.

IV. **Clinical presentation:** Majority of patients are asymptomatic; the profunda femoral artery provides important flow to the thigh musculature and through collaterals can sustain near-normal activity. Other presentations are as follows:

A. **Intermittent claudication:** crampy calf pain with ambulation; intensity of symptoms depends on severity of disease

B. **Critical limb ischemia:** ischemic rest pain, nonhealing ulcer, or gangrene

1. **Rest pain:** Pain that occurs with no activity; patients usually describe pain in the more dependent areas such as the toes or on the dorsum of the foot.

2. **Most common complaint:** pain that occurs at night and is relieved by dangling the leg from the bed

Quick Cut
Rest pain, ulcers, and gangrene are signs of imminent limb loss, and intervention to restore flow is needed urgently.

V. **Physical examination:** In contrast to patients with AIOD, they have palpable femoral pulses but diminished popliteal and pedal pulses. Some patients with severe limb ischemia may have leg pallor on foot elevation and develop rubor in the dependent position.

Diagnostic Studies

I. **Noninvasive vascular studies:** include the following:

A. **ABI:** Pressure drop of greater than 20 mm Hg indicates significant hemodynamic arterial obstruction.

B. **Exercise treadmill testing:** can be used in patients with claudication with normal resting ABI

C. **Waveform analysis:** Doppler waveforms and PVR

Quick Cut
In healthy patients, ankle pressure should remain normal or increase after exercise.

II. **DSA:** usually reserved for patients as part of planned intervention and gives excellent detail of the target lumen (Fig. 7-3)

A. **Procedure:** Contrast media is injected using catheters placed either by transfemoral or the transbrachial percutaneous approach. Images are recorded under fluoroscopy.

B. **Associated complications:** include dye-associated nephrotoxicity, allergy, and site complications as listed earlier

III. **CTA of abdomen and pelvis with extremity runoff:** gives near-equal static information, especially with new three-dimensional (3D) reconstruction techniques; however, there is no dynamic information. Avoids the access site complications associated with DSA and is especially good to delineate calcium within vessels

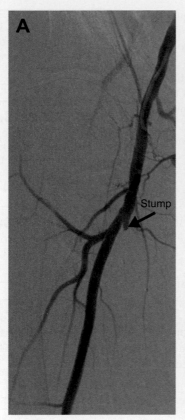
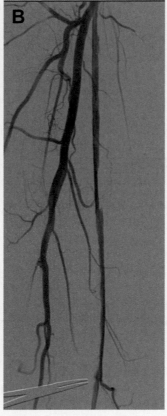
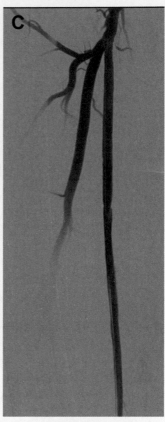

Figure 7-3: A: Baseline angiography of the right superficial femoral artery (SFA) revealing a complete occlusion at the ostium with a short stump. **B:** Angiography following laser atherectomy with restoration of flow. The SFA was then postdilated with a 5.0-mm balloon at low pressure. **C:** Final SFA angiography revealing a widely patent SFA with no evidence of dissection or need for stenting. (From Casserly IP, Sachar R, Yadav JS. *Practical Peripheral Vascular Intervention*, 2nd ed. Philadelphia: Lippincott Williams & Wilkins; 2011.)

Treatment Options

I. **Best medical therapy:** See earlier discussion (e.g., smoking cessation, lipid control, cilostazol).

II. **Percutaneous interventions:** Angioplasty and stenting convey a good outcome and durability (up to 80% patency over 3 years).

III. **Open surgical options:** can involve endarterectomy or bypass
   A. **Local endarterectomy of the common femoral and profunda with patch angioplasty:** highly effective in patients with severe focal lesions
   B. **Bypass:** Five-year primary patency of femoropopliteal above and below knee bypass with greater saphenous vein is 70%–90%.
      1. **Inflow:** common femoral artery
      2. **Outflow:** typically the popliteal artery above or below the knee
      3. **Conduit:** As a rule, autogenous vein bypass is preferred over prosthetic bypass; prosthetic grafts have overall poor patency when used for below-knee vessels.

> **Quick Cut**
> The adequacy of inflow, the suitability of the outflow, and the type and quality of the conduit all influence the outcome of the procedure.

> **Quick Cut**
> In general, patency rates are better for above-the-knee procedures than below knee.

◆ INFRAGENICULATE TIBIAL DISEASE

General Aspects

I. **Clinical presentation and anatomic extent:** usually multisegmental; patients are usually high risk due to other associated medical comorbidities
   A. **Characteristics:** commonly seen with DM and end-stage renal disease
   B. **Presentation: Patients typically present with foot ulcers or gangrene.**

II. Treatment: For selected patients, endovascular interventions can achieve wound healing.

   A. Bypass: For rest pain or tissue loss, open bypass is the procedure of choice.

      1. Distal target: any of the three tibial arteries (anterior tibial, posterior tibial, or peroneal) or to the pedal arteries of the foot

      2. Tibial bypasses: Autogenous vein conduit has superior patency rate as compared to prosthetic graft.

   B. DSA: important to identify the appropriate inflow and outflow vessel

Quick Cut
Toe pressure of greater than 40 mm Hg is needed to heal a foot wound.

ACUTE ARTERIAL INSUFFICIENCY

Etiologies

I. Embolism: Debris (thrombus, lipid, tumor, etc.) dislodges from proximal source and obstructs a distal artery. Majority have a cardiac origin.

   A. Cardiac origins: mural thrombus in patients with atrial fibrillation, ventricular thrombus after myocardial infarction (MI), rheumatic valvular abnormalities, vegetations on prosthetic valves, atrial myxoma

   B. Noncardiac embolic sources: atherosclerotic or aneurysmal, peripheral artery aneurysm (popliteal artery), thoracic outlet syndrome, iatrogenic atheroembolization after percutaneous vascular interventions

II. Thrombosis: In situ thrombosis in patients with atherosclerotic arterial disease can produce acute ischemia.

III. Hypercoagulable states: can cause in situ thrombosis in the absence of atherosclerosis

IV. Aortic or arterial dissection: Extension of a dissection can cause acute arterial insufficiency.

V. Other: acute occlusion of previously patent bypass graft

Quick Cut
The ultimate goal of peripheral bypass is to provide inline flow to the distal foot.

Quick Cut
The most common cause of late graft failure is neointimal hyperplasia.

Quick Cut
Acute arterial insufficiency is a vascular emergency, as rapid restoration of blood flow is required to prevent irreversible tissue loss, limb loss, and even death.

Quick Cut
Thrombosis is the most common cause of acute arterial insufficiency.

Clinical Presentation

I. Symptoms: depend on the size of the artery occluded and the presence of collateral circulation

II. Large or macroembolus: usually gets lodged at bifurcation sites such as the common femoral artery (superficial femoral/profunda bifurcation) or popliteal artery (tibioperoneal/anterior tibial bifurcation)

III. Microemboli: usually affect more distal tibial or digital vessels, and patients present with blue toe syndrome

Evaluation

I. Prompt physical examination: helps determine the level of occlusion

II. CTA with runoff: can provide useful information about the level of the occlusion and about options for revascularization

III. Duplex: operator dependent but can be used to make a quick diagnosis (i.e., to locate a thrombus at the femoral bifurcation)

Quick Cut
Comparison with the contralateral extremity and identification of motor and sensory deficits are important parts of the vascular exam.

IV. On-table angiography: used when endovascular intervention needs to be performed and to confirm patency after any intervention

Management

I. Anticoagulation: always the first step in critical limb ischemia; IV heparin is the drug of choice

II. Percutaneous thrombectomy and thrombolysis: preferred in acute limb ischemia patients with intact motor and sensory function

   A. Absolute contraindications to thrombolytic therapy: recent stroke or brain surgery within 2 months, major surgery within 2 weeks, and patients at significant risk of bleeding

   B. Timing: Thrombolytic therapy frequently takes more than 24 hours for effect.

III. **Open thrombectomy/embolectomy:** Performed using Fogarty catheters that are advanced into the artery through the embolus, and balloon is inflated. As the catheter is withdrawn with the inflated balloon, the thrombus is extracted.

IV. **Combined endovascular and open procedures:** Recently, an open approach combined with endovascular adjuncts such as angioplasty or stenting. Initial angiography can be followed by an open embolectomy, culminating with stenting of inflow, direct infusion of tissue plasminogen activator (tPA) into the artery, and a bypass to below-the-knee arterial target.

V. **Compartment syndrome:** Results from reperfusion injury to the ischemic muscle. Postrevascularization patients need to be watched closely for myoglobinuria and associated nephrotoxicity.

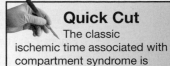

Quick Cut
The classic ischemic time associated with compartment syndrome is 6 hours.

   A. **Presentation:** pain on passive stretch, calf tenderness, and loss of sensation in the first web space
   B. **Untreated:** can lead to permanent neurologic sequelae such as foot drop
   C. **Fasciotomy:** therapeutic and based on clinical suspicion

AMPUTATIONS

General Aspects

I. **Indications:** nonambulatory bed-bound patients, nonreconstructible disease, extensive tissue loss, medical comorbidities that make revascularization procedures risky, wet gangrene with sepsis

II. **Technical considerations:** Amputation level must maximize the rehabilitation potential of each individual patient.

Quick Cut
Primary amputation is offered to patients with critical limb ischemia as first-line therapy when bypass is not possible or not desirable.

   A. **Goal:** to remove all the infected or necrotic tissue and to achieve a healing stump of appropriate length so as to fit prosthesis
   B. **Level of amputation:** determined by the patient's preoperative functional status and the involved extremity's underlying arterial circulation

Specific Amputations

I. **Toe amputation:** Can be performed across a phalanx or metatarsal bone (ray amputation). Associated with minimal gait disturbance.

II. **Transmetatarsal amputation:** involves transection of all five metatarsal bones midshaft with a posteriorly based flap

III. **Below-knee amputation:** Tibia and fibula are transected 10 cm below tibial tuberosity and coverage obtained by a longer posterior flap. Energy expenditure for ambulation is increased 10%–40% over bipedal gait.

Quick Cut
Ambulation requires progressively more energy with more proximal levels of amputation.

IV. **Above-knee amputation:** Femur is transected at distal one third of shaft. Energy expenditure for ambulation is increased 50%–70% over bipedal gait.

EXTRACRANIAL CEREBROVASCULAR DISEASE

General Aspects

I. **Incidence and etiology:** Stroke is the third leading cause of death in the United States. Atherosclerosis of extracranial carotid arteries usually affects the carotid bifurcation and the origin of the internal carotid artery and may predispose to stroke (Fig. 7-4).

II. **Asymptomatic:** Patients are evaluated on the basis of their degree of stenosis. Patients may have an incidental carotid bruit.

III. **Symptomatic:** Clinical symptoms are as follows.
   A. **Amaurosis fugax:** Transient monocular blindness due to embolization to retinal artery. Hollenhorst plaques (cholesterol atheroemboli) in retinal artery on funduscopy are diagnostic.
   B. **Transient ischemic attack (TIA):** sudden onset neurologic event lasting less than 24 hours with complete resolution

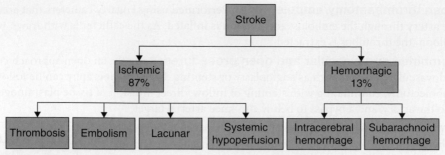

Figure 7-4: The etiologies of stroke (cerebrovascular accident).

C. Reversible ischemic neurologic deficit (RIND): focal neurologic deficit lasting more than 24 hours but resolving within a week

D. Stroke: infarction of brain tissue resulting in permanent neurologic deficit

E. Vertebrobasilar insufficiency: Symptoms are due to ischemia in brain supplied by vertebral arteries (posterior circulation) and may produce loss of vision, ataxia, gait disturbances, or vertigo.

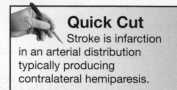

Quick Cut
Stroke is infarction in an arterial distribution typically producing contralateral hemiparesis.

Diagnostic Studies

I. **Main objectives:** to identify the precise location of the defect and its mechanism of origin

II. **Types:** include the following:

A. **Computed tomography (CT) of the head without contrast:** initial test of choice to be obtained in any symptomatic patient to identify the mechanism (i.e., ischemic or hemorrhagic)

B. **Magnetic resonance imaging (MRI):** more sensitive in detecting early ischemic changes but time-consuming and may induce claustrophobic reactions

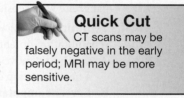

Quick Cut
CT scans may be falsely negative in the early period; MRI may be more sensitive.

C. **Cerebrovascular duplex:** primary screening modality for detecting and grading the severity of lesions in extracranial carotid and vertebral arteries

D. **Cerebral angiography:** defines the vessel defect and can be used as the first step for interventions to remove thrombus using interventional methods

E. **Echocardiography:** useful in evaluation of a cardiac source of embolism

Management

I. **Medical management:** aspirin, statin therapy, strict control of HTN and DM, and smoking cessation

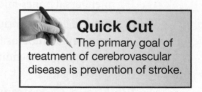

Quick Cut
The primary goal of treatment of cerebrovascular disease is prevention of stroke.

II. **Surgical repair:** Indications depend on whether the patient is symptomatic or asymptomatic and on the degree of stenosis determined by preoperative testing.

A. **Asymptomatic:** Asymptomatic carotid atherosclerosis study (ACAS) has demonstrated 5.9% risk reduction over 5 years in stroke incidence in asymptomatic patients with 60%–99% stenosis who underwent carotid endarterectomy (CEA) and best medical management compared to medical management alone.

B. **Symptomatic:** North American symptomatic endarterectomy trial (NASCET) demonstrated a 2-year decrease in stroke incidence from 26% to 9% in symptomatic patients with greater than 70% stenosis with CEA and best medical management compared to medical management alone.

C. **Contraindications:** disabling stroke with altered level of consciousness, occluded internal carotid artery, presence of medical comorbidities with short life expectancy

Quick Cut
Routine practice is to offer CEA to patient who are symptomatic and have at least 50% carotid stenosis.

D. **CEA:** involves removal of atherosclerotic plaque from within the distal common, internal, and external carotid arteries

1. **Procedure:** Can be performed under local anesthesia with regional cervical block or general anesthesia. Done with or without a shunt depending on assessment of collateralization of cerebral blood flow (stump pressure, neuromonitoring, patient response).

2. **Patch:** Patch closure is more durable than CEA without patch.
3. **Complications:** stroke, TIA, bleeding, cranial nerve injury (vagus and hypoglossal)
E. **Carotid angioplasty and stent:** Indications include surgically inaccessible lesion (skull base), previous carotid surgery (restenosis), irradiated neck, and severe comorbid cardiopulmonary conditions that preclude open carotid repair. Currently has a higher rate of complications than CEA.

AORTIC DISSECTION

General Aspects

I. **Pathophysiology:** Tear in the intima resulting in blood to flow in between the layers of aortic wall. True lumen and false lumen are created with formation of intimal flap. Thoracic aortic aneurysms tend to dissect; abdominal aortic aneurysms do not.

> **Quick Cut**
> Dissection occurs when the blood can flow between the layers of the vessel wall rather than inside the lumen.

II. **Classification based on timing:** acute or chronic
A. **Acute:** within 2 weeks from the onset of symptoms
  1. **Complicated:** must include the presence of rupture, impending rupture, or evidence of end-organ ischemia and is a *surgical emergency*
  2. **Uncomplicated:** No evidence of ischemia or rupture. Standard of care is medical management and tight blood pressure control.
B. **Chronic:** diagnosis more than 2 weeks after symptom onset

> **Quick Cut**
> Acute dissection is a life-threatening emergency and requires immediate intervention.

III. **Classification based on anatomy:** Figure 7-5
A. **DeBakey classification:** based on location of tear and extent of involvement of aorta with dissection
  1. **DeBakey type I:** involves the entire aorta from the root down into the descending aorta and is a *surgical emergency*
  2. **DeBakey type II:** involves the ascending aorta and is a *surgical emergency*
  3. **DeBakey type III:** Starts distal to the subclavian artery. Treatment is dictated by occurrence of complications.
B. **Stanford:** based on location of entry tear only
  1. **Stanford type A:** entry tear located in ascending aorta and is a *surgical emergency*
  2. **Stanford type B:** entry tear located distal to origin of left subclavian artery; medical management

IV. **Risk factors:** HTN (main), aortic wall structural anomalies, bicuspid aortic valve, hereditary conditions (e.g., Marfan syndrome), cocaine abuse

V. **Clinical presentation:** usually have significant HTN
A. **Pain:** Severe, "tearing" chest, back, or abdominal pain. Patients usually describe "worst ever" pain. Misdiagnosis is common, as other causes (MI, pulmonary embolism) are usually ruled out first.

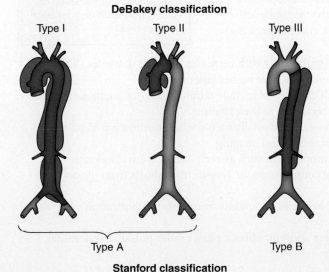

DeBakey classification

Type I   Type II   Type III

Type A   Type B

Stanford classification

Figure 7-5: DeBakey and Stanford classification systems for aortic dissection.

B. End-organ hypoperfusion: may cause symptoms when the dissection compromises blood flow through branch vessels

Diagnosis and Management

I. **CTA of chest abdomen and pelvis:** gold standard diagnostic modality of choice

II. **Transesophageal echocardiography (TEE):** excellent to delineate anatomy and extent of involvement of the ascending aorta, arch, coronaries, and aortic valve with type A dissection

III. **Type A dissections:** Urgent open surgical repair of ascending aorta with prosthetic graft replacement is treatment of choice.

IV. **Uncomplicated type B aortic dissection:** Medical management with strict blood pressure control with IV antihypertensive medications in intensive care setting (goal: mean blood pressure = 60–70 mm Hg) is treatment of choice.

V. **Indications for type B dissection:** presence of end-organ malperfusion, progression of dissection despite best medical management, impending rupture, or increase in size of aneurysm

> **Quick Cut**
> The most important late complication of chronic aortic dissection is aneurysmal dilation.

VI. **Thoracic endovascular aortic repair (TEVAR):** has become the technique of choice for surgical repair of type B aortic dissections (when indicated)

ARTERIAL ANEURYSMS

General Aspects

I. **Definition:** Permanent localized dilation of an artery. Aneurysmal degeneration can affect any artery of human body.

> **Quick Cut**
> Aneurysms have a diameter at least 50% greater than the native artery.

II. **Classification:** Aneurysms can be classified according to location, morphology, or etiology.
   A. **Location:** infrarenal aortic aneurysm, thoracoabdominal aortic aneurysm, splenic artery aneurysm, popliteal artery aneurysm, etc.
   B. **Morphology:** fusiform (involving the entire circumference of artery), saccular (outpouching along one wall of the artery)
   C. **Etiology:** inflammatory, infectious, congenital, degenerative, post-traumatic

III. **Abdominal aortic aneurysm (AAA):** Infrarenal degenerative fusiform aneurysm is the most common type and is considered aneurysmal when diameter is greater than 3 cm.
   A. **Complications:** include rupture, embolization to the lower extremities (blue toe syndrome), dissection within an existing aneurysm, and fistulization to adjacent structures (viscera, ureters)
   B. **Growth:** on average, rate of 0.2–0.3 cm per year
   C. **Risk factors:** Advanced age, male gender, smoking, family history. Other less consistent risk factors are HTN, coronary artery disease (CAD), white race, and hypercholesterolemia.
   D. **AAA rupture:** Risk factors include HTN, chronic obstructive pulmonary disease (COPD), female gender, current smoking status, and current steroid use.

> **Quick Cut**
> Rupture is the most feared complication of aneurysms, as it may result in sudden death.

   1. **AAA diameter:** Rupture risk increases significantly with increases in aortic diameter (Table 7-2).
   2. **Shape:** Eccentric or saccular-shaped aneurysms have higher risk of rupture.
   E. **Screening:** Criteria for one-time abdominal ultrasound include family history of aneurysm or males aged 65–75 years who smoked at least 100 cigarettes in their lifetime.
   F. **Asymptomatic:** Most aneurysms are diagnosed incidentally on physical examination as palpable pulsatile mass in periumbilical region or on abdominal imaging.
   G. **Symptomatic:** may have symptoms from compression such as early satiety from duodenal compression, hydronephrosis from ureteral compression, or venous thrombosis from iliocaval compression
   1. **Small aneurysms:** may present with LE ischemic symptoms from distal embolization of thrombus present within the aneurysm sac
   2. **Ruptured aneurysms:** present with severe abdominal/back pain, tender pulsatile abdominal mass, and signs of shock

Table 7-2: Abdominal Aortic Aneurysm Rupture Risk

AAA Diameter (cm)	Rupture Risk (%/year)
<4	0
4–5	0.5–5
5–6	3–15
6–7	10–20
7–8	20–40
>8	30–50

AAA, abdominal aortic aneurysm.

H. Diagnosis: includes MRI and the following:
1. **Abdominal x-ray:** may show "egg shell sign" due to calcification of the aneurysm wall
2. **Abdominal ultrasound:** Valuable noninvasive tool for diagnosis, screening, and monitoring AAA. It is *not* useful in cases of ruptured aneurysm.
3. **Abdominal CT scan with contrast:** Gold standard diagnostic test; it accurately identifies the presence, size, and extent of aneurysm.

I. Indications for repair: any symptomatic AAA (irrespective of size), AAA with size 5.5 cm or greater (in female patients and those with Marfan syndrome, the size cutoff is 5 cm), and rapidly expanding aneurysm (i.e., >5 mm growth in 6 months)

J. Types of surgical repair: include the following:
1. **Endovascular repair:** performed via percutaneous access or femoral cutdown and requires the following specific anatomic criteria:
   a. **Aortic neck:** length (>15 mm), diameter that provides appropriate proximal sealing zone, and angle less than 60 degrees
   b. **Diameter of access arteries:** Common and external iliac artery should be sufficient to pass the delivery system.
   c. **Calcification:** should be less than 50% of aortic circumference in the proximal and distal seal zone to prevent endoleak (persistent blood flow outside the endoluminal graft but inside the walls of aneurysm sac)
2. **Open surgical repair:** can be performed either via midline transperitoneal or left retroperitoneal approach and involves opening the aneurysm sac and suturing the prosthetic graft to normal aorta. The aneurysm wall is then wrapped around the graft.

K. Postoperative complications: include the following:
1. **Acute renal failure:** Depending on the position of the clamp in open repair, risk is higher if clamp is supra- or juxtarenal. For all patients, also related to the administration of contrast dye.
2. **Acute LE ischemia:** Caused most commonly by distal embolization in open and access site complications in endovascular repair. *Requires emergent repair.*
3. **Ischemic colitis:** More commonly seen in sigmoid following ruptured AAA repair. Every attempt should be made to preserve the large inferior mesenteric artery (IMA). Can also occur with coverage of IMA during endovascular repair.
4. **Spinal cord ischemia:** Incidence is very low after infrarenal aortic aneurysm repair but higher with thoracoabdominal aortic aneurysm repair. Some factors related to spinal cord ischemia are duration of aortic cross-clamping, episodes of hypotension, and cholesterol embolization.

Quick Cut
All patients with an endovascular repair require lifelong surveillance.

Quick Cut
Endovascular repair has lower perioperative mortality as compared to open AAA repair.

Quick Cut
Bloody diarrhea after AAA repair is ischemic colitis until proven otherwise. Perform sigmoidoscopy to confirm and resect nonviable bowel promptly.

Quick Cut
Spinal cord ischemia may be related to interruption of the artery of Adamkiewicz, which arises between T8 and T12.

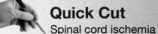

5. **Sexual dysfunction:** from injury to sympathetic nerves near aortic bifurcation
6. **Pelvic ischemia and gluteal claudication:** May be seen if both hypogastric arteries are ligated or covered with graft. Perfusion to one of the hypogastric arteries must be preserved.
7. **Endograft migration and endoleak:** associated with endovascular repair and can lead to increase in aneurysm size and eventual rupture.
8. **Aortic graft infection:** usually a late complication; may present decades after surgery
   a. **Presentation:** dull abdominal pain, fever, leukocytosis
   b. **Diagnosis:** CT scan shows presence of air and fluid collection around the graft.
   c. **Treatment:** consists of broad-spectrum antibiotics, removal of infected graft via open surgery, and reconstruction via extra-anatomic bypass

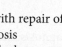
Quick Cut
The most common organism in aortic graft infection is *Staphylococcus aureus.*

9. **Aortoenteric fistula:** presents as gastrointestinal bleeding
   a. **Diagnosis:** endoscopy
   b. **Treatment:** graft explant and extra-anatomic bypass along with repair of enteric fistula
10. **Aneurysm or pseudoaneurysm:** at proximal or distal anastomosis
11. **Patients with open repair:** may have complications related to the laparotomy, such as adhesive small bowel obstruction or hernia formation

IV. **Splenic artery aneurysm:** Risk factors include female gender, multiple pregnancies, and portal HTN.
   A. **Clinical presentation:** Majority of patients are asymptomatic. Patients with rupture usually present with sharp pain, abdominal distension, and hemorrhagic shock. The aneurysm usually first ruptures in lesser sac followed by free intraperitoneal rupture (double rupture phenomenon).
   B. **Indications for repair:** symptomatic or ruptured aneurysm, size greater than 2 cm, and any size in a women of childbearing age
   C. **Endovascular treatment:** coil embolization or stenting across the aneurysm
   D. **Open surgical repair:** Proximal and distal ligation of splenic artery with or without aneurysmectomy; for aneurysms located in distal splenic artery, splenectomy is performed.

Quick Cut
Splenic artery aneurysms are the most common visceral aneurysms.

Quick Cut
The rate of splenic artery aneurysm rupture is greater than 90% with pregnancy.

V. **Popliteal artery aneurysms:** Mostly seen in men; 2.50% are bilateral.
   A. **Asymptomatic clinical presentation:** palpable pulsatile mass behind knee
   B. **Symptomatic:** Popliteal aneurysms can cause distal embolization, can compress nearby structures, or can acutely thrombose, resulting in acute lower leg ischemia.
   C. **Indications for repair:** symptomatic aneurysm of any size; asymptomatic aneurysm greater than 2.5 cm in diameter
   D. **Mode of repair:** Patients who present with acute limb ischemia are started on therapeutic anticoagulation. *Emergent arteriography is performed.*
   1. **Open repair:** ligation of aneurysm and arterial bypass or excision of aneurysm and interposition graft to restore distal circulation
   2. **Endovascular repair:** Newer treatment option when anatomy is feasible; most surgeons reserve this form of treatment for patients who are high operative risk.
   3. **Thrombolysis:** Consider in stable patient with intact sensory and motor function but must be followed by staged, definitive repair.

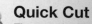
Quick Cut
One third of patients with popliteal aneurysms also have AAA.

MESENTERIC VASCULAR DISEASE

Anatomy
I. **Main blood supply:** celiac axis, superior mesenteric artery (SMA), IMA
II. **Collateral circulation:** pancreaticoduodenal between celiac and SMA; marginal artery between IMA and SMA

Quick Cut
The marginal artery of Drummond and the arc of Riolan are the collateral arcades between the SMA and the IMA.

Acute Mesenteric Ischemia

I. **Epidemiology:** Patients tend to be elderly with significant comorbidities.

II. **Classification:** based on etiology

A. **Cardiac source (atrial fibrillation):** most common cause of embolic occlusion of mesenteric vessels. The emboli usually lodge distal to the origin of proximal jejunal branches and middle colic artery, which spares the proximal jejunum and ascending colon.

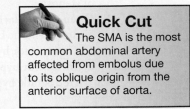

Quick Cut
The SMA is the most common abdominal artery affected from embolus due to its oblique origin from the anterior surface of aorta.

B. **Acute thrombosis:** In 20% of cases, pre-existing severe atherosclerotic stenotic lesion thrombosis is seen. The entire small and large bowel supplied by SMA is affected, as the origin of vessel is occluded.

C. **Nonocclusive mesenteric ischemia:** Due to diffuse mesenteric vasospasm in absence of arterial or venous occlusion. Most commonly seen in patients with severe cardiopulmonary insufficiency and shock.

D. **Mesenteric venous thrombosis:** Involves thrombosis of superior mesenteric vein with or without extension into portal or splenic vein. It can be spontaneous or secondary to abdominal injury, hypercoaguable states, inflammation, or infection.

III. **Clinical presentation:** Peritonitis is seen late once infarction of bowel occurs.

IV. **Diagnosis:** High index of suspicion along with prompt treatment before bowel infarction sets in is key to prevent mortality.

Quick Cut
Pain out of proportion is the classic physical examination finding in mesenteric ischemia.

A. **Plain abdominal x-rays:** may show ileus in early cases of mesenteric ischemia or pneumatosis in advanced cases

B. **Duplex ultrasound of mesenteric vessels:** Useful in identifying stenoses of celiac and SMA. It is mostly used in chronic mesenteric ischemia.

C. **CTA:** good to assess the patency of mesenteric arteries and vein and also useful in assessing the state of the bowel and other intra-abdominal pathology

D. **Mesenteric angiogram:** provides diagnosis and potential treatment such as angioplasty and stent, thrombolysis, or injection of vasodilator agents

V. **Treatment:** depends on the etiology of acute mesenteric ischemia

A. **Bowel infarction:** All patients need exploratory laparotomy and resection of nonviable bowel. Usually, a second look laparotomy is performed within 24 hours to ensure viability of residual bowel.

B. **Embolism:** Embolectomy is performed; postprocedure, therapeutic anticoagulation is mandatory.

C. **Acute arterial thrombosis:** Aortomesenteric bypass is performed.

D. **Nonocclusive mesenteric ischemia:** usually treated with supportive care including bowel rest, antibiotics, and fluid resuscitation. Surgical exploration is indicated if peritonitis develops.

E. **Mesenteric venous thrombosis:** systemic anticoagulation; operation if bowel necrosis occurs

Chronic Mesenteric Ischemia

I. **Etiology:** Seen in patients with slowly progressive stenosis/occlusion of origin of mesenteric vessels. Atherosclerosis is the most common etiology.

II. **Pathophysiology:** In normal individuals, blood flow to intestine increases 30–90 minutes after food ingestion. This increased blood flow is required for metabolism and absorption.

Quick Cut
In chronic mesenteric ischemia, the postprandial hyperemic response is attenuated, resulting in "mesenteric angina."

III. **Clinical presentation:** Most commonly seen in middle-aged women with a long history of smoking. Patients are usually cachectic with typical symptoms of postprandial epigastric pain, fear of food, and weight loss.

IV. **Diagnosis:** Modalities include the following:

A. **Mesenteric duplex ultrasound:** screening tool with greater than 80% sensitivity and specificity

B. **CTA:** diagnostic modality of choice for chronic mesenteric ischemia

C. **Mesenteric angiogram:** Gold standard diagnostic tool. If a stenosis is amenable to endovascular intervention, it can be performed at same time.

V. **Treatment:** All patients with chronic mesenteric ischemia must undergo revascularization to prevent bowel infarction and to improve nutritional status.
   A. **Endovascular revascularization:** involves balloon angioplasty and stent placement across the area of stenosis
   B. **Open revascularization:** performed either by transaortic mesenteric endarterectomy or by aortomesenteric bypass
      1. **Conduit for bypass procedure:** can be prosthetic graft or greater saphenous vein
      2. **Inflow for bypass:** Can be supraceliac aorta (antegrade bypass) or infrarenal aorta or iliacs (retrograde bypass). Usually both celiac and SMA are bypassed beyond the area of occlusion.

RENAL ARTERY STENOSIS

General Aspects

I. **Definition:** Renovascular HTN is defined as systemic HTN resulting from renal arterial compromise.

II. **Diagnosis:** Renal artery stenosis (RAS) is suspected as cause with abrupt onset or exacerbation of chronic HTN, adults on multiple antihypertensive medications with modest control of blood pressure, angiotensin-converting enzyme (ACE) inhibitor–induced azotemia, flash pulmonary edema out of proportion to left ventricular failure, and HTN in children.

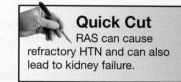

Quick Cut
RAS can cause refractory HTN and can also lead to kidney failure.

III. **Pathophysiology of renovascular HTN:** Stenosis at the level of the renal artery is sensed by receptors in kidney, which secretes renin. Renin increases angiotensin, which causes vasoconstriction and also stimulates the adrenal cortex to secrete aldosterone. Aldosterone increases blood volume and increase blood pressure (Fig. 7-6).

IV. **Etiology of RAS:** associated risk factors for atherosclerosis
   A. **Atherosclerosis:** involves the ostium or proximal one third of renal artery; bilateral involvement, males greater than females
   B. **Fibromuscular dysplasia:** Younger women; involves middle or distal portion of renal artery. Right side greater than left side; 30% of cases bilateral. These lesions respond very well to endovascular intervention, with greater than 75% cure of HTN at 1 year.

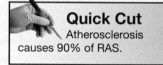

Quick Cut
Atherosclerosis causes 90% of RAS.

   C. **Other causes:** traumatic or spontaneous dissection or disruption, vasculitis, thromboembolic disease, renal artery aneurysm, extrinsic compression, radiation injury

V. **Clinical presentation:** Asymptomatic RAS is diagnosed incidentally; symptomatic presents with sudden worsening of renal failure, sudden worsening of previously controlled HTN, or sudden-onset HTN.

Diagnosis and Treatment

I. **Functional tests:** include the following:
   A. **Captopril scintigraphy:** noninvasive test that uses technetium-99m–labeled diethylene triamine pentaacetic acid (DTPA) along with administration of the ACE inhibitor, captopril; sensitivity = 75% and specificity = 90%

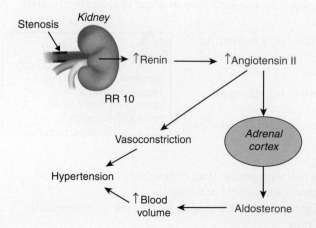

Figure 7-6: Pathophysiology of renovascular hypertension. Renal artery stenosis activates the renin-angiotensin system, which produces aldosterone. Elevated blood volume and vasoconstriction translate into elevated blood pressures.

B. **Renal vein renin assay:** invasive test that documents the contribution of each kidney to plasma renin

II. **Anatomic imaging tests:** include the following:
  A. **Duplex ultrasound evaluation of renal arteries:** Initial diagnostic modality of choice. Painless, noninvasive, no exposure to ionizing radiation or nephrotoxic contrast agent, low cost, and had sensitivity of 85% and specificity of greater than 90%.
  B. **CTA and MRA:** Less invasive, expensive, need for IV contrast. CTA carries the risk of radiation exposure, and MRA overestimates the degree of stenosis.
  C. **Conventional renal angiography:** Gold standard test of choice for diagnosis of RAS. Invasive procedure with need for IV contrast and potential contrast-induced nephropathy. Has an advantage that therapeutic intervention can be performed at same time.

III. **Treatment:** include the following:
  A. **Percutaneous angioplasty and stent placement:** Minimally invasive procedure for treatment of stenosis located at proximal or midportion of renal artery. The preferred mode of treatment when applicable. May require bilateral treatment for effective cure of HTN.

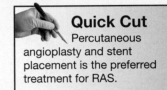

Quick Cut
Percutaneous angioplasty and stent placement is the preferred treatment for RAS.

  B. **Aortorenal bypass:** using either autogenous (reversed saphenous vein) or prosthetic conduit (e.g., PTFE)
  C. **Thromboendarterectomy of renal artery:** old technique; seldom used
  D. **Nephrectomy:** in patients with unilateral disease (small and nonfunctioning kidney) and functional contralateral kidney

MISCELLANEOUS

Raynaud Phenomenon

I. **Characteristics:** Episodic, exaggerated vasospastic response to cold or emotional stimuli, typically seen in fingers. Affected digits show a classic series of color changes, initial pallor (due to vasospasm), followed by cyanosis (due to deoxygenation of the static blood), and then by rubor (due to reactive hyperemia from restoration of blood flow).

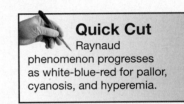

Quick Cut
Raynaud phenomenon progresses as white-blue-red for pallor, cyanosis, and hyperemia.

  A. **Primary Raynaud phenomenon (Raynaud disease):** seen in an otherwise healthy individual with no underlying disease
  B. **Secondary Raynaud phenomenon:** associated with an underlying systemic disease (mostly autoimmune disorders like scleroderma, systemic lupus erythematosus, giant cell arteritis, etc.)

II. **Management:** Lifestyle modification includes avoidance of cold and emotional stress, smoking cessation, and discontinuation of vasoconstricting substances such as caffeine and cocaine.
  A. **Medical treatment:** includes calcium channel blockers
  B. **Surgical sympathectomy:** limited to severe or refractory cases

Giant Cell Arteritis (Temporal Arteritis)

I. **Characteristics:** Large vessel vasculitis affecting the aorta and the extracranial branches of the carotid artery. Typically affects older women of northern European descent.

II. **Clinical presentation:** Constitutional symptoms such as fever and fatigue; jaw claudication is characteristic symptom and may have ocular symptoms.

III. **Diagnosis:** Temporal artery biopsy is the standard.

IV. **Treatment:** medical with corticosteroids

Takayasu Disease

I. **Characteristics:** Large vessel vasculitis affecting aorta and its major branches and pulmonary artery. Affects young females; commonly seen among Asians.

II. **Clinical presentation:** constitutional symptoms such as fever, myalgia, and weight loss; vessel inflammation resulting in vessel pain/tenderness and vessel fibrosis and aneurysmal degeneration

   III. Diagnosis: DSA is the gold standard.

   IV. Medical management: consists of immunosuppression with corticosteroids as first line of treatment

   V. Revascularization: should be performed when disease activity is minimal

Thromboangiitis Obliterans/Buerger Disease

   I. Characteristics: Affects small- and medium-sized arteries and veins of extremities; characterized by normal proximal pulses but diminished distal pulses. Strong association with smoking and more commonly seen in young males.

   II. Presentation: Patient presents with ischemic symptoms such as claudication or paresthesias.

   III. Angiography: Corkscrew collaterals around the area of occlusion may be seen.

   IV. Treatment: Main effective therapy is smoking cessation.

Chapter 8

Venous and Lymphatic Disease

Edwin Kendrick and Rajabrata Sarkar

ACUTE DEEP VENOUS THROMBOSIS

Epidemiology

I. **Incidence:** Cases of recurrent, fatal, and nonfatal deep venous thrombosis (DVT) exceed 900,000 cases annually in the United States.
   A. **Untreated proximal DVT:** associated with a 30%–50% risk for pulmonary embolism (PE) and a 12% mortality rate
   B. **DVT without prophylaxis:** Overall incidence is <20% in general surgical patients, 25% in elective neurosurgical patients, and nearly 50%–60% in patients undergoing orthopedic surgery.

II. **Pathophysiology:** Virchow triad
   A. **Hemodynamic changes:** stasis or turbulence
   B. **Hypercoagulability**
   C. **Endothelial abnormality**

> **Quick Cut**
> 30% of DVT patients experience a recurrence in a 10-year time span.

> **Quick Cut**
> Almost 1 million DVT are diagnosed in the United States annually.

Clinical Findings

I. **Signs and symptoms:** lower extremity pain, pain on passive dorsiflexion (Homans sign), edema, erythema, local warmth, prominent superficial veins, and peripheral cyanosis

II. **Locations of thrombosis:** include iliofemoral, calf, and upper limb deep veins as well as ovarian, renal, mesenteric, hepatic, and retinal veins; vena cava; and cerebral venous thrombosis

> **Quick Cut**
> The Virchow triad is stasis, coagulopathy, and endothelial injury.

> **Quick Cut**
> Up to 50% of DVT patients are asymptomatic, and DVT may be unidentifiable with imaging.

Diagnostic Tests

I. **Duplex ultrasonography (US):** replaced contrast venography (CV) as the diagnostic test of choice
   A. **Function:** It may distinguish among vascular and nonvascular pathologies (i.e., adenopathy, Baker cyst, and hematoma).
   B. **Benefits:** lack of radiation, portability, noninvasiveness, and relative cost-effectiveness

II. **D-dimers:** Degradation products of cross-linked fibrin. Its high sensitivity makes its major clinical usage *exclusion* of a DVT diagnosis on the basis of a negative result. An elevated D-dimer is nonspecific.

> **Quick Cut**
> D-dimer may be used as a screening test for DVT.

III. **Magnetic resonance venography (MRV):** Has the greatest sensitivity and specificity in imaging iliac, pelvic, and central vein thrombosis compared to CV or US. Disadvantages include

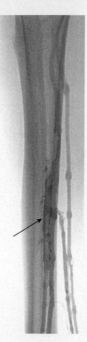

Figure 8-1: DVT, contrast venogram. Intraluminal filling defect outlined by contrast (*arrow*) diagnostic for acute DVT on a lower extremity venogram. (From Geschwind JF, Dake MD. *Abrams' Angiography*, 3rd ed. Philadelphia: Lippincott Williams & Wilkins; 2013.)

relative cost, patient cooperation (claustrophobia), study time required, and gadolinium-associated nephrogenic systemic fibrosis (seen in renal failure patients).

IV. **CV:** Figure 8-1
  A. **Uses:** used historically as a "golden backup" in cases of initial diagnostic uncertainty
  B. **Disadvantages:** include radiation exposure, contrast nephrotoxicity, allergic reactions, radiation exposure, phlebitis, and increased cost

Initial Treatment

I. **Objective:** prevent PE and propagation of the DVT

II. **Anticoagulation:** Acute DVTs should be treated with low-molecular-weight heparin (LMWH), fondaparinux, or unfractionated heparin (UFH) and warfarin as soon as the diagnosis is confirmed by objective imaging techniques or until the diagnosis can be confirmed if clinical suspicion is very high.

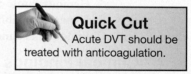

Quick Cut
Acute DVT should be treated with anticoagulation.

  A. **After a 5- to 10-day overlap of anticoagulation:** Warfarin remains the sole therapy when the international normalized ratio (INR) is within the target (2.0–3.0) for at least 24 hours.
  B. **Anticoagulation 3 months with compression therapy:** recommended if it is the first DVT, a proximal DVT, a surgery-provoked DVT, or due to a nonsurgical transient risk factor
  C. **Longer therapy:** recommended for an unprovoked DVT, recurrent DVT, prior PE, or active cancer (use LMWH)
  D. **Disadvantage:** Bleeding risk is associated with usage of all anticoagulants. Approximate bleeding risks with LMWH include postoperative bleeding (6%), major hemorrhage (3%), and wound hematoma (4%).

III. **Inferior vena cava (IVC) filter:** Figure 8-2
  A. **Uses:** In patients with DVT who cannot be anticoagulated (e.g., recent neurologic surgery, ongoing bleeding, etc.), place a filter immediately to prevent PE.

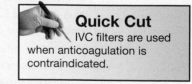

Quick Cut
IVC filters are used when anticoagulation is contraindicated.

  B. **Retrieval:** Consideration should be given to placement of a retrievable filter, which can be removed once the risk of PE is subsequently decreased.

Additional Therapy

I. **Goal:** directed at removal of the thrombus to preserve venous valve function and prevent long-term complications such as post-thrombotic syndrome (PTS). This therapy is reserved for good risk, active younger patients without contraindications to thrombolytic therapy (e.g., recent surgery or bleeding).

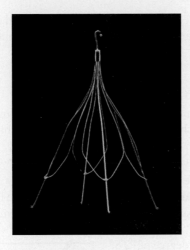

Figure 8-2: Retrievable IVC filter. Note the retrieval at the upper end of the filter. The filter has four "petals" for centering in the IVC.

II. **Thrombolysis**
A. **Catheter-directed thrombolysis (CDT) with tissue plasminogen activator agents:** indicated for iliofemoral DVTs (Fig. 8-3)
B. **Pharmacomechanical thrombolysis (CDT with mechanical thrombectomy):** effective option with an anticipated 75%–90% success rate of rapid recanalization of the venous system. Disadvantages include bleeding (5%–11%) and the need for anticoagulation to prevent immediate rethrombosis.

III. **Operative venous thrombectomy:** Infrainguinal balloon catheter thrombectomy is used in patients with worsening venous edema or venous gangrene in whom thrombolysis is not possible. Disadvantages include invasiveness of the procedure with general anesthesia and the need for anticoagulation to prevent immediate rethrombosis.

Prevention

I. **Leg elevation:** has a dual physiologic effect; it reduces swelling (improving venous return) and venous pressure (gravitational effect)

II. **Mechanical**
A. **Graduated compression stockings:** reduce the cross-sectional area of the veins and increase the velocity of venous blood flow (50% reduction in PTS development)
B. **Intermittent pneumatic compression (IPC):** improves venous hemodynamics and stimulates fibrinolytic activity
C. **Foot compression devices:** indicated in patients with a high risk for venous thromboembolism (VTE) in whom the use of anticoagulants and IPCs are contraindicated

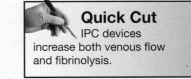

Quick Cut
IPC devices increase both venous flow and fibrinolysis.

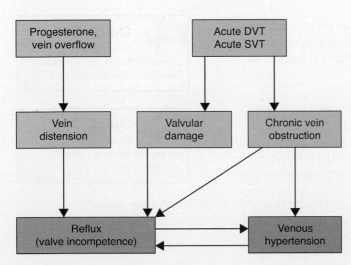

Figure 8-3: Post-thrombotic syndrome. Etiopathogeny of chronic venous insufficiency and its relation to post-thrombotic syndrome. (From Geschwind JF, Dake MD. *Abrams' Angiography*, 3rd ed. Philadelphia: Lippincott Williams & Wilkins; 2013.)

III. Pharmacologic: Anticoagulation with LMWH, UFH, or fondaparinux is the standard of care for VTE prevention in surgical and medical patients. Rivaroxaban is now licensed in the United States for VTE prevention after hip or knee arthroplasty.

Complications

I. **Acute complications**
   A. **Phlegmasia alba dolens: nonischemic limb** with massive pitting edema and blanching
   B. **Phlegmasia cerulea dolens:** reversible phase of ischemic venous occlusion (painful blue leg) with predisposition for limb loss
   C. **Venous gangrene:** irreversible phase of ischemic venous occlusion

II. **Chronic complication:** Post Thrombotic Syndrome (PTS)
   A. **Clinical manifestations of venous hypertension and valvular dysfunction:** include limb swelling, limb fatigue or pain, venous claudication, pigmentation (dermatoliposclerosis), eczema, erythema, or frank ulceration of the skin
   B. **Incidence:** <40% of DVT patients will have some degree of PTS, and 4% will develop severe manifestations with ulceration.
   C. **Consequences:** decreased physical activity abilities and a lower quality of life

Quick Cut
Severe PTS may be treated with iliac vein stenting.

   D. **Therapy:** includes elevation of extremity at rest/night, pain management, compression therapy, wound care, and angioplasty/stenting of iliac vein stenosis (present in 50%–75% of PTS patients)

Anticoagulation Therapy Complications

I. **Heparin-induced thrombocytopenia:** antibody response against neoantigens expressed on platelet factor 4 (PF4) upon binding to heparin
   A. **Clinical diagnosis:** thrombocytopenia, thrombosis, or both during or immediately after heparin use
   B. **Laboratory diagnosis:** heparin-induced platelet aggregation assays, heparin antibody test, and serotonin release assay
   C. **Treatment:** immediate cessation of *all forms* of heparin and rapid initiation of a direct thrombin inhibitor (e.g., argatroban, lepirudin, or bivalirudin) for anticoagulation

Quick Cut
Heparin is so commonly used that it may be overlooked, such as in intravenous flushes.

Quick Cut
Caution—warfarin alone is not protective for HIT and can result in severe thrombotic complications.

II. **Bleeding risk:** See the sections "Anticoagulation" and "Thrombolysis."

III. **Osteoporosis:** LMWH and UFH

◆ ACUTE PULMONARY EMBOLISM

Epidemiology and Etiology

I. **Incidence:** Occurs in <650,000 American patients annually and accounts for up to 15% of all in-hospital deaths. Approximately 50%–80% of symptomatic DVT patients have evidence of an asymptomatic PE.

Quick Cut
The initial presentation of PE is sudden death in 25% of cases.

II. **Etiology**
   A. **Thrombotic embolism:** Approximately 90% arise from the lower extremity veins; major risk factors include previous VTE, surgery, trauma, malignancy, chemotherapy, chronic heart or respiratory failure, paralytic stroke, hypercoagulability, pregnancy, and hormone/contraceptive therapy.

Quick Cut
Most pulmonary emboli arise from lower extremity veins.

   B. **Nonthrombotic PE:** With the exception of severe air and fat embolism, the hemodynamic consequences are usually mild. Treatment is mostly supportive but may differ according to the type of embolic material and clinical severity.

Clinical Findings

I. **Asymptomatic PE:** reported in high frequency in DVT patients

II. **Symptomatic PE:** Severity depends on the amount of occluded pulmonary circulation and the patient's underlying cardiopulmonary reserve.

III. **Poor prognostic indicators:** marked dyspnea, anxiety, and low oxygen saturation; elevated troponin (indicating right ventricular [RV] microinfarction, RV dysfunction on echocardiography, or RV enlargement on chest computed tomography [CT] scan)

IV. **Hemodynamic compromise and death:** results from an increase in pulmonary artery pressure with acute RV failure; decreased left ventricular stroke volume, cardiac output, and organ perfusion; and hypotension

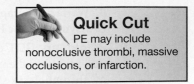

Quick Cut
PE may include nonocclusive thrombi, massive occlusions, or infarction.

Diagnostic Tests

I. **D-dimer:** Negative D-dimer safely excludes PE in patients with a low or moderate clinical probability (99% negative predictive); an elevated D-dimer is nonspecific.

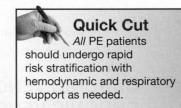

Quick Cut
As with DVT, a negative D-dimer virtually excludes a diagnosis of PE.

II. **CT:** Multidetector computed tomography (MDCT) or computed tomography angiography (CTA) showing a thrombus up to the segmental level can be taken as adequate evidence of PE in most instances (Fig. 8-4). In patients with a low or moderate clinical probability, a negative MDCT or CTA should be combined with a compression ultrasonography.

III. **Compression ultrasonography (CUS):** Lower extremity CUS is used to reduce the overall false-negative rate of CT in suspected PE patients. CUS yields a positive proximal DVT result in <20% of patients with PE.

IV. **Ventilation-perfusion scintigraphy (V/Q scan):** Normal perfusion scan is safe for excluding PE. A high-probability V/Q scan may establish the diagnosis of PE in patients with a high degree of suspicion.

V. **Pulmonary angiography:** reliable but invasive clinically useful test when MDCT/CTA and CUS results are both negative in patients with a high suspicion for PE

VI. **Echocardiography:** helpful in emergency situations such as shock or hypotension; it serves for further prognostic stratification but is not diagnostic for PE

Initial Treatment

I. **Anticoagulation:** initiated without delay in patients with confirmed acute PE and those with a high or intermediate clinical probability of an acute PE while the diagnostic workup continues

Quick Cut
All PE patients should undergo rapid risk stratification with hemodynamic and respiratory support as needed.

A. **Initial treatment with LMWH, UFH, or fondaparinux and warfarin:** should continue for at least 5 days and until the INR is greater than or equal to 2.0 for at least 24 hours

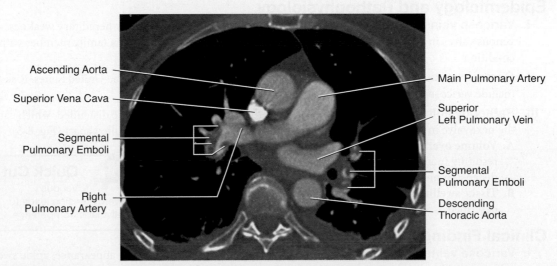

Figure 8-4: Pulmonary embolism. CT axial images of pulmonary embolus.

    B. Warfarin therapy: should continue for at least 3 months

    C. Asymptomatic PE: Identical initial and long-term anticoagulation is recommended.

  II. **Pulmonary CDT or systemic thrombolysis:** first-line treatment in hemodynamic compromised patients unless there are major contraindications

    A. Thrombolysis: should not be delayed because irreversible cardiogenic shock may ensue

    B. Risks: invasiveness, major bleeding (13%), and intracranial/fatal hemorrhage (1.8%)

  III. **Percutaneous catheter embolectomy:** mechanical embolectomy or fragmentation of proximal pulmonary arterial clots; recommended in hemodynamic compromised patients with contraindications for thrombolysis or when thrombolysis failed

  IV. **Surgical pulmonary embolectomy:** recommended in hemodynamic compromised patients with contraindications for thrombolysis or when thrombolysis failed

Prevention

  I. **IVC filters:** should not be placed routinely in patients receiving anticoagulant therapy

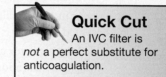

Quick Cut
An IVC filter is *not* a perfect substitute for anticoagulation.

    A. Anticoagulant therapy contraindicated: Filters may be placed in these patients with acute PE.

    B. If the risk of bleeding resolves: Patients with filters should receive a conventional course of anticoagulant therapy.

  II **Risks**

    A. Early complications: insertion site thrombosis (10%), bleeding, and vessel perforation

    B. Late complications: recurrent DVT (20%), PTS (40%), and vena cava occlusion in 33% of patients in 10 years, regardless of the use and duration of anticoagulation

Chronic Complication

  I. **Chronic thromboembolic pulmonary hypertension (CTEPH):** Pulmonary vascular remodeling may cause severe pulmonary hypertension out of proportion to pulmonary vascular thrombosis (a severe and rare consequence of PE).

  II. **Medical management:** associated with poor outcomes

  III. **Pulmonary thromboendarterectomy:** provides excellent results and should be considered as first-line treatment whenever possible

  IV **Management:** Patients should have lifelong anticoagulant treatment targeted to an INR of 2.0–3.0.

CHRONIC VENOUS DISORDERS: VARICOSE VEINS AND CHRONIC VENOUS INSUFFICIENCY

Epidemiology and Pathophysiology

  I. **Varicose veins:** Prevalence is 5%–30% in the adult population; caused by hereditary weakness of the venous valves in the superficial veins of the legs. Most patients can identify a family member with the condition.

  II. **Chronic venous insufficiency (CVI)** Present in <5 million people in the United States. Risk factors include varicose veins, family history of varicose veins, and prior DVT.

  III. **Pathophysiology:** With venous valve failure, the superficial veins become distended, which causes the next valve in the vein to become incompetent as the valve leaflets are pulled apart (Fig. 8-5).

    A. Volume overload: causes distention of the deep system, with resulting incompetence of the deep venous valves by the same distension process

Quick Cut
Venous overdistension leads to valvular incompetence.

    B. Tissue swelling: irritates adjacent nerves, causing pain, commonly described as a throbbing ache relieved by elevation of the limb

Clinical Findings

  I. **Varicose veins:** Most common complaints are a cosmetically displeasing appearance, ankle swelling, calf vein and localized cutaneous pigmentation, eczema, and limb heaviness or ache that occurs after prolonged standing.

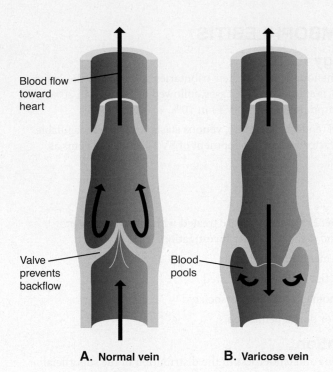

A. Normal vein   **B. Varicose vein**

Blood flow toward heart

Valve prevents backflow

Blood pools

Figure 8-5: Varicose veins. Many older people, particularly women, have varicose veins. **A:** In a healthy vein, the valves help blood to flow back toward the heart and prevent it from pooling. **B:** In varicose veins, the valves no longer function properly, allowing the blood to pool. (From Carter PJ. *Lippincott Textbook for Nursing Assistants*, 3rd ed. Philadelphia: Lippincott Williams & Wilkins; 2011.)

II **Phlebitis:** Stasis in the varicose veins predisposes to phlebitis, which causes pain, swelling, and discomfort; it does not embolize to cause PE, but ascending phlebitis of the greater or short saphenous vein can propagate into the deep venous system and cause DVT.

III. **CVI:** Patients may be incapacitated by venous claudication or have severe skin pigmentation changes and ulceration.

Diagnosis

I. **Physical examination:** Examining the great saphenous vein (GSV) and small saphenous vein (SSV) in the standing and Trendelenburg positions accurately identifies the presence of venous disease in the vast majority of patients.

II. **Duplex US:** used for detection of venous reflux disease in chronic venous disorder patients; widely adopted as a standard of care because of its precision and reproducibility

III. **Ambulatory venous pressure (AVP):** Venous pressure in a dorsal foot vein is measured after the execution of 10 tiptoe maneuvers in a standing position.

IV. **Plethysmography:** noninvasive method of estimating changes in volume in an extremity when assessing for CVI

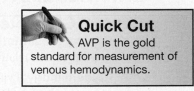

Quick Cut
AVP is the gold standard for measurement of venous hemodynamics.

Treatment and Prevention

I. **CEAP (clinical, etiologic, anatomic, pathophysiologic) classification:** standardized system for evaluating venous insufficiency

II. **Primary benefit:** Venous interventions can confer long-term improvement in symptoms and ulcer recurrence.

III. **Therapeutic options:** based on clinical assessment and classification

A. **No treatment**

B. **Traditional therapy:** conservative management with compression stockings, skin care, and lifestyle changes

C. **Surgical therapy:** Endovenous ablation (i.e., laser or thermal); sclerotherapy; a combination of venous ligation, axial stripping, and stab phlebectomy. Venous angioplasty and stenting is performed in selected patients with advanced CVI who have recurrent ulceration or swelling with severe and disabling symptoms.

SUPERFICIAL VENOUS THROMBOPHLEBITIS

Epidemiology and Pathophysiology

I. **Etiology:** most commonly occurs in the saphenous veins and their tributaries, followed by the upper extremity cephalic and basilic veins. The GSV is affected in 70% cases, followed by the SSV in 20% and bilateral lower extremity superficial venous thrombophlebitis (SVT) in 10%.

II. **Pathophysiology:** Related to Virchow triad (endothelial injury, venous stasis, and hypercoagulable states). The most common predisposing risk factor for the development of SVT is varicose veins as discussed earlier.

Clinical Types

I. **SVT with varicose veins**

II. **SVT of superficial extremity veins:** Upper extremity SVT are treated with NSAIDs. Lower extremity SVT raise the possibility of DVT, and demand further investigation.

III. **Traumatic thrombophlebitis:** catheter or medication induced

IV. **Septic and suppurative thrombophlebitis:** infection associated

V. **Migratory thrombophlebitis:** often carcinoma or vasculitis associated

VI. **Mondor disease:** SVT of the breast, chest, or dorsal penile vein

Diagnosis, Treatment, and Prevention

I. **Diagnosis:** based on the presence of erythema and tenderness in the distribution of the superficial veins with a palpable cord (thrombosis)

II. **Therapy:** aimed at preventing potential serious complications such as propagation to DVT/PE, preventing recurrence of SVT, and decreasing pain and acute inflammation

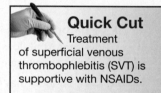

Quick Cut
Treatment of superficial venous thrombophlebitis (SVT) is supportive with NSAIDs.

   A. **Traditional treatment:** ambulation, warm soaks, and nonsteroidal anti-inflammatory drugs (NSAIDs)

   B. **Serial duplex scans:** used in patients with phlebitis of the GSV or SSV where the possibility of proximal propagation to DVT is possible

   C. **Anticoagulation:** indicated in extensive SVT or SVT in the GSV or SSV that is ascending toward the deep system

   D. **Surgical excision:** plays a role in suppurative thrombophlebitis where infection is suspected or confirmed

LYMPHEDEMA

General Characteristics

I. **Clinical presentation:** characterized by the interstitial accumulation of protein-enriched fluid as a consequence of relative impairment of lymphatic drainage

II **Epidemiology:** Lymphatic outflow dysfunction may result from either primary or acquired (secondary) anomalies.

   A. **Primary lymphedema:** Females are affected 2- to 10-fold more commonly than males. Peaks are classified based on genetics (familial vs. sporadic) and time of onset (congenital, praecox, tarda).

   1. **Congenital:** Onset is before age 1 year and may be familial (**Milroy disease**) or nonfamilial.

   2. **Lymphedema praecox:** Onset is from age 1 to 35 years and may be familial (**Meige disease**) or nonfamilial.

   3. **Lymphedema tarda:** Onset is after age 35 years.

   B. **Secondary lymphedema:** most common form of lymphatic disease

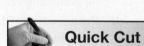

Quick Cut
Lymphedema secondary to intervention or infection is far more common than primary lymphatic disease.

   1. **Developed countries:** Iatrogenic causes predominate as consequence of lymphatic trauma or dissection, cancer, or radiotherapy for cancer (e.g., breast cancer). Other causes include large burns, pregnancy, and bacterial and fungal infections.

   2. **Developing countries:** Filariasis (parasitic infestation with the *Wuchereria bancrofti*) is the most frequent cause of secondary lymphedema (**elephantiasis**).

III. **Pathophysiology:** Lymphatic circulation provides the normal conduit for return of interstitial fluid and protein to the central circulation. Lymphedema will ensue if the production of lymph exceeds the maximal transport capacity of the lymphatic conduits. Accumulation of protein and cellular metabolites in the extracellular space generates water accumulation, collagen deposition, and elevated interstitial pressure.

IV. **Clinical findings:** depend largely on the duration and severity of the disease
   A. **Edema:** extends to the distal aspects of the feet, resulting in "**square toes**" (**Stemmer sign**), which is pathognomonic for the loss of cutaneous elasticity with an inability to tent the skin of the interdigital web space
   B. **Skin changes**
      1. **Acute:** Skin is usually a pinkish red color with a mildly elevated temperature.
      2. **Chronic:** results in thickened skin with areas of hyperkeratosis, lichenification, and development of *peau d'orange*
   C. **Pain:** Aching or heaviness of the limb is the most frequent complaint; significant pain is rare.

Diagnosis

I. **Clinical presentation, history, and physical findings:** Often establish the diagnosis. Diagnosis is difficult in the early stages when edema is mild or intermittent.

II. **Physical examination:** inspection for cutaneous and subcutaneous fibrosis, *peau d'orange*, and Stemmer sign

III. **Lymphoscintigraphy:** reliable and reproducible method to confirm the diagnosis. A radiolabeled macromolecular tracer is injected within one of the interdigital spaces of the affected limb.

Treatment, Prevention, and Complications

I. **Treatment:** Nonsurgical management options should be considered initially.
   A. **Mechanical reduction:** elevation, therapeutic exercise, manual massage, and compression therapy (i.e., wraps, pumps, or garments)
   B. **Surgical therapy:** should be considered only after a trial of conservative therapy

II. **Preventive measures:** skin hygiene, clothing precautions, trauma avoidance, and infection control

III. **Complications:** infection, malnutrition and immunodeficiency (loss of protein, triglycerides, lymphocytes, etc.), and malignancy (i.e., development of lymphangiosarcoma after radiation therapy in breast cancer patients with resultant long-standing arm edema)

Study Questions for Part III

Directions: *Each of the numbered items in this section is followed by several possible answers. Select the ONE lettered answer that is BEST in each case.*

1. A 65-year-old woman with a long history of atrial fibrillation presents to the emergency department with a history of sudden onset of severe, constant abdominal pain. After the onset of pain, she vomited once and had a large bowel movement. No flatus has been passed since that time. Physical examination reveals a mildly distended abdomen, which is diffusely tender, although peritoneal signs are absent. Ten years ago, she underwent an abdominal hysterectomy. What is the most likely diagnosis in this patient?

   A. Acute cholecystitis
   B. Perforated duodenal ulcer
   C. Acute diverticulitis
   D. Acute embolic mesenteric ischemia
   E. Small bowel obstruction secondary to adhesions

2. A 60-year-old woman develops weakness in her right arm and leg, and she has some difficulty speaking. This condition resolves after 5 minutes, and she has no residual symptoms. Her physician does not hear a carotid bruit, and her electrocardiogram is normal. A carotid duplex ultrasound shows a 75% stenosis of the left carotid artery and an 80% stenosis of the right carotid artery; both are confirmed by a carotid arteriogram. What should be the next step in the management of this patient?

   A. Right carotid endarterectomy
   B. Left carotid endarterectomy
   C. Superficial temporal artery to middle cerebral artery bypass
   D. Percutaneous transluminal angioplasty of the left carotid artery
   E. Bilateral carotid endarterectomy

Questions 3–4

A 70-year-old man who is a new patient presents with a history of insulin-dependent diabetes mellitus; renal insufficiency (serum creatinine, 2.5); chronic obstructive pulmonary disease; and two myocardial infarctions, the most recent being 1 year ago. His ejection fraction is 35%, and he has a right below-the-knee amputation, which he says was secondary to "peripheral vascular disease." Now, the patient has a large pulsatile nontender abdominal mass.

3. All of the following studies would be appropriate *except*:

   A. CT scan of the abdomen
   B. Pulmonary function tests
   C. Arteriogram
   D. Colonoscopy
   E. Persantine thallium scan

His workup demonstrates a 6-cm infrarenal abdominal aortic aneurysm with a 4-cm left common iliac artery aneurysm and normal renal arteries. He has normal external iliac arteries bilaterally, with relatively normal femoral vessels. Pulmonary function tests indicate a forced expiratory volume in 1 second (FEV_1) to be 75% of the predicted value. The Persantine thallium scan shows an old scar but no reperfusion defect.

4. What is the next step in this patient's management?

    A. Letting the patient live with the aneurysm because he is too high a surgical risk for elective surgery

    B. Checking the size of the aneurysm with ultrasound every year until it starts to enlarge

    C. Not performing surgery until he develops back pain because he is currently asymptomatic

    D. Performing an aortobiiliac bypass

    E. Repairing the abdominal aortic aneurysm with a tube graft

5. A 67-year-old woman notices a swollen right leg following a 6-hour plane flight. Which of the following would be a reasonable next step for the treating physician?

    A. Prescribe compression stockings and leg elevation.

    B. Start 6 months of warfarin anticoagulation.

    C. Prescribe one baby aspirin per day.

    D. Order a venous duplex evaluation.

    E. Order a pelvic CT scan to look for lymphadenopathy.

Questions 6–8

A 59-year-old patient undergoes a craniotomy for a benign meningioma. On the 10th postoperative day, he is noted to have a swollen left calf and thigh.

6. What is the *least* accurate method to diagnose the cause of the swollen leg?

    A. Physical examination

    B. Left leg venogram

    C. ^{125}I Fibrinogen scan

    D. Impedance plethysmography

    E. Duplex US

7. If DVT is documented, initial treatment should include which of the following?

    A. Subcutaneous unfractionated heparin therapy

    B. Intravenous heparin therapy

    C. Thrombolytic therapy with urokinase

    D. Aspirin therapy

    E. Warfarin treatment

8. After recovery from the acute illness, the patient returns in 6 months, complaining of persistent leg swelling. Which of the following would be the optimal long-term management as initial treatment?

    A. Chronic diuretic therapy

    B. Venous thrombectomy

    C. Venous bypass using an autologous vein

    D. Venous bypass using a prosthetic graft

    E. Support hose

9. A 24-year-old woman presents to your office. She is a heavy smoker, approximately 2½ packs per day. She complains of pain in the left thigh with exercise. On exam, she has a normal left leg, with diminished pulses on the left compared to the right. An ankle-brachial index (ABI) is 0.8 on the left, 1.0 on the right. The best initial management is:

   A. Aortobifemoral bypass grafting
   B. Aortoiliac bypass with reversed saphenous vein
   C. Tissue plasminogen activator (tPA)
   D. Therapeutic heparin
   E. Smoking cessation

10. The same patient in the aforementioned scenario returns to your office after 2 years with worsening symptoms. In fact, the patient reports constant pain, even without exercise. Repeat ABI on the left is 0.4, 1.0 on the right. The most appropriate intervention is:

    A. Aspirin, 325 mg/day
    B. tPA
    C. Angiography with stent placement
    D. Aortoiliac bypass with polytetrafluoroethylene
    E. LMWH

11. A 68-year-old man without past medical history is found to have an incidental carotid bruit on routine physical examination. Physical examination is otherwise benign, and the patient denies any symptoms. An ultrasound of the neck demonstrates a unilateral 80% stenosis at the junction of the common carotid and internal carotid arteries. What is the best management for this patient?

    A. Carotid endarterectomy with patch angioplasty
    B. Carotid angiography with stent placement
    C. Aspirin, 325 mg
    D. Carotid endarterectomy with primary repair
    E. Cilostazol

12. A 75-year-old woman has progressive weight loss over the past year since the death of her spouse. She has also some baseline abdominal pain, which is worsened with large meals. Her physical exam is benign, but the patient complains of abdominal pain during the exam. The best single test for this patient is:

    A. Upper gastrointestinal (GI) series
    B. CT angiogram
    C. Mesenteric angiography
    D. Right upper quadrant ultrasound
    E. Magnetic resonance imaging (MRI) of the abdomen

13. A 41-year-old woman undergoes an uneventful right hemicolectomy for stage II cecal cancer. On the third postoperative day, she develops new, unilateral leg swelling; local warmth; and pain with passive dorsiflexion. What is the most appropriate initial management?

    A. Warfarin
    B. Aspirin (325 mg)
    C. LMWH
    D. Retrievable IVC filter
    E. Unfractionated subcutaneous heparin

14. A 60-year-old man has an acute DVT at the time of repair of a femur fracture. After treatment, he has complete resolution of symptoms. Three years later, he returns with swelling of the same leg, local pain, and some skin ulceration. A D-dimer level is normal. The most likely diagnosis is:

A. Acute DVT
B. Heparin-induced thrombocytopenia
C. Pulmonary embolus
D. Post-thrombotic syndrome
E. Phlegmasia alba dolens

15. A 28-year-old woman undergoes left modified radical mastectomy for locally advanced breast cancer. Two weeks later, she develops pain and swelling of her left arm. On exam, her arm appears diffusely swollen. The skin is pink and radial pulses are strong and equal bilaterally. The best initial test is:

A. US
B. Lymphoscintigraphy
C. Magnetic resonance angiography (MRA)
D. Contrast angiography
E. CT of the chest

Answers and Explanations

1. **The answer is D** (Chapter 7, Mesenteric Vascular Disease, Acute Mesenteric Ischemia, III). The triad of a cardiac arrhythmia, the sudden onset of severe abdominal pain, and gut emptying is a classic indicator of embolic mesenteric ischemia. This combination constitutes a surgical emergency, and the patient should be treated promptly with vigorous rehydration followed by arteriography to confirm the diagnosis. Rapid embolectomy of the superior mesenteric artery could save this patient, provided that no delay occurs in her definitive surgical treatment.

   Cholecystitis usually presents with right upper quadrant pain and diverticulitis with left lower quadrant pain. A perforated ulcer will have associated diffuse abdominal tenderness but also will have signs of peritoneal irritation (guarding and rebound). A small bowel obstruction usually presents with colic or intermittent pain.

2. **The answer is B** (Chapter 7, Extracranial Cerebrovascular Disease, Management II). The symptomatic artery is usually repaired first because it carries the highest risk of stroke. Percutaneous transluminal angioplasty of the carotid artery is presently under investigation as an alternative to carotid endarterectomy, but it is not considered to be the standard of care at this point. Percutaneous transluminal angioplasty is sometimes used for smooth, regular lesions associated with fibromuscular dysplasia. The superficial temporal artery to middle cerebral artery bypass has not been shown to be effective for this patient's disease. Bilateral carotid endarterectomy is usually not performed because of the risk of recurrent laryngeal nerve trauma, which, if bilateral, could result in a tracheostomy.

3–4. **The answers are 3-D** (Chapter 7, Arterial Aneurysms, General Aspects, III H), **and 4-D** (Chapter 7, Arterial Aneurysms, General Aspects, III I). Colonoscopy is not indicated if the patient's stool is heme negative. CT can help to evaluate the proximal extent of the aneurysm. Pulmonary function tests can help to assess risk and to help plan perioperative care. An arteriogram acts as a road map, showing the renal arteries in relation to the aneurysm and the extent of occlusive disease in the iliac and femoral arteries. A Persantine thallium scan helps to define perioperative cardiac risk.

   Elective repair of an abdominal aortic aneurysm (AAA) can be performed with a mortality rate lower than 5%. The leading cause of death in these patients with AAA is rupture. A 6-cm AAA has a 35% rupture rate, and surgery should be recommended unless the patient has a life expectancy of less than 1 year. Rate of enlargement is not a safe predictor of risk of rupture. Patients with symptomatic or rupturing AAA have a 75% mortality rate when operated on as an emergency. An aortobiiliac graft is the appropriate procedure in this patient, rather than a tube graft, to repair the associated iliac aneurysm. With no iliac occlusive disease, an aortoiliac bypass avoids groin incisions.

5. **The answer is D** (Chapter 8, Acute Deep Venous Thrombosis, Diagnostic Tests, I). A swollen leg following a period of immobilization is a typical history leading to a DVT. Although lymphedema or other causes can also lead to leg swelling, a pelvic CT scan would not be the next step for this patient. Physical examination is reliable only 50% of the time for DVT, so an accurate diagnostic study such as a venous duplex ultrasound is needed before starting long-term anticoagulation. If no other reason for the swelling can be found, a pelvic CT scan may be reasonable. Leg elevation is helpful to reduce swelling, but compression stockings are not recommended in the acute phase for fear of dislodging the clot. Aspirin is of no proven benefit in treating DVT.

6–8. **The answers are 6-A** (Chapter 8, Acute Deep Venous Thrombosis, Clinical Findings, I, Diagnostic Tests, I–IV), **7-B** (Chapter 8, Acute Deep Venous Thrombosis, Initial Treatment, II), **and 8-E** (Chapter 8, Acute Deep Venous Thrombosis, Complications, II D). Physical examination is the least likely method to diagnose the cause of acute leg swelling. Currently, such a patient would undergo duplex US or venography to confirm the presumed diagnosis of DVT. Impedance plethysmography can detect increased resistance to venous flow but does not identify the cause. ^{125}I Fibrinogen scanning can identify ongoing thrombosis, but the scan takes 24 hours to complete and is therefore not useful in acute situations.

Intravenous heparin therapy is the most appropriate initial treatment. Subcutaneous unfractionated heparin therapy in its current form is not acceptable treatment for DVT. Thrombolytic therapy would be contraindicated in a patient with a recent craniotomy because it would increase the risk of hemorrhage. Aspirin therapy has no role in the treatment of DVT. Warfarin can be used once the patient is discharged but not as the initial treatment. Transition from intravenous heparin to warfarin therapy should occur on the fourth or fifth day of heparin administration.

Support hose is the mainstay of treatment for patients with chronic postphlebitic syndrome. Thrombectomies have been unsuccessful, and the efficacy of venous bypass has yet to be established. There is interest in transplanting venous valves and segments of a vein to replace short-segment thromboses, but this area is still experimental. Prosthetic grafts have no role in venous reconstruction. Chronic diuretic therapy may be useful for short-term therapy but is certainly not optimal long-term management for this problem.

9. **The answer is E** (Chapter 7, Lower Extremity Arterial Occlusive Disease, Classification, II A; Aortoiliac Occlusive Disease, Treatment, I–II). The best initial treatment for claudication is control of risk factors. For this patient, smoking cessation is the first line of treatment but also promotes success should any other intervention need to be undertaken. The patient does not require anticoagulation or thrombolysis but may benefit from antiplatelet therapy and a graduated exercise program. Bypass is premature.

10. **The answer is C** (Chapter 7, Aortoiliac Occlusive Disease, Treatment, III A). The patient appears to have a hemodynamically significant unilateral lesion. In this instance, iliac stenting produces effective relief and durable results. Bypass is an option, but the overall complication rate is higher for open surgery than for the endovascular approach. Aspirin is useful as an adjunct but not as primary therapy for a patient with rest pain. tPA and heparin does not have a role unless there is an acute thrombosis.

11. **The answer is A** (Chapter 7, Extracranial Cerebrovascular Disease, Management, II). The patient meets criteria for endarterectomy, as it has been shown to have a reduced risk of stroke versus maximum medical therapy. Patch angioplasty is preferred over primary repair to minimize risk of recurrence. Angiography and stenting has not yet produced equivalent results. Either stenting or medical therapy such as aspirin may be beneficial in the patient who is not a candidate for surgery.

12. **The answer is B** (Chapter 7, Mesenteric Vascular Disease, Chronic Mesenteric Ischemia, IV). The patient has high suspicion for chronic mesenteric ischemia. Although mesenteric duplex is a reasonable screening test, CT angiogram is the definitive test of choice. An upper GI series is unlikely to provide specific information in this case, and a right upper quadrant ultrasound is too focused to suggest hypoperfusion of the gut. MRI may yield static information on the character of the bowel but not necessarily the vessels.

13. **The answer is C** (Chapter 8, Acute Deep Venous Thrombosis, Initial Treatment). The patient presents with signs and symptoms of an acute DVT, for which the treatment is anticoagulation. Warfarin is useful in the long-term but is never started first due to the potential complication of skin necrosis. Aspirin and other NSAIDs may be used for superficial venous thrombosis but is insufficient for DVT. IVC filters have a role in those who cannot be anticoagulated but are not primary therapy. Subcutaneous heparin is used in prophylaxis, not treatment.

14. **The answer is D** (Chapter 8, Acute Deep Venous Thrombosis, Complications, II). The patient presents with the long-term sequelae of DVT, known as *post-thrombotic syndrome*. Skin ulceration would not be expected in an acute DVT. The timing of heparin-induced thrombocytopenia is in close association with the dosing of heparin. PE should present with respiratory symptoms. Phlegmasia is an acute complication of DVT, and phlegmasia alba dolens would present with pitting edema and blanching.

15. **The answer is B** (Chapter 8, Lymphedema, Diagnosis, III). The patient is presenting with signs and symptoms of lymphedema secondary to disruption of the axillary lymphatics. The test of choice is lymphoscintigraphy. US is reasonable to rule out a DVT, but this is less likely in the clinical scenario. MRA and conventional angiography are used to assess the arterial system, which seems normal in this patient. CT of the chest is unlikely to be useful in this instance.

Part IV
Gastrointestinal Disorders
Chapter Cuts and Caveats

CHAPTER 9

Esophagus:

◆ Every patient with dysphagia should undergo EGD to rule out carcinoma. Squamous cell cancer is most common in the upper and middle third of the esophagus, adenocarcinoma in the lower third.

◆ Esophageal reflux is remarkably common. Most patients respond to acid suppression therapy, and those that do not can be treated with minimally invasive surgery. Fundoplication is effective at re-establishing a physiologic barrier to reflux. Preoperative manometry to ensure good esophageal motility is essential in these patients.

◆ Barrett esophagus is replacement of distal squamous epithelium with columnar epithelium that can undergo malignant transformation. It should be monitored for degree of dysplasia. Severe dysplasia and carcinoma in situ should be resected. Barrett is associated with chronic GERD but is not cured by an antireflux procedure.

◆ Carcinoma of the esophagus is treated with multimodal protocols, with surgery reserved for early stages.

◆ Achalasia is the most common motility disorder, associated with dysphagia and regurgitation. Its findings are dilated esophagus, loss of peristalsis, and increased LES tone showing a bird's beak on barium swallow and treated by endoscopic dilation or surgical transection of the LES (Heller myotomy).

CHAPTER 10

Stomach and Duodenum:

◆ The management of peptic ulcer disease is initially medical: acid suppression therapy and treatment for *H. pylori* will cure most patients.

◆ Prophylaxis with PPIs to *prevent* stress ulcer and UGI bleeding should be considered for patients with mechanical ventilation, coagulopathy, sepsis, multiorgan failure, prior UGI bleed, and neurologic trauma, among others.

◆ Gastric ulcers are associated with the risk of cancer. Gastric cancer is usually diagnosed late due to nonspecific symptoms.

◆ Reconstructions after gastrectomy cause unique physiologic problems such as dumping syndrome.

◆ A duodenal ulcer that has recently bled and has a visible artery in its base has a high risk for rebleeding.

◆ GISTs are common in the stomach and treated by resection to grossly negative margins.

◆ MALT lymphoma is the only malignancy successfully treated with antibiotics.

CHAPTER 11

Small Intestine:

◆ Many small bowel obstructions are due to adhesions and will resolve with bowel rest, correction of fluid and electrolytes, and time. Partial small bowel obstruction is usually best managed conservatively with NG decompression and IV fluid support. Surgery is usually indicated if it fails to resolve or if certain clinical findings are present, such as localized abdominal tenderness, a hernia, fever, markedly elevated WBC, acidosis, large fluid requirements, or a closed loop obstruction on radiograph. Tumors of the small bowel such as carcinoid tumor can present with obstruction.

◆ Ischemic bowel is a difficult diagnosis and should be suspected when atrial fibrillation, acute MI, hypercoagulable state, low-flow state, or an abdominal bruit is present with severe abdominal pain.

◆ The common complications of IBD that may lead to surgical intervention include obstruction, bleeding, fistula formation, and failure of medical therapy.

CHAPTER 12

Colon, Rectum, and Anus:

◆ UC has an increasing risk for dysplasia and colonic malignancy with active disease over 10 years. Cancer develops in flat areas in contrast to the polyp–cancer progression in the usual colon cancers.

◆ A retrocecal appendix may not exhibit the usual clinical course of RLQ pain.

◆ Adenomatous polyps lead to colon cancer if unchecked—most polyps are initially amenable to endoscopic resection. Colorectal cancer is the third leading cause of cancer death, and screening with fecal occult blood testing or endoscopy allows early detection. Adjuvant chemotherapy improves survival in stage III colon cancer.

◆ Rectal cancer has a high risk of local recurrence at the site of resection. Rectal cancers respond to radiation therapy, whereas colonic cancers do not.

◆ Diverticulitis typically involves the sigmoid colon. Initial uncomplicated attacks are usually treated medically with antibiotics, but most complicated cases ultimately require surgical resection. Patients with clinical diverticulitis must have colon cancer ruled out.

◆ The site of lower GI bleeding must be confirmed before surgery. Massive lower GI bleed is usually secondary to diverticulosis or AV malformations of the cecum.

◆ *C. difficile* is a common cause of antibiotic-associated diarrhea; it is detected by PCR and treated with metronidazole.

CHAPTER 13

Liver, Gallbladder, and Biliary Tree:

◆ Liver failure has an elevated INR due to deficiency of factors II, VII, IX, and X, which is corrected with FFP in an acute bleed and vitamin K. It also is associated with thrombocytopenia due to hypersplenism.

◆ The natural history of asymptomatic gallstones is benign, and cholecystectomy is not recommended. Symptomatic gallstones are treated with laparoscopic cholecystectomy.

◆ Biliary obstruction due to stones may present as painful jaundice and should be treated with removal of the stones by ERCP in most cases followed by cholecystectomy or operative common duct exploration at the time of cholecystectomy.

◆ Acute cholecystitis should be treated with antibiotics followed by cholecystectomy in several days in most cases.

◆ Painless jaundice is associated with distal biliary obstruction from tumors. Resected ampullary cancer has the best long-term survival of the pancreatobiliary cancers obstructing the distal CBD.

◆ Cystic liver lesions are usually simple cysts, are not usually symptomatic, and do not require surgery.

◆ In the presence of fever and sepsis, the cystic structure may have internal echoes on US and represent an abscess, which is usually drained percutaneously.

◆ The most common solid liver masses are hemangiomas, which do not require surgery.

◆ The most common malignant tumor of the liver is metastatic carcinoma. The primary should be sought. Resection of metastatic colonic carcinoma to the liver with no metastasis outside the liver as demonstrated by PET scan can result in long-term survival.

◆ Hepatocellular carcinoma is the most common primary liver cancer and is associated with cirrhosis of any cause as well as elevated serum alpha-fetoglobulin.

◆ Most blunt liver trauma can be managed nonoperatively.
◆ Portal hypertension may lead to bleeding esophageal varices, which may be lethal.

CHAPTER 14

Pancreas:

◆ Pancreatitis may produce both exocrine and endocrine deficiency. Ranson criteria mark the severity of the pancreatitis. The most common etiologies are alcohol and gallstones, but it may be a result of viral infection, drug reactions, or other causes. Supportive care is the rule.
◆ Gallstone pancreatitis is best treated by alleviating the obstruction, fluid resuscitation, and antibiotics. Surgery is reserved for cases of pancreatic necrosis.
◆ Small pseudocysts may resolve spontaneously; large pseudocysts often require internal drainage.
◆ Most pancreatic cancer occurs in the head of the pancreas presents late as painless jaundice. The usual treatment is the Whipple operation. Pancreatic resections are complex and have the potential for high morbidity.

CHAPTER 15

Spleen:

◆ The spleen functions both in hematology (RBC and platelet clearance) as well as immunology (removal of encapsulated organisms).
◆ ITP is the most common reason for elective splenectomy. All patients should be immunized for meningococcus, pneumococcus, and H. influenza prior to splenectomy.
◆ Accessory spleens occur commonly and may result in recurrence of disease.
◆ The pancreatic tail may be injured during splenectomy, resulting in pancreatic fistula.
◆ The spleen is frequently injured during blunt trauma and often can be salvaged with nonoperative management.

Chapter 9

Esophagus

Jonathan P. Pearl

INTRODUCTION

Anatomy (Fig. 9-1)

I. **Location:** The esophagus is <24 cm in length, extending from vertebral level C6 to T11.

   A. **Upper esophageal sphincter:** at esophageal origin, composed of the cricopharyngeal muscle; courses behind the aortic arch and descends into the thorax on the right

   B. **Esophageal hiatus:** Esophagus deviates anteriorly and enters the abdomen through the hiatus.

   C. **Gastroesophageal junction (GEJ):** The tubular esophagus meets the saccular stomach here (<40 cm from the incisors), where it is anchored by the phrenoesophageal ligament.

II. **Histology**

   A. **Esophageal mucosa:** consists of squamous epithelium except for the distal 1–2 cm, which is columnar epithelium

   B. **Two layers of muscle line the esophagus:** An inner circular and outer longitudinal layer. The upper one third is striated muscle, whereas smooth muscle predominates in the lower two thirds.

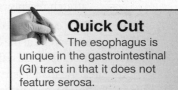

> **Quick Cut**
> The esophagus is unique in the gastrointestinal (GI) tract in that it does not feature serosa.

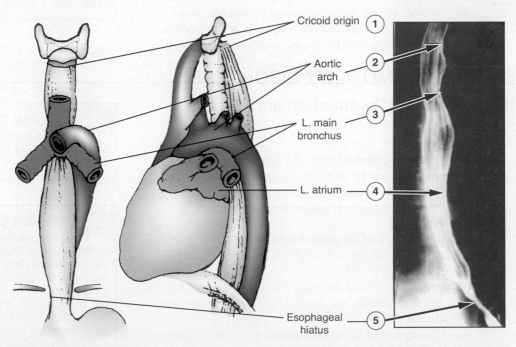

Figure 9-1: Esophageal anatomy. (From Dudek RW. *High-Yield Gross Anatomy*, 4th ed. Baltimore: Lippincott Williams & Wilkins; 2010.)

Vasculature

I. **Arteries:** Arterial supply to the esophagus is from branches of the inferior thyroid; the bronchial, intercostal, inferior phrenic, and left gastric arteries; and direct esophageal branches from the aorta.

II. **Veins:** An extensive subepithelial venous plexus empties superiorly into the hypopharyngeal veins and inferiorly into the gastric veins. Segmental drainage occurs also via the azygous and hemiazygous systems.

III. **Lymphatic drainage (to the nearest lymph nodes):** Upper esophageal lymphatics drain into the cervical or mediastinal nodes, whereas distal esophageal drainage is often to the celiac nodes.

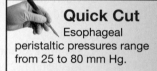
Quick Cut
The venous system is more variable than the arterial system.

Innervation

I. **Sympathetic and parasympathetic systems:** The esophagus is supplied by the pharyngeal plexus, vagus, upper and lower cervical sympathetic, and splanchnic nerves.

II. **Auerbach (myenteric) and Meissner (submucosal) plexuses:** influence esophageal motility

Physiology

I. **Upper esophageal sphincter (UES):** This 3–5 cm high-pressure zone at the esophageal upper border is composed primarily of the cricopharyngeus muscle and relaxes during swallowing to allow food bolus passage.

II. **Peristalsis:** These wavelike movements in the central portion of the esophagus pass down the body of the esophagus and become stronger toward the lower portion.
   A. **Primary peristalsis:** propels food down the esophagus
   B. **Secondary peristalsis:** If a food bolus fails to progress, local stretch receptors trigger secondary peristalsis to move it.

III. **Lower esophageal sphincter (LES):** This 3–5-cm high-pressure zone at the esophageal lower portion functions to prevent gastroesophageal reflux (GER). No distinct sphincter muscle exists in this area, but manometry readily demonstrates the physiologic high-pressure zone. LES pressure is influenced by several factors and substances.
   A. **LES pressure increase:** occurs with a protein meal, stomach alkalinization, gastrin, vasopressin, and cholinergic drugs
   B. **LES pressure decrease:** occurs with secretin, nitroglycerine, glucagon, chocolate, fatty meals, and gastric acidification

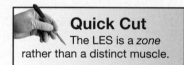
Quick Cut
Esophageal peristaltic pressures range from 25 to 80 mm Hg.

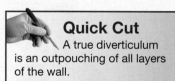
Quick Cut
The LES is a *zone* rather than a distinct muscle.

 # ESOPHAGEAL MOTILITY DISORDERS

Cricopharyngeal Dysfunction and Zenker Diverticulum

I. **Pathophysiology**
   A. **Cricopharyngeal dysfunction:** UES fails to relax properly.
      1. The problem may be an incoordination between UES relaxation and simultaneous pharyngeal contraction.
      2. This may result in **pharyngoesophageal (Zenker) diverticulum**.
   B. **Pharyngoesophageal (Zenker) diverticulum**
      1. "False" diverticula consist only of mucosa rather than the entire esophageal wall.
      2. **Symptoms:** dysphagia, halitosis, undigested food regurgitation, nocturnal aspiration, and recurrent aspiration pneumonia
      3. **Diagnosis**
         a. **History and physical examination:** raise the suspicion for Zenker diverticulum
         b. **Esophagram:** Using water-soluble contrast can provide the diagnosis.

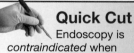
Quick Cut
A true diverticulum is an outpouching of all layers of the wall.

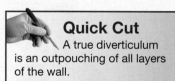
Quick Cut
Endoscopy is *contraindicated* when Zenker diverticulum has been documented radiographically because the risk of perforation is high. If a diverticulum is *not* seen on contrast studies, then endoscopy is indicated to rule out other esophageal disorders.

4. **Treatment**
   a. **Cricopharyngeal myotomy:** through a neck incision
   b. **Endoscopic stapler:** This alternative to open surgery divides the diverticulum wall.
   c. **Diverticulopexy:** Large diverticula may require myotomy combined with suspension of the diverticulum to prevent foodstuff from entering the residual sac.

Achalasia

I. **Pathophysiology:** unknown etiology
   A. Coordinated peristalsis is absent in the body of the esophagus.
   B. Resting LES pressure is high, and the LES fails to relax during swallowing.
   C. The body of the esophagus becomes dilated, and the muscle hypertrophies in an attempt to force material through the dysfunctional LES.

II. **Symptoms:** Dysphagia, regurgitation, and weight loss. Respiratory symptoms caused by aspiration may be present.

III. **Diagnosis**
   A. **Radiographic studies:** typically reveal a dilated midesophagus with a "bird's beak" appearance of the lower esophagus (Fig. 9-2)
   B. **Esophageal manometry:** shows absence of peristalsis
   C. **Esophagoscopy:** Required to rule out cancer and to document the extent of esophagitis. Retained food is commonly found at endoscopy, and the LES may be difficult to traverse.

Quick Cut
Zenker diverticulum is treated surgically.

Quick Cut
The primary problem in achalasia is the failure of the LES to relax. Contractions may be low or high amplitude depending on where the patient is in the course of the disease.

Quick Cut
Chagas disease, which is caused by the organism *Trypanosoma cruzi,* causes a symptom complex similar to achalasia.

Quick Cut
The sine qua non of achalasia is absence of peristalsis on esophageal manometry.

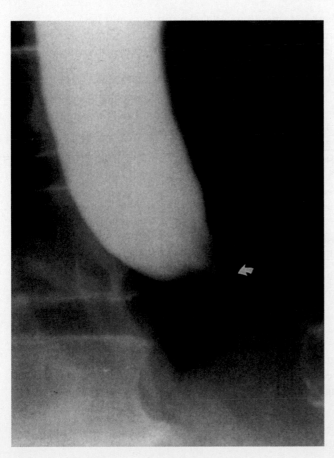

Figure 9-2: Barium swallow study demonstrating classic "bird's beak" appearance (*arrow*) of achalasia. (From Eisenberg RL. *Gastrointestinal Radiology: A Pattern Approach*, 3rd ed. Philadelphia: Lippincott-Raven Publishers; 1996.)

IV. **Treatment:** aims to disrupt the lower esophageal musculature to allow unimpeded food passage into the stomach

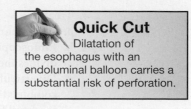

Quick Cut
Dilatation of the esophagus with an endoluminal balloon carries a substantial risk of perforation.

   A. **Nonsurgical**
      1. **Pneumatic dilatation:** A high-pressure endoluminal balloon dilates the lower esophagus.
      2. **Botulinum toxin:** injected into the lower esophageal musculature to provide temporary relaxation
   B. **Surgical (Heller myotomy):** This involves division of the outer longitudinal and inner circular layers of the distal 6 cm of esophagus. The myotomy is carried onto the proximal 3 cm of the stomach.
      1. **Myotomy:** relieves dysphagia in 80%–90% of patients
      2. **Esophagomyotomy:** usually combined with an anterior **Dor** fundoplication or a partial posterior **Toupet** fundoplication to ameliorate postoperative reflux
   C. **Peroral endoscopic myotomy (POEM):** Endoscopically divides the inner circular layer of musculature. Early data are encouraging.

Diffuse Esophageal Spasm

I. **Pathophysiology**
   A. Characterized by **strong nonperistaltic contractions**
   B. Normal sphincteric relaxation and may be associated with GER

II. **Symptoms:** may be spontaneous or may be induced by cold or hot liquids, stress, or carbonated beverages

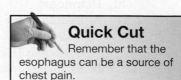

Quick Cut
Remember that the esophagus can be a source of chest pain.

   A. **Chest pain:** may be confused with angina pectoris
   B. **Dysphagia:** to liquids and solids

III. **Diagnosis**
   A. **Manometry:** reveals high-amplitude simultaneous contractions with a normal sphincteric response to swallowing
   B. **Contrast esophagram:** may show a corkscrew appearance of the esophagus

IV. **Treatment**
   A. **Medical therapy:** calcium channel blockers and smooth muscle relaxants (e.g., nitrates)
   B. **Endoscopic therapy:** Botulinum toxin injected into the spastic segment may provide relief.
   C. **Surgery:** indicated in patients who continue to have chest pain and dysphagia after medical therapy or who have an associated pathologic entity (e.g., a diverticulum)

Esophageal Reflux

I. **Etiology:** Common—may affect up to 80% of the population to varying degrees. The normal barrier against reflux is provided by multiple factors.
   A. **LES:** normally provides a high-pressure zone
   B. **Esophagogastric junction:** normally rests within the abdominal cavity, and the positive intra-abdominal pressure adds tone to the LES
   C. **Angle of His (acute angle created between the junction of the lower esophagus and the cardia of the stomach):** When the angle is disrupted, as with a hiatal hernia (Fig. 9-3), gastric contents more easily traverse the LES.
   D. **Esophageal motility:** Some reflux is physiologic, but a normally functioning esophagus clears the refluxate. In cases of esophageal dysmotility, peristalsis is not adequate to clear the refluxed secretions.

II. **Symptoms:** Substernal pain, heartburn, and regurgitation. Extraesophageal symptoms include sore throat, hoarse voice, halitosis, and dental caries.

Quick Cut
Typical reflux symptoms are heartburn and chest pain.

III. **Diagnosis**
   A. **History and physical**
   B. **Esophagoscopy:** may reveal varying degrees of esophagitis
   C. **24-hour pH probes:** placed in the lower esophageal area to measure exposure of the esophagus to acid
   D. **Intraesophageal impedance monitoring:** detects nonacid reflux

IV. **Treatment**
   A. **Lifestyle modifications:** weight loss, head-of-the-bed elevation during sleep, Avoiding carbonated beverages, and abstinence from smoking and alcohol

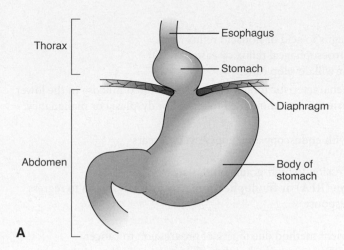

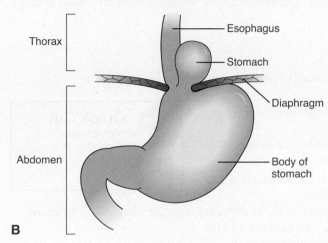

Figure 9-3: Major types of paraesophageal hernia. (From Porth CM. *Essentials of Pathophysiology: Concepts of Altered Health States*, 3rd ed. Baltimore: Lippincott Williams & Wilkins; 2010.)

   B. **Medical management**
      1. **Acid-suppressing medications:** include proton pump inhibitors and histamine receptor blockers
      2. **Baclofen (gamma-aminobutyric acid receptor agonist):** may diminish transient LES relaxation and reduce symptoms in patients with refractory reflux
   C. **Surgical treatment**
      1. **Indications**
         a. Symptoms refractory to medical treatment
         b. Patient desires to avoid lifelong pharmacotherapy, even if responsive to medication.
         c. Less common indications include laryngopharyngeal symptoms, esophageal strictures, or Barrett esophagus (see next section).
      2. **Antireflux operations:** designed to mechanically restore the barrier to reflux and involve wrapping the lower esophagus with gastric fundus and restoring the distal esophagus to its original intra-abdominal position with the GEJ below the diaphragm. The following are most common.
         a. **Nissen fundoplication (360-degree wrap of the gastric fundus around the distal esophagus):** usually performed laparoscopically with favorable results
         b. **Belsey Mark IV operation (270-degree wrap):** performed through a left thoracotomy
         c. **Hill posterior gastropexy (includes a posterior 180-degree fundoplication, which is then anchored to the arcuate ligament of the diaphragm):** emphasizes restoration of the LES to the intra-abdominal position

Barrett Esophagus
   I. **Definition**
      A. **Intestinal metaplasia:** occurs in the distal esophagus
      B. **Columnar intestinal mucosa:** replaces the normal squamous mucosa

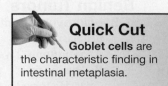

Quick Cut
Goblet cells are the characteristic finding in intestinal metaplasia.

II. **Etiology**
  A. Caused by exposure of the lower esophagus to acid or nonacid reflux
  B. Occurs in 5%–20% of patients with gastroesophageal reflux disease (GERD)
  C. Approximately 0.5% of patients per year will develop cancer.

III. **Diagnosis:** Detected at **endoscopy** by its characteristic tongues of salmon-colored mucosa in the lower esophagus. When suspected, multiple biopsies are recommended to assess for dysplasia or malignancy.

IV. **Management**
  A. **Barrett without dysplasia:** surveilled with endoscopy and biopsy every 3 years
  B. **Low-grade dysplasia**
    1. Can be surveilled annually for progression to high-grade dysplasia
    2. **Endoscopic radiofrequency ablation (RFA) or fundoplication:** may cause dysplasia to regress but there has been an inconsistent response
  C. **High-grade dysplasia**
    1. **Esophagectomy:** common management method due to risk of progression to cancer
    2. **Endoscopic mucosal resection and RFA:** aggressive, but these therapies are in their nascent stages

ESOPHAGEAL STRICTURES

Caustic Stricture

I. **Etiology:** caused by ingesting caustic agents, such as lye, drain openers, and oven cleaners

II. **Diagnosis**
  A. **History: caustic ingestion** and complaints of chest pain, cough, drooling, or shortness of breath
  B. **Endoscopy:** indicated within 24 hours to determine damage extent

III. **Treatment**
  A. **Supportive therapy:** This mainstay of treatment includes broad-spectrum antibiotics and respiratory support.
  B. **Esophageal contrast radiographs:** performed at 10–14 days after ingestion to assess for stricutres
    1. Strictures occur in 5%–10% of patients who have ingested lye.
    2. **Endoscopic dilatation:** begins 3–4 weeks after ingestion
  C. **Surgery:** reserved for cases of perforation or chronic stricture refractory to dilation

> **Quick Cut**
> With a history of caustic ingestion, it is important to identify airway compromise early.

Strictures Secondary to Esophagitis and Reflux

I. **Pathophysiology:** recurrent alternating pattern of mucosal destruction most often in the distal esophagus due to gastric acid reflux and subsequent healing
  A. **Schatzki rings:** benign strictures of the lower esophagus likely caused by reflux but may have a congenital component
  B. Cases of long-standing uncontrolled reflux may cause a long, narrow stricture.

II. **Diagnosis**
  A. **History:** Reflux symptoms with dysphagia development suggests strictures.
  B. **Esophagoscopy (with stricture biopsy):** determines disease extent and can rule out malignancy
  C. **Radiographs:** confirm the diagnosis

III. **Treatment**
  A. **Esophageal dilatation:** first-line treatment
  B. **Corticosteroids:** Some strictures respond to injections.
  C. **Antireflux operations:** may eliminate the inciting factors, and, in some cases, the stricture may recede
  D. **Esophagectomy:** indicated if dilatation and an antireflux operation do not relieve the obstruction

ESOPHAGEAL TUMORS

Benign Tumors

I. **Leiomyomas:** intramural smooth muscle tumors that account for two thirds of all esophageal benign neoplasms
  A. **Symptoms:** Dysphagia occurs with lesions over 5cm as they grow within the muscular wall.
  B. **Diagnosis**
    1. **History:** Dysphagia is typical.
    2. **Barium swallow:** reveals a localized smooth filling defect in the esophageal wall

3. **Esophagoscopy:** confirms the diagnosis if there is a bulge into the esophagus with normal overlying mucosa
4. **Biopsy:** contraindicated because it violates the mucosa, making subsequent surgical therapy more difficult
5. **Endoscopic ultrasound (EUS):** helpful to confirm the intramural location of the lesion

C. **Surgical treatment:** *rarely indicated* for leiomyomas
1. **Tumor enucleation (in symptomatic patients):** occurs without mucosa violation
2. **Limited esophageal resection:** indicated if the tumor lies in the lower esophagus and cannot be enucleated

II. **Benign intraluminal tumors:** usually **mucosal polyps, lipomas, fibrolipomas,** or **myxofibromas**
A. **Symptoms:** dysphagia, occasional regurgitation, and weight loss
B. **Diagnosis**
1. **Radiographs:** suggest the diagnosis
2. **Esophagoscopy:** confirms the diagnosis and can rule out malignancy
C. **Surgical treatment:** Esophagotomy, tumor removal, and esophagotomy repair comprise the surgical treatment.

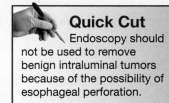

Quick Cut
Endoscopy should not be used to remove benign intraluminal tumors because of the possibility of esophageal perforation.

Malignant Tumors

I. **Incidence and prevalence:** Annual incidence in the United States is 4.5 cases per 100,000 people.
A. Esophageal cancer accounts for 1% of all malignancies in the United States.
B. In 2013, there were an estimated 18,000 cases with 15,000 deaths attributed to the disease.

II. **Etiology (unknown):** Associated factors are tobacco use, excessive alcohol ingestion, nitrosamines, poor dental hygiene, and hot beverages. Certain pre-existing conditions also increase the likelihood of developing esophageal cancer (e.g., Barrett esophagus).

III. **Pathology**
A. **Types**
1. **Adenocarcinoma:** Accounts for 60% of cases in the United States; GERD is the primary risk factor. Barrett metaplasia progresses to low-grade dysplasia then high-grade dysplasia and cancer.
2. **Squamous cell carcinoma:** Most common form worldwide. Risk factors include smoking, alcohol ingestion, and nitrate ingestion.

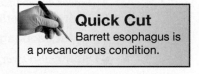

Quick Cut
Barrett esophagus is a precancerous condition.

B. **Tumor spread:** Esophageal malignancies metastasize through both the lymphatic system and the bloodstream, with metastases occurring in liver, bone, and brain.

IV. **Diagnosis**
A. **History:** Dysphagia and weight loss are almost always present.
B. **Contrast study of the esophagus:** may demonstrate tumor location and extent
C. **Esophagoscopy:** essential for tissue diagnosis and determining tumor extent
D. **Computed tomography (CT) scan of the chest and abdomen:** done to evaluate local lymphatic spread and to search for distant metastases
E. **EUS:** done to assess the depth of the invasion and for staging
F. **Bronchoscopy (in patients with proximal esophageal lesions):** done to assess the possibility of tracheobronchial tree invasion

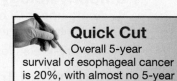

Quick Cut
Overall 5-year survival of esophageal cancer is 20%, with almost no 5-year survivors of stage IV disease.

V. **Treatment:** Survival is poor and depends on stage.
A. **Surgical therapy**
1. **Transhiatal esophagectomy (through a laparotomy and cervical incisions):** A complete thoracic esophagectomy is performed bluntly with reconstruction of GI continuity with the stomach.
2. **Ivor Lewis esophagectomy (through a right thoracotomy and laparotomy):** Reconstruction is also accomplished with the stomach.

B. **Neoadjuvant therapy (with radiation and chemotherapy prior to surgery):** Considered standard treatment by many experts. The effects on outcomes and survival are not fully understood.
   1. **Chemotherapy:** May shrink tumor size and treat micrometastases. Most tumors respond to cisplatin-based regimens, but complete responses are rare.
   2. **Radiotherapy:** May improve local control of disease at the expense of higher rates of postoperative complications. There may be little effect on overall survival.
   3. **Palliation (in patients who have advanced disease with either invasion of the tracheobronchial tree or advanced metastases):** Endoscopically placed metallic stents may allow swallowing of saliva and soft foods.

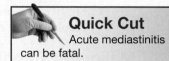

Quick Cut
The esophagus may be replaced with stomach, or even a segment of colon, after esophagectomy.

ESOPHAGEAL PERFORATION

Etiology

I. **Causes**
   A. **Iatrogenic:** Instrumentation (e.g., esophagoscopy or dilatation) accounts for 50% of all esophageal perforations.
   B. **Trauma (blunt or penetrating):** causes 20%
   C. **Boerhaave syndrome (postemetic esophageal rupture):** causes 15%

II. **Esophageal rupture:** results in acute mediastinitis

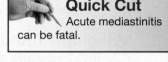

Quick Cut
Acute mediastinitis can be fatal.

Diagnosis

I. **History:** Patients give a recent history of instrumentation of the esophagus or severe vomiting. Almost all patients complain of severe chest pain.

II. **Physical examination**
   A. **Crepitus (in the neck):** results from mediastinal air
   B. **Hamman sign (crunching sound heard over the heart):** caused by mediastinal air behind the heart

III. **Chest radiography:** reveals mediastinal air and, possibly, a widened mediastinum
   A. **Lower esophageal perforation:** Air may be present under the diaphragm.
   B. **Hydropneumothorax (usually left side):** may be present if the pleura has been violated

IV. **Contrast esophagram:** study performed if perforation is suspected

V. **CT scan:** also a very useful diagnostic modality

Quick Cut
Contrast esophagram is preferred over esophagoscopy for identifying a perforation.

Treatment

I. Perform primary repair with tissue buttress reinforcement, combined with wide mediastinal and pleural drainage

II. **Surgical approach**
   A. **Upper esophageal perforations:** approached through the **left neck**
   B. **Midesophageal perforations:** repaired through the **right chest**
   C. **Lower perforations:** treated via **left thoracotomy** or **laparotomy**

MALLORY-WEISS SYNDROME

Pathophysiology

I. **Acute upper GI hemorrhage (presenting sign):** Bleeding results from a partial-thickness tear in the lower esophagus near the esophagogastric junction.

II. **Mallory-Weiss lesions:** may result from retching or vomiting

Diagnosis and Treatment

I. **Endoscopy:** locates the tear and rules out other causes of bleeding

II. **Treatment:** begins with standard resuscitation
   A. **Endoscopy with hemostasis:** mainstay of treatment and effective in most cases
   B. **Surgery (rarely indicated):** If endoscopy is not effective, a laparotomy with anterior gastrotomy and suture ligation of the mucosal tear will stop the bleeding.

Chapter 10

Stomach and Duodenum

Cherif Boutros, Ernest L. Rosato, and Francis E. Rosato Jr.

 STOMACH

Function and Embryology

I. **Functions:** storage, emulsification, initial digestion by acidification and salivary amylase, and food transmission to the duodenum

II. **Development**
  A. **Rotation:** causes the left vagus to lie in the anterior position and the right vagus to lie in the posterior position
  B. **Mesentery:** Ventral and dorsal mesenteries of the foregut become the lesser and greater omentums, respectively.

> **Quick Cut**
> The rate of growth of the stomach left wall outpaces the right, forming the greater and lesser curvatures.

Surgical Anatomy

I. **Histology:** Mucosal morphology is composed of distinctly different types of glands by stomach region (cardia, fundus, body, and antrum).
  A. **Fundus and body:** contain gastric glands with specialized cell types
    1. **Mucous cells:** provide an alkaline coating for the epithelium, which facilitates food passage and provides mucosal protection
    2. **Chief cells:** Secrete **pepsinogen**, the precursor to **pepsin**, which aids in protein digestion. Chief cells are stimulated by cholinergic impulses, gastrin, and secretin.
    3. **Oxyntic (parietal) cells:** stimulated by gastrin to produce **hydrochloric acid** and **intrinsic factor**
  B. **Antrum:** Contains **G cells**, which secrete gastrin and are part of the amine precursor uptake and decarboxylase system of endocrine cells. Gastrin stimulates hydrochloric acid and pepsinogen secretion and gastric motility.

> **Quick Cut**
> The stomach can be divided into a proximal region that mainly produces acid and pepsin and a distal stomach that mainly secretes gastrin.

II. **Stomach divisions:** four divisions (Fig. 10-1)
  A. **Cardia:** most proximal portion of the stomach, where it attaches to the esophagus, and containing the **gastroesophageal junction (GEJ)**, which is typically found 2–3 cm below the diaphragmatic hiatus and contains the lower esophageal sphincter (LES)
  B. **Fundus:** most cephalad extension of the stomach, bounded by the diaphragm superiorly and the spleen laterally
  C. **Body (corpus):** Largest portion of the stomach and consisting of the lesser and greater curves. The **incisura angularis** creates an abrupt angle along the lesser curvature and marks the beginning of the antrum.
  D. **Antrum:** distal 25% of the stomach that begins at the incisura angularis and ends at the pylorus

> **Quick Cut**
> The angle created by the fundus and the left lateral border of the esophagus is referred to as the **angle of His**.

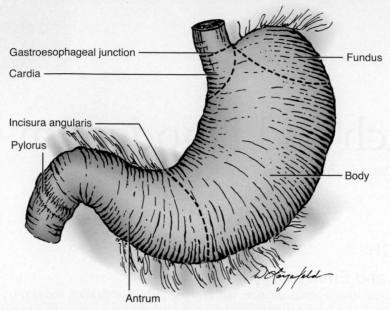

Figure 10-1: Anatomy of the stomach.

III. Stomach sphincters: two sphincter mechanisms
  A. LES (physiologic sphincter): high-pressure zone of muscular activity in the distal esophagus
  B. Pylorus (anatomic sphincter): controls food flow from the stomach into the duodenum

IV. Arterial supply: extremely rich blood supply provided mainly by two arcades running along the lesser and the greater curvature (Fig 10-2)
  A. Lesser curvature arcade: consists of the right (branch of the common hepatic artery) and left gastric (branch of the celiac trunk)
  B. Greater curvature arcade: consists of the right gastroepiploic (branch of the gastroduodenal artery) and the left gastroepiploic artery (branch of the splenic artery)
  C. Short gastric arteries (from the splenic artery): supply directly the gastric fundus

V. Venous drainage: in general, parallels the arterial supply
  A. Left gastric vein (coronary vein): drains into the portal system and has multiple anastomoses with the lower esophageal venous plexus
  B. Portal hypertension: Venous connections provide a detour for blood and form esophageal varices that may lead to massive upper gastrointestinal (UGI) hemorrhage.

VI. Vagal innervation *(parasympathetic system)*: The vagus nerve stimulates parietal cell secretion, gastrin release, and gastric motility.
  A. Left vagus nerve: lies anterior to and left of the esophagus and gives a hepatic branch to the liver, gallbladder, and biliary tree, and a fundal branch
  B. Right vagus nerve: lies posterior to and right of the esophagus and supplies branches to the posterior stomach and a celiac branch to the pancreas, small bowel, and right colon
  C. Truncal vagotomy: Division of the main trunk of vagus nerves has the best chance to control acid production by eliminating all gastric branches; however, it is associated with gallstone formation (impaired gallbladder motility with loss of the hepatic branches of the left vagus) and diarrhea (loss of the celiac branches from right vagus).

Quick Cut
Failure of the LES to relax results in achalasia; failure to remain contracted results in reflux.

Quick Cut
Sacrificing three of the four main arteries can still leave a viable stomach.

Quick Cut
Acetylcholine is the primary neurotransmitter used by the efferent vagal fibers.

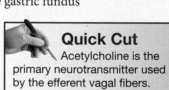

Quick Cut
The **criminal nerve of Grassi** is a proximal branch of the right posterior vagus. It can be easily missed, and may lead to ulcer recurrence if not divided.

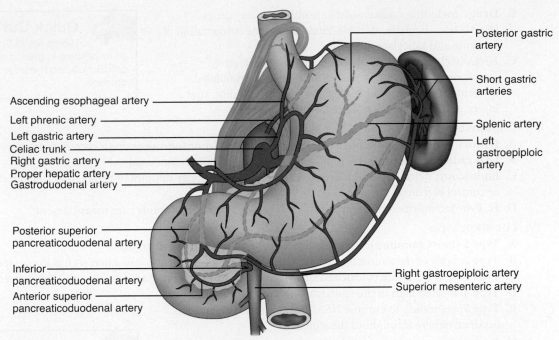

Figure 10-2: Arterial supply and venous drainage of the stomach. (From McKenney MG, Mangonon PC, Moylan JP, eds. *Understanding Surgical Disease.* Philadelphia: Lippincott–Raven Publishers; 1998:118. Used by permission of Lippincott Williams & Wilkins.)

VII. Lymphatic drainage: extensive but can be divided into four general zones
   A. Zones: superior gastric, pancreaticolienal, suprapyloric, and inferior gastric
   B. Oncology: Lymph node dissection for gastric cancer is classified in three categories (D1–D3).
      1. D1: en bloc gastric resection with surrounding gastric lymph nodes
      2. D2: en bloc gastric resection with lymph nodes at the origin of the arteries supplying the stomach
      3. D3: further dissection of lymph nodes beyond D2 (e.g., para-aortic)

Quick Cut
In cancer operations, "D" refers to the extent of lymph node dissection.

PEPTIC ULCER DISEASE

Gastric and Duodenal Digestion

   I. Gastric acid secretion: mediated by a complex interplay of neuronal and hormonal influences; the secretory response during eating is divided into three phases
      A. Cephalic phase: initiated by the sight, smell, and thought of food
      B. Gastric phase: initiated by mechanical distention of the antrum, with additional gastrin release
      C. Intestinal phase (not well understood): Intestinal factors, such as **cholecystokinin**, are mild stimulators of acid production.

   II. Negative acid feedback mechanisms: include a decline in vagal stimulation, increased acid content, and duodenal negative feedback. An antral pH of 2 inhibits gastrin release. Acid chyme in the duodenum stimulates secretin release, which further inhibits gastrin secretion.

Quick Cut
Ulcers result from an imbalance between acid production and mucosal defense.

Gastric Ulcers

   I. Incidence: more common in men, the elderly, and lower socioeconomic groups
   II. Etiology: Damage to the gastric mucosal barrier appears to be the most important factor, which can be secondary to the following.
      A. Bile reflux to the stomach

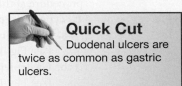

Quick Cut
Duodenal ulcers are twice as common as gastric ulcers.

B. **Drugs:** including nonsteroidal anti-inflammatory drugs (NSAIDs), salicylates, steroids, ethanol, and the combination of smoking and salicylate ingestion

C. *Helicobacter pylori* **infection:** weakens the protective gastric mucous barrier, increases the basal and stimulated concentrations of gastrin, and impedes gastric healing after injury, resulting in gastric ulcer formation

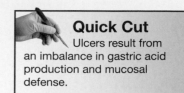

Quick Cut
Ulcers result from an imbalance in gastric acid production and mucosal defense.

III. Diagnosis

A. **History of burning midepigastric pain (stimulated by or follows eating):** common presentation

B. **UGI radiographs:** shows barium in an ulcer crater but is seldom used

C. **Endoscopy:** detects 90% of ulcers and allows multiple biopsy samples to be taken to rule out cancer or control bleeding

D. *H. pylori:* confirmed by urease breath test, tissue biopsy, or antibody titer measurement

IV. Location/type

A. **Type 1 (most common):** along the lesser curve at the incisura angularis

B. **Type 2:** body of the stomach in combination with duodenal ulcers; associated with acid oversecretion

C. **Type 3:** develop in the pyloric channel within 3 cm of the pylorus; associated with acid oversecretion

D. **Type 4:** located high in the stomach adjacent to the esophagus

E. **Type 5:** secondary to chronic NSAID and aspirin use and can occur anywhere throughout the stomach

V. Malignancy

A. **Gastric cancer will ulcerate in 25% of cases:** making it mandatory to prove by biopsy that an ulceration is not carcinoma

B. **A gastric ulcer and carcincoma are two separate entities:** A gastric ulcer does not degenerate into carcinoma

Quick Cut
Ten percent of gastric ulcers are malignancies with ulceration.

VI. Treatment

A. **Medical treatment:** Used initially; most ulcers will heal in 8–12 weeks.

1. **Eliminate irritants of the gastric mucosa:** Avoid ethanol, tobacco, and drugs.

2. **Sucralfate:** sulfated sucrose that binds to the ulcer crater and enhances the mucosal barrier

3. **Histamine (H$_2$) blockers:** effectively reduce gastric output

4. **Proton pump inhibitors (PPIs):** block the enzyme involved in the parietal cell secretion of acid

5. *H. pylori* **treatment:** Requires antisecretory agents, antibiotics (amoxicillin or clarithromycin and metronidazole), and/or bismuth; 90% cure rates are reported with dual antibiotic and omeprazole treatment ("triple therapy") and have decreased ulcer recurrence.

Quick Cut
Antisecretory medications (H$_2$ blockers and PPIs) are among the most commonly prescribed drugs worldwide.

B. **Surgical treatment:** indicated in the following situations:

1. **Intractability:** Ulcer fails to heal after 3 months of medical therapy or recurs within a year despite adequate therapy.

2. **Bleeding:** not controlled by endoscopy or medical therapy

3. **Perforation:** Definitive ulcer surgery should be performed if no preoperative shock, no life-threatening comorbidities, perforation less than 48 hours, known *H. pylori* negative, and failed medical treatment.

4. **Gastric outlet obstruction**

5. **Malignancy:** Biopsy proven, or if unable to exclude

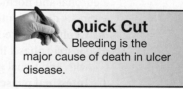

Quick Cut
Bleeding is the major cause of death in ulcer disease.

C. **Surgical procedures:** Type of ulcer, location, and condition of the patient determines the operative procedure at the time of surgery (Fig. 10-3).

1. **Type 1 ulcer:** distal gastrectomy with reconstruction

   a. **Gastroduodenal anastomosis (Billroth I gastrectomy):** if the duodenum can be mobilized (see Fig. 10-3A)

   b. **Gastrojejunal anastomosis (Billroth II gastrectomy):** if the duodenum cannot be mobilized (see Fig. 10-3B)

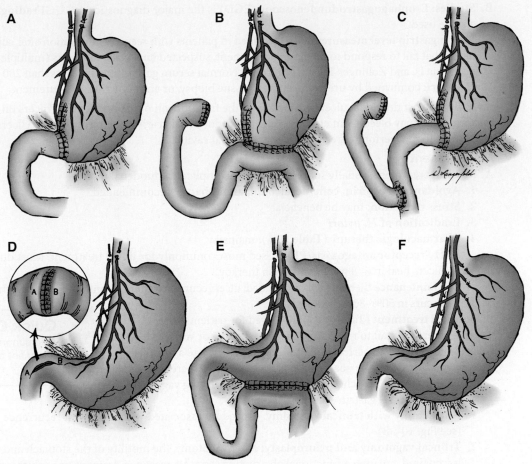

Figure 10-3: Common gastric surgical procedures: **(A)** vagotomy and antrectomy (Billroth I), **(B)** vagotomy and antrectomy (Billroth II), **(C)** Roux-en-Y gastrojejunostomy, **(D)** vagotomy and pyloroplasty, **(E)** vagotomy and gastrojejunostomy, and **(F)** parietal cell vagotomy.

2. **Types 2 and 3 ulcers:** vagotomy with antrectomy with extension to include excision of the ulcer
3. **Type 4 ulcer**
    a. **Antrectomy with extension of resection to include the ulcer:** for ulcers greater than 2 cm from GEJ
    b. **Csendes procedure:** For ulcers less than 2 cm from the GEJ, resection of the gastric antrum and body up to the GEJ (subtotal gastrectomy). **Roux-en-Y gastrojejunostomy** is done along the resection line (see Fig. 10-3C).
4. **Type 5 ulcer:** Surgical intervention is reserved for emergency situations (i.e., perforation or hemorrhage). Primary closure, omental patch, or wedge excision combined with cessation of NSAIDs and acetylsalicylic acid (ASA) are standard treatments.

Duodenal Ulcers
I. **Etiology:** may result from inappropriate gastrin secretion from a tumor mass (gastrinoma)
    A. **Mucosal resistance:** may be altered by bacteria (*H. pylori*) and is the most common etiology of ulceration
    B. **Gastrinoma also called Zollinger-Ellison syndrome:** usually (70%–90%) present in a triangular area (gastrinoma triangle) formed by the junction of second and third portion of the duodenum, cystic duct and common bile duct junction, and the pancreatic neck

II. **Diagnosis:** Gastrinoma is diagnosed by inappropriately high gastrin level (150–1,000 pg/mL) while not taking PPI therapy. A secretin test (rise of gastrin level 200 pg/mL after secretin infusion) confirms the diagnosis.
    A. **History of epigastric pain (radiating to the back):** Usual presentation; pain is relieved by food and typically wakes the patient at night.

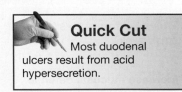

Quick Cut
Most duodenal ulcers result from acid hypersecretion.

B. **Studies: Esophagogastroduodenoscopy (EGD)** is the major diagnostic tool. **UGI radiographs** may also be used.

C. **Serum gastrin level measurements:** Obtained in patients with recurrent ulceration after surgery, ulcers that fail to respond to medical management, suspected endocrine disorders (multiple endocrine neoplasia I), and Zollinger-Ellison syndrome. Normal serum gastrin levels are less than 200 pg/mL.

D. ***H. pylori:*** confirmed by urease breath test, tissue biopsy, or antibody titer measurement

III. **Location:** Most duodenal ulcers are located in the first portion of the duodenum. Ulcers on the posterior wall may bleed from erosion of the gastroduodenal artery penetrating ulcers. Ulcers on the anterior wall may perforate freely into the abdominal cavity.

IV. **Management**

A. **Medical treatment:** usually successful with uncomplicated duodenal ulcer

1. **Avoidance of aspirin, caffeine, alcohol, and tobacco:** recommended

2. **Stress reduction:** may be beneficial

3. **Eradication of *H. pylori***

4. **Pharmacologic therapy (Table 10-1):** mainstay

   a. **H$_2$-receptor antagonists/PPIs:** Used most commonly for initial treatment. Most duodenal ulcers heal in 6–8 weeks with such therapy.

   b. **Maintenance therapy:** Recommended; ulcer recurrence after discontinuing medical therapy occurs in 50%–80% of patients.

B. **Surgical treatment (Table 10-2):** Reserved for patients who have ulcers that fail to respond to medical therapy or who have complications (e.g., perforation or bleeding). There are a number of surgical options; the goal of each is to reduce acid secretion; therefore, most approaches concentrate on interrupting vagal stimulation, antral gastrin secretion, or both.

> **Quick Cut**
> Acid suppression is the initial treatment of most ulcer disease.

1. **Antrectomy with truncal vagotomy:** procedure associated with the lowest recurrence rate (see Fig. 10-3B)

2. **Truncal vagotomy and pyloroplasty:** After vagotomy, the motility of the stomach and pylorus is impaired, creating a functional obstruction. For this reason, a drainage procedure, such as a **pyloroplasty** (see Fig. 10-3D) or **gastrojejunostomy** (see Fig. 10-3E), is required.

3. **Parietal cell vagotomy (highly selective vagotomy):** Only the gastric branches of the vagus nerve are divided (see Fig. 10-3F).

   a. **Drainage:** Because innervation of the pylorus is maintained, a drainage procedure is not necessary.

Table 10-1: Therapy of Peptic Ulcer Disease

Agent	Effect	Advantages and Disadvantages
Decrease gastric acidity		
Antacids	Neutralize gastric acid; also may increase mucosal resistance	Inexpensive; readily available
H$_2$-receptor antagonists (e.g., cimetidine)	Inhibit histamine receptor on parietal cell, which decreases acid output	Excellent results; mainstay therapy; once daily evening Dosing for maintenance therapy
Proton pump inhibitors (e.g., omeprazole)	Inhibit ATPase proton pump, which is final step in acid secretion from parietal cell	Quicker healing but more expensive than preceding agents
Increase mucosal defense		
Cytoprotective topical agent (e.g., sucralfate)	Binds to proteins in ulcer to form protective barrier	Not proven for gastric ulcers
Antibiotics (e.g., amoxicillin)	Eradicate *Helicobacter pylori*	Inexpensive; important in preventing recurrences in patients with *H. pylori*

ATPase, adenosine triphosphatase.

Table 10-2: Comparison of Morbidity and Mortality Rates of Different Surgical Options of Peptic Ulcer Surgeries

Morbidity	Antrectomy and Truncal Vagotomy	Truncal Vagotomy and Pyloroplasty	Highly Selective Vagotomy
Ulcer recurrence rate	1%–2%	10%	10%–30%
Dumping syndrome	10%–15%	10%	<5%
Mortality	1%–2%	0.5%–1%	0%

    b. Recurrence rates: Somewhat higher (>10%) but the morbidity is less as compared with truncal vagotomy with antrectomy. This procedure is often performed laparoscopically, further decreasing its morbidity.

C. Complications: include perforation, hemorrhage, and obstruction

    1. Perforations: Occur most commonly with ulcers on the anterior surface of the duodenum. Gastric perforations are less common.

        a. Typical symptoms: include sudden onset of severe abdominal pain, pain radiating to the shoulder, nausea, and vomiting

        b. Signs: Include a rigid, boardlike abdomen and shock. An upright chest x-ray commonly demonstrates free air under the diaphragm.

        c. Treatment

            (1) Observation: May be occasionally used if the patient is hemodynamically stable and the initial event occurred several hours previously. A monitored setting, antibiotics, and intravenous (IV) fluids are required.

            (2) Simple operative closure (often with a patch of omentum [Graham patch]): usual treatment

            (3) Definitive treatment (e.g., by vagotomy with antrectomy): may be indicated in low-risk patients with minimal spillage of the peritoneal cavity, especially if they give a long history (~3 months) of ulcer symptoms—or proven failure of the medical treatment

    2. Hemorrhage: Occurs in ~15%–20% of patients with ulcers. Medical management controls the hemorrhage in most cases.

        a. Endoscopy: Necessary to evaluate the site of the hemorrhage. Thermal techniques using electrocoagulation, laser, or heater probe or injection of sclerosing or vasoconstrictive agents may also be used endoscopically.

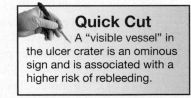

Quick Cut
A "visible vessel" in the ulcer crater is an ominous sign and is associated with a higher risk of rebleeding.

        b. Surgery: Surgical intervention is usually needed to control **massive hemorrhage,** defined as blood loss >2 liters, hemodynamically unstable despite resuscitation, or continued blood loss requiring more than 6 units of transfused blood in a 24 hour period.

            (1) Control of the bleeding vessel: Oversewing of the bleeding point is done via a longitudinal opening through the pylorus.

            (2) Gastroduodenal artery ligation: if oversewing fails to control the vessel

            (3) Truncal vagotomy (division of the two main vagal trunks): also done to reduce acid stimulation (see Fig. 10-3C)

            (4) Pyloroplasty (widening of the pylorus): Pyloric incision is closed transversely after ligation. (see Fig 10-3D)

Quick Cut
Pyloroplasty after vagotomy is used to aid in stomach emptying because the vagotomy changes the mechanical function of the pylorus.

            (5) Vagotomy with antrectomy: option in low-risk patients

    3. Gastric outlet obstruction: may be caused by chronic scarring of the pyloric channel due to prepyloric ulcers

        a. Symptoms: Obstruction causes symptoms of crampy abdominal pain, nausea, and vomiting.

        b. Signs: Stomach is usually markedly dilated. Prolonged vomiting due to obstruction can lead to electrolyte disorders, particularly hypokalemic metabolic alkalosis from the large hydrochloric acid losses.

c. **Initial treatment:** several days of nasogastric suction to allow the stomach to decompress

d. **Surgery: Vagotomy with antrectomy** or **vagotomy with drainage** is the standard procedure.

GASTRIC CANCER

Gastric Adenocarcinoma

I. **Epidemiology and etiology:** Leading cause of cancer-related death worldwide in the 20th century, gastric adenocarcinoma is now ranked second only to lung cancer. The overall incidence may be decreasing.

II. **Risk factors**
   A. **Preventable factors**
      1. **Nutritional factors:** food preparation (smoked, salt cured); foods low in vitamin A and C and high in salt
      2. **Occupational factors:** exposure to rubber, coal, or radiation
      3. **Habits:** cigarette smoking
      4. **Infection:** *H. pylori*, Epstein-Barr virus
      5. **Precancerous lesions:** adenomatous polyps, chronic atrophic gastritis, dysplasia, intestinal metaplasia, Ménétrier disease
   B. **Genetic factors:** type A blood, pernicious anemia, family history, hereditary nonpolyposis colorectal cancer (HNPCC; Lynch syndrome), Li-Fraumeni syndrome
   C. **History:** previous gastric resection

III. **Pathology:** classified according to its histologic characteristics
   A. **Intestinal type:** well-differentiated, glandular tumor found most commonly in the distal stomach
   B. **Diffuse type:** poorly differentiated, small cell infiltrating tumor with submucosal infiltration and found most commonly in the proximal stomach

IV. **Clinical presentation and workup**
   A. **Symptoms:** Include epigastric pain, anorexia, fatigue, vomiting, and weight loss. Proximal tumors can present with dysphagia, whereas more distal tumors may present as gastric outlet obstruction. Symptoms tend to occur late in the course of the disease.
   B. **Signs:** include palpable supraclavicular (Virchow) or periumbilical (Sister Mary Joseph) lymph nodes
   C. **Diagnosis:** Upper endoscopy with biopsy is considered the best test.
   D. **Preoperative evaluation:** aims to assess local spread to adjacent organs (e.g., spleen, diaphragm, omentum, colon), "drop metastases" to the ovary (Krukenberg tumor) or the pelvis (Blumer shelf on rectal exam), or distant disease (e.g., to liver, lung)
      1. **Computed tomography (CT) scan:** to look for local extension, ascites, and distant metastases
      2. **Endoscopic ultrasound:** has been shown to be useful in determining depth of penetration and in detecting nodal metastases
      3. **Whole body positron emission tomography:** applied increasingly to identify metastatic or recurrent disease
      4. **Staging laparoscopy:** may detect small peritoneal metastases and is required before most neoadjuvant protocols

V. **Staging:** Uniform and accurate staging is essential to dictate treatment options and predict prognosis and assess outcome. The most commonly used is the American Joint Committee on Cancer based on tumor-node-metastasis classification (Table 10-3).

VI. **Treatment:** Gastric carcinoma is better managed in a multidisciplinary approach to discuss management of each patient according to the disease stage, patient comorbidities, and available resources.
   A. **General approach**
      1. **Early disease (Tis and T1a):** can be offered endoscopic mucosal resection with close endoscopic surveillance
      2. **Local disease limited to (T1b N0):** should be offered surgical resection with regional lymph node dissection in a fit patient

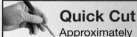

Quick Cut
Approximately 90%–95% of gastric tumors are malignant, and of the malignancies, 95% are adenocarcinomas. Other histologic types include squamous cell, carcinoid, gastrointestinal stromal tumor (GIST), and lymphoma.

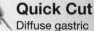

Quick Cut
Diffuse gastric carcinoma has a higher incidence of lymph node metastasis than does the intestinal type.

Quick Cut
Gastric cancer symptoms are vague and nonspecific, so most patients are diagnosed at advanced stage.

Table 10-3: American Joint Committee on Cancer TNM Classification

Gastric adenocarcinoma that extends to the GEJ is classified and managed as esophageal cancer.

Primary tumor (T)	Stage 0	Tis	N0	M0
Tx Cannot be assessed	Stage IA	T1	N0	M0
T0 No evidence of tumor	Stage IB	T2	N0	M0
Tis No invasion of the lamina propria		T1	N1	M0
T1a Tumor invades lamina propria	Stage IIA	T3	N0	M0
T1b Invades the submucosa		T2	N1	M0
T2 Invades the muscular layer		T1	N2	M0
T3 Invades subserosal connective tissue	Stage IIB	T4a	N0	M0
T4a Invades the serosa		T3	N1	M0
T4b Invades adjacent structures		T2	N2	M0
		T1	N3	M0
Regional lymph nodes (N)	Stage IIIA	T4b	N1	M0
Nx Cannot be assessed		T3	N2	M0
N0 No LN metastasis		T2	N3	M0
N1 Metastasis in 1–2 regional LNs	Stage IIIB	T4b	N0	M0
N2 3–6 LN metastasis		T4b	N1	M0
N3a 7–15 LN metastasis		T4a	N2	M0
N3b >16 LN metastasis		T3	N3	M0
Distant metastasis (M)	Stage IIIC	T4b	N2	M0
M0 No distant metastasis		T4b	N3	M0
M1 Distant metastasis		T4a	N3	M0
	Stage IV	Any T	Any N	M1

TNM, tumor-node-metastasis; GEJ, gastroesophageal junction; LN, lymph node.
Used with permission from American Joint Committee on Cancer. Exocrine and endocrine pancreas. In: Edge SB, Byrd DR, Compton CC, et al, eds. *AJCC Cancer Staging Manual*, 7th ed. New York: Springer; 2010.

3. **Locally advanced disease (T2 or with regional lymph node metastasis):** should be managed by multidisciplinary approach with possible neoadjuvant chemotherapy or chemoradiation therapy
4. **Metastatic disease:** should be offered palliative chemotherapy

B. **Surgical resection with curative intent**
1. **Subtotal or total gastrectomy:** depending on tumor location
2. **Wide margins (~5 cm on the stomach):** Necessary because extensive submucosal tumor spread can occur. Lesions of the fundus and cardia may require resection of the spleen, pancreas, or transverse colon to completely remove the cancer.
3. **Lymphadenectomy:** Extent is controversial. Removal of the omentum and its nodes is included. Radical lymphadenectomy that includes distant nodal basins has not been shown to improve survival and may increase morbidity.

C. **Palliative resections:** Indicated in the presence of obstructing or bleeding gastric cancers. Treatment may include resection, bypass alone, or either one in conjunction with adjuvant therapies.

D. **Adjuvant chemotherapy (5-fluorouracil/leucovorin or taxane and radiation therapy):** after potentially curative resection improves median survival and is the current standard of care

VII. **Prognosis:** depends largely on the depth of invasion of the gastric wall, involvement of regional nodes, and presence of distant metastases but still remains poor
A. **Survival:** decreases dramatically if the tumor is through the serosa or into regional nodes
B. **Recurrence rates after gastric resection:** high, ranging from 40% to 80%

Gastric Lymphoma
I. **Etiology:** The stomach is the most common site of **primary intestinal lymphoma**; however, gastric lymphoma is relatively uncommon. Patients at risk for developing lymphomas are those who are immunocompromised or have an *H. pylori* infection.

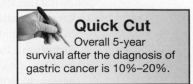
Quick Cut
Overall 5-year survival after the diagnosis of gastric cancer is 10%–20%.

II. **Diagnosis:** Endoscopy with biopsy and endoscopic ultrasound for staging. As with all lymphomas, assessment of distant disease should include bone marrow biopsy; CT of chest, abdomen, and pelvis; and an upper airway exam. *H. pylori* testing should be done.

III. **Treatment**
   A. **Medical treatment:** Combining chemotherapy and radiation is now the most accepted therapy.
      1. **Chemotherapy:** Most common combination is cyclophosphamide, hydroxydaunomycin, vincristine, and prednisone (CHOP).
      2. **Mucosa-associated lymphoid tissue (MALT) lymphoma:** treated effectively by the eradication of *H. pylori* infection alone
   B. **Surgical treatment:** reserved for residual disease or complications

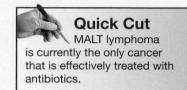

Quick Cut
MALT lymphoma is currently the only cancer that is effectively treated with antibiotics.

Gastric Sarcomas

I. **Etiology:** arise from the mesenchymal cells of the gastric wall and constitute 3% of all gastric cancers

II. **GISTs:** Most common; arise from mesenchymal cells of the gastrointestinal (GI) tract, usually the pacemaker cell of Cajal. GISTs are found predominately in the stomach.

III. **Histologic diagnosis:** confirmed by immunohistochemical staining for **CD 117**, a cell surface antigen

IV. **Presentation:** varies from incidental findings to symptomatic large tumors causing obstruction, pain, bleeding, or metastases

V. **Treatment:** complete surgical removal with negative margins; no need for lymph node dissection
   A. **Clinical behavior and malignant potential:** based on several factors, including mitotic count greater than 5 per 50 high-power fields; size greater than 5 cm; and cellular atypia, necrosis, or local invasion
   B. **Tumor recurrence or unresectable disease:** Can be treated by **imatinib mesylate**, which inhibits the **c-KIT gene**–associated tyrosine kinase receptor responsible for tumor growth. Patients with tumors with high malignant potential are offered adjuvant imatinib therapy.

POSTGASTRECTOMY SYNDROMES

Alkaline Reflux Gastritis

I. **Etiology:** most common problem postgastrectomy, occurring in <25% of all patients

II. **Symptoms:** postprandial epigastric pain, nausea, vomiting, and weight loss

III. **Diagnosis:** endoscopy demonstrates the gastritis and a free reflux of bile

IV. **Treatment:** conversion of the Billroth I or II gastrectomy (see Fig. 10-3A,B) to a Roux-en-Y anastomosis (see Fig. 10-3C)

Afferent Loop Syndrome

I. **Etiology:** caused by intermittent mechanical obstruction of the afferent loop of a gastrojejunostomy

II. **Symptoms:** include early postprandial distention, pain, and nausea, which are relieved by vomiting of bilious material not mixed with food

III. **Treatment:** Provide good drainage of the afferent loop, usually by conversion to a Roux-en-Y anastomosis.

Dumping Syndrome

I. **Etiology:** Affects most postgastrectomy patients but is a significant problem in only a few. It exists in either an early or late form with the early form being more common.

Quick Cut
Dumping syndromes are caused by rapid emptying of nutrients into the small bowel.

   A. **Early dumping syndrome:** occurs within 20–30 minutes following ingestion of a meal
      1. **Characteristics:** More common after partial gastrectomy with Billroth II reconstruction. It results from the rapid movement of a hypertonic food bolus into the small intestine.
      2. **Symptoms:** Rapid fluid shifts into the small bowel cause distention and a subsequent autonomic response along with the release of several humoral agents responsible for GI symptoms such as nausea, bloating, abdominal cramps, and explosive diarrhea.

B. **Late dumping syndrome:** Occurs 2–3 hours after a meal and is far less common, causing mostly vasomotor symptoms. The large carbohydrate load passed into the small intestine causes on over-release of insulin resulting in profound hypoglycemia.

II. **Treatment**

A. **Conservative nonsurgical measures:** Change of dietary habits control symptoms in the majority of cases. Patients are advised to avoid a high-carbohydrate diet and not to drink fluids with meals. Octreotide may be used to control symptoms.

B. **Surgical treatment:** If conservative management fails, surgery aims to delay gastric emptying, including interposition of an antiperistaltic jejunal loop between the stomach and small bowel or conversion to a long limb Roux-en-Y reconstruction.

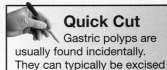

Quick Cut
These symptom complexes can be disabling—the tendency to pass out when attempting to ingest meals can change every aspect of eating habits.

Postvagotomy Diarrhea

I. **Characteristics:** common in its mild form but seldom is a disabling problem

II. **Symptoms:** usually improve during the first year after surgery

BENIGN STOMACH LESIONS

Gastric Polyps

I. **Hyperplastic polyps:** Most common gastric polyp and arise most often in the setting of chronic atrophic gastritis. They are non-neoplastic, and treatment consists of polypectomy.

II. **Adenomatous polyps:** Associated with a 20% risk of malignancy, especially if greater than 1.5 cm. Treatment consists of endoscopic polypectomy. Surgery is required for evidence of invasion on polypectomy specimen, for sessile lesions more than 2 cm, and for polyps with symptoms of bleeding or pain.

Quick Cut
Gastric polyps are usually found incidentally. They can typically be excised via endoscopy.

Dieulafoy Gastric Lesion

I. **Etiology:** an abnormally large tortuous artery located in the submucosa

II. **Classic presentation:** sudden onset of massive upper GI bleeding with associated hypotension

III. **Treatment:** Endoscopy is both diagnostic and therapeutic; surgery is rarely needed.

Bezoars

I. **Definition:** agglutinated masses of hair (**trichobezoars** occur most commonly in young, neurotic women), vegetable matter (**phytobezoars**), or a combination of the two forms within the stomach

II. **Symptoms:** include nausea, vomiting, weight loss, and abdominal pain

III. **Complications:** include obstruction and ulceration

Quick Cut
Bezoars are collections of material that remain in the stomach.

IV. **Treatment:** generally requires endoscopic or surgical removal, although enzymatic dissolution of some bezoars has been successful

GASTRITIS

Uncomplicated Acute Gastritis

I. **Etiology:** Likely due to a number of irritating agents, particularly aspirin and ethanol. **Hemorrhage** can occur and be massive.

II. **Treatment:** Removal of the inciting agent and antacid therapy usually result in prompt healing.

Stress Ulceration

I. **Etiology:** Ischemia of the gastric mucosa is the inciting event. The injury is compounded by the effect of the intraluminal acid. Although stress ulceration is common in critically ill patients, only 5% develop significant gastric bleeding.

II. **Location:** Characteristically shallow mucosal lesions start in the fundus. They then spread distally and can involve the entire stomach.

III. **Clinical presentation:** Affected patients frequently have sepsis, multiple organ system failure, severe trauma, a complicated postoperative course or are on assisted ventilation.

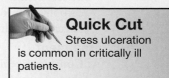

Quick Cut
Stress ulceration is common in critically ill patients.

   A. **Curling ulcer:** stress ulceration that occurs in burn patients

   B. **Cushing ulcer:** stress ulceration occurring in patients with head injury

IV. **Treatment**

   A. **Prophylaxis:** Antacids given as needed to keep the gastric pH greater than 5. H_2-receptor antagonists and PPIs are equally effective at maintaining an adequate gastric pH.

   B. **Medical treatment:** Correcting the underlying problems (e.g., sepsis) and vigorous use of antacids. Cimetidine is not helpful once bleeding has occurred.

   C. **Surgical treatment:** Rarely necessary and associated with a high mortality. In the case of uncontrollable bleeding, near total gastrectomy is usually the best option.

   D. **Radiographic embolization:** done to identify and control the main artery bleeding

Chapter 11

Small Intestine

Katherine G. Lamond

 INTRODUCTION

Anatomy

I. **Structure:** The small intestine extends from the pylorus to the cecum (Fig. 11-1).

    A. **Duodenum:** most proximal portion, which extends from the pylorus to the ligament of Treitz

    B. **Jejunum:** begins just beyond the ligament of Treitz

    C. **Ileum:** most distal portion of the small bowel

    D. The duodenum is considered *retroperitoneal*, whereas the jejunum and ileum are *intraperitoneal*.

    E. **Length:** Total ~3 m; the duodenum measures 30 cm, the jejunum is 110 cm, and the ileum is 160 cm.

II. **Vasculature:** Arterial supply to the small intestine stems primarily from the **superior mesenteric artery (SMA)**, which branches into the jejunal and ileal arteries. The duodenum is also supplied by branches of the celiac axis.

    A. **Jejunal mesenteric arteries:** have only one or two arcades with *long* **vasa recta** (small arteries directly adjacent to the bowel wall)

    B. **Ileal arteries:** have multiple arcades that extend closer to the bowel with *short* **vasa recta**

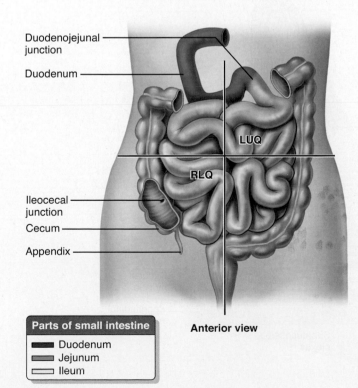

Duodenojejunal junction
Duodenum
LUQ
RLQ
Ileocecal junction
Cecum
Appendix

Parts of small intestine
Duodenum
Jejunum
Ileum

Anterior view

Figure 11-1: Jejunum and ileum. LUQ, left upper quadrant; RLQ, right lower quadrant. (From Moore KL, Agur AMR, Dalley AF. *Clinically Oriented Anatomy*, 7th ed. Baltimore: Lippincott Williams & Wilkins; 2013.)

III. **Small intestine wall layers (four):** as shown in Figure 11-2
   A. **Mucosa:** Consists mostly of **absorptive columnar epithelium** and **mucus-producing goblet cells.** Nutrient absorption takes place via epithelial cells.
      1. **Villi:** have a surface area of ~500 m²
      2. **Mucosal cells:** proliferate rapidly with a life span of 5 days
   B. **Submucosa:** strongest layer; contains nerves, **Meissner plexus**, blood vessels, lymphoid tissue (**Peyer patches**), and fibrous and elastic tissue
   C. **Muscularis:** consists of two muscle layers with the **Auerbach plexus** sandwiched in between
      1. **Outer layer:** runs longitudinally along bowel length
      2. **Inner layer:** circular
   D. **Serosa:** outermost layer and derived embryologically from the **peritoneum**

IV. **Internal structure**
   A. **Plicae circulares:** These spiral folds of mucosa and submucosa are more prominent proximally; they may help delineate the small bowel on a plain x-ray.
   B. **Jejunum:** larger in diameter, thicker walled, and has more prominent plicae circulares and less mesenteric fat than the ileum
   C. **Peyer patches (or lymphoid tissue):** more prominent distally in the ileum

> **Quick Cut**
> The submucosa is the layer that provides strength in intestinal anastomosis.

Physiology

I. **Function:** The primary functions of the small intestine are **digestion** and **absorption.** Food, fluid, and secretions from the stomach, liver, and pancreas reach the small intestine. The total volume may reach 9 L/day, and all except 1–2 L will be absorbed.

II. **Motility**
   A. Two types of **contractions** occur after a meal.
      1. **To-and-fro motion:** mixes **chyme** with digestive juices, which prolongs exposure to the absorptive mucosa
      2. **Peristalsis:** moves all intestinal contents distally

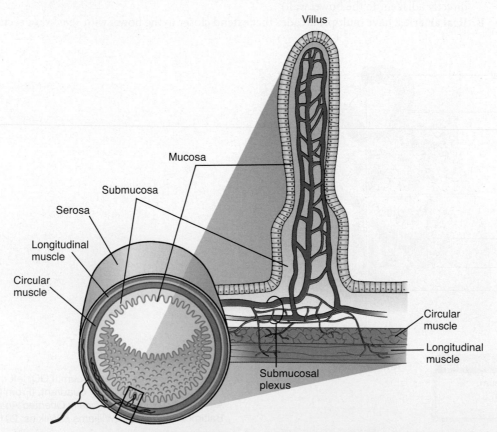

Figure 11-2: Vasculature of the small intestine. (From Rhoades RA, Bell DR. *Medical Physiology: Principles for Clinical Medicine*, 4th ed. Baltimore: Lippincott Williams & Wilkins; 2012.)

B. **Migrating motor complex (MMC):** When fasting, strong contractions occur in the duodenum every 2 hours to empty residual food.

C. *Parasympathetic stimulation* promotes contractions and digestion, whereas *sympathetic stimulation* is inhibitory.

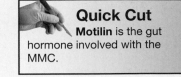

Quick Cut
Motilin is the gut hormone involved with the MMC.

III. **Absorption:** Vitamins, fat, protein, carbohydrates, water, and electrolytes are all absorbed in the small intestine.

A. **Water:** Absorbed by *passive* absorption and osmosis throughout the small intestine: Jejunum > ileum > duodenum.

B. **Electrolytes**

1. **Potassium:** absorbed by *passive* diffusion through intercellular pores in the jejunum

2. **Sodium:** absorbed and *actively* transported, whereas **chloride** follows *passively*

3. **Calcium:** *actively* transported in the jejunum and enhanced by vitamin D and parathyroid hormone

4. **Iron:** mainly absorbed in the duodenum and enhanced by an acid environment

   a. The ferric form (Fe^{3+}) must be reduced into the ferrous ion Fe^{2+}.

   b. Vitamin C (ascorbic acid) can assist with the *active* transport of iron.

C. **Fat:** Absorption occurs mainly in the jejunum.

1. **Pancreatic lipase:** digests fat, which becomes emulsified in bile salt micelles

2. **Micelles:** release fatty acids and monoglycerides to the epithelial cells

3. **Epithelial cells:** After absorption, these cells resynthesize triglycerides, which are assembled into chylomicrons and transported directly to the lymphatics.

4. All other nutrients are transported directly into the portal venous system.

D. **Carbohydrates:** digested by **salivary** and **pancreatic amylase**

1. Enzymes of the mucosal cell surface further reduce sugars to the **monosaccharides**.

2. **Galactose and glucose:** absorbed by *active* transport

3. **Fructose:** absorbed by *diffusion*

E. **Protein**

1. **Pepsin:** Digestion begins in the stomach with this enzyme and continues in the small bowel by **pancreatic proteases**.

2. **Brush border:** Digestion is completed here, yielding tripeptides, dipeptides, and amino acids; all are absorbed by *active* transport.

F. **Fat-soluble vitamins:** A, D, E, and K are absorbed from micelles by the mucosa.

G. **Vitamin B$_{12}$ (or cobalamin):** complexed with intrinsic factor and absorbed in the terminal ileum

H. **Vitamin C, thiamine, and folic acid:** *Actively* transported; the remaining water-soluble vitamins are absorbed by *passive* diffusion.

DISEASES

Small Bowel Obstruction

I. **Causes**

A. **Adhesions (scar tissue):** cause obstruction through mechanical kinking

B. **Hernias (including ventral, incisional, umbilical, and direct and indirect inguinal):** Femoral hernias are particularly prone to incarceration and bowel necrosis.

Quick Cut
Adhesions are the principal cause of small bowel obstruction (SBO) in the United States.

C. **Malignancy:** adenocarcinoma or lymphoma

D. **Less likely causes:** gallstone ileus (obstruction of the terminal ileum by a gallstone), Crohn disease (see Crohn Disease), intussusception, and volvulus

II. **Symptoms:** crampy abdominal pain, nausea, vomiting, and distention; may lack flatus or bowel movements

III. **Diagnosis**

A. **History and physical:** Focused evaluation must include a surgical history, and physical exam must rule out hernias.

B. **Radiology:** Abdominal x-rays show dilated loops of small bowel on supine films and air-fluid levels on upright films (Fig. 11-3). Small bowel follow-through or computed tomography (CT) scan can also be used to find the obstruction or determine the nature of the lesion.

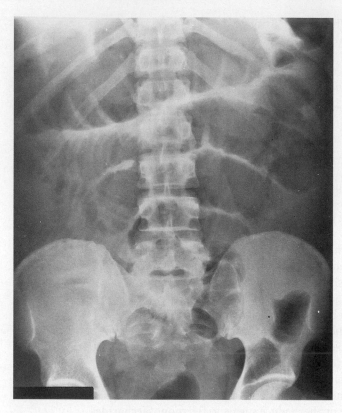

Figure 11-3: Small bowel obstruction, plain film. (From Daffner RH. *Clinical Radiology: The Essentials*, 3rd ed. Philadelphia: Lippincott Williams & Wilkins; 2007.)

IV. **Treatment:** resuscitation with intravenous (IV) fluids, nasogastric tube decompression, and urinary catheter placement to monitor urine output

A. **Abdominal exploration:** performed in patients with peritoneal signs, leukocytosis, fever, hypotension, acidosis, a hernia or failure of resolution of obstructive symptoms

B. **Partial SBO:** may be treated with the aforementioned therapies and monitoring, and may not require surgery unless it progresses to **complete SBO**

C. **Complete bowel obstruction:** more likely to require operative intervention. Evidence of a closed loop obstruction, or vascular compromise and impending perforation, demands immediate operation.

Tumors

I. **Benign neoplasms:** usually asymptomatic and rare

A. **Surgery:** indicated for bleeding, obstruction, or intussusception

B. **Adenomas:** rare in small intestine, yet **10 times** more common than malignant tumors (autopsy data)

1. **Duodenum:** most common site
2. **Three types: tubular**, **villous** (highest malignancy potential), and **Brunner gland**
3. Usually discovered **incidentally** or as a source of gastrointestinal (GI) **bleeding**, **obstruction**, or **intussusception**
4. **Treatment:** endoscopic or surgical resection

B. **Hamartomatous polyps:** found in patients with **Peutz-Jeghers syndrome** (mucocutaneous pigmentation accompanied by widespread intestinal polyposis, with little malignant potential)

C. **Juvenile (retention) polyps:** benign hamartomas and not true neoplasms; more common in the rectum and may autoamputate

Quick Cut
 If a patient with bowel obstruction does not have hypotension, fever, acidosis, leukocytosis, a hernia or a closed loop obstruction, they may be watched with supportive care for 1-2 days.

Quick Cut
Complete bowel obstruction is more likely to need surgery in the same admission

Quick Cut
 Surgery is indicated for *symptomatic* benign lesions.

D. **Gastrointestinal stromal tumors (GIST):** mesenchymal neoplasms of the small bowel, formerly called *leiomyomas*
   1. Most commonly benign and present with bleeding, obstruction, or intussusception
   2. **Origin: cells of Cajal**, which stain positive for **CD 117** on immunohistochemical analysis
   3. **Ileum:** most common site
   4. **Treatment:** wide surgical resection
      a. **Metastases:** debulked (if possible) for palliation
      b. **Imatinib mesylate:** Tyrosine kinase inhibitors may be effective for patients with unresectable or metastatic GIST.
E. **Other: lipomas, hemangiomas, fibromas,** and **neurofibromas,** which may present with bleeding, obstruction, or abdominal pain

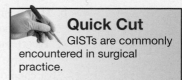

Quick Cut
GISTs are commonly encountered in surgical practice.

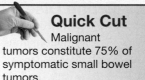

Quick Cut
Between 10% and 30% of GISTs are malignant, based on tumor size greater than 5 cm, greater than 5 mitotic figures per 50 high-power fields, necrosis, and/or the presence of metastases.

II. **Malignant neoplasms**
A. **Overview**
   1. **Incidence: adenocarcinoma** (40%), **carcinoid** (30%), **lymphoma** (20%), and **sarcoma**
      a. Metastases from other intra-abdominal malignancies are also possible, especially with peritoneal carcinomatosis.
      b. Metastases from extra-abdominal malignancies are rare except for malignant **melanoma**.
   2. **Symptoms:** bleeding, diarrhea, perforation, or obstruction (which may be caused by intussusception)
   3. **Diagnosis:** commonly made late in the course of disease because symptoms are often subtle and insidious in onset
   4. **Imaging:** enteroscope or capsule endoscopy
   5. **Treatment:** segmental resection with adequate margins and mesenteric lymphadenectomy

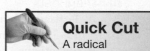

Quick Cut
Malignant tumors constitute 75% of symptomatic small bowel tumors.

B. **Adenocarcinoma:** most common in the duodenum and proximal jejunum
   1. **Pancreaticoduodenectomy (when located in the first and second portions of the duodenum):** Unresectable tumors at this location can be palliated by gastrojejunostomy or an intraluminal stent.
   2. **Tumors of the distal duodenum and small bowel:** wide local bowel resection
   3. **Metastases to surrounding lymph nodes:** often found at presentation
      a. **Node-negative disease:** Five-year survival may be as high as 80%.
      b. **Node-positive disease:** Five-year survival is only 10% as there is no effective adjuvant therapy.

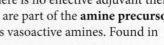

Quick Cut
A radical pancreaticoduodenectomy is also called a *Whipple operation*.

C. **Carcinoid tumors:** Derived from **enterochromaffin cells**, which are part of the **amine precursor uptake and decarboxylation (APUD)** system and secrete various vasoactive amines. Found in Appendix > Ileum > Rectum.
   1. **Prognosis and treatment:** related to tumor size and the presence of metastases at diagnosis
      a. **Small bowel Tumors smaller than 1 cm (75%):** 2% incidence of metastases
      b. **Small bowel Tumors larger than 1 cm (20%):** 50% rate of metastases
      c. **Small bowel Tumors larger than 2 cm (5%):** 80%–90% rate of metastases
   2. Only small bowel carcinoids tend to be multicentric (30%). Early on, they tend to be pedunculated, and may cause intermittent small bowel obstruction
   3. **Appendiceal carcinoid treatment:** these carcinoid tumors have an excellent prognosis.
      a. **Tumor less than 2 cm at tip of appendix:** appendectomy
      b. **Tumor 2 cm or larger or involving base of appendix:** right hemicolectomy
   4. **Carcinoid syndrome:** Serotonin secreted by **Kulchitsky cells** (enterochromaffin cells) causes flushing, diarrhea, and bronchoconstriction and may progress to tricuspid and pulmonary valvular disease.
      a. Only occurs in patients with liver metastases (10%) because the liver otherwise clears these substances via portal venous drainage

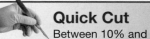

Quick Cut
Carcinoid syndrome indicates metastatic disease to the liver.

      b. Diagnosis: confirmed by elevated urinary levels of 5-hydroxyindoleacetic acid (5-HIAA), the breakdown product of serotonin

      c. Treatment: Resection of the primary tumor and metastases. Liver metastases may require palliative therapies, such as alpha blockers (flushing), octreotide, intra-arterial chemotherapy, or chemoembolization.

      d. Prognosis: Overall 5-year survival rate is 70%. If liver metastases are present at diagnosis, the 5-year survival rate is 20%.

    D. Small bowel lymphomas: usually arise in the ileum

      1. Non-Hodgkin B-cell lymphomas: most primary lesions

      2. Increased incidence: with Crohn and Wegener diseases, systemic lupus erythematosus, AIDS, and celiac sprue

      3. Symptoms: abdominal pain, fatigue, and weight loss

      4. Complications: bowel perforation, hemorrhage, obstruction, and intussusception

      5. Treatment: Wide local resection, radiation, and chemotherapy. Liver biopsy and distant nodal biopsies are done for accurate staging.

      6. Overall 5-year survival rates: 20%–40%

    E. Leiomyosarcoma: most common of the small bowel sarcomas

      1. Difficult to differentiate from leiomyoma

      2. Treatment: resection

Crohn Disease

   I. Definition: also called **regional enteritis** and **granulomatous ileitis**; chronic, transmural granulomatous inflammatory disease that can involve any area of the GI tract (mouth to anus)

  II. Distribution: The small bowel alone is involved in 25% of patients, both the small and the large bowel in 50%, and the colon alone in 25%. The distal ileum is involved in 70% of all cases and may also be called **terminal ileitis.**

 III. Diagnosis

    A. Peak age of onset: Between the second and fourth decades, ages 15–35 years. Incidence is higher in Ashkenazi Jews.

    B. Symptoms: Abdominal pain, diarrhea (usually not bloody), lethargy, fever, weight loss, and anorectal disease. Anal fissures, fistulas, ulcers, or perirectal abscesses are seen in 50% of patients with colonic involvement and in 20% of patients with small bowel disease.

> **Quick Cut**
> An enterocutaneous fistula in an otherwise healthy young patient is likely to signal Crohn disease.

    C. Signs: Abdominal mass, anemia, and malnutrition. Extraintestinal manifestations include inflammatory ocular (uveitis, iritis), joint (arthralgias, arthritis), skin (erythema nodosum, pyoderma gangrenosum), and biliary (primary sclerosing cholangitis) conditions.

    D. Radiographic findings: Contrast study may include areas of stricture separated by "skip areas" of uninvolved bowel (**string sign**).

    E. Endoscopic findings: "cobblestone" appearance and skip lesions of the mucosa and possible fistulas

    F. Gross appearance: thickened, shortened mesentery, grayish pink to purple discoloration of the bowel, and **creeping fat** (circumferential growth of mesenteric fat around the bowel wall)

    G. Pathology: mucosal ulceration that progresses to **transmural inflammation** and noncaseating granulomas in the bowel wall and lymph nodes

 IV. Differential diagnosis: ulcerative colitis (limited to colon), lymphoma, and infectious enteritides (tuberculosis, amebiasis, *Yersinia, Campylobacter, Salmonella*)

  V. Medical treatment: Combination of 5-aminosalicyclic acid, sulfasalazine, prednisone, antispasmodics, low-residue diet, and intermittent antibiotics may improve symptoms.

    A. Total parenteral nutrition (TPN): may induce remission and can lead to fistula closure

    B. Infliximab: Tumor necrosis factor-alpha inhibitor helps enterocutaneous fistulas close and may provide short-term remission.

 VI. Surgical treatment: Reserved for **complications** but may be necessary in 80% of patients. Goals of surgery are to resect as little bowel as possible; margins of resection need only be to grossly uninvolved bowel. If resection is hazardous, bypass or exclusion of the involved segment may be necessary.

    A. Surgical indications: obstruction, abscess, megacolon, hemorrhage, fissures, enterocutaneous fistula

    B. Intestinal obstruction: Usually caused by stricture and inflammation. Short strictures can be repaired by a stricturoplasty to avoid bowel resection.

C. **Abscesses and fistulas:** Common. Abscesses may be intra- or retroperitoneal. Fistulas may form from bowel to skin, bladder, vagina, urethra, or other loops of bowel.

D. **Perianal disease:** Oral (PO) metronidazole therapy. In general, surgery should be limited because wound healing is poor.
  1. **Perirectal abscesses:** require drainage
  2. **Anal fistulas and fissures:** may require surgery if severe

E. **Perforation, hemorrhage, intractable symptoms, cancer, and growth retardation (in children):** less common indications for surgery

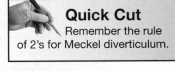

Quick Cut
Use anti-inflammatory medicine for the treatment of Crohn disease and surgery for the treatment of *complications* of Crohn disease.

VII. **Prognosis:** <50% of patients who require surgery will require another procedure again within 5 years.

VIII. **Cancer risk:** somewhat increased risk of small bowel and colon adenocarcinoma associated with the severity and chronicity of inflammation

Diverticular Disease

I. **Duodenal diverticula**
  A. **Relatively common** (seen on 10%–20% of upper GI radiographs), but most are asymptomatic
  B. **Periampullary diverticula (~70%):** can impair the emptying of bile through the ampulla, resulting in cholangitis, pancreatitis, and common bile duct stones

II. **Jejunoileal diverticula:** rare
  A. May cause obstruction (from intussusception), bleeding, or perforation
  B. May also cause malabsorption from bacterial overgrowth within the diverticulum

III. **Meckel diverticulum:** most common diverticulum of the GI tract
  A. **The rule of 2's:** incidence = **2%** of the population, location ~**2 feet** from the ileocecal valve, male/female ratio = **2:1**, age at diagnosis = first **2 years** of life (if bleeding), and length ~**2 cm**

Quick Cut
Remember the rule of 2's for Meckel diverticulum.

  B. **True diverticula:** involves all layers of bowel wall
  C. **Bleeding:** Due to heterotopic gastric mucosa in the diverticulum, which causes ulceration in adjacent ileal mucosa. Pancreatic mucosa may also be found.
  D. **Complications:** bowel obstruction (from intussusception), bleeding, and acute inflammation, which may be indistinguishable from appendicitis
  E. **Surgery:** If found incidentally, relative indications for resection include patient age younger than 40 years, diverticulum larger than 2 cm in length, and fibrous bands between the diverticulum and the umbilicus or mesentery.

Short Gut Syndrome

I. **Definition:** Complication of extensive small bowel resection due to volvulus, vascular accident, or repeated surgical resections. Diagnosis is made based on symptoms, not a specific bowel length.

II. **Symptoms:** diarrhea, steatorrhea, weight loss, and nutritional deficiencies

III. **Treatment**
  A. **TPN:** Small bowel hypertrophy occurs while on TPN, and allows increased PO intake. A PO regimen should include the following:
    1. High-calorie, low-fat, low-residue, or elemental diet
    2. H_2-receptor blockers or proton pump inhibitors to reduce acid
    3. Vitamin supplementation including B_{12} if the distal ileum is absent
    4. **Length:** likely need at least 75 cm to survive without of TPN or 50 cm of bowel with a competent ileocecal valve

Quick Cut
Short gut syndrome is associated with less than 100 cm of functional small bowel.

  B. **Surgical therapy (rarely performed):** Reversal of a short segment of distal small bowel to slow intestinal transit time. Small bowel transplant in extreme cases.

Radiation Injury (Two Phases)

I. **Acute-phase injury:** Caused by mucosal injury; symptoms include nausea, vomiting, and diarrhea and are transient. Bleeding or perforation is rare.

II. **Chronic injury:** caused by obliterative vasculitis, which appears months to years after exposure
  A. **Minor symptoms:** abdominal pain, malabsorption, and diarrhea
  B. **Major complications:** Bowel obstruction, perforation, abscess, fistula, and hemorrhage. All of these may require surgery.
  C. Surgery is technically difficult owing to fibrosis and scarring.

Chapter 12

Colon, Rectum, and Anus

Julia Terhune and Andrea C. Bafford

◆ INTRODUCTION

Anatomy

I. **Colon (large intestine):** ~3–5 ft in length and divided into several parts: the **cecum**, **ascending colon**, **transverse colon**, **descending colon**, and **sigmoid colon**

   A. **Arterial blood supply, venous drainage, and lymphatic channels:** based on embryologic origin

      1. **Arterial blood supply (Fig. 12-1)**

         a. **Superior mesenteric artery (SMA):** branches supply **midgut** structures (cecum, ascending colon, and proximal transverse colon)

         b. **Inferior mesenteric artery (IMA):** branches supply **hindgut** structures (distal transverse, descending, and sigmoid colon)

         c. **Splenic flexure:** watershed area susceptible to **ischemia** with hypotension and therefore an undesirable location for an anastomosis

      2. Venous drainage

         a. **Superior mesenteric vein:** drains the right colon and joins the splenic vein to form the portal vein

         b. **Inferior mesenteric vein:** carries blood from the left colon to the splenic vein

      3. **Lymphatic drainage:** Lymphatics follow the arteries.

> **Quick Cut**
> Colonic blood supply to the midgut (cecum to midtransverse colon) comes from the SMA and to the hindgut (midtransverse colon to sigmoid) from the IMA.

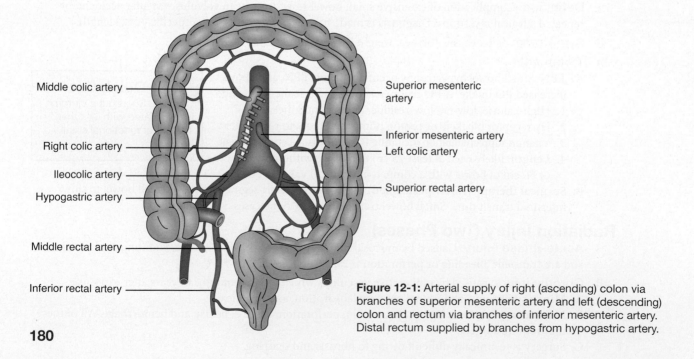

Middle colic artery

Right colic artery

Ileocolic artery

Hypogastric artery

Middle rectal artery

Inferior rectal artery

Superior mesenteric artery

Inferior mesenteric artery

Left colic artery

Superior rectal artery

Figure 12-1: Arterial supply of right (ascending) colon via branches of superior mesenteric artery and left (descending) colon and rectum via branches of inferior mesenteric artery. Distal rectum supplied by branches from hypogastric artery.

B. **Bowel wall**
1. **Layers:** mucosa, submucosa, muscularis, and visceral peritoneum (serosa)
2. **Crypts of Lieberkühn:** distinguishing histologic feature of the colonic mucosa; there are no villi
3. **Tenia coli:** three distinct bands that form the outer longitudinal muscle of the colon, which is incomplete
4. **Haustra:** outpouchings of the colonic wall between the tenia coli

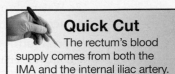

> **Quick Cut**
> Metastases from colon cancers generally spread through lymphatic paths in progressive fashion with closer nodes involved first.

II. **Rectum:** extends from the sigmoid colon to the anus and is ∼15 cm in length
A. **Arterial blood supply:** See Figure 12-1.
1. **Superior rectal artery (IMA's terminal branch):** supplies the upper and middle rectum
2. **Middle and inferior rectal arteries (branches from the internal iliac artery):** supply lower rectum

> **Quick Cut**
> The rectum's blood supply comes from both the IMA and the internal iliac artery.

B. **Venous drainage**
1. **Superior rectal veins:** drain the upper and middle rectum, emptying into the portal vein via the inferior mesenteric vein
2. **Middle and inferior rectal veins:** drain the lower rectum and anal canal via the internal iliacs to the inferior vena cava
3. **Lower rectal and anal cancers:** drain to the inguinal and iliac systems.

> **Quick Cut**
> Because rectal veins ultimately drain to both the portal vein and the vena cava through the internal iliac or femoral systems, rectal tumors can metastasize into either the portal or the systemic circulation.

C. **Lymphatic drainage**
1. **Inferior mesenteric nodes:** Filter lymph from the upper and middle rectum channels that parallel the arterial supply.
2. **Iliac nodes:** Filter lymph from the distal rectum channels adjacent to the middle and inferior rectal arteries.
3. **Inguinal nodes:** May be involved in lower rectal and anal cancers

D. **Bowel wall**
1. In contrast to the colon, *complete* layers of inner circular and outer longitudinal muscle line the rectum.
2. The proximal one third of the rectum is covered with peritoneum; the lower one third is extraperitoneal.
3. **Valves of Houston:** three mucosal folds that project into the rectal lumen

> **Quick Cut**
> The rectum has *complete* layers of inner circular and outer longitudinal muscle and *no tenia coli*.

III. **Anus:** Terminal portion of the intestinal tract surrounded by the anal sphincters, which regulate continence and defecation. The **levator ani** is palpable as the **anorectal ring**.
A. **Epithelial lining**
1. **Anal margin:** normal squamous hair-bearing skin around the anus
2. **Anal verge:** junction between the anal canal and the perianal skin
3. **Anatomic anal canal:** Begins at the anal verge and ends at the dentate line. It is lined by **anoderm**, a modified squamous epithelium devoid of skin appendages.
4. **Dentate line:** located ∼1–2 cm above the anal verge
   a. **Structures cephalad to the dentate line:** endodermal in origin, supplied by the autonomic nervous system, and drained via the systemic circulation
   b. **Structures below the dentate line:** ectodermal in origin, supplied by the somatic nervous system, and drained via the portal circulation

> **Quick Cut**
> Areas cephalad to the dentate line are insensate.

5. **Transitional zone (6–12 mm):** resides above the dentate line and is where squamous epithelium gradually changes to cuboidal epithelium and then to columnar epithelium
B. **Columns of Morgagni:** longitudinal mucosal folds located just above the dentate line, where they meet to form the **anal crypts**
C. **Anal glands (small):** exist beneath the anoderm between the internal and external sphincters and communicate with the anal crypts via **anal ducts**

D. **Anal canal:** surrounded by two muscular sphincters, which provide continence
   1. **Internal sphincter (continuation of the rectum's inner circular muscle):** smooth muscle with involuntary control and autonomic innervation
   2. **External sphincter:** striated muscle under voluntary control with somatic innervation

Physiology

I. **Water and electrolyte absorption**
   A. **Ileal chyme:** The colon receives 900–1,500 mL each day, of which all but 100–200 mL is absorbed.
      1. **Sodium:** actively absorbed across the colonic mucosa
      2. **Water:** absorbed passively, accompanying Na^+ molecules across the mucosa

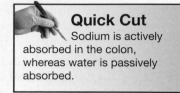

Quick Cut
Sodium is actively absorbed in the colon, whereas water is passively absorbed.

II. **Bacterial fermentation (of undigested carbohydrates):** produces **short-chain fatty acids,** which provide energy for the colonic mucosa

III. **Feces storage**
   A. **Nondigestible waste:** stored in the colon until voluntary evacuation occurs
   B. **Bacteria:** comprises ~90% of the dry weight of feces, each gram containing 10^{11} to 10^{12} bacteria, with anaerobes being predominant
      1. *Bacteroides:* anaerobic bacterium; the most common colonic organism
      2. *Escherichia coli:* most common colonic aerobe

IV. **Colonic gas:** Comes from intraluminal bacterial fermentation and from swallowed air; five gases constitute 98%: **nitrogen**, **oxygen**, **carbon dioxide**, **hydrogen**, and **methane.**

EVALUATION

History

I. **Symptoms**
   A. **Change in bowel habits:** including incontinence
   B. **Bleeding:** passage of bright red blood (**hematochezia**) or dark, tarry stools (**melena**)
   C. **Pain:** abdominal or anal

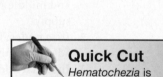

Quick Cut
Hematochezia is bright red blood per rectum. *Melena* is dark, tarry stools.

II. **Signs**
   A. **Rectal discharge:** anal or perianal
   B. **Presence of a mass:** anal or perianal

III. **Cancer, colorectal polyps, or inflammatory bowel disease (IBD):** personal or family

Physical Examination

I. **Patient complaint driven:** The patient with severe anal pain may not be able to tolerate digital or anoscopic examination, and if the cause of pain is not revealed by simple inspection (e.g., fissure or thrombosed hemorrhoid), examination under anesthesia may be necessary.

II. **Anorectal examination:** usually performed with the patient in prone jackknife or left lateral position
   A. **Inspection:** Skin abnormalities, masses, protrusions, and drainage sites should be noted.
   B. **Palpation:** The perineum, anal canal, and lower rectum should be gently palpated with a gloved, well-lubricated index finger. Sphincter tone, areas of tenderness, and any masses should be noted.
   C. **Anoscopy:** best method to evaluate hemorrhoids and other anal canal lesions
   D. **Proctosigmoidoscopy:** Rigid proctosigmoidoscope is used to inspect the mucosa for any abnormalities, such as inflammation or tumors.

Radiographic Studies

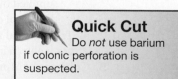

Quick Cut
Do *not* use barium if colonic perforation is suspected.

I. **Barium enema:** cost-effective but cannot reliably detect small tumors or other abnormalities and has been surpassed by computed tomography (CT) scans and by flexible endoscopy, which permit detection and treatment

II. **Water-soluble contrast enema:** If colonic perforation is suspected, barium enema is *contraindicated* because extravasation of barium and feces can cause severe peritonitis. Water-soluble material is safer, although quickly diluted, giving these studies lesser diagnostic quality than barium studies.

III. **CT scan:** Can demonstrate bowel wall thickening, pericolic inflammation, and/or fistulas/abscesses. CT scan is also useful in large bowel obstructions and for detecting metastases in patients with known colorectal cancer (CRC).

IV. **Magnetic resonance imaging (MRI):** offers little advantage over CT scans for colonic disease evaluation but is useful for assessing anorectal fistulas/abscesses and rectal cancer staging

V. **Positron emission tomography (PET):** Typically used for staging after recurrence to detect metastatic disease after the primary is resected. Occasionally used initially in cases of suspected metastatic disease.

VI. **Defecography:** Dynamic radiologic study used to evaluate defecation. The distal colon and rectum are imaged as the patient eliminates barium.

Flexible Endoscopy

I. **Flexible sigmoidoscopy:** A 65-cm flexible tool examines the distal colon and rectum.

II. **Colonoscopy**
   A. Enables evaluation of the entire colorectal mucosa in greater than 90% of patients with a 160- or 185-cm flexible instrument. Lesions can be biopsied and polyps removed.
   B. **Indications**
      1. **IBD:** evaluation and surveillance
      2. **Differentiation:** between benign conditions (e.g., **diverticulitis**) and **cancer**
      3. **CRC:** screening and surveillance
      4. **Precancerous polyps:** detection and removal
      5. **Gastrointestinal (GI) symptoms:** bleeding, abdominal pain, iron deficiency anemia
      6. **Acute lower GI bleeding:** localization and treatments
      7. **Sigmoid volvulus:** reduction

Quick Cut
Flexible endoscopy permits a more extensive evaluation of the bowel than is possible with short, rigid instruments and allows detection of small lesions or mucosal irregularities.

Quick Cut
Flexible sigmoidoscopy evaluates the distal colon and rectum, whereas colonoscopy evaluates the entire colon and rectum.

Fecal Occult Blood

I. **Determination**
   A. Stool is placed on guaiac-impregnated paper. If hemoglobin is present, a blue color appears when a peroxide-containing developer is added.
   B. A daily GI blood loss of ∼20 mL produces a positive result.

II. **False-positives:** Some foods (red meat, radishes, tomatoes) and medications (aspirin, nonsteroidal anti-inflammatory drugs [NSAIDs]) may cause false-positive results.

III. **False-negatives:** Others (e.g., vitamin C [ascorbic acid]) can produce false-negatives.

Quick Cut
A positive fecal occult blood test requires investigation to determine the cause.

Physiologic Studies

I. **Anorectal manometry:** describes anal sphincter function in the workup of fecal incontinence and constipation. It can also detect the **rectoanal inhibitory reflex,** which is absent in **Hirschsprung disease**.

II. **Electromyography (pudendal nerve conduction velocity):** demonstrates injury to the pudendal nerves that supply the anal sphincter

Endorectal Ultrasound

I. **Rectal cancer:** shows depth of invasion into the bowel wall and adjacent lymph nodes

II. **Anal sphincter injury:** reveals site in the incontinent patient

III. **Complicated anal fistulas:** shows their paths

BOWEL PREPARATION

Diet, Purgatives, and Enemas

I. **Diet:** Clear liquids for 24 hours before the procedure

II. **Purgatives**
   A. **Cathartics or laxatives:** used to purge the large intestine of stool
   B. **Mannitol, castor oil, and bisacodyl tablets:** largely abandoned due to complications and poor patient tolerance
   C. **Polyethylene glycol (PEG):** isotonic lavage solution that acts as an osmotic purgative; 4 L, ingested within 4 hours, is recommended for adequate cleansing
   D. **Sodium phosphate solution:** previously favored over PEG due to the smaller volume needed
      1. Concern over an association with kidney damage has reduced its usage.
      2. Taking the two doses at least 6 hours apart minimizes this risk.

III. **Enemas:** cleanse the distal colon and rectum; made up of **saline, sodium phosphate solution,** or **soap suds**

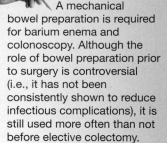

Quick Cut
A mechanical bowel preparation is required for barium enema and colonoscopy. Although the role of bowel preparation prior to surgery is controversial (i.e., it has not been consistently shown to reduce infectious complications), it is still used more often than not before elective colectomy.

Antibiotics

I. **Neomycin and erythromycin base (typical regimen):** Oral antibiotics are sometimes given the day before surgery to reduce the bacterial count in the large intestines.

II. **Broad-spectrum intravenous (IV) antibiotic:** administered within 60 minutes of the start of most colorectal procedures

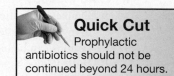

Quick Cut
Prophylactic antibiotics should not be continued beyond 24 hours.

BENIGN AND MALIGNANT COLORECTAL TUMORS

Polyps

I. **Definition:** any abnormal projection from the surface of the intestinal mucosa
   A. **Pedunculated polyps:** attached to the bowel wall by a stalk
   B. **Sessile polyps:** flat growths

II. **Benign polyps**
   A. **Hyperplastic polyps (most common):** Small (90% are <3 mm) lesions of thickened mucosa without cellular atypia. They are not premalignant but are often removed in order to rule out adenomatous changes.
   B. **Hamartomatous polyps:** Non-neoplastic growths that consist of an abnormal mixture of normal tissue. **Juvenile polyps** are rare hamartomas that occur more frequently in children and may cause GI bleeding or intussusception.
   C. **Inflammatory polyps:** non-neoplastic growths resulting from tissue reaction to inflammation, such as **pseudopolyps** in ulcerative colitis and benign **lymphoid polyps**

III. **Neoplastic polyps**
   A. **Adenomatous polyps (three types):** precancerous neoplasms of the colonic mucosa without invasion beyond the basement membrane
      1. **Tubular adenomas (75%–85%):** branched glands often on a stalk
      2. **Villous adenomas (5%–10%):** long, frondlike projections
      3. **Tubulovillous adenomas (10%–25%):** elements of both tubular and villous adenomas
   B. **Adenoma–carcinoma sequence:** Evidence has shown that adenomatous polyps can progress from benign neoplasia to malignancy.
      1. **Synchronous adenomatous polyps:** seen in CRC patients
      2. **Histopathology:** shows 10-year transition from adenoma to carcinoma
         a. **Peak incidence (discovery):** age 50 years
         b. **Peak incidence (cancer development):** age 60 years
   C. **Familial adenomatous polyposis (FAP):** progresses to colon cancer if not treated

Quick Cut
Pedunculated polyps are on stalks ("peduncles"), whereas *sessile* polyps are flat.

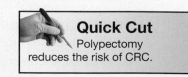

Quick Cut
Polypectomy reduces the risk of CRC.

D. **Molecular genetic studies:** show four main genetic alterations in colorectal adenomas and carcinomas (*ras mutations* and deletions from chromosomes 5, 17, and 18)

E. **Malignant potential:** More than 95% of CRCs arise from neoplastic polyps.
   1. **Size:** Risk increases with size (<1 cm, 1%; 1–2 cm, 10%; >2 cm, 50%).
   2. **Histology:** tubular, 5%; tubulovillous, 20%; villous, 40%
   3. **Sessile appearance**

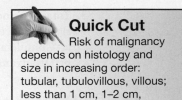

Quick Cut
Risk of malignancy depends on histology and size in increasing order: tubular, tubulovillous, villous; less than 1 cm, 1–2 cm, greater than 2 cm.

IV. **Treatment:** Neoplastic polyps should be removed because of their malignant potential.
   A. **Endoscopic polypectomy:** Ideal for pedunculated polyps. A *malignant polyp* may be treated by endoscopic polypectomy if *all* of the following characteristics are present.
      1. The polyp is pedunculated.
      2. The cancer is confined to the head (i.e., does not invade the stalk).
      3. Venous and lymphatic channels have not been invaded.
      4. The polyp is moderately or well differentiated histologically.
   B. **Transanal polypectomy:** Rectal polyps may be removed surgically through the anus.
   C. **Segmental colectomy with regional lymphadenectomy:** Required for polyps that cannot be excised endoscopically and show positive resection margins and submucosal invasion. Removal of the polyp through a **colotomy**, or a surgically made opening in the colon, is a historical procedure that has no place in polyp disease treatment.

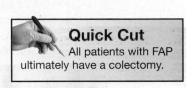

Quick Cut
Peutz-Jeghers syndrome produces hyperpigmented skin spots and GI tract hamartomas.

Polyposis Syndromes

I. **Peutz-Jeghers syndrome:** autosomal dominant disorder characterized by **hyperpigmented spots** on the lips, buccal mucosa, face, and digits and **hamartomas** throughout the GI tract
   A. **Complications:** Polyps may cause GI bleeding and intussusception.
   B. **Cancer risk:** increased risk of malignancy of the intestine (typically the duodenum, and not at the hamartoma) and other organs
   C. **Treatment:** Symptomatic polyps should be removed, preserving as much intestine as possible. Regular endoscopic surveillance is also necessary.

Quick Cut
All patients with FAP ultimately have a colectomy.

II. **FAP:** Patients develop hundreds of adenomatous polyps as early as puberty and will ultimately develop CRC, usually by age 40 years.
   A. **Genetic transmission:** autosomal dominant syndrome with high penetrance
      1. Almost all cases are caused by germline mutations of the **adenomatous polyposis coli (APC) gene**, a tumor suppressor gene on chromosome 5.
      2. No family history of the disease in one third of patients.
   B. **Clinical presentation:** Polyps are not present at birth; 50% of patients develop adenomas by age 15 years and 95% by age 35 years.
      1. **Other complications:** Polyps may cause bleeding or, rarely, intussusception.
      2. **Extraintestinal manifestations:** common; include epidermoid cysts, osteomas, abdomen and mesentery desmoid tumors, retinal pigmentation, and periampullary and thyroid carcinoma
   C. **Screening:** First-degree relatives should be tested for APC gene mutation and begin annual endoscopic screening at age 10–12 years.
   D. **Treatment:** If untreated, virtually all patients will develop colon cancer on average at age 34–43 years.
      1. **Total proctocolectomy with ileostomy:** removes all colorectal mucosa, and the patient must wear an appliance
      2. **Colectomy with ileorectal anastomosis (relative rectal sparing):** The ileum is anastomosed to the rectum.
         a. Patients are examined by proctoscopy every 6–12 months, and all rectal polyps must be removed.
         b. **Celecoxib (selective cyclooxygenase-2 inhibitor):** causes polyp regression in some FAP patients

3. **Total proctocolectomy with ileal pouch–anal anastomosis:** removes all colorectal mucosa at risk for cancer without requiring frequent proctoscopic examinations
   a. **Complications:** Sepsis and impotence are more likely with this procedure.
   b. **Disadvantages:** more frequent stools and higher incidence of anal incontinence and nocturnal seepage

III. **Gardner syndrome:** FAP with osteomatosis, epidermoid cysts, and skin fibromas

IV. **Turcot syndrome:** FAP with central nervous system malignancies

Colorectal Carcinoma

I. **Incidence:** CRC is the most common malignancy of the GI tract and the second most common nonskin cancer in men and women.

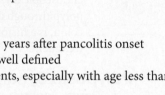

Quick Cut
CRC is the third most lethal cancer in men *and* women.

   A. **Women:** third most lethal cancer after lung and breast
   B. **Men:** third most lethal cancer after lung and prostate
   C. Americans have an ~5% probability of developing CRC.
   D. **Incidence rises with age:** Most cancers are detected after age 50 years.

II. **Site:** Incidence of cancers in the right colon as compared to the left has increased; therefore, screening should be of the entire colon and not just the rectosigmoid.

III. **Etiology:** A number of factors are considered important in CRC development.
   A. **Polyp–cancer sequence**
   B. **IBD**
      1. **Ulcerative colitis (UC):** causes increased CRC risk, ~18% at 30 years after pancolitis onset
      2. **Crohn colitis:** causes increased CRC risk, but the degree is not well defined
   C. **Genetics:** increased incidence in first-degree relatives of CRC patients, especially with age less than 50 years at diagnosis
      1. **FAP**

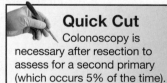

Quick Cut
HNPCC is the most common inherited CRC syndrome, caused by DNA mismatch repair gene.

      2. **Hereditary nonpolyposis colorectal carcinoma (HNPCC):** most common hereditary CRC syndrome and accounts for 3%–5% of all CRC
         a. **Characteristics**
            (1) Autosomal dominant inheritance
            (2) Proximal colon cancers predominate.
            (3) Increased risk of both synchronous and metachronous colon cancers
            (4) Early age of onset (average age is 44 years)
            (5) Increased incidence of mucinous or poorly differentiated carcinomas
            (6) Improved survival stage for stage compared with those who have sporadic tumors
         b. **Extracolonic malignancies:** increased incidence of endometrium, ovary, breast, stomach, hematopoietic, small bowel, and skin cancers
         c. **DNA mismatch repair gene mutation:** Mismatch repair genes include hMSH2, hMLH1, hPMS1, hPMS2, and hMSH6. Alterations in these genes lead to **microsatellite instability (MSI).**
         d. **Clinical diagnosis:** based on the **Amsterdam criteria**
            (1) Three or more relatives with CRC, spanning two generations, one of whom is a first-degree relative
            (2) One or more CRC cases diagnosed before age 50 years

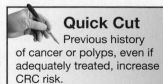

Quick Cut
Colonoscopy is necessary after resection to assess for a second primary (which occurs 5% of the time).

         e. **Screening recommendations:** Individuals should undergo colonoscopy every 1–2 years beginning at age 20 years and yearly past the age 35–40 years or 10 years younger than the age at which the relative was diagnosed.
   D. **CRC risk factors**
      1. **Family CRC history:** With a first-degree relative who has had CRC, the risk for developing CRC is three to nine times that of the general population.
      2. **Race:** African Americans have a higher risk than do people of other races.
      3. **Personal CRC or polyp history:** Even if adequately treated, they increase the likelihood of developing new cancers.

Quick Cut
Previous history of cancer or polyps, even if adequately treated, increase CRC risk.

4. **Personal IBD history**
5. **Age:** More than 90% of people found to have CRC are older than age 50 years.
6. **Diet:** High-fat (especially from animal sources), low-fiber diets may increase CRC risk.
7. **Activity level:** Sedentary individuals have a higher risk of developing CRC.
8. **Obesity:** Risk of dying of CRC is increased in overweight people.
9. **Diabetes**: increases risk of developing CRC
10. **Alcohol intake and smoking:** CRC has been linked to alcohol and tobacco use.

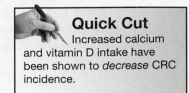

Quick Cut
Increased calcium and vitamin D intake have been shown to *decrease* CRC incidence.

IV. **Clinical presentation:** depends on the location, size, and extent of the tumor
   A. **Right-sided cancers:** present with melenic stools, fatigue, and iron deficiency anemia
   B. **Left-sided cancers:** present as a change in bowel habits, hematochezia, and/or cramping abdominal pain (caused by partial obstruction)

Quick Cut
Right-sided lesions are notable for melena and anemia, whereas left-sided lesions produce a change in bowel habits and hematochezia.

V. **Patient evaluation:** includes abdominal and rectal examinations and studies
   A. **Digital examination:** useful to assess the location, size, and extent of tumor invasion of the distal rectum
      1. Firm lesions suggest carcinoma, whereas soft polyps are likely benign.
      2. If a tumor feels fixed or "tethered" to the adjacent pararectal tissues, malignant invasion of the bowel wall is likely.
   B. **Rigid proctosigmoidoscopy:** determines the distance of a rectal tumor from the anal verge
   C. **Endorectal ultrasound:** provides information concerning the depth of invasion into the bowel wall by a rectal tumor and involvement of lymph nodes
   D. **Colonoscopy (with biopsy of the lesion and inspection of the remaining colon):** necessary to confirm the diagnosis and exclude synchronous lesions
   E. **Laboratory studies:** include **carcinoembryonic antigen (CEA)**, liver enzymes, and hemoglobin/hematocrit
   F. **Imaging:** CT scan is used to evaluate the chest and abdomen for metastases. MRI is used to stage rectal cancers and to evaluate the liver for metastases.

VI. **Staging:** The American College of Surgeons' Commission on Cancer has urged adoption of the **TNM staging system (Tables 12-1 and 12-2)**, which identifies the depth of tumor invasion (**T**), regional lymph node status (**N**), and the presence of distant metastases (**M**).

VII. **Treatment:** Surgical resection is necessary for most CRC cases. Important aspects of surgery include the following.
   A. Thorough abdominal exploration to search for metastases
   B. Removing the colon segment containing the tumor with the lymphovascular pedicle, which contains the lymph nodes that drain the cancer
   C. **Anastomosis** without tension between segments of bowel with satisfactory blood supply
   D. **Rectal cancer operations:** require special considerations

Quick Cut
Surgical treatment of rectal cancer: upper and middle third, LAR; lower third, APR or TATA.

   1. **Upper third (10–15 cm above the anus) and middle third (5–10 cm above the anus) tumors:** can be treated by resection through the abdomen with anastomosis between the left colon and the remaining rectum, or low anterior resection (**LAR**)
   2. **Lower third lesions:** Several options may be considered.
      a. **Resection of the rectum, anus, and anal sphincters (by a combined abdominal and perineal approach):** requires construction of a colostomy abdominoperineal resection (**APR**, also called the **Miles procedure**).
      b. **Resection of the rectum with coloanal anastomosis:** May require distal rectal mobilization and anastomosis via a transanal approach (transabdominal, transanal or **TATA** resection). A temporary diverting ileostomy allows the anastomosis to heal without the risk of sepsis from uncontrolled anastomotic leak.

Table 12-1: TNM Classification of Colorectal Cancer

TNM Classification	Abbreviation	Definition
Primary tumor (T)	TX	Primary tumor that cannot be assessed
	T0	No evidence of primary tumor
	Tis	Carcinoma in situ
	T1	Tumor that invades submucosa
	T2	Tumor that invades muscularis propria
	T3	Tumor that invades the muscularis propria into the subserosa or into nonperitonealized pericolic or perirectal tissues
	T4	Tumor that perforates the visceral peritoneum (a) or directly invades other organs (b)
Regional lymph nodes (N)	NX	Regional lymph nodes that cannot be assessed
	N0	No regional lymph node metastasis
	N1	Metastasis in one to three pericolic or perirectal lymph nodes
	N2	Metastasis in four or more pericolic or perirectal lymph nodes
	N3	Metastasis in any node along the course of a named vascular trunk
Distant metastasis (M)	MX	Presence of distant metastases not able to be assessed
	M1	No distant metastases
	M2	Distant metastases

TNM, tumor-node-metastasis.

c. **Local excision:** used for select, very favorable rectal cancers (small [<3–4 cm], T1N0, moderately or well-differentiated tumors, without lymphovascular invasion)

F. **Adjuvant therapy**

1. **Colon cancer:** Chemotherapy, often as combinations of **5-fluorouracil (5-FU)** and **leucovorin** with **oxaliplatin (FOLFOX)** or **irinotecan (FOLFIRI)**, is currently recommended for stage II poor prognostic histologic characteristics or III disease patients with inadequate lymph node sampling.

2. **Rectal cancer:** Neoadjuvant chemoradiation as well as adjuvant chemotherapy is recommended for stages II and III rectal cancers. Preoperative radiation therapy may shrink tumors and reduce local recurrence.

3. **Monoclonal antibodies (e.g., bevacizumab, cetuximab):** have shown clinical efficacy in patients with metastatic CRC, both alone and in combination with FOLFOX

VIII. **Prognosis:** determined by 5-year survival and clearly related to disease stage (Table 12-2)

IX. **Follow-up**

A. **Physical examination:** seldom reveals early tumor recurrences

B. **Colonoscopy:** Done 1 year after surgery to assess for local recurrence and to detect any new polyps. After a negative colonoscopy, the examination should be repeated every 3–5 years to detect any new polyps.

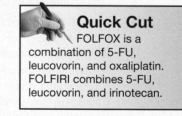

Quick Cut
FOLFOX is a combination of 5-FU, leucovorin, and oxaliplatin. FOLFIRI combines 5-FU, leucovorin, and irinotecan.

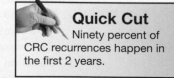

Quick Cut
Ninety percent of CRC recurrences happen in the first 2 years.

Table 12-2: Stage and Prognosis of Colorectal Cancer

Stage	Dukes Classification	T Level	N Level	M Level	Cure Rate
0	—	Tis	N0	M0	100%
I	A	T1 or T2	N0	M0	90%
II	B	T3 or T4	N0	M0	80%
III	C	Any T	N1, N2, or N3	M0	60%
IV	D	Any T	Any N	M1	5%

T, tumor; N, regional lymph nodes; M, distant metastases.

C. **CEA:** most sensitive indicator of recurrent CRC the incidence of a second CRC occurring after the first is as high as 5%, with most occurring within five years
   1. CEA may also be elevated in patients with cirrhosis, pancreatitis, renal failure, UC, and other types of cancer and can also be influenced by smoking.
   2. Most surgeons recommend obtaining CEA levels every 3 months during the first 2 postoperative years, every 6 months during the third to fifth postoperative years, and annually thereafter.
   3. **Rising CEA level:** indication for further workup (often a PET scan)
D. **Early recurrence detection:** could improve survival
   1. **Isolated hepatic metastases:** may be resected with a 25% 5-year survival
   2. **Solitary pulmonary metastases:** may be resected with a 20% 5-year survival
E. **Chemotherapy and radiation therapy:** palliative for recurrent nonresectable CRC

Carcinoid Tumors

I. **Etiology:** Arise from neuroectodermal cells and have the ability to incorporate and store amine precursor (5-hydroxytryptophan) and to decarboxylate this substrate, which produces several biologically active amines (e.g., **amine precursor uptake and decarboxylation [APUD]** tumors). The GI tract is the most common site, and (in decreasing order of frequency) carcinoids arise in the appendix, ileum, rectum, stomach, and colon. The tumors are usually small, submucosal nodules.

II. **Colon carcinoids:** account for less than 2% of GI carcinoids; they may be multicentric, and they may cause **carcinoid syndrome** from liver metastases

III. **Rectal carcinoids:** account for ~15% of GI carcinoids; they are usually solitary, and they do not cause carcinoid syndrome

IV. **Treatment:** related to tumor size
   A. **Tumors <2 cm:** seldom metastasize and can be locally excised
   B. **Tumors ≥2 cm:** usually malignant and should be treated by radical resection

DIVERTICULAR DISEASE

Terminology

I. **Diverticulum:** abnormal sac or pouch protruding from the wall of a hollow organ
   A. **True diverticulum:** diverticulum composed of all layers of bowel wall (rare in the colon)
   B. **False diverticulum:** diverticulum lacking a portion of the bowel wall (common in the colon)

II. **Diverticulosis:** presence of diverticula

III. **Diverticulitis:** inflammation associated with diverticula

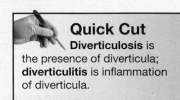

Quick Cut
Diverticulosis is the presence of diverticula; **diverticulitis** is inflammation of diverticula.

Diverticulosis

I. **Etiology:** unclear

II. **Epidemiology:** Incidence of this acquired disorder increases with age.
  A. Common in Western societies and rare in unindustrialized nations
  B. Populations who eat high-fiber, low-sugar foods (e.g., sub-Saharan Africans) have a low incidence of diverticulosis.
  C. Rare in persons younger than age 30 years
  D. Present in 75% of people older than age 80 years

III. **Pathogenesis:** herniations of mucosa through the colonic wall
  A. Diverticula occur at sites where arterioles traverse the wall.
  B. They usually lack a muscular layer (i.e., they are false diverticula).

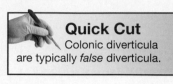

Quick Cut
Colonic diverticula are typically *false* diverticula.

IV. **Sigmoid colon:** most common site for diverticula; it is rare for diverticula to occur in the rectum

V. **Increased intraluminal pressure (in the colon):** thought to be associated with a low-fiber diet and has been proposed as the cause of mucosal herniation
  A. **Segmentation (of isolated areas of colon):** can produce high pressures
  B. Highest pressure across the colon wall occurs in the sigmoid colon, which is the region where diverticulosis occurs

VI. **Muscular hypertrophy (of the colon wall):** often accompanies diverticula and is especially common in the involved sigmoid colon

Diverticulitis

I. **Pericolic infection:** Perforation of one or more diverticula causes extravasation of colonic bacteria, leading to a wide spectrum of disease.
  A. **Pericolic phlegmon:** localized inflammation
  B. **Intra-abdominal abscess**
  C. **Generalized purulent peritonitis:** from ruptured abscess
  D. **Feculent peritonitis:** persistent fecal leakage from the perforation
  E. **Fistula formation:** including fistulas from the colon to the bladder, vagina, skin, and other sites

II. **Clinical presentation:** variable, depends on perforation site and infection extent
  A. **Left lower quadrant (LLQ) abdominal pain:** most common symptom and may radiate to the suprapubic area, groin, or back
  B. **Abdominal or pelvic mass:** may be caused by a phlegmon or abscess
  C. **Fever** and **leukocytosis:** common
  D. **Associated ileus:** may cause small bowel distention and vomiting
  E. **Generalized peritonitis:** may be present in severe cases
  F. **Colovesical fistula:** may cause pneumaturia, dysuria, pyuria, or fecaluria or may lead to vaginal drainage of pus or stool

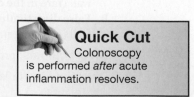

Quick Cut
LLQ pain is most common symptom of diverticulitis.

III. **Initial evaluation:** CT scan of the abdomen and pelvis is the most helpful test to confirm the suspected diagnosis and/or extent of diverticulitis.
  A. **IV contrast:** given before the CT scan to simultaneously evaluate the kidneys and ureters, making intravenous pyelography (IVP) unnecessary
  B. **CT-guided percutaneous drainage:** to drain an abscess
  C. **Air in the bladder:** suggests a **colovesical fistula**
  D. **Contrast enema:** Avoided if diverticulitis is suspected; hydrostatic pressure can worsen the extravasation of contrast and feces through the perforation.
  E. **Leukocyte count:** Obtain initially as a baseline and serially to evaluate the response to treatment.
  F. **Frequent abdominal examinations:** determine disease activity

IV. **Subsequent evaluation:** Colonoscopy is indicated to exclude cancer as the cause of the perforation.
  A. **Barium enema:** less useful than colonoscopy because small tumors may be masked by diverticula
  B. **Cystoscopy:** can be performed if a colovesical fistula is suspected to rule out a bladder cancer

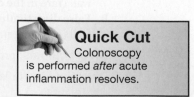

Quick Cut
Colonoscopy is performed *after* acute inflammation resolves.

V. **Treatment:** depends on disease severity, number of previous attacks, presence of complications, and the patient's overall condition

    A. **Phlegmon of the sigmoid colon:** Initial treatment includes IV fluids, bowel rest (with nasogastric tube decompression if ileus is present), and broad-spectrum IV antibiotics.

    B. **Intra-abdominal abscess:** Treatment is as above plus CT-guided percutaneous abscess drainage.

        1. Immediate surgery for acute diverticulitis with abscess carries an increased likelihood of complications and need for colostomy.

        2. If the abscess can be successfully drained, the patient usually recovers sufficiently to permit an elective single-stage sigmoidectomy with colorectal anastomosis.

    C. **Purulent** or **feculent peritonitis:** includes IV fluids, nothing orally, broad-spectrum IV antibiotics, and *urgent surgical resection*

        1. **Hartmann procedure:** resection of the diseased segment of bowel, **rectal stump closure, and colostomy** creation, as it is not safe to make an anastomosis in the presence of severe infection

        2. The colostomy can be taken down and the colon anastomosed to the rectum, when the patient has recovered, usually after at least 12 weeks .

    D. **Fistulas caused by diverticulitis:** same as for uncomplicated diverticulitis plus surgical resection after the acute inflammation has subsided

        1. **Sigmoidectomy and primary colorectal anastomosis:** usually possible if acute inflammation has resolved

        2. The structure at the other end of the fistula is repaired primarily.

    E. **Sigmoidectomy and primary colorectal anastomosis:** Can be done *after* recurrent attacks of diverticulitis following recovery from the acute episode. However, considerable clinical judgment is required to determine indications.

        1. After one attack, approximately one third of patients will have a second attack, after which another one third will have a third episode.

        2. **Younger patients:** Longer life span means a higher cumulative risk for recurrent diverticulitis; therefore, surgery may be recommended earlier.

        3. **Elective colon resection:** typically advised if an episode of complicated diverticulitis is treated nonoperatively

> **Quick Cut**
> The usual indication for surgery is a complication of diverticulitis (perforation or abscess, hemorrhage, or stricture). Uncomplicated diverticulitis may not need to be resected.

    F. **Additional surgical considerations:** Removing all colon containing diverticula is unnecessary; remove only the portion with hypertrophied muscular segment.

        1. **With significant pelvic inflammation:** Ureteral catheters may be placed prior to surgery to aid in identifying a ureteral injury should one occur.

        2. **Anastomosis:** In order to avoid recurrence, anastomose at the level of the rectum; the distal sigmoid colon almost always has a hypertrophied muscular wall.

> **Quick Cut**
> In resections for diverticulitis, the proximal line of resection is uninvolved bowel; the distal line is the rectum, which is safe to use because diverticulitis does not involve the rectum.

Hemorrhage

I. **Another major complication of diverticular disease:** An arteriole adjacent to a diverticulum may rupture, causing massive bleeding.

II. **Presentation:** Abdominal pain is rare; patients usually pass large amounts of bright red blood via the rectum. Rapid blood loss may result in shock.

> **Quick Cut**
> Diverticular bleeds are typically single episodes of brisk, bright red bleeding.

III. **Diagnostic tests:** accompany resuscitation

    A. **Immediate patient stabilization:** IV crystalloids and blood products if necessary. A nasogastric tube is inserted to rule out gastroduodenal hemorrhage; anoscopy is done to rule out an anorectal source of bleeding.

    B. **Laboratory studies:** baseline complete blood count and coagulation studies

    C. **Nuclear scan (labeled red blood cell scan):** done if the patient's condition permits

    D. **Colonoscopy:** Useful for bleeding localization and treatment. Endoscopic clipping and epinephrine injection are examples of hemostasis techniques.

 E. **Mesenteric arteriogram:** used if the nuclear scan or colonoscopy indicates the bleeding site and in patients with brisk bleeding
  1. With a known site, the branch can be embolized or **vasopressin** infused to constrict the mesenteric artery and lower portal pressure.
  2. **Segmental colectomy:** indicated if bleeding persists and angiography or colonoscopy has identified the hemorrhage site
  3. **Total abdominal colectomy with ileostomy:** indicated if bleeding persists and the site cannot be detected by arteriography

ANGIODYSPLASIA

General Considerations

 I. **Characteristics:** This **acquired vascular lesion** is also a major cause of colonic hemorrhage. Other names include *angiectasis, arteriovenous malformation,* and *vascular ectasias.*
  A. **Site:** Lesions occur most commonly in the right colon.
  B. **Incidence:** increases in frequency with age
   1. Occur rarely in persons younger than 40 years
   2. Lesions are probably present in most people older than 70 years.
  C. **Cause:** may be the result of chronic, intermittent submucosal vein obstruction
  D. Hemorrhage tends to be slower than that from diverticulosis. Stools may be melenic or bright red, depending on the rate of hemorrhage.

>
> **Quick Cut**
> Angiodysplasias are more common in patients of advanced age than in younger patients, and are most frequent in the cecum. They can cause massive lower GI bleeding.

 II. **Evaluation and treatment:** Similar to that for patients with bleeding diverticulosis. However, angiodysplasias tend to bleed intermittently, in contrast to diverticular bleeds, which tend to be a single episode of massive bleeding.
  A. **Colonoscopy:** Some angiodysplastic lesions can be detected as **"cherry red spots"** on the mucosa and can be eradicated by endoscopic electrocoagulation.
  B. **Segmental colectomy:** indicated with persistent or recurrent bleeding that can be isolated to a colonic segment by nuclear scans, arteriography, or colonoscopy
  C. **Total abdominal colectomy with ileostomy:** may be required as a lifesaving measure if bleeding persists and the site cannot be identified

INFLAMMATORY BOWEL DISEASE

General Considerations

 I. **Presentation:** Two major types of IBD can cause colitis, **Crohn disease (CD)** and **UC,** and their presentations overlap considerably (Table 12-3). In ~15% of cases, neither pathologic nor clinical distinction can be made and is called **indeterminate colitis.**

 II. **Etiology:** remains unknown for both diseases
  A. Genetic, environmental, infectious, and autoimmune mechanisms have been suggested, but a clearly defined cause has not been identified.
  B. Both diseases can occur at any age but tend to present in young adults.

>
> **Quick Cut**
> Distinguishing between CD and UC (when possible) is important because the medical and surgical treatments are different for each.

 III. **Serologic markers:** can help distinguish between CD and UC

Ulcerative Colitis

 I. **Inflammation:** Limited to the mucosa. The rectum is virtually always involved, with inflammation extending proximally for variable distances. Inflammation is **continuous.**

 II. **Involvement:** No perianal disease or small bowel involvement exists with UC.

 III. **Histology:** Crypt abscesses may be present but not granulomas. **Pseudopolyps** may be present.

>
> **Quick Cut**
> UC demonstrates mucosal inflammation only, *not* full-thickness inflammation. Perianal or small bowel involvement is absent.

Table 12-3: Inflammatory Disease of the Colon

Characteristics	Ulcerative Colitis	Crohn Colitis
Usual location	Rectum, left colon	Any segment of colon; ileocolic disease most common
Rectal bleeding	Common, continuous	Less common, intermittent
Rectal involvement	Almost always	~50%
Fistula	Rare	Common
Ulcers	Shaggy, irregular, continuous distribution	Linear with transverse fissures ("cobblestone")
Bowel stricture	Rare; should raise suspicion of cancer	Common
Carcinoma	Significantly increased incidence	Mildly increased incidence
perinuclear antineutrophil cytoplasmic antibodies (pANCA)	60%–70%	5%–10%
anti–*Saccharomyces cerevisiae* antibodies (ASCA)	10%–15%	60%–70%

UC, ulcerative colitis.

IV. **Extraintestinal manifestations:** include ankylosing spondylitis and sacroiliitis, peripheral arthritis, erythema nodosum and pyoderma gangrenosum, aphthous stomatitis, iritis and episcleritis, and primary sclerosing cholangitis

V. **Risk for colon cancer:** occurs with chronic disease
   A. The risk is minimal until 10 years after onset, and then it increases by ~1% per year thereafter.
   B. The risk is highest in patients with pancolitis.
   C. **Dysplasia (of the mucosa):** associated with an increased risk of cancer. Cancer in UC does not follow the usual polyp-carcinoma sequence and occurs in the flat areas.
   D. **Surveillance colonoscopy (with multiple mucosal biopsies to search for dysplasia):** done annually in patients who have had UC more than 10 years

VI. **Clinical presentation:** Disease severity ranges from occasional episodes of diarrhea to fulminant colitis.
   A. **Bloody diarrhea** is the most common symptom. Rarely, bleeding can be massive and life threatening.
   B. **Mucus and pus:** may accompany the passage of loose stools
   C. **Cramping abdominal pain, malaise, fever, weight loss, and anemia:** common
   D. **Fulminant colitis:** severe disease characterized by the following:
      1. Dilatation of the colon
      2. Abdominal pain, tenderness, and distention
      3. Fever, leukocytosis, and hypoalbuminemia
      4. Significant risk of colonic perforation

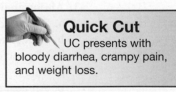

Quick Cut
UC presents with bloody diarrhea, crampy pain, and weight loss.

VII. **Evaluation:** Depends on disease severity. Mild cases can be evaluated on an outpatient basis, whereas fulminant colitis with toxic megacolon is a life-threatening situation requiring hospitalization, intensive medical treatment, and emergency surgery if medical treatment fails.
   A. **Proctoscopy:** most valuable test to establish the diagnosis
      1. **Continuous mucosal inflammation (beginning at the level of the dentate line):** highly suggestive of UC
      2. **Mucosal biopsies:** confirm the diagnosis and/or exclude Crohn and infectious colitis

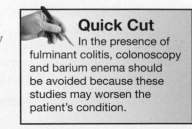

Quick Cut
In the presence of fulminant colitis, colonoscopy and barium enema should be avoided because these studies may worsen the patient's condition.

B. **Stool samples:** Culture for pathogens and examine for ova and parasites to rule out infectious colitis.

C. **Serologic markers:** for IBD (mainly perinuclear antineutrophil cytoplasmic antibody); see Table 12-4

D. **Colonoscopy:** used to evaluate entire colon if symptoms are mild

E. **Small bowel contrast studies or enterography:** obtained to rule out small bowel involvement, which would indicate CD

VIII. **Medical treatment:** A "step-up" approach based on disease severity and extent is used.

A. **Oral and topical aminosalicylates (5-aminosalicylic acid [5-ASA], mesalamine):** Used as primary therapy in patients with mild to moderate UC. These avoid the toxicity of sulfapyridine, which is present in sulfasalazine.

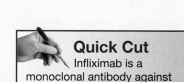

Quick Cut
Aminosalicylates (5-ASA and mesalamine) are first-line treatments for UC.

B. **Immunomodulating agents:** used for more severe, medically resistant disease

1. **Steroids:** effective for short-term treatment, but side effects prevent their long-term use
2. **IV cyclosporine:** more commonly used to induce, rather than maintain remission
3. **Others:** 6-mercaptopurine/azathioprine, methotrexate (same effects as for CD)

C. **Biologics:** Monoclonal antibodies to the proinflammatory cytokine tumor necrosis factor (TNF), such as **infliximab**, are effective in inducing remission in patients with refractory UC.

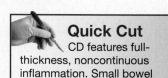

Quick Cut
Infliximab is a monoclonal antibody against TNF.

D. **Broad-spectrum antibiotics:** indicated for fulminant colitis

IX. **Surgical treatment**

A. **Indications:** hemorrhage, fulminant colitis or toxic megacolon unresponsive to intensive medical treatment, medically refractory disease, colonic stricture (at least 30% incidence of cancer), and dysplasia or cancer

B. **Procedures**

1. **Total proctocolectomy with a permanent ileostomy**
2. **Restorative proctocolectomy:** proctocolectomy with anal sphincter preservation and ileal pouch anal anastomosis (IPAA)
   a. Most common operation for UC and usually accompanied by a temporary ileostomy, which is closed 8–12 weeks after the initial operation
   b. Rarely used in patients with CD because of the risk of recurrent disease in the ileal pouch
3. **Abdominal colectomy with closure of the rectal stump:** Hartmann procedure
   a. Indicated with fulminant colitis
   b. Completion proctectomy and IPAA can be performed at a later time.
4. **Total proctocolectomy with continent ileostomy:** Kock pouch
   a. Due to incidence of complications, this procedure has been largely replaced by IPAA.
   b. An ileal pouch is fashioned with a nipple valve that is attached to the abdominal wall and requires intubation to evacuate the ileum several times daily.

Crohn (Granulomatous) Colitis

I. **Inflammation:** important feature of CD

A. **Transmural inflammation:** Full thickness of the bowel wall is inflamed.

B. **Noncontinuous inflammation:** "Skip areas" of normal bowel may separate inflamed regions.

Quick Cut
CD features full-thickness, noncontinuous inflammation. Small bowel and perianal involvement is common.

II. **Involvement:** The small bowel is frequently involved (especially the terminal ileum). Anal or perianal disease (e.g., fistulas, abscesses, fissures) is present in approximately one third of patients. Rectal sparing may be present.

III. **Histology:** Granulomas are present in ~50% of surgical specimens.

IV. **Endoscopic findings:** Linear ulcers may join transverse fissures to give a "**cobblestone**" appearance to the mucosa.

V. **Extraintestinal manifestations:** generally the same as for UC, except that sclerosing cholangitis is less common

VI. **Cancer risk:** increased in the diseased segments but less defined than with UC

VII. **Clinical presentation:** typically, abdominal pain, diarrhea, and weight loss

    A. **Malaise, fever, and leukocytosis:** common

    B. **Abdominal abscesses and fistulas:** may occur (fistulas between the involved bowel and the bladder, vagina, skin, or other segments of intestine)

    C. **Fulminant colitis:** may be as severe as with UC

        1. **Megacolon:** The colon usually does not dilate with fulminant CD, which is thought to be because of the transmural inflammation with wall thickening.

        2. **Perforation risk:** Same as in UC; therefore, patients must be treated with the same vigor.

VIII. **Evaluation:** As with UC, evaluation depends on disease severity.

    A. **Physical exam:** abdominal examination to evaluate areas of tenderness or mass and anorectal examination to detect abscesses, fissures, or fistulas

    B. **Laboratory studies:** include serologic markers for IBD, mainly anti–*Saccharomyces cerevisiae* antibody (see Table 12-4), and stool sample for culture, ova, and parasite to rule out infectious causes of colitis

    C. **Radiographic studies:** Upper GI series with small bowel follow-through or enterography is important to evaluate small bowel involvement and/or CT scan if an abscess or perforation is suspected.

    D. **Endoscopy:** Proctoscopy is important; if rectal mucosa is not involved, UC is essentially excluded. Colonoscopy is the most sensitive diagnostic modality for colonic involvement.

IX. **Medical treatment**

    A. **Budesonide, 5-ASA agents, and antibiotics:** common treatments for mild to moderate CD

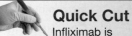
Quick Cut
Budesonide, a glucocorticoid with high topical activity and first-pass metabolism in the liver, has been shown to be as effective as traditional steroids with less adrenal suppression.

    B. **Immunomodulating agents:** more severe, refractory disease

        1. **Steroids:** helpful for acute disease but have many well-established side effects

        2. **6 Mercaptopurine/azathioprine:** have a slow onset of action and are therefore most useful for maintaining disease remission

        3. **Methotrexate:** contraindicated in pregnancy

        4. **IV cyclosporine:** may be helpful, but most patients on therapy ultimately come to colectomy

    C. **Biologics:** Anti-TNF agents are increasingly being used to induce and maintain remission in patients with steroid-dependent or refractory CD. These agents are particularly effective in treating patients with fistulizing disease.

Quick Cut
Infliximab is particularly effective for fistulizing CD.

    D. **Total parenteral nutrition (TPN):** Permits bowel rest and induces remission in some patients with significant CD. This remission rate is much higher than the rate for patients with severe UC treated by TPN.

    E. **Metronidazole and ciprofloxacin:** beneficial for perianal disease

X. **Surgical treatment**

    A. **Indications:** intestinal obstruction, abdominal abscesses and fistulas, perforation, debilitating disease refractory to medical treatment, fulminant colitis, hemorrhage (rare), and cancer (less common than with UC)

Quick Cut
Anorectal abscesses or fistulas require special surgical considerations (pus should be drained, but large incisions are avoided to prevent sphincter injury).

    B. **Surgical considerations:** High recurrence rate (~50% within 10 years) follows intestinal resection. The most likely site of recurrence is at the anastomosis from the previous operation.

        1. **Surgery goal:** Conserve bowel.

            a. Only grossly involved bowel should be resected.

            b. **Stricturoplasty:** To conserve bowel, this is done rather than resection to relieve obstruction in short strictures.

Quick Cut
Bowel conservation in CD surgery is critical because recurrence is common and numerous resections can lead to short gut syndrome.

        2. **Abdominal abscesses:** drained percutaneously prior to surgery

3. **Total proctocolectomy with ileostomy:** May be required for severe rectal disease. IPAA is used rarely due to the risk of disease recurrence.

4. **TPN:** allows bowel rest for 7–10 days preoperatively to promote resolution of intra-abdominal inflammation and potentially reduce the risk of injury to adjacent organs

PSEUDOMEMBRANOUS COLITIS (ANTIBIOTIC-ASSOCIATED COLITIS)

Epidemiology and Clinical Presentation

I. **Acute diarrhea associated with the use of antibiotics:** Clindamycin and ampicillin are most often implicated, but almost every antibiotic has been implicated. Frequently, the antibiotic has been discontinued before diarrhea development.

II. **Common in hospitals and nursing homes:** Epidemics have been reported and also after intestinal operations, especially when antibiotic bowel preparations have been used.

Pathogenesis and Presentation

I. **Antibiotics alter the normal colonic bacterial population.**

II. *Clostridium difficile*: Normally suppressed by colonic bacteria, this pathogen emerges and causes mild diarrhea to severe life-threatening colitis.

A. **Exotoxins:** *C. difficile* elaborates two exotoxins, enterotoxin A and cytotoxin B.

B. **Pseudomembranes:** Yellow plaques may cover the mucosa.

1. Pseudomembranes are composed of fibrin and debris from cells and bacteria.

2. The absence of pseudomembranes does not rule out infection.

Diagnosis

I. **History:** History of diarrhea after treatment with an antibiotic is suspicious.

II. **Stool sample:** for *C. difficile* toxin titer or real-time PCR

III. **Proctoscopy or colonoscopy:** may reveal pseudomembranes, which are diagnostic

Treatment

I. **Causative antibiotic:** Discontinue.

II. **Metronidazole (oral or IV) and vancomycin (oral):** equally effective; however, the daily cost for metronidazole treatment is much lower

III. **Constipating agents (e.g., loperamide):** Avoid constipating agents.

IV. **Recurrence:** common (25%) and requires retreatment with metronidazole, vancomycin, or newer agents such as rifaximin

V. **Abdominal colectomy with ileostomy:** often necessary for rare fulminant cases

ISCHEMIC COLITIS

Etiology

I. **Watershed areas:** Points of communication between collateral arteries are theoretically at increased risk for ischemia. These points include the **splenic flexure** and the **midsigmoid colon**; however, any segment of the colon may be involved. Rectal involvement is very rare.

II. **Predisposing factors:** include the following:

A. **Surgery:** especially aortic surgery with IMA ligation

B. **Vascular disease:** atherosclerosis, vasculitis, and collagen vascular diseases

C. **Hypercoagulable states:** such as polycythemia vera

D. **Low-flow states:** particularly in the setting of myocardial infarction, sepsis, or congestive heart failure

E. **Medications:** digitalis, oral contraceptives, antihypertensive medications, and vasopressors

Quick Cut
Ischemic colitis occurs most commonly at the splenic flexure and midsigmoid colon because they are watershed areas of the vascular supply.

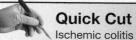

Quick Cut
Ischemic colitis may result in dusky, mildly ischemic mucosa, partial thickness injury with moderate ischemia, or full-thickness necrosis.

Table 12-4: Colonic Ischemia

Phase of Ischemia	Transient Ischemia	Chronic or Partial-Thickness Ischemia	Gangrene
Defining features	Involves only mucosa, which often looks dusky and hemorrhagic on endoscopy	Often results in stricture formation	Entire bowel wall is nonviable.
Symptoms	Cramping abdominal pain with passage of small amount of blood	More severe abdominal pain with tenderness, fever, leukocytosis	Severe abdominal pain frequently with peritonitis, acidosis, sepsis
Treatment	Supportive care with treatment and/or correction of causative factors	More intensive monitoring, intravenous fluids, and broad-spectrum antibiotics. Surgical resection if symptomatic stricture develops.	Emergent resection of any nonviable bowel is necessary and almost always requires a colostomy.

Pathogenesis and Treatment

I. **Supportive care:** IV fluids, antibiotics

II. **Surgical resection for nonviable bowel (see Table 12-4)**

◆ VOLVULUS

Overview

I. **Definition:** twist or torsion of an organ on its pedicle

II. **Symptoms:** produced by occluding the bowel lumen (obstruction) or occluding the blood supply (ischemia)

III. **Incidence:** Low in the United States. It is the most common cause of colon obstruction in Africa, where there is a significantly lower rate of diverticular disease, perhaps related to dietary fiber intake.

Sigmoid Volvulus

I. **Etiology:** Sigmoid volvulus accounts for more than 80% of cases of colonic volvulus.
   A. **Patient characteristics:** Average age is 60 years. Patients with this condition often reside in nursing homes or mental institutions.
   B. **Predisposing conditions:** include an elongated sigmoid colon with an ample, freely mobile mesentery and a narrow point of fixation about which the colon can twist

II. **Pathogenesis:** The sigmoid colon usually twists counterclockwise around the axis of the mesentery. Together, this causes obstruction of the colon lumen and may also cause vascular compromise leading to ischemic bowel.

Quick Cut
Twisting of the bowel and mesentery in volvulus obstructs the lumen and can compromise blood supply.

Cecal Volvulus

I. **Etiology:** occurs much less frequently than sigmoid volvulus
   A. **Patient characteristics:** more common in women, and patients are often younger than 40 years
   B. **Cause:** incomplete peritoneal fixation of the right colon (for axial torsion) or a redundant cecum that can flop into the left upper quadrant (LUQ) in the cecal bascule

II. **Other contributing factors:** may include cancer of the distal colon, malrotation, prior surgery, and pregnancy

III. **Pathogenesis:** The cecum and ascending colon usually twist clockwise. Bowel and vascular obstruction occurs in a manner similar to that described for sigmoid volvulus.

Diagnosis

I. **History:** usually indicates increasing abdominal distention, discomfort, and obstipation

II. **Physical examination:** Reveals abdominal distention and tympany; rebound tenderness suggests gangrenous bowel.

III. Abdominal radiographs
  A. **Sigmoid volvulus:** Massively distended sigmoid colon, with both ends in the pelvis and the bow near the diaphragm in the right upper quadrant (**"bent inner tube sign"**) is seen.
  B. **Cecal volvulus:** often reveals a large distended cecum that occupies the LUQ (**"coffee bean"** or **"kidney"** shape)

IV. Barium enema: reveals the pathognomonic obstructing twist (**"bird's beak deformity"**)

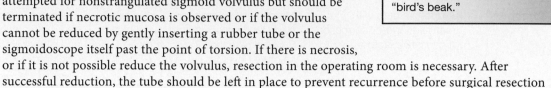

Quick Cut
Radiology key words: Sigmoid volvulus looks like a "bent inner tube"; cecal volvulus looks like a "coffee bean." Volvulus on a barium enema resembles a "bird's beak."

Treatment
  I. **Sigmoid volvulus:** Endoscopic decompression should be attempted for nonstrangulated sigmoid volvulus but should be terminated if necrotic mucosa is observed or if the volvulus cannot be reduced by gently inserting a rubber tube or the sigmoidoscope itself past the point of torsion. If there is necrosis, or if it is not possible reduce the volvulus, resection in the operating room is necessary. After successful reduction, the tube should be left in place to prevent recurrence before surgical resection is performed.
  A. **Elective sigmoidectomy with colorectal anastomosis:** recommended after successful decompression, typically during the same hospital admission
  B. **Sigmoidectomy with colostomy (Hartmann operation):** indicated if decompression cannot be achieved or if there is gangrenous bowel

  II. **Cecal volvulus:** Colonoscopic decompression is risky and rarely successful; therefore, surgical resection is necessary to prevent recurrences.
  A. **Right colectomy with primary anastomosis:** generally indicated if the bowel is viable
  B. **Cecopexy:** rarely performed due to high recurrence rates

ANORECTAL DYSFUNCTION

Incontinence
  I. **Etiology:** inability to control elimination of rectal contents
  A. **Anal sphincter mechanical defects:** include iatrogenic injury (e.g., episiotomy or previous fistulotomy) and anorectal trauma (e.g., impalement injuries)
  B. **Neurogenic causes:** include pudendal nerve injury due to prolonged labor and systemic neurologic disease (e.g., multiple sclerosis)
  C. **Systemic disease:** including that affecting the sphincters (e.g., scleroderma, diabetes)
  D. **Causes unrelated to the anal sphincter:** include severe diarrhea, severe proctitis with decreased rectal capacity, fecal impaction with overflow incontinence, and large rectal tumors

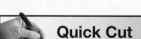

Quick Cut
Incontinence can be due to causes unrelated to the sphincters (e.g., diarrhea, fecal impaction with overflow, severe proctitis, etc.).

  II. **Evaluation:** History and anorectal examination often suffice to establish the diagnosis.
  A. **Anterior sphincter defect and patulous anus:** may be confirmed by a thorough examination and endorectal ultrasound of the anal musculature, if necessary
  B. **Physiologic evaluation:** helpful if the cause of incontinence is not obvious
  1. **Anal manometry:** documents resting and squeeze pressures, sphincter length, and minimal sensory volume of the rectum
  2. **Pudendal nerve terminal motor latency:** detects neurogenic impairment

  III. **Surgical treatment:** Sphincter defects may be surgically corrected by **overlapping sphincter repair** with some success.
  A. **Gracilis muscle transposition or artificial anal sphincter implantation:** for more extensive loss of the anal sphincter; however, complication rates are high
  B. **Sacral nerve stimulation and injectable biomaterials:** newer methods
  C. **Colostomy:** may be required for severe sphincter injuries or for neurogenic or systemic causes of incontinence

Obstructed Defecation (Pelvic Floor–Outlet Obstruction)

I. **Anal stenosis:** May be caused by circumferential hemorrhoidectomy, trauma, or radiation. Treatment generally entails repeated dilatation or advancing full-thickness skin pedicles into the anal canal.

II. **Puborectalis (anismus) nonrelaxation:** functional disorder characterized by paradoxical contraction of the puborectalis muscle at the time of defecation
  A. **Symptoms:** include a sense of incomplete evacuation and severe straining during defecation
  B. **Incidence:** occurs in women nine times more often than in men
  C. **Normal colonic transit time:** measured by radiopaque marker tracking through the colon (**Sitz marker study**)
  D. **Diagnosis:** confirmed by defecography and manometry, which demonstrate the failure of the muscle to relax appropriately
  E. **Treatment:** Nonsurgical; **biofeedback** is the treatment of choice.

III. **Internal intussusception (internal rectal prolapse):** Characterized by the distal rectum telescoping into itself, causing partial obstruction. Patients complain of urge to defecate, rectal fullness, and pelvic pain.
  A. **Solitary rectal ulcer:** Often seen in this syndrome, located in the anterior rectal wall. Chronically, it may cause ischemia resulting in **colitis cystica profunda**, which is the entrapment of mucin-secreting glands beneath the mucosa. It is important to distinguish this benign lesion from cancer.
  B. **Abnormal rectal fixation:** accompanies intussusception and permits the rectum to descend
  C. **Medical treatment:** suffices for most patients and consists of increased dietary fiber, stool softeners, and glycerine suppositories or enemas
  D. **Surgical treatment:** Rectopexy with or without rectosigmoid resection. Indications include the following.
    1. **Debilitating symptoms:** despite maximum medical therapy
    2. **Impending anal incontinence:** due to stretch injury to the pudendal nerves caused by constant straining and perineal descent
    3. **Chronic bleeding:** from a solitary rectal ulcer

IV. **Rectal prolapse:** Protrusion of the full thickness of the rectum (and occasionally the sigmoid colon) through the anus in *concentric* mucosal folds should be distinguished from **prolapsed internal hemorrhoids**, which have *radial* folds in the prolapsing mucosa.
  A. **Etiology:** Patients frequently have diastasis of levator ani, a deep cul-de-sac, redundant sigmoid colon, patulous anal sphincters, and/or loss of rectal sacral attachments.
  B. **Epidemiology:** increased incidence in patients in mental institutions, women who have had a hysterectomy, and elderly women
  C. **Symptoms:** include mucosa-lined bowel protruding through the anus, bleeding, anal pain, mucous discharge, and fecal incontinence caused by stretch of the anal sphincters or the pudendal nerves
  D. **Treatment:** Surgical; incarceration and strangulation are rare but can occur.
    1. **Rectopexy with or without rectosigmoid resection:** treatment of choice for patients in satisfactory health and with satisfactory anal continence
    2. **Perineal proctectomy (Altemeier procedure):** For patients with significant comorbidities, an abdominal incision is avoided; however, recurrence rates are higher.
    3. **Anal encircling:** Placing a band of synthetic material (wire or mesh) subcutaneously around the anus is of historical interest only.
    4. **Colostomy:** for total incontinence

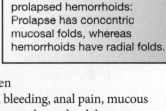

> **Quick Cut**
> Rectal prolapse must be distinguished from prolapsed hemorrhoids: Prolapse has concentric mucosal folds, whereas hemorrhoids have radial folds.

BENIGN ANORECTAL DISEASE

Hemorrhoids

I. **Etiology:** Cushions of vascular and connective tissue develop, which are thought to protect the sphincter during defecation and permit complete closure of the anus during rest.
  A. **Vascular tissue engorgement:** causes these cushions/complexes to enlarge
  B. **Hemorrhoidal enlargement:** Prolonged straining during defecation and increased abdominal pressure are thought to produce symptoms.

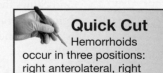

> **Quick Cut**
> Hemorrhoids occur in three positions: right anterolateral, right posterolateral, and left lateral.

II. Classification

A. **Internal hemorrhoids** are located above the dentate line and are covered by rectal mucosa; therefore, they are typically not painful. Internal hemorrhoids are graded as follows:
1. **First degree:** bleed, but do not prolapse
2. **Second degree:** bleed and prolapse, but reduce spontaneously
3. **Third degree:** bleed and prolapse, and must be manually reduced
4. **Fourth degree:** protrude through the anus and cannot be reduced

B. **External hemorrhoids** reside below the anal verge and are lined by squamous epithelium. A thrombosis within an external hemorrhoid may cause acute swelling and anal pain.

III. Symptoms:
Bleeding and prolapse are the predominant symptoms of internal hemorrhoids. Acutely prolapsed and incarcerated internal hemorrhoids may cause pain. External hemorrhoids cause discomfort, pruritus, and pain if thrombosed.

IV. Treatment:
depends on the symptoms

A. **Medical therapy:** includes increasing dietary fiber and fluid, stool softeners, and avoidance of straining

B. **Rubber band ligation:** often used to treat first-, second-, and third-degree hemorrhoids and selected cases of fourth-degree hemorrhoids
1. The rubber bands must be placed above the dentate line or severe pain will result.
2. Caution must be exercised to avoid unintentional ligation of full-thickness rectal tissue, which can result in life-threatening sepsis.

> **Quick Cut**
> Rubber band ligation is the most common treatment for internal hemorrhoids and can *only* be used for internal hemorrhoids.

C. **Sclerotherapy and infrared photocoagulation:** less frequently used for first-, second-, and third-degree hemorrhoids

D. **Hemorrhoidectomy:** May be required for refractory hemorrhoids and most fourth-degree hemorrhoids. Options include the following.
1. **Surgical excision:** of one or more hemorrhoidal columns with the mucosa left open or sutured closed
2. **Stapled hemorrhoidectomy:** Excises a ring of mucosa and submucosa above the hemorrhoids and returns the anal cushions to their anatomic position. This procedure has been associated with chronic postoperative pain and is therefore seldom used today.

E. **Thrombosed hemorrhoids:** May require excision for pain relief if patient presents within 48–72 hours of thrombosis, when pain is most intense. However, most cases resolve within 2 weeks without any specific therapy.

Anal Fissure

I. Definition:
An anal fissure is a tear in the anoderm, commonly caused by constipation. Approximately 90% of fissures are in the posterior midline, where anal perfusion is the lowest, and ~10% are in the anterior midline.

II. Symptoms:
anal pain and bleeding associated with defecation

III. Physical findings:
may include the following:

A. **Fissure or ulcer:** distal to the dentate line with underlying exposed internal sphincter muscle

B. **Sentinel skin tag:** externally and/or hypertrophied anal papilla internally

C. **Spasm or hypertrophy of the internal sphincter:** in chronic cases

IV. Treatment:
Most fissures will heal with medical treatment.

A. **Medical:** Stool softeners, increased dietary fiber, and warm sitz baths are beneficial.
1. **Nitroglycerin or diltiazem:** Topical application has been shown to increase blood flow to the ischemic internal sphincter muscle and facilitate fissure closure.
2. **Botulinum toxin:** Injection into the internal sphincter muscle temporarily paralyzes the muscle and allows the fissure to heal.

B. **Surgical: Lateral internal sphincterotomy** may be done for fissures refractory to medical therapy. This can be done via an open or a closed technique and is highly curative.

Anorectal Abscess and Fistula

I. Pathogenesis:
Abscess is the acute stage and **fistula** is the chronic stage of the same disease process.

A. **Cryptoglandular infections:** They begin in the anal glands that empty into the anal crypts.

> **Quick Cut**
> Anorectal abscess is acute infection; anorectal fistulas are the sequelae of chronic infection.

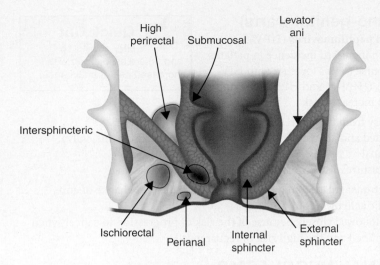

Figure 12-2: Perirectal abscesses develop from fistulous tracts that begin in rectal ulcers of anorectal glands. These fistulae extend into the intersphincteric space and then follow tissue planes to a variety of pelvic locations where abscesses may form. (From Yamada T, Alpers DH, Kaplowitz N, et al. *Textbook of Gastroenterology*, 4th ed. Philadelphia: Lippincott Williams & Wilkins; 2003.)

    B. Intersphincteric abscesses: Most abscesses originate between the internal and external sphincters (Fig. 12-2).

        1. Perianal abscess: downward extension

        2. Ischiorectal fossa abscess: lateral extension through the external sphincter

        3. Supralevator abscess: upward extension (rare)

  II. Signs and symptoms: anorectal pain, usually referred to as throbbing pain, frequently with fever and leukocytosis

    A. Swelling and fluctuance: late signs

    B. Pus and blood drainage: signifies spontaneous rupture and is usually associated with pain relief

  III. Treatment: Incision and drainage (I&D) should be performed promptly after the diagnosis is made.

    A. Ischiorectal fossa: may contain a large volume of pus before fluctuance is obvious

    B. Antibiotics: required only if immune status is compromised (e.g., diabetes, leukemia) or there is extensive cellulitis

> **Quick Cut**
> Despite adequate drainage, nearly 50% of patients will develop anorectal fistula.

  IV. Anorectal fistula: communication between the anorectal lumen and the perianal skin

    A. Internal opening: must be identified to allow proper treatment

        1. Posterior anal crypt: most common site of the internal opening

        2. Goodsall rule: Envision a transverse line that bisects the anus. External openings that are posterior to this line will curve and connect to the posterior midline crypt, whereas external openings anterior will communicate to an anterior crypt by a short, radial tract.

    B. Fistulotomy: Used to treat simple anal fistula. Both openings are identified and the tract unroofed.

    C. Complicated fistulas (involve significant sphincter muscle): Require procedures that eradicate the internal opening; fistulotomy would likely cause incontinence.

Pilonidal Disease

  I. Pathophysiology: Exact mechanism is unclear, although it is characterized by hair from the skin of the postsacral superior gluteal cleft becoming trapped below the surface, leading to foreign body reaction and acutely causing local infection (i.e., abscess) or chronically draining sinuses.

  II. Treatment: I&D for acute abscess and excision with closure by primary or secondary intent for a chronic sinus tract. Complex flap procedures may be necessary for recurrence after these measures.

Hidradenitis Suppurativa

  I. Pathophysiology: infection of the apocrine sweat glands

    A. Subcutaneous sinus tracts: form from infected glands and can spread to the perineum, scrotum, or labia

    B. Distinguish from cryptoglandular disease: does not involve the anal canal, whereas cryptoglandular disease originates there

  II. Clinical presentation: varies from acute sinus tracts to complicated fistulas and abscesses

  III. Treatment: Excision of involved skin, frequently without primary closure. Recurrence is common.

Condyloma Acuminatum (Ano-genital warts)

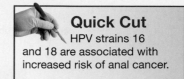

I. **Etiology:** Causative agent is **human papillomavirus (HPV).**
   A. **Transmission:** usually sexual, with increased incidence in patients who practice anoreceptive intercourse travels together with HIV
   B. **Anal cancer:** Certain viral strains (HPV-16 and HPV-18) found in condyloma are associated with increased risk.
II. **Clinical presentation:** Lesions vary from tiny excrescences to cauliflowerlike masses.
   A. **Site:** may be sessile or pedunculated and are usually located on the perianal skin, penis, vulva, vagina, or cervix or in the anal canal
   B. **Symptoms:** pruritus, perianal moisture, discomfort, and the presence of masses
III. **Treatment:** Local excision and electrocoagulation may be done and offer the best chance of cure.
   A. **Topical treatments:** bichloroacetic acid or imiquimod
   B. **Surveillance:** Patients should be followed closely because of the risk of progression to cancer when carcinogenic viral strains are identified and the high risk of recurrence.

PERIANAL AND ANAL CANAL NEOPLASMS

Anal Margin (below Dentate Line)

I. **Neoplasms:** include squamous cell carcinoma, basal cell carcinoma, Bowen disease, and perianal Paget disease
II. **Presentation and treatment:** Table 12-5

Anal Canal (above Dentate Line)

I. **Epidermoid carcinoma:** includes squamous cell, basaloid, cloacogenic, and mucoepidermoid carcinoma
   A. **Clinical presentation:** may be bleeding, pain, or anal mass
   B. **Diagnosis and evaluation:** includes physical examination to assess tumor size, depth of invasion, ulceration, and regional lymph nodes and anoscopy and/or proctoscopy with biopsy, endorectal ultrasound, and CT scan of the pelvis and liver

   C. **Treatment:** Most lesions require combined modality therapy consisting of 5-FU and mitomycin C with external beam radiation.
      1. **Superficial early-stage lesions:** can be effectively treated with local excision only
      2. **APR:** reserved for treatment failures with greater than 50% 5-year survival
   D. **Prognosis:** Combined treatment has an overall response rate of 90% and a 5-year survival rate greater than 80%.

Table 12-5: Anal Margin Neoplasms

Tumor Type	Presentation	Treatment
Squamous cell carcinoma	Polypoid, fungating, or ulcerated mass; pruritus; bleeding	Local excision or radiation if large or recurrent
Basal cell carcinoma	Central ulceration with irregular, raised pearly borders	Local excision; radiation or abdominal perineal resection for rare, advanced lesions
Bowen disease (squamous cell carcinoma in situ)	Variable skin changes: erythematous, crusty, scaly plaques; itching; burning; bleeding; 10% develop squamous cell carcinoma	Wide local excision or topical 5-FU
Perianal Paget disease (intraepithelial adenocarcinoma)	Erythematous, eczematous rash with white ulcerations; intractable pruritus; high incidence of visceral carcinoma	Wide local excision or topical retinoic acid; if underlying rectal cancer— abdominoperineal resection

5-FU, 5-fluorouracil.

II. **Adenocarcinoma:** most commonly an extension from cancer in the distal rectum

A. **Cancer arises from anal glands and ducts:** It may manifest outside the lumen of the anal canal and present as an anal fistula.

B. **Treatment:** generally similar to that for rectal cancer, with preoperative chemoradiation followed by APR

III. **Melanoma:** The anal canal is the third most common site (after skin and eyes). Not all anal melanomas are darkly pigmented (i.e., some are amelanotic).

A. **Symptoms and presentation:** Anal mass, pain, and bleeding are most common. Regional lymphatic and distant metastases are common at diagnosis.

B. **Treatment:** APR versus wide local excision is controversial, although the key to surgical treatment is a *complete excision*. The 5-year survival rate is less than 15%.

Chapter 13

Liver, Gallbladder, and Biliary Tree

Daniel Medina and Srinevas K. Reddy

GENERAL ASPECTS

Anatomy and Physiology

I. **Hepatobiliary embryology:** Hepatic diverticulum forms as an embryologic outpouching of the foregut.
   A. **Cranial portion:** forms the liver and the larger branches of the intrahepatic ducts
   B. **Caudal portion:** forms the gallbladder, cystic duct, and common bile duct

II. **Liver:** weighs <2% of total body weight and is composed of two lobes (left and right), each subdivided into multiple segments (Fig. 13-1)
   A. **Hepatic lobes:** divided by the interlobar fissure, an invisible line between the gallbladder fossa anteriorly and the inferior vena cava posteriorly
   B. **Falciform ligament:** marks the segmental fissure between the median and lateral segments of the left lobe and is the only externally visible boundary
   C. **Arterial supply:** emanates from the common hepatic artery, which is a branch of the celiac axis
      1. **Left hepatic artery:** arises from the left gastric artery in 20% of the population
      2. **Right hepatic artery:** arises from the superior mesenteric artery (SMA) in ~20% of the population
   D. **Venous supply:** emanates from the portal vein, which carries partially oxygenated blood from the splanchnic circulation
      1. **Route:** Like the arterial supply, the portal supply also follows the hepatic segmental anatomy.
      2. **Venous drainage:** occurs through left, middle, and right hepatic veins emptying into the inferior vena cava at the level of the diaphragm

III. **Biliary tree:** Bile produced by the liver drains into left and right hepatic ducts, whose confluence forms the common hepatic duct (Fig. 13-2).
   A. **Common bile duct:** formed by the cystic and common hepatic ducts
   B. **Pancreatic duct:** typically joins the common bile duct before they enter the duodenum through the ampulla of Vater, surrounded by the sphincter of Oddi, which controls bile flow

IV. **Gallbladder:** located on the inferior aspect of the liver and divided into the fundus, body, infundibulum, and the neck
   A. **Histology:** Wall is composed of smooth muscle and fibrous tissue; the lumen is lined with high columnar epithelium.
   B. **Arterial supply:** through the cystic artery, which is usually a branch of the right hepatic artery

Quick Cut
The segmental anatomy of the liver is determined by the vascular supply and biliary tree and does not have obvious external landmarks.

Quick Cut
The oxygenated blood supply to the liver is 25% arterial and 75% portal.

Quick Cut
A replaced right hepatic artery arises from the SMA instead of the proper hepatic artery.

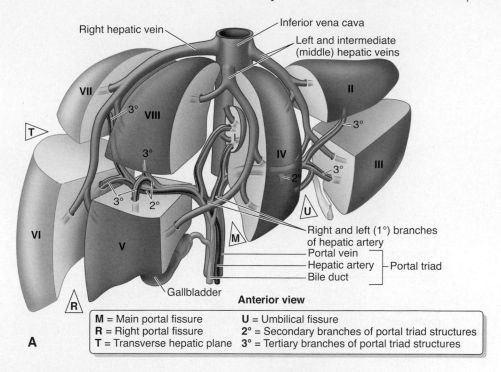

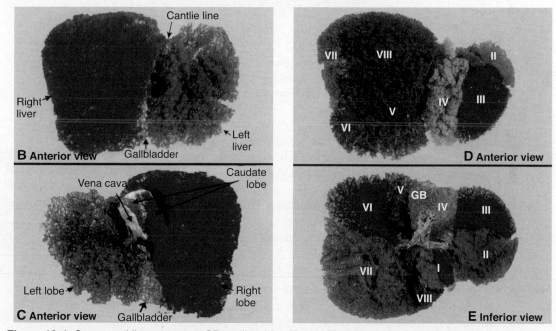

Figure 13-1: Segmental liver anatomy. GB, gallbladder. (From Moore KL, Agur AMR, Dalley AF. *Clinically Oriented Anatomy*, 7th ed. Baltimore: Lippincott Williams & Wilkins; 2013.)

    C. Venous return: via cystic veins that drain to the portal vein and directly into the liver

    D. Lymphatic drainage: goes both to the liver and to hilar nodes

    E. Innervation: from the celiac plexus

V. Physiology: Generally, the function of the liver may be classified in the following categories.

    A. Metabolic: detoxification, glycogenolysis, ammonia conversion, drug processing, recycling of byproducts, gluconeogenesis, lipogenesis, and cholesterol synthesis

    B. Neurologic: Liver failure leads to encephalopathy due to increased toxin level (e.g., ammonia).

    C. Cardiovascular: angiotensinogen synthesis

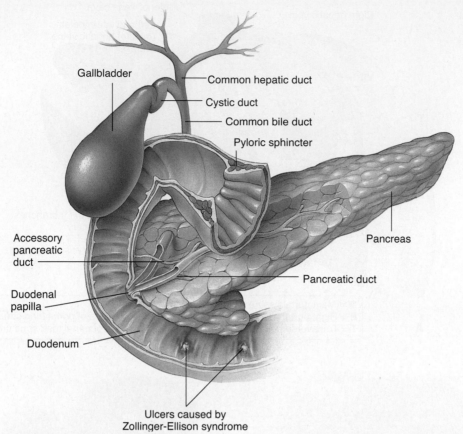

Figure 13-2: Biliary anatomy. (From Escott-Stump S. *Nutrition and Diagnosis-Related Care*, 7th ed. Baltimore: Lippincott Williams & Wilkins; 2011.)

D. Gastrointestinal (GI): bile production, fat emulsification, and absorption of essential molecules from the GI tract

E. Endocrine: thrombopoietin and insulinlike growth factor 1 synthesis and insulin metabolism

F. Hematologic: fetal erythrocyte production; synthesis of coagulation and anticoagulation factors

G. Immunologic: acute phase reactants, complement synthesis, and part of the reticuloendothelial system

> **Quick Cut**
> The function of the hepatobiliary system is quite complex, and overall function cannot yet be replaced by artificial means.

VI. Bile production: Approximately 600 mL of bile are produced daily (normal range: 250–1,000 mL/day).

A. Composition: electrolytes and water, bile pigments, protein, lipids, phospholipids (e.g., lecithin), cholesterol, and chenodeoxycholic acid conjugated with taurine and glycine primarily

B. Storage: gallbladder, which absorbs water and electrolytes de facto, concentrating bile by 10-fold

C. Release: Coordinated release of bile requires simultaneous contraction of the gallbladder and relaxation of the sphincter of Oddi. The process is predominantly under humoral control, via cholecystokinin (CCK), but vagal and splanchnic nerves also play a role.

> **Quick Cut**
> The sphincter of Oddi is tonically contracted, which allows bile to enter the gallbladder by backfilling through the cystic duct.

Hepatobiliary Studies

I. Liver function tests (LFTs): reflect the following:

A. Synthetic function: albumin, fibrinogen, clotting factors

B. Clearance: ammonia, indirect bilirubin

C. Excretory function and patency of the biliary tree: direct bilirubin, alkaline phosphatase

D. Hepatocyte injury: direct bilirubin, transaminases

II. **Hepatobiliary imaging:** assesses hepatic, biliary, and extrahepatobiliary lesions; overall function; and biliary obstruction

A. **Sulfur-colloid liver-spleen scan:** Visualizes the reticuloendothelial system (i.e., differentiates adenoma from focal nodular hyperplasia). Rarely performed.

B. **Ultrasound:** detects parenchymal lesions and assesses hepatic vascular flow, gallbladder calculi, biliary ductal dilation, gallbladder wall thickening, and the presence of pericholecystic fluid

C. **Computed tomography (CT) and magnetic resonance imaging (MRI):** Visualize parenchyma and adjacent tissues with great clarity and are useful in the delineation of tumors as well as resection planning. Gadoxetate sodium is a contrast agent used in MRI that is highly specific for focal nodular hyperplasia (FNH).

D. **Arteriography:** defines arterial supply usually prior to lesion embolization

E. **Hepatobiliary iminodiacetic acid (HIDA) scan (cholescintigraphy):** employs technetium 99m (^{99m}Tc), which is excreted in the bile

1. **HIDA scan:** provides images of the liver, the biliary tree, and the intestinal transit of bile

2. **Diagnostic:** useful in diagnosing acute cholecystitis, choledochal cyst, bile leaks (after cholecystectomy), and common bile duct obstruction

3. **In conjunction with CCK injection:** HIDA scan helps diagnose biliary dyskinesia and acalculous cholecystitis.

> **Quick Cut**
> The normal ejection fraction of the gallbladder is 35%.

F. **Magnetic resonance cholangiopancreatography (MRCP):** provides the highest resolution of the hepatobiliary and pancreatic structures

G. **Endoscopic retrograde cholangiopancreatography (ERCP):** Combines endoscopic and fluoroscopic techniques directed at the biliopancreatic tree. Typically performed for biopsy, stenting (e.g., common bile duct and pancreatic duct obstruction), stone extraction, papillotomy, and sphincterotomy.

H. **Endoscopic ultrasound (EUS):** lymph node visualization and biopsy

III. **Needle biopsy:** provides liver tissue for histology and cultures

HEPATIC TUMORS

Benign Tumors

I. **Hemangioma:** Usually asymptomatic and discovered incidentally. May cause symptoms by compressing adjacent structures or distending the liver capsule (Fig. 13-3). They are rarely resected except when they are clearly symptomatic.

> **Quick Cut**
> Hemangioma is the most common benign hepatic tumor.

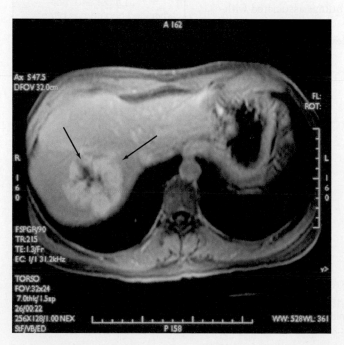

Figure 13-3: MRI of hemangioma (*arrows*). (From Smith WL. *Radiology 101*, 4th ed. Baltimore: Lippincott Williams & Wilkins; 2013, courtesy of Alan Stolpen, MD.)

II. Hepatocellular adenoma (hepatic adenoma): uncommon benign tumor usually seen in women using oral contraceptives (OCPs); also found in men and women who take anabolic (androgenic) steroids

    A. Symptoms: Usually found incidentally, may cause symptoms by compressing adjacent structures but may hemorrhage into the peritoneal cavity. The mortality rate for rupture is ~9%.

    B. Pathology: Soft tumors with sharply circumscribed edges, no true capsule, and histologically normal hepatocytes. MRI is the diagnostic test of choice.

    C. Treatment: includes avoidance of OCPs, anabolic steroids, and pregnancy

        1. Large adenomas: should be resected, particularly in anticipation of pregnancy

        2. In case of rupture: Treatment is embolization or operation (for resection or hepatic artery ligation), depending on patient stability.

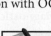
Quick Cut
Thirty percent of patients with hepatocellular adenoma (hepatic adenoma) present with spontaneous rupture.

III. FNH: common; occurs more often in women and has a weak association with OCPs

    A. Symptoms: Usually incidentally diagnosed; spontaneous rupture is rare. FNH is notorious for the presence of central scarring and radiating septations.

    B. Histology: Contains hyperplastic hepatocytes with inflammatory (Kupffer) cells. Bile duct epithelium is a prominent finding.

    C. Diagnosis and treatment: similar to those for hepatocellular adenoma

Quick Cut
On MRI with gadoxetate, FNH is easily distinguished from normal parenchyma.

Malignant Tumors

I. Hepatocellular carcinoma (hepatoma): Hepatoma is the most common primary malignant liver tumor (Fig. 13-4).

    A. Incidence: Highest in Africa and Asia. Male/female ratio is 2:1.

    B. Etiology: associated with chronic hepatitis B virus/hepatitis C virus, cirrhosis from any etiology, hemochromatosis, schistosomiasis, and carcinogens such as chlorinated hydrocarbons, nitrosamines, polyvinyl chloride, organochloride pesticides, aflatoxins

    C. Symptoms: Small hepatocellular carcinomas are usually asymptomatic.

        1. If symptomatic: Malaise, fever, and jaundice may also be present.

        2. Signs: include hepatomegaly (88%), weight loss (85%), a tender abdominal mass (50%), or findings associated with cirrhosis (60%)

    D. Diagnosis: includes abnormal LFTs, elevated alpha-fetoprotein, and cross-sectional imaging

Quick Cut
Primary hepatic malignant tumors account for 0.7% of all cancers. In men, 90% of primary liver tumors are malignant; in women, only about 40% are malignant (due to the higher prevalence of hepatic adenoma and FNH).

Quick Cut
Larger and more advanced hepatomas often present as a dull, aching pain in the right upper quadrant (RUQ).

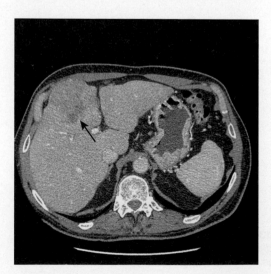

Figure 13-4: CT scan demonstrating hepatoma (*arrow*) . (From Erkonen WE, Smith WL. *Radiology 101*, 3th ed. Baltimore: Lippincott Williams & Wilkins; 2009.)

    E. **Definitive treatment:** consists of resection or transplantation
      1. **Survival:** Resection among eligible patients has a 5-year survival ~40%.
      2. **Other:** Chemotherapy and ablation are usually palliative measures.
II. **Intrahepatic cholangiocarcinoma:** arises from the bile duct epithelium and represents 5%–30% of all primary hepatic malignancies
    A. **Presentation:** Patients have RUQ pain, jaundice, hepatomegaly, and occasionally a palpable mass.
    B. **Etiology:** associated with parasitic infections (e.g., *Clonorchis sinensis*), primary sclerosing cholangitis
    C. **Treatment:** Resection when possible; otherwise, survival is poor.

Metastatic Malignant Tumors

I. **Overview:** Liver is the second most common site of metastasis (exceeded only by regional lymph nodes) for all primary cancers of the abdomen. The ratio of metastatic to primary liver tumors is 20:1.

> **Quick Cut**
> One third of all abdominal cancers ultimately spread to the liver, which is the most common site of hematogenous spread.

II. **Diagnosis:** may be difficult because liver metastases are often asymptomatic
    A. **Tests:** No single laboratory blood test predicts liver metastases in patients with subclinical disease. Currently, LFTs and carcinoembryonic antigen have been used albeit with low specificity.
    B. **Imaging techniques:** These are expensive as screening tests, but are currently the most reliable nonsurgical method of detecting liver metastases.

III. **Treatment:** Depends on the type of primary tumor. Because colorectal cancer has generated the most reliable statistics, those figures are cited here.
    A. **Chemotherapy with 5-fluorouracil therapy:** 10%–30% response rate and a median survival less than 1 year
    B. **Hepatic arterial infusion:** has not improved patient survival
    C. **Radiation and cryoablation:** palliative
    D. **Resection:** Most effective mode of therapy but is limited to patients who have unilobar liver lesions and no evidence of extrahepatic disease; 5-year survival rate approaches 40% in patients meeting these criteria.

> **Quick Cut**
> Many cancers metastasize to the liver. Only colorectal metastasis to the liver are potentially resectable (if they are anatomically favorable and there is no extrahepatic disease)

HEPATIC ABSCESSES AND CYSTS

Abscesses

I. **Bacterial abscesses:** most common
    A. **Common organisms:** *Escherichia coli, Bacteroides, Streptococcus,* and *Enterococcus*
    B. **Clinical presentation:** includes sepsis, fever and chills, leukocytosis, anemia, abnormal LFTs, RUQ tenderness, and occasionally hemobilia
    C. **Treatment:** Drainage and antibiotics usually suffice; surgical intervention is rarely required.

> **Quick Cut**
> Bacterial abscesses of the liver are typically secondary to intra-abdominal infection, such as cholangitis, appendicitis, or diverticulitis.

II. **Amebic abscess:** second most common hepatic abscess and the most common abscess in the developing world
    A. **Organism:** Infection with *Entamoeba histolytica* reaches the portal vein from intestinal amebiasis.
    B. **Clinical presentation:** includes fever, leukocytosis, hepatomegaly, RUQ pain
    C. **Diagnosis:** Occasionally, liver enzyme levels are elevated. Indirect hemagglutination titers for *Entamoeba* are elevated in most patients with intestinal infestation and in 98% with hepatic abscess. Trophozoites (the active stage) are occasionally present in the periphery of the abscess.
    D. **Treatment:** Metronidazole; surgical drainage is not usually necessary.

> **Quick Cut**
> Amebic abscess is usually sterile on routine culture and is treated by metronidazole.

Hydatid Cysts

I. **Overview:** Result from infection with the parasite *Echinococcus granulosus*, which is endemic in southern Europe, Middle East, Australia, and South America. Dogs are the definitive host.

II. **Clinical presentation:** Cysts can develop anywhere in the body, but two thirds occur in the liver and one half in the lungs. They rupture into the peritoneal cavity, resulting in urticaria, eosinophilia, and anaphylactic shock. Symptoms include hepatomegaly, RUQ pain, and eosinophilia.

III. **Diagnosis:** history, imaging, and a positive serum antigen

IV. **Treatment:** Symptomatic cysts require surgical removal. The surgical approach consists of careful isolation of the operative field, followed by aspiration of the cyst. The site should be sterilized with 0.5% silver nitrate solution or hypertonic saline.

Hepatic Trauma

I. **Mortality:** Due to its high blood flow, proximity to the inferior vena cava (IVC), nearby vital structures, and propensity to develop infections, overall mortality is 10%–20%.

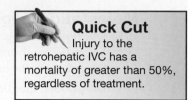

Quick Cut
Injury to the retrohepatic IVC has a mortality of greater than 50%, regardless of treatment.

II. **Diagnosis:** By imaging and mechanism. Injuries are classified in five levels based on the degree of parenchymal injury seen on cross-sectional imaging.

III. **Nonsurgical management:** In a hemodynamically stable patient with evidence of bleeding, the source can be visualized angiographically and embolized.

Quick Cut
Most patients with low-grade to moderate liver injuries can be safely admitted and observed and do not need liver-specific intervention.

IV. **Surgical management:** At surgery, hemostasis is usually obtained via packing. Less common methods to control bleeding include tractotomy, resectional debridement, anatomic resection, and hepatic artery ligation.

V. **Late complications:** Subcapsular and intrahepatic hematomas can be carefully observed, but many ultimately require drainage.

A. **Perihepatic collections:** usually become infected whether of blood or bile and must be drained

B. **Biliary fistulas:** May track to the skin or into the chest (biliopleural, bronchobiliary fistula). Treatment is similar to that for GI fistulas.

C. **Traumatic arteriovenous fistulas (AVFs):** Result usually from penetrating trauma. Large fistulas are best treated by arterial embolization.

D. **Arteriobiliary fistulas:** treated via arteriography and embolization

Portal Hypertension

I. **Pathophysiology:** abnormal elevation of portal venous pressure greater than 5–6 mm Hg

Quick Cut
In portal hypertension, submucosal varices are likely to hemorrhage (esophageal varices, hemorrhoidal bleeding).

A. **Increase in portal pressure:** leads to collateral development to decompress the portal system into the systemic circulation

B. **Dilated veins or varices:** likely to develop when pressure is greater than 20 mm Hg

II. **Intrahepatic etiology:** most common

A. **Cirrhosis (alcohol and hepatitis C virus):** causes 85% of portal hypertension in the United States

B. **Schistosomiasis:** Common cause worldwide. Portal hypertension develops when parasitic ova in small portal venules cause a presinusoidal block.

C. **Other:** Wilson disease, hepatic fibrosis, and hemochromatosis are occasional causes.

III. **Prehepatic etiology:** rare; more commonly encountered in children (e.g., portal vein obstruction due to thrombosis, congenital atresia, or stenosis from extrinsic compression)

IV. **Posthepatic etiology:** also rare

A. **Budd-Chiari syndrome:** characterized by hepatic vein thrombosis; may be idiopathic or secondary to a hypercoagulable state as occurs with tumors, hematologic disorders, OCP use, and trauma

B. **Other:** Any process leading to severe right ventricular failure, splenic disease, and splenic AVFs/shunts also lead to posthepatic portal hypertension.

V. **Clinical presentation:** includes encephalopathy, GI hemorrhage, malnutrition, and ascites

VI. **Medical management of acute variceal hemorrhage:** includes the following

A. **Esophagogastroduodenoscopy (EGD):** Should be performed as soon as possible to find the site of bleeding and determine the presence of varices. Upper GI hemorrhage in cirrhotic patients results from varices (35%), erosive gastritis (40%), peptic ulcer disease (15%), and esophageal tears (Mallory-Weiss syndrome, 10%).

1. **Variceal banding with small rubber bands:** treatment of choice
2. **Sclerotherapy:** controls bleeding temporarily in 80%–90% of patients and is associated with minimal mortality

B. **Pharmacotherapy:** vasopressin (vasoconstricts the splanchnic circulation), nitroglycerin (lowers portal pressure independently), somatostatin (splanchnic vasoconstriction)

C. **Sengstaken-Blakemore tube:** nasogastric tube with esophageal and gastric balloons for tamponade of varices

D. **Transjugular intrahepatic portosystemic shunt (TIPS):** now the preferred procedure for controlling variceal bleeding (Fig. 13-5)

VII. **Surgical management:** Acute massive bleeding refractory to nonsurgical maneuvers requires emergency intervention. However, emergent surgical procedures are rarely performed currently due to high mortality.

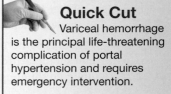

Quick Cut
Variceal hemorrhage is the principal life-threatening complication of portal hypertension and requires emergency intervention.

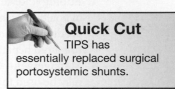

Quick Cut
TIPS has essentially replaced surgical portosystemic shunts.

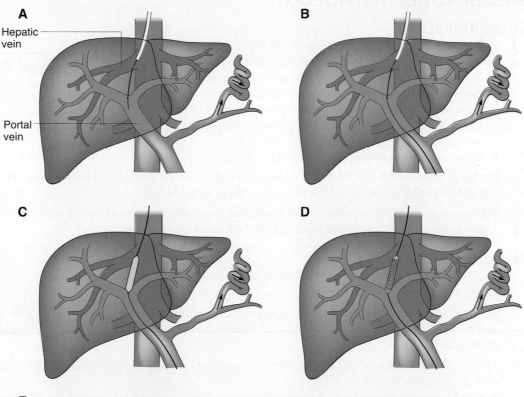

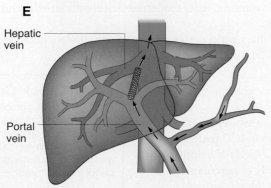

Figure 13-5: Transjugular intrahepatic portosystemic shunt. A wire is passed through an hepatic vein branch, across the liver parenchyma, and into a portal vein branch. The parenchymal path is dilated and a stent is placed across it to maintain patency of the newly created venous conduit. This conduit allows the portal blood to flow freely into the systemic venous system, thus lowering portal pressure and the propensity to bleed from esophageal varices. (From Mulholland MW, Lillemoe KD, Doherty GM, et al. *Greenfield's Surgery*, 4th ed. Baltimore: Lippincott Williams & Wilkins; 2005.)

VIII. **Elective management:** aims at preventing rebleeding
    A. **Nonoperative management:** TIPS, EGD banding/sclerosing
    B. **Operative shunts:** rarely performed
        1. **Nonselective portosystemic shunts:** portacaval, mesocaval, and their variations
        2. **Selective portosystemic shunts:** distal splenorenal (Warren)
    C. **Liver transplantation:** only therapy that addresses the underlying liver disease and restores the patient's hepatic functional reserve to normal

IX. **Hypersplenism:** Common in patients with portal hypertension and should be treated nonoperatively; <50% of patients who undergo shunting show improvement.

> **Quick Cut**
> Splenectomy for hypersplenism should be performed only in cases of splenic vein thrombosis.

X. **Ascites:** complication of hepatic disease/cirrhosis
    A. **Etiology:** Results from sinusoidal hypertension, hypoalbuminemia, abnormal hepatic and abdominal lymph production, and abnormal salt and water retention by the kidneys. Impaired hepatic metabolism of aldosterone leads to salt and water retention.
    B. **Management:** Consists of salt/water restriction and diuretics; peritoneal-jugular shunting and TIPS may be used to treat refractory ascites.

GALLBLADDER PATHOLOGY

Cholelithiasis

I. **Gallstones:** Form as a result of bile precipitation. Most stones (70%) are made up of cholesterol, bilirubin, and calcium.
    A. **Stone type:** cholesterol stones (increase in the cholesterol to bile salts or lecithin ratio predisposes to stone formation), pigmented stones (bilirubin; associated with hemolysis and hemoglobinopathies), calcium bilirubinate stones (associated with infection or inflammation of the biliary tree)
    B. **Prophylactic treatment:** scant evidence to justify

> **Quick Cut**
> Symptomatic cholelithiasis usually requires cholecystectomy.

II. **Surgical treatment:** Calcified or porcelain gallbladder should be removed because the risk of malignancy, although the incidence is less than 5% in recent series.

III. **Complications of cholecystectomy:** retained stone (which can be extracted with ERCP) and common bile duct injury (which requires surgical hepatobiliary reconstruction)

Cholecystitis

I. **Gallbladder inflammation:** In 85%–90% of patients, cholecystitis is caused by calculi, bile stasis, and bacteria.

II. **Chronic cholecystitis:** Complaints include nausea, vomiting, and intermittent RUQ pain. Symptoms may be associated with eating fatty foods. Laboratory studies are generally normal; treatment is elective cholecystectomy.

III. **Acute cholecystitis:** Most cases are due to an impacted stone in the gallbladder neck/cystic duct with resultant obstruction.
    A. **Clinical presentation:** Fever, nausea and vomiting, RUQ tenderness with/without rebound tenderness, and Murphy sign are common.
    B. **Diagnosis and treatment:** Ultrasound is diagnostic; perform laparoscopic cholecystectomy, if possible, either immediately (i.e., within 72 hours) or as interval surgery (4–6 weeks).

IV. **Acalculous cholecystitis:** acute or chronic cholecystitis in the absence of stones
    A. **Acute form:** occurs as a complication of burns, sepsis, trauma, or collagen vascular disease. Typically occurs in ICU patients.
    B. **Diagnosis and treatment:** HIDA scan is especially helpful with the diagnosis; treatment is cholecystectomy or percutaneous cholecystostomy if the patient is too ill to tolerate surgery.

> **Quick Cut**
> Some complications of cholecystitis/cholelithiasis require urgent surgery including emphysematous/gangrenous gallbladder and perforated gallbladder.

Gallbladder Trauma

I. **Treatment:** usually managed with cholecystectomy during exploratory laparotomy

II. **Associated visceral injuries:** common; most frequently involve the liver

BILIARY TREE PATHOLOGY

Choledocholithiasis

I. **Stones in the common bile duct:** can be single or multiple and are found in 10%–20% of patients who undergo cholecystectomy

II. **Clinical presentation:** RUQ pain that radiates to the back and right shoulder, intermittent obstructive jaundice, acholic stools, or bilirubinuria

III. **Definitive diagnosis:** ultrasonography, ERCP, and labs

IV. **Treatment:** ERCP before or after cholecystectomy, intraoperative cholangiogram, biliary-enteric connection (e.g., choledochoduodenostomy or choledochojejunostomy)

Quick Cut
Most stones found in the ducts are formed in the gallbladder.

Quick Cut
Common bile duct stones post cholecystectomy are arbitrarily defined as retained stones if they present within a year. After one year, they are thought to be primarily occuring and not retained.

Cholangitis

I. **Etiology:** ascending infection of the bile ducts, associated with obstruction due to stones or benign stricture

II. **Clinical presentation:** Charcot triad of fever, jaundice, and RUQ pain is present in 70% of cases.

III. **Treatment:** includes antibiotics, resuscitation with fluids/electrolytes, and relief of the obstruction

Quick Cut
E. coli is the most commonly cultured organism in cholangitis.

Primary Sclerosing Cholangitis

I. **Etiology:** Disease of unknown etiology that affects the biliary tract, resulting in stenosis or obstruction of the ductal system. PSC is associated with ulcerative colitis. Progressive obstruction results in biliary cirrhosis and liver failure.

II. **Clinical presentation:** Symptoms include RUQ or painless jaundice, usually without fever/chills, pruritus, fatigue, and nausea; associated with ulcerative colitis.

III. **Diagnosis:** ERCP or a transhepatic cholangiogram

IV. **Treatment:** includes internal biliary drainage (stenting), hepatobiliary reconstruction, T-tube, and orthotopic liver transplantation

Biliary Neoplasms

I. **Overview:** Benign tumors of the gallbladder are rare (papilloma, adenomyoma, fibroma, lipoma, myoma, myxoma, and carcinoid).

II. **Carcinoma of the gallbladder:** Accounts for 4% of all carcinomas; ~80% of these are adenocarcinomas.

Quick Cut
The only truly curable gallbladder carcinoma is when the tumor is found incidentally at cholecystectomy.

A. **Clinical presentation:** Patient usually complains of pruritus, anorexia, weight loss, and RUQ pain. Jaundice occurs late.

B. **Treatment:** Generally surgical, although less than 10% are resectable. If gallbladder cancer is found in a specimen removed for benign disease, proceed as follows.

1. **Confined to the mucosa (T1):** No further treatment is necessary.

2. **Invasive disease (>T1):** Partial hepatectomy after appropriate imaging workup is indicated.

III. **Cancer of the bile ducts**

A. **Risk factors:** sclerosing cholangitis, chronic parasitic infection of the bile ducts, gallstones (present in 18%–65% of cases), and exposure to Thorotrast (a contrast agent used in the 1950's)

B. **Diagnosis:** may be made by percutaneous transhepatic cholangiography, ERCP, CT, or MRI

1. **Location:** Tumor may be in the distal common bile duct, common hepatic duct, cystic duct, or the right or left hepatic duct (most common location).

2. **Metastasis:** initially to the regional lymph nodes (16%), spreads by direct extension into the liver (14%), or metastasizes to the liver (10%)

C. **Treatment:** Proximal lesions require hepatic resection and biliary reconstruction. Distal tumors usually require a Whipple operation.

> **Quick Cut**
> Cholangiocarcinoma of the confluence of the hepatic ducts is termed a *Klatskin tumor.*

Choledochal Cysts

I. **Overview:** Congenital malformations of the pancreaticobiliary tree. Diagnosis is with ultrasound, ERCP, and MRCP.

II. **Classification:** as follows

A. **Type I:** Fusiform dilatation of the common bile duct. Treated with cholecystectomy, cyst excision, and a Roux-en-Y choledochojejunostomy.

B. **Type II:** Diverticulum of the common bile duct. Treated by excision of the common bile duct diverticulum.

C. **Type III:** Choledochocele involving the intraduodenal portion of the common bile duct. Treated by cyst excision and choledochoduodenostomy or by transduodenal sphincteroplasty.

D. **Type IV:** Cystic involvement of the intrahepatic bile ducts (Caroli disease); may be fatal. Patients require liver transplantation.

> **Quick Cut**
> The most common presenting symptom of a choledochal cyst is intermittent jaundice.

III. **Treatment:** In adults, all choledochal cysts are removed due to the 5% risk of developing malignancy.

Other

I. **Biliary tree trauma:** Most extrahepatic bile duct injuries are iatrogenic, occurring during cholecystectomy. Diagnosis by ERCP. Treatment with end-to-end (duct-to-duct) anastomosis may be done at the time of initial injury; otherwise, a Roux-en-Y choledochojejunostomy is necessary.

> **Quick Cut**
> Only 15% of intraoperative biliary injuries are diagnosed at the time of surgery.

II. **Intraperitoneal extravasation of bile:** Extravasation of sterile bile results in chemical peritonitis. Infected intraperitoneal bile induces a fulminant and frequently fatal peritonitis.

Hepatic Resection

I. **Right or left hepatic lobectomy:** The right and left lobes are divided by the interlobar fissure, a plane running between the gallbladder fossa and the IVC

> **Quick Cut**
> Hepatic resections rely on the hepatic segmental anatomy.

II. **Trisegmentectomy:** removes the entire right lobe and the median segment of the left lobe across the anatomic division of the falciform ligament (leaving only the left lateral segment)

III. **Left lateral segmentectomy:** removes the segment of liver to the left of the falciform ligament

IV. **Wedge resections:** Performed for small lesions near the liver surface that do not require a full lobectomy. These resections do not adhere to anatomic boundaries but are safe because a limited amount of tissue is transected.

Chapter 14

Pancreas

H. Richard Alexander, Peter E. Darwin, and Ronald J. Weigel

 ANATOMY AND PHYSIOLOGY

Characteristics

I. **Orientation:** The pancreas is a 12–15-cm long solid organ that lies in a slightly oblique transverse orientation in retroperitoneum of the upper abdomen (Fig. 14-1). The anterior border of the pancreas is covered by a smooth glistening membrane, the visceral peritoneum, which must be divided to gain access to the gland.

> **Quick Cut**
> The pancreas has a light pink color distinct from adjacent retroperitoneal fat.

II. **Divisions:** four anatomic portions of the gland
   A. **Head:** lies in the right upper quadrant (RUQ) and is nested into the medial border of the duodenum
   B. **Neck:** lies directly over the superior mesenteric vein (SMV)
   C. **Body:** lies to the left of the SMV
   D. **Tail:** lies adjacent to the hilum of the spleen in the left upper quadrant

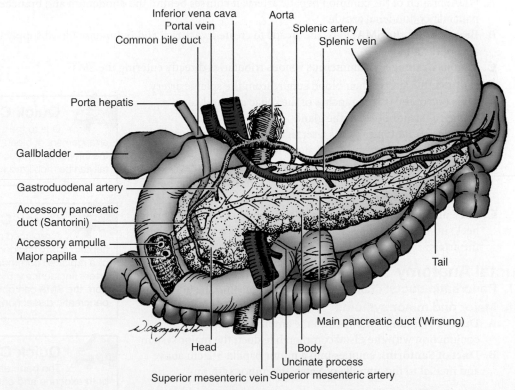

Figure 14-1: Anatomy of the pancreas. The normal anteroposterior thickness of the head is less than 2.5 cm; the neck, 1.5 cm; the body, 2 cm; and the tail, 2.5 cm.

Important Anatomic Relationships

I. **Head:** Head is slightly lower (caudal) than the tail; it lies over the aorta and is fused to the medial wall of the duodenal C-loop. Just cephalad to the head are the porta hepatis structures including the common bile duct, portal vein, and proper hepatic artery.

A. **Common bile duct and pancreatic duct:** Course through the head of the pancreas and enter through a common channel into the medial wall of the duodenum via the ampulla of Vater. Flow through the common channel is regulated by the sphincter of Oddi.

B. **Nomenclature inconsistency:** Within the head of the pancreas, the *distal* common bile duct and the *proximal* pancreatic duct are adjacent to each other. The pancreatic duct contains multiple side branches at regular intervals.

C. **Pancreatic head:** has a common blood supply with the medial wall of the **duodenal C-loop**

D. **Body and tail:** derive their blood supply from the splenic artery

> **Quick Cut**
> There is a close proximity (sometimes with a common channel) between the pancreatic duct and the common bile duct. Pathology affecting one duct may secondarily affect the other.

II. **Uncinate process:** small portion of the head that lies posteriorly to the SMV

III. **Neck:** lies over the SMV, which joins the splenic vein at the superior border of the pancreas to form the portal vein

IV. **Body:** lies adjacent to the posterior wall of the stomach, forming the posterior border of the lesser omental bursa or lesser sac

V. **Tail:** close to the splenic hilum

Vasculature

I. **General:** Well-vascularized organ that derives most of its blood supply from the celiac axis branches. Venous drainage is exclusively through the portal venous system to the liver. Inflammatory and neoplastic conditions of the pancreas can result in thrombosis or encasement of adjacent vascular structures.

II. **Head and neck:** derive their blood supply from the gastroduodenal artery (GDA) and a branch from the superior mesenteric artery (SMA)

A. **GDA:** branch of the common hepatic artery; it courses behind the duodenum and branches into the pancreaticoduodenal arcade

B. **Branch from the SMA:** joins the arcade to create a very rich and redundant blood supply to this area of the gland

C. **Venous drainage:** via numerous venous tributaries directly entering the SMV

III. **Body and tail:** derive their blood supply from the splenic artery, which is one of the three branches of the celiac axis and courses along the superior border of the gland

A. **Splenic artery:** typically has a serpiginous course, and numerous small branches enter the gland along its superior border

B. **Venous drainage:** via the splenic vein, which is slightly caudal to the artery and typically contained more or less within the body of the gland

C. **SMV and SMA:** Vein lies at the inferior border of the pancreatic neck; immediately adjacent and slightly posterior to the left lies the artery.

> **Quick Cut**
> Due to the arrangement of blood vessels, the inferior pancreatic body and tail can be mobilized with ease.

> **Quick Cut**
> A replaced right hepatic artery (incidence 25%) or a replaced common hepatic artery (incidence 2.5%) arising from the SMA can complicate pancreatic dissection.

Ductal Anatomy

I. **Pancreatic ducts:** drain pancreatic secretions into the duodenum

II. **Major and minor systems**

A. **Duct of Wirsung:** empties into the ampulla of Vater in conjunction with the distal common bile duct; the major system

B. **Duct of Santorini:** empties into a minor papilla ~2 cm above and medial to the ampulla of Vater; the minor system

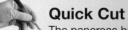

> **Quick Cut**
> The pancreas has both exocrine and endocrine functions.

Physiologic Functions

I. **Exocrine pancreas:** Makes ~800–1,000 mL daily of alkaline bicarbonate-rich fluid (pH 8) that contains proteases, lipases, and other enzymes for digestion. Under pathologic conditions, the integrity of the exocrine ductal system may be breached; leakage of enzyme-rich fluid into the retroperitoneum can result in sepsis, hemorrhage, and inflammation with secondary shifts in fluids.

II. **Endocrine pancreas:** Synthesizes various hormones; most important are the islet cells that produce various peptide hormones such as insulin.

PANCREATITIS

Definition and Classification

I. **Pancreatitis:** inflammatory process in the pancreas

II. **Classification:** divided into four categories to clarify the different syndromes that are found and to improve the standardization of treatment and prognosis
   A. **Acute pancreatitis**
      1. **Characteristics:** arises in a previously asymptomatic patient and subsides with appropriate treatment; it can involve other regional tissues or remote organ systems
      2. **Clinically based classification:** from the International Symposium on Acute Pancreatitis
         a. Severe acute pancreatitis
         b. Mild acute pancreatitis
         c. Acute fluid collection
         d. Pancreatic necrosis
         e. Acute pseudocysts
         f. Pancreatic abscess
   B. **Acute relapsing pancreatitis:** series of recurrent episodes of acute pancreatitis in an otherwise asymptomatic patient
   C. **Chronic relapsing pancreatitis:** chronic inflammation with chemical evidence of pancreatitis, which fluctuates in its intensity without a period of resolution
   D. **Chronic pancreatitis:** Shows unrelenting symptoms due to pancreatic inflammation and fibrosis; the pancreatic duct and parenchyma may show calcification.

Quick Cut
Chronic pancreatitis can be associated with exocrine insufficiency (malabsorption), endocrine insufficiency (diabetes), or both.

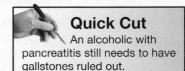

Quick Cut
An alcoholic with pancreatitis still needs to have gallstones ruled out.

Etiology

I. **Acute:** Approximately 75% of pancreatitis cases can be explained on the basis of biliary tract disease or alcohol abuse, although the exact mechanism for the production of pancreatitis remains theoretical.
   A. **Gallstone pancreatitis:** Thought to be induced by the inflammation that results from passage of stones into the common bile duct. Most often, the gallstone has passed by the time the patient is studied.
      1. **Pancreatic duct and bile duct:** empty into a common papilla
      2. **Obstruction:** Entire common channel can be obstructed if a large calculus becomes impacted in the papilla.
      3. **Reflux:** Bile flows into the pancreatic duct. Experiments have shown that reflux can induce pancreatitis; however, it is unclear whether this reflux occurs in humans.
   B. **Alcohol-induced pancreatitis:** may be the result of various mechanisms
      1. **Alcohol:** implicated in the direct damage of acinar cells and the increased enzyme concentration in pancreatic secretion
      2. **Stones:** development encouraged by high-protein concentration with calcium carbonate precipitation in the protein-filled spaces
      3. **Inflammation and fibrosis:** Multifocal ductal obstruction and increased intraductal pressure along with increased permeability caused by alcohol destroys parenchyma.
   C. **Congenital abnormalities and hereditary pancreatitis:** Duct strictures, pancreas divisum, and metabolic disorders (e.g., hypertriglyceridemia and hypercalcemia) are factors in a small percentage of cases.
   D. **Iatrogenic:** Pancreatitis can be caused by instrumentation (e.g., endoscopic retrograde cholangiopancreatography [ERCP]), trauma, or certain drugs (steroids, sulfonamides, furosemide, and thiazides).

E. **Infectious:** Mumps, coxsackievirus, cytomegalovirus, herpes simplex virus, mycoplasma, legionella, salmonella, fungi, and parasites have been implicated.

F. **Malignancy:** Pancreatic ductal obstruction from cancer may present as acute pancreatitis.

G. **Duodenal ulcer:** Penetrating ulcer may manifest as acute pancreatitis.

H. **Idiopathic:** Up to 20% of cases have no identifiable cause.

II. **Chronic**

A. **Toxic-metabolic:** Alcohol, tobacco smoking, occupational hydrocarbon exposure, hypercalcemia, and hyperlipidemia are factors that may contribute to inflammation/fibrosis.

B. **Genetic:** Cystic fibrosis transmembrane regulator (*CFTR*) and other genetic mutations (*PRSS1* and *SPINK*) are associated with chronic pancreatitis.

C. **Idiopathic:** Majority of cases worldwide have no definable etiology.

D. **Autoimmune:** Immunoglobulin G4–related pancreatitis may present as either acute or chronic disease. Associated focal pancreatic enlargement and biliary obstruction may mimic pancreatic carcinoma.

Acute Pancreatitis

I. **Clinical presentation:** varies from mild abdominal discomfort to profound shock with hypotension and hypoxemia, depending on the severity of the inflammatory process

A. **Pain:** Most patients have mild to moderate abdominal tenderness, classically epigastric pain radiating to the back.

B. **Severe cases:** Rigid abdomen with epigastric guarding, rebound tenderness, and marked abdominal pain may be present.

C. **Retroperitoneal hemorrhage:** caused by severe pancreatic inflammation and necrosis, which can lead to large third-space fluid losses, hypotension, tachycardia, and shock with blood dissection (i.e., the blood extravasates between tissue planes)

1. **Turner sign:** Blood dissection extends to the flank, resulting in flank ecchymoses.

2. **Cullen sign:** Blood dissects up the falciform ligament and creates a periumbilical ecchymosis.

II. **History:** Patient commonly mentions recent consumption of a heavy meal, many times with generous quantities of alcoholic beverages. The pain typically begins 1–4 hours after a meal and is often less severe when the patient is slumped forward.

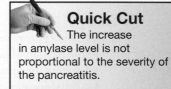

Quick Cut
The increase in amylase level is not proportional to the severity of the pancreatitis.

III. **Diagnosis:** aided by the following studies:

A. **Serum amylase level:** increased in 95% of patients with acute pancreatitis

1. **False-positives:** Approximately 5% of all amylase determinations; 75% of patients with abdominal pain and an increased amylase level have pancreatitis.

2. **Advantages:** Some inferences can be made from the amylase level. Higher amylase levels (usually over 1,000 Somogyi units) may indicate gallstone pancreatitis

3. **Origin:** Some circulating amylase is not of pancreatic origin; major alternative source is the salivary glands.

B. **Amylase-to-creatinine clearance ratio:** Amylase determinations are more sensitive identifiers when the amylase clearance rate is compared with the creatinine clearance rate and a ratio is established.

Quick Cut
The pancreas must be intact and functional to synthesize amylase and release it into the circulation; therefore, patients with acute pancreatitis superimposed on chronic pancreatitis may not show an increase in serum amylase.

1. **Amylase-to-creatinine greater than 5:** strongly suggestive of pancreatitis

2. **Rapid renal clearance of amylase:** Using the ratio avoids this problem, which tends to reduce serum levels below the point where a simple serum amylase determination would be positive.

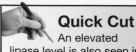

Quick Cut
An elevated lipase level is also seen in pancreatitis.

3. **Impaired renal function:** Affects the creatinine clearance rate sooner than the amylase clearance rate. Even in this situation, however, the amylase-to-creatinine clearance ratio appears to be more sensitive than the serum amylase level.

C. **Radiographic imaging**
1. **Upper abdominal plain films:** Relatively insensitive for diagnosis. Significant findings include the following.
    a. **Calcification (in the area of the lesser sac and pancreas):** may indicate chronic pancreatitis, which is most often found in association with alcoholism
    b. **Gas collection (in the lesser sac):** suggests abscess formation in or around the pancreas
    c. **"Cutoff" sign:** Area of colonic spasm adjacent to an inflamed pancreas causes the gas in the transverse colon to end abruptly.
2. **Barium studies:** may show upper gastrointestinal (GI) abnormalities
    a. **Duodenal C-loop:** may be widened by pancreatic edema
    b. **Hypotonic duodenography:** may show the **"pad" sign**, a smoothing out of the duodenal mucosal folds by the edematous pancreas and the inflammatory response on the medial aspect of the C-loop
3. **Angiography:** Useful for delineating pancreatic and hepatic blood supply before radical surgery. Largely superseded by spiral computed tomography (CT) scan and magnetic resonance imaging (MRI).
D. **Ultrasound (US) imaging:** especially useful in the diagnosis of pancreatitis

> **Quick Cut**
> US may be particularly useful in the initial workup of pancreatitis to rule out gallstones.

1. **Anatomic and vascular landmark changes:** can be delineated
    a. **Acute pancreatitis:** suggested by swelling greater than the normal anteroposterior thickness and loss of tissue planes between the pancreas and the splenic vein
    b. **Other pancreatic anomalies:** may also be found (e.g., a change in duct size or calcification)
    c. **Chronic pancreatitis:** often manifested by the presence of calcification or pseudocysts containing fluid or showing a complex cystic structure
    d. **Ascites (easily diagnosed by US):** may or may not be present in chronic pancreatitis
2. **Echogenicity:** affected by various pancreatic disorders
    a. **Decreased:** Most diseases decrease the echogenicity because they include edema and inflammation.
    b. **Increased:** generally due to gas or calcification
3. **Fluid densities:** lying within the pancreas indicate cysts, abscesses, or possibly lymphoma
4. **Cholelithiasis:** May be identified, suggesting gallstone pancreatitis. US may also show the presence of cholecystitis or a dilated common bile duct.
5. **US limitation:** cannot be performed when excessive bowel gas is present, as with an ileus
E. **Pancreatic CT scan:** extremely helpful; provides higher resolution than US, and it is not limited by the masking effect of intestinal gas

> **Quick Cut**
> Dynamic CT can be used to diagnose pancreatic necrosis.

1. **Advantages:** Improvements in availability, speed, and resolution in CT have made it the most important imaging modality in initial diagnosis and treatment of pancreatitis.
2. **CT severity index (including percent gland necrosis):** provides valuable prognostic information and allows exclusion of addition pathology and complications (Table 14-1)
F. **Magnetic resonance (MR)**
1. **MR pancreatograms and cholangiograms:** Widely available and are very useful for delineating anatomy before surgery. They can provide excellent detail of the pancreatic duct and bile ducts.
2. **MR angiography:** increasingly available and has replaced invasive angiography for planned pancreatic surgery
G. **ERCP:** In the first 5 days of severe acute pancreatitis, use is dangerous and is associated with an increased mortality rate. However, patients with acute biliary pancreatic and concurrent cholangitis benefit from urgent endoscopic intervention (Table 14-2).

IV. **Prognosis:** aided by certain signs that are associated with a higher mortality rate and, therefore, are useful prognostic indicators
A. **Prognostic indicators (Ranson signs):** Table 14-3
B. **Other: Acute Physiology and Chronic Health Evaluation II** (APACHE II) score (Table 14-4), Atlanta classification for severe acute pancreatitis, Balthazar score, and CT severity index assist in identifying those at high risk for morbidity and mortality.

Table 14-1: Radiologic Severity Assessment

Balthazar Computed Tomography Score	
Grade	**Computed Tomography Findings**
A	Normal
B	Focal or diffuse enlargement of pancreas
C	B + peripancreatic inflammation
D	C + single fluid collection
E	D + two or more fluid collections and/or presence of gas

Computed Tomography Severity Index			
Computed Tomography Grade	**Assigned Score**	**Percent Necrosis**	**Assigned Score**
A	0	None	0
B	1	<30	2
C	2	30–50	4
D	3	>50	6
E	4		

Maximum score = 10 points
- **Conflicting data regarding extent of necrosis and clinical outcome**
  Retrospective study of 268 patients, CTSI >5:
  - **8× more likely to die**
  - **17× more likely to have prolonged hospital stay**
  - **10× more likely to need necrosectomy**

CTSI, computed tomography severity index.

V. Treatment: Certain measures are considered standard, but not all of them are indicated in each case. The patient's symptoms dictate much of the treatment.
  A. Nasogastric suction: Used to control nausea and vomiting, decrease pancreatic stimulation, and decrease GI distention from an ileus. This suction also makes the patient more comfortable, although it does not appear to shorten the hospital stay.
  B. Intravenous (IV) fluids: Used to replace the third-space fluid loss from edema and extravasation into the peripancreatic spaces. Crystalloid solutions are usually adequate.
    1. Patient monitoring: Include strict input/output measurement (with a Foley catheter).
    2. Severe cases with unstable hemodynamics: Invasive hemodynamic monitoring is used.

Table 14-2: Role of Endoscopic Retrograde Cholangiopancreatography

	Pancreatitis				
	Acute	**Persistent**	**Complicated**	**Convalescent**	**Recurrent**
Diagnosis	Cause is in question	Status of main duct; indication for surgery	Assessment of pseudocysts and fistulas	Cause is in question (e.g., lymphoma)	Anatomic assessment (e.g., pancreatic divisum)
Treatment	Sphincterotomy for biliary obstruction	Sphincterotomy; stone extraction	Stent or internal drainage	Sphincterotomy in selected high-risk patients	Sphincterotomy or stent in selected patients

Reprinted with permission from Neoptolemos JP. In: Bradley EL III, ed. *Acute Pancreatitis: Diagnosis and Therapy*. New York: Raven Press; 1994:75.

Table 14-3: Ranson's 11 Criteria for Determining the Severity of Pancreatitis

On Admission	Initial 48 Hours
Age >55 years	HCT decrease >10 percentage points
WBC >16,000/mm^3	BUN increase >5 mg/dL
Glucose >200 mg/dL	Ca^{2+} <8 μg/dL
LDH >350 IU/L	Pao_2 <60 mm Hg
SGOT >250 SF units %	Base deficit >4 mEq/l Estimate fluid >6,000 mL

WBC, white blood cell count; LDH, lactate dehydrogenase; SGOT, serum glutamine-oxaloacetic transaminase; HCT, hematocrit; BUN, blood urea nitrogen; Ca^{2+}, calcium ion; Pao_2, partial pressure of oxygen in arterial blood.

C. Antibiotics: May reduce the risk of abscess formation and of lesser sac collections, which often progress to abscess formation. Prophylactic antibiotics are usually reserved for those cases with necrosis in an attempt to maintain sterile tissue.

D. Pao_2 monitoring and serial chest radiographs: For patients who have severe pancreatitis, respiratory distress is common, as are **pleural effusions**, which are more often on the left and contain high concentrations of amylase.

E. Withhold oral feedings: Until laboratory test results return to normal and pain is gone for 48 hours. In cases without severe ileus, enteral elemental feedings are preferred to parenteral nutrition.

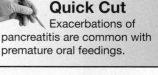

Quick Cut
Exacerbations of pancreatitis are common with premature oral feedings.

F. Surgery
1. **Indications**
   a. **To confirm the diagnosis:** In severe cases that do not respond to medical management. Symptoms can be mimicked by visceral perforation, mesenteric arterial occlusion, and other intra-abdominal catastrophes.
   b. **To relieve biliary or pancreatic duct obstruction**
      (1) **Early biliary tract operation:** May increase mortality in patients who have severe pancreatitis. If possible, surgery should be delayed until the pancreatitis has subsided.
      (2) **Continued patient status deterioration: Surgical exploration may become necessary.**
      (3) **Endoscopic clearance of common bile duct stones: most often the preferred route**

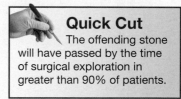

Quick Cut
The offending stone will have passed by the time of surgical exploration in greater than 90% of patients.

   c. **To drain the lesser sac:** Drainage increases morbidity and should be performed only after septic complications have occurred. It is not effective as a prophylactic measure.
      (1) **Indication:** improves prognosis when sepsis has already occurred and lesser sac collections and pancreatic necrosis are present
      (2) **Established lesser sac abscesses:** Drains can be inserted after opening the lesser omentum widely.
      (3) **Irrigation catheters:** can also be used as part of the therapeutic plan
      (4) **Dependent drainage through the transverse mesocolon:** useful approach when the upper abdomen is obliterated by inflammation and adhesions

Quick Cut
Pancreatic collections occur in patients with extensive necrosis. The approach is to sample them endoscopically or percutaneously, but drainage is only performed for pus.

2. **Operative procedures**
   a. **Cholecystectomy:** may be required in patients who have gallstone pancreatitis and persistent acute pancreatitis that does not respond to supportive measures
   b. **Resection (for acute pancreatitis):** Dangerous and not indicated. Removing necrotic pancreas (nonanatomic dissection) may be required in pancreatic abscess. These operations have a high mortality rate.

Table 14-4: APACHE II Score

Physiologic Variable	High Abnormal Range				0	Low Abnormal Range				Points
	+4	+3	+2	+1		+1	+2	+3	+4	
Temperature (°C)	≥41	39–40.9	—	38.5–38.9	36–38.4	34–35.9	32–33.9	30–31.9	≤29.9	—
MAP mm Hg	≥160	130–159	110–129	—	70–109	—	50–69	—	≥49	—
Heart rate	≥180	140–179	110–139	—	70–109	—	55–69	40–54	≥39	—
Respiratory rate	≥50	35–49	—	25–34	12–24	10–11	6–9	—	≤5	—
Oxygenation: A-aDo$_2$ or Pao$_2$	≥500	350–499	200–349	—	<200 Po$_2$ >70	Po$_2$ 61–70	—	Po$_2$ 55–60	Po$_2$ <55	—
Arterial pH or Serum HCO$_3$	≥7.7 / ≥52	7.6–7.69 / 41–51.9	—	7.5–7.59 / 32–40.9	7.33–7.49 / 22–31.9	—	7.25–7.32 / 18–21.9	7.15–7.24 / 15–17.9	<7.15 / <15	—
Serum Na (mEq/L)	≥180	160–179	155–159	150–154	130–149	—	120–129	111–119	≥110	—
Serum K (mEq/L)	≥7	6–6.9	—	5.5–5.9	2.5–5.4	3–3.4	2.5–2.9	—	<2.5	—
Serum Cr (mg/dL) Double-point score for ARF	≥3.5	2–3.4	1.5–1.9	—	0.6–1.4	—	<0.6	—	—	—
Hct (%)	≥60	—	50–59.9	46–49.9	30–45.9	—	20–29.9	—	<20	—
WBC in 1,000's	≥40	—	20–39.9	15–19.9	3–14.9	—	1–2.9	—	<1	—
GCS score					15–GCS					

A. Total acute psychology score (sum of above 12 points)
B. Age points (years) ≥44 = 0, 45–54 = 2, 55–64 = 3, 65–74 = 5, ≥75 = 6
C. Chronic health points (see below)
   Total APACHE II score (A+B+C)

Chronic health points—assign 5 points for pre-existing organ insufficiency or immunocompromised state.
- **Liver:** cirrhosis, portal hypertensive GI bleed, or hepatic encephalopathy
- **Cardiovascular:** NYHA class IV heart failure
- **Respiratory:** severe exercise restriction (unable to climb stairs or perform household duties), chronic hypoxia, chronic hypercapnia, severe pulmonary hypertension (>40 mm Hg), secondary polycythemia, respirator dependency
- **Renal:** chronic hemodialysis
- **Immunocompromised:** immunosuppression, chemotherapy, radiation, leukemia/lymphoma, AIDS

APACHE, Acute Physiology and Chronic Health Evaluation; MAP, mean arterial pressure; A-aDo$_2$, alveolar-arterial oxygen gradient; Pao$_2$, partial pressure of oxygen in arterial blood; HCO$_3$, bicarbonate; Na, sodium; K, potassium; Cr, creatinine; ARF, acute renal failure; Hct, hematocrit; WBC, white blood cell count; GCS, Glasgow Coma Scale; GI, gastrointestinal; NYHA, New York Heart Association.

c. **Peritoneal lavage:** can be useful in excluding other severe intra-abdominal processes and can be therapeutic in severe pancreatitis
- **Catheters:** can be placed percutaneously, and antibiotics can be included in the lavage solution
- **Laparotomy:** When performed for diagnosis and lesser sac exploration, accompanying peritoneal lavage can be undertaken.
- **Complications:** include a deterioration of pulmonary function, which can be compromised by abdominal distention from the dialysis solutions. A high glucose load in the dialysis solution can induce severe hyperglycemia.

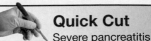

Quick Cut
Severe pancreatitis is usually managed non-operatively except for persistent biliary obstruction due to stones, abscess or sepsis, or failure to improve.

Relapsing Pancreatitis

I. **Etiology:** commonly occurs in nonalcoholic patients and results from biliary tract disease—either calculi in the ducts or inflammation and spasm of the sphincter of Oddi

II. **Diagnosis:** can be made by demonstrating the presence of biliary stones or biliary sphincter dysfunction
   A. **US:** useful for diagnosing biliary calculi
   B. **Microscopic examination of the bile:** Bile is aspirated through a suction tube placed in the duodenum and examined for white blood cells (WBCs), cholesterol crystals, and microspheroliths.

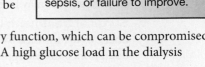

Quick Cut
Relapsing pancreatitis can result from stones or inflammation causing spasm of the sphincter of Oddi.

III. **Treatment:** based on the cause
   A. **Patient with biliary calculi:** Procedures include cholecystectomy, common bile duct exploration, biliary manometry, and sphincteroplasty plus pancreaticobiliary septum resection.
   B. **Perisphincteric disease:** gallbladder removal and a wide sphincteroplasty that includes the pancreaticobiliary septum
   C. **Postcholecystectomy patients:** Often have a positive provocative test and can be treated successfully by sphincteroplasty. A negative provocative test requires workup, including ERCP. Alcoholism should be ruled out.
   D. **Patients with severe intrinsic disease:** respond poorly to sphincteroplasty

Chronic Pancreatitis

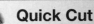

Quick Cut
Calcification of the pancreas indicates chronic pancreatitis.

I. **Pathologic findings:** include fibrosis and calcification throughout the gland
   A. **Early changes:** plugging of the small pancreatic ducts with proteinaceous material containing eosinophils
   B. **With disease progression:** Calcification becomes prominent; multiple areas of ductal dilatation can result.
   C. **Ductal dilatation:** in its end stages, produces a "chain-of-lakes" appearance
   D. **Common bile duct obstruction or duodenal obstruction:** can occur in advanced cases as a result of inflammation in surrounding areas

II. **Cause:** Almost always alcohol related. However, certain congenital anomalies can produce chronic ductal obstruction and chronic pancreatitis.

III. **Clinical presentation**
   A. **History of unrelenting pain:** usually the major indication for surgical intervention
   B. **Endocrine insufficiency:** Damage may be severe enough to cause impaired glucose tolerance or true diabetes.
   C. **Exocrine pancreatic insufficiency:** results in malabsorption, with consequent weight loss and steatorrhea
   D. **Plain films:** may show the calcifications in the ductal system or may aid in delineating neighboring areas that are caught in the inflammatory process
   E. **Severe disease (in the head of the pancreas):** can mimic carcinoma and cause bile duct obstruction
   F. **Splenic vein thrombosis:** may cause upper GI bleeding

IV. Medical treatment: Analgesia and endocrine replacement as needed are typical.

A. Exocrine replacement with pancreatic enzymes:
Pancrelipase or pancreozymin in high doses (i.e., 5 g four
times daily) can suppress pancreatic secretion by the feedback
phenomenon.

B. General nutritional measures: including alcohol avoidance

C. Octreotide: may be of benefit in select cases

> **Quick Cut**
> Surgery for chronic
> pancreatitis is considered
> when there is a dominant
> stricture, or refractory pain.

V. Surgical treatment: Depends on the condition of the pancreatic
ducts, as determined by ERCP (Fig. 14-2). If ERCP is not possible and the patient must undergo an
operation, pancreatograms can be obtained.

A. Puestow operation: Dilated chain-of-lakes duct is treated by wide unroofing of the duct and
dilated ductules, with drainage of the entire open pancreas into a defunctionalized jejunal loop.
A side-to-side procedure may be used, or the surgeon may choose an invagination in which the
pancreas is placed into the jejunal loop.

B. Distal pancreatectomy: used to treat a distal ductal obstruction

C. Duval operation: Proximal ductal obstruction can be treated by amputating the tail of the pancreas
and draining the pancreas retrograde into a defunctionalized jejunal loop. This is not as effective or
long lasting as lateral pancreaticojejunostomy.

D. Patient with severe pain and a fibrotic, nondilated duct: Possible surgical procedures include the
following.

1. Child operation: 95% pancreatectomy

2. Splanchnicectomy: either abdominal or thoracic

a. Technique: This procedure serves only to relieve the pain of pancreatitis by dividing the
splanchnic nerves, with no direct effect on the underlying disorder.

b. Disadvantage: also eradicates the pain from appendicitis and other intra-abdominal
problems, which may delay diagnosis of an abdominal emergency

3. Duodenum-sparing pancreatic head resection: Approach has become a popular option for
patients who have had failed sphincteroplasties.

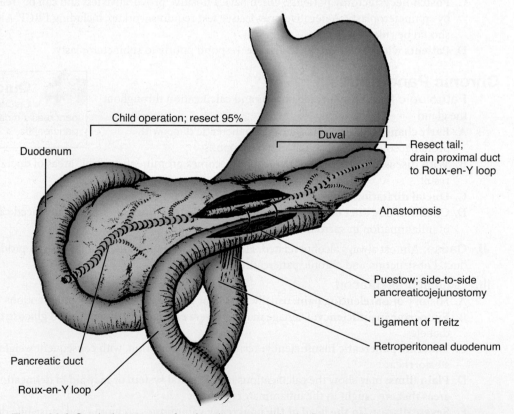

Figure 14-2: Surgical treatments for chronic pancreatitis: the Puestow, Duval, and Child operations.

4. **Total pancreatectomy and islet cell transplant:** limited to select patients with hereditary relapsing pancreatitis and preserved endocrine function

Pseudocyst

I. **Pathologic findings**

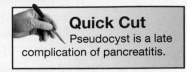
Quick Cut
Pseudocyst is a late complication of pancreatitis.

A. **Lesser sac collection:** Pseudocyst forms as a result of fibrosis, thickening, and organization of the organs bordering the collection.

B. **Not lined by epithelium:** Pseudocyst consists only of the inflammatory response of the neighboring organs.

C. **Related organs:** Stomach, duodenum, colon, and transverse mesocolon form the walls. The major organ involved is generally the stomach, which forms the anterior surface of the pseudocyst.

D. **Maturation (3–5 weeks):** not truly formed until the walls are sufficiently organized to become firm anatomic structures

E. **Natural history:** Depends on its size. Small pseudocysts may resolve; large pseudocysts with mature organized walls generally do not resolve.

II. **Clinical presentation**

A. **Maturation phase:** Patient recovers from a bout of pancreatitis but develops a persistent increase of amylase, a low-grade fever, a minimally increased WBC count, and chronic pain.

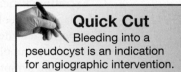
Quick Cut
Bleeding into a pseudocyst is an indication for angiographic intervention.

B. **Continuous minor bleeding:** Causes a gradual decrease in hemoglobin. More significant bleeds are associated with acute pain or hemorrhagic shock.

III. **Diagnosis:** Pseudocysts are usually diagnosed by US or CT scan.

IV. **Treatment:** Goal is to allow the maturation phase to continue until the walls of the pseudocyst have matured.

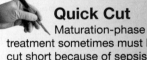
Quick Cut
Maturation-phase treatment sometimes must be cut short because of sepsis or hemorrhage within the pseudocyst.

A. **Diet:** total parenteral nutrition (TPN) or an elemental diet for 3–4 weeks until maturation has occurred

B. **Surgical treatment of mature pseudocysts**

1. **Internal drainage:** Best approach is through the anterior stomach wall to locate the firm connection that usually exists between the posterior stomach and the pseudocyst.

   a. **Aspirate the cyst through the stomach wall:** First step; after which, an opening is made between the stomach and the pseudocyst and is sutured for hemostasis.

   b. **Resolution:** Pseudocyst then drains into the stomach and generally resolves.

2. **Defunctionalized (Roux-en-Y) loop of jejunum:** If the pseudocyst is not fixed to an organ that lends itself to internal drainage, suture a loop of jejunum to the pseudocyst wall to establish internal drainage.

3. **External drainage:** Used if the pseudocyst is not found to be mature and if suturing of the pseudocyst wall is not safe. The external drainage results in a pancreatic fistula, which usually heals with continued TPN. Pancreatic fistula may be quite difficult to treat.

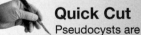
Quick Cut
Pseudocysts are best drained internally; abscesses (infected pseudocysts) are drained externally.

4. **Excision:** rare; however, may be indicated if the pseudocyst is small and is located distally in the tail of the pancreas

C. **Endoscopic drainage:** Mature collections within 1 cm of the stomach or duodenum can be drained internally via endoscopic ultrasound (EUS) guidance.

PANCREATIC MALIGNANCIES

Pancreatic Adenocarcinoma

Quick Cut
Pancreatic cancer has a five-year survival rate less than 5%.

I. **Incidence:** Approximately 43,000 new cases of pancreatic adenocarcinoma in 2009; incidence is 11.4 per 100,000 and has not changed in ~10 years. African Americans have a higher rate than the white population.

A. **Mortality:** Fourth most common cause of cancer death in the United States. Most patients have advanced disease at diagnosis, and the 5-year survival for all patients diagnosed with the disease is only 5%.

B. **Median age (in the United States):** Age 72 years; only 10% of patients are age younger than 50 years.

C. **Risk factors**

1. **Environmental factors:** most notably tobacco, as well as chlorinated hydrocarbon solvents and organochlorine insecticides

2. **Patient-related factors:** diabetes mellitus, obesity, and the chronic inflammatory conditions cirrhosis or pancreatitis

II. **Clinical presentation**

A. **Symptoms:** Vague and nonspecific, including anorexia, weight loss, and fatigue. Back pain is an ominous symptom that frequently indicates a locally advanced condition with malignant infiltration of the retroperitoneal splanchnic nerve plexus.

> **Quick Cut**
> About 80% of pancreatic cancers occur in the head; therefore, painless jaundice from distal bile duct obstruction is a common presenting symptom.

B. **Obstructive jaundice:** Patients will typically also experience acholic stools and dark urine. When jaundice is severe, patients will complain of severe pruritus and often present with excoriation of the skin from nocturnal scratching.

C. **Excretion:** Patients may report loose malodorous stools that float in the bowl secondary to malabsorption of fat from exocrine insufficiency.

D. **Superficial or deep thrombophlebitis (Trousseau sign):** May be the initial presentation. It is migratory and ultimately develops in as many as 10% of patients.

E. **Location:** Symptoms at the time of presentation are related to tumor location within the pancreas.

1. **Head:** Most common site; tumors here produce weight loss and obstructive jaundice in 75% of patients.

   a. **Jaundice:** Usually painless; skin excoriation related to pruritus may be present.

   b. **Pain:** when present, is usually upper abdominal and radiates to the back

   c. **Physical exam:** Usually normal outside of jaundice. Ascites, hepatic mass or hepatomegaly, and palpable lymphadenopathy in the left supraclavicular region (Virchow node) or periumbilical (Sister Mary Joseph nodes) are physical findings consistent with metastatic disease.

   d. **Courvoisier gallbladder:** RUQ nontender mass may represent a passively dilated gallbladder secondary to bile duct obstruction.

2. **Body or tail:** less common and generally present at a more advanced stage because tumors do not produce local symptoms

III. **Diagnosis:** Routine screening of asymptomatic populations is currently not feasible. Progress in serologic testing for tumor markers provides hope for the future.

> **Quick Cut**
> Pancreatic head cancer may involve the SMV because the vein is immediately adjacent to the head of the pancreas posteriorly.

A. **Abdominal ultrasonography:** Commonly used as the first test to assess the etiology of jaundice. Uniformly dilated ductal system without evidence of cholelithiasis or choledocholithiasis is consistent with malignant obstruction.

B. **Pancreatic protocol contrast-enhanced CT:** definitive imaging test to assess for resectability of the primary tumor and for the presence of metastases

C. **Percutaneous fine-needle aspiration (FNA) under CT guidance:** can diagnose malignancy but should only be done rarely due to the risk of disseminating cancerous cells

D. **ERCP:** Flexible side-viewing duodenoscope cannulates the pancreatic duct. Contrast medium is injected, and radiographs are taken.

1. **Advantages:** Small pancreatic cancers can be found, and specimens via brushing can be collected from the pancreatic duct for cytologic examination.

2. **Successful cannulation:** Requires a skilled endoscopist. A stent is usually placed to relieve the biliary obstruction.

3. **EUS with FNA:** preferred technique for obtaining tissue for diagnosis

   a. **Advantages:** Yields very precise information regarding relationship of the primary tumor to surrounding structures such as the hepatic artery or SMV. This provides very high resolution of small lesions and can allow transduodenal needle biopsies.

   b. It is less specific for staging of lymph node metastases.

E. **Percutaneous transhepatic cholangiography:** evaluation of patients who have obstructive jaundice and who cannot undergo ERCP

1. **Procedure:** With the patient under local anesthesia, a long small-bore needle is inserted through the liver into a dilated hepatic duct, and contrast medium is injected to identify the site of obstruction.

2. **Jaundice:** relieved preoperatively by passing a catheter through the site of obstruction

3. **Potential complications:** bleeding from the needle track in the liver and sepsis

> **Quick Cut**
> The value of EUS in tumor staging is in determining vascular invasion and local lymph nodes. It does not detect liver or peritoneal metastases, or other findings of unresectable cancer.

IV. Treatment

A. **Pancreaticoduodenectomy (Whipple procedure):** standard surgical treatment for adenocarcinoma of the head of the pancreas when the lesion is curable by resection (Fig. 14-3)

1. **Resectability:** Many patients are deemed unresectable, as evidenced by metastatic disease identified by abdominal imaging and confirmed by percutaneous biopsy. Resectability is confirmed at operation using several criteria.

a. **Metastases:** No metastases in the abdominal cavity; favored sites of metastatic disease include liver and peritoneal dissemination.

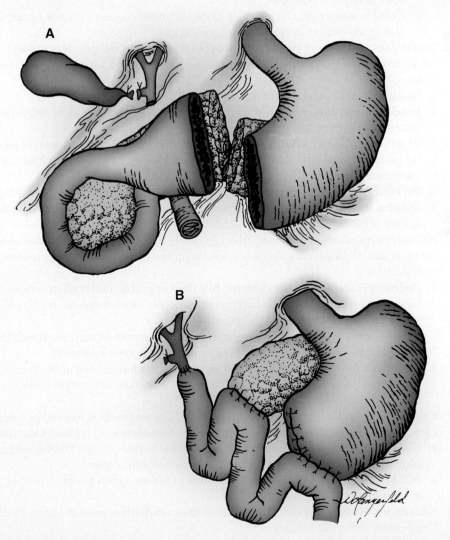

Figure 14-3: Whipple procedure. **A:** The head of the pancreas, distal common bile duct, gastric antrum, and duodenum are removed. **B:** The GI tract, pancreatic duct, and bile duct are reconstructed.

b. **Porta hepatis structures intact:** Tumor has not invaded this area including the hepatic artery or SMV as it passes behind the neck of the pancreas.

c. **Laparoscopy:** Increased use to rule out peritoneal seeding before proceeding with laparotomy in selected patients. This procedure is indicated in patients with tumors involving the body and tail of the pancreas and in patients with a cancer antigen 19-9 level 400 ng/mL or more.

2. **Tissue diagnosis:** not required before definitive resection in patients who have a high suspicion of cancer; however, in cases of a question regarding the diagnosis or the mass cannot be immediately resected, tissue is required before definitive nonoperative treatment can be initiated

3. **"Classic" Whipple procedure:** Removal of the head of the pancreas, duodenum, distal common bile duct, gallbladder, and distal stomach. An alternative is the pylorus-preserving Whipple in which the transection of the GI tract is across the duodenum just distal to the pylorus.

> **Quick Cut**
> The Whipple procedure is a radical pancreaticoduodenectomy.

a. **GI tract reconstruction:** creation of a gastrojejunostomy (or duodenojejunostomy), choledochojejunostomy, and pancreaticojejunostomy

b. **Operative mortality rate:** Should be 2% or lower in centers where this operation is frequently performed. According to recent publications, the lower mortality rate is realized in institutions doing at least 20 of these procedures annually.

c. **Complication rate:** Considerable (25%); the most common include hemorrhage, abscess, and leakage (fistula) at the pancreaticojejunostomy.

B. **Distal pancreatectomy (usually with splenectomy and lymphadenectomy):** performed for carcinoma of the midbody and tail of the pancreas and for benign mucinous pancreatic tumors

1. **Staging:** should include laparoscopy

2. **In selected patients:** Procedure can be laparoscopically or robotically although data do not show better patient outcomes with minimally invasive techniques.

C. **Total pancreatectomy:** proposed but not commonly done for the treatment of pancreatic cancer

1. **Advantages:** removal of a possible multicentric tumor and avoidance of pancreatic duct anastomotic leaks

2. **Survival rates:** not markedly better, and the operation has not been widely adopted

3. **Disadvantage:** In addition, it has resulted in a particularly brittle type of diabetes, thus decreasing quality of life.

D. **Palliative procedures:** Performed more frequently than curative ones because so many patients are incurable. With advances in endoscopic techniques, most palliative procedures can be offered nonoperatively.

1. **Endoscopic stenting of the common bile duct or gastric outlet obstruction:** Because survival for patients with unresectable or recurrent cancer is short, these are usually effective in relieving symptoms for the life span of the patient.

2. **Percutaneous transhepatic biliary stents:** can sometimes be used to provide internal biliary drainage for obstructive jaundice, thereby avoiding a major operation

3. **Celiac axis block:** Combined alcohol and lidocaine administered in the periaortic soft tissues just adjacent to the celiac axis can relieve pain from malignant infiltration of the sensory splanchnic nerves.

E. **Chemotherapy:** Has been used in the treatment of patients with advanced pancreatic adenocarcinoma. Even with active treatment, the overall survival is usually less than 1 year.

1. **Gemcitabine:** Most commonly used; antimetabolite that inhibits DNA synthesis. It can be combined with erlotinib, an epidermal growth factor inhibitor.

2. **FOLFIRINOX:** Recently adopted combination of four agents has been used in patients with a modest improvement in survival.

F. **Neoadjuvant (treatment before operation) chemoradiation:** used in selected patients who have "borderline" resectable tumors

1. **Adjuvant therapy (after surgery):** Chemotherapy, radiation, or a combination of the two is offered to patients at risk of recurrence.

2. **Overall survival:** modest improvement compared to surgery alone; typically only a few months

V. **Prognosis: extremely poor**
   A. **Overall:** Five-year survival rate is less than 5%, and cures are extremely rare. The median survival after resection and neoadjuvant or adjuvant therapy is 20–22 months.
   B. **Unresectable tumors or metastases:** Median length of survival is 6 months.
   C. **Resectable tumors (few):** Results of surgery are not good; ~20% of patients who undergo resection will live 5 years.

Other Pancreatic Malignancies

I. Cystic and solid lesions of the pancreas are not rare, but most are not malignant.

II. Serous cystic neoplasms are slow growing, with low malignant potential. When asymptomatic, they may be followed radiographically.

III. Mucinous cystic neoplasms commonly harbor carcinoma and should be resected.

IV. Intraductal papillary mucin-producing neoplasia (IPMN) is characterized by mucin production through the pancreatic duct and into the ampulla. Main duct lesions have as poor a prognosis as pancreatic adenocarcinoma.

> **Quick Cut**
> The poor prognosis is due in part to the difficulty in making a diagnosis while the tumor is at an early stage: Only ~10% of pancreatic adenocarcinomas are resectable at the time of diagnosis.

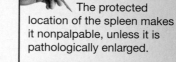

Spleen

Daniel E. Mansour, Mayur Narayan, and Ajay Jain

 INTRODUCTION

Anatomy

I. **Location:** Largest secondary lymphoid organ in the body, the spleen is located in the left upper quadrant of the abdomen (left hypochondrium), below the diaphragm, and is protected by the 8th–11th ribs.

> **Quick Cut**
> The protected location of the spleen makes it nonpalpable, unless it is pathologically enlarged.

A. **Borders:** bordered by the left kidney posteriorly, the diaphragm superiorly, and the fundus of the stomach and the splenic flexure of the colon anteriorly; also closely approximates the tail of the pancreas

B. **Major ligaments**
1. **Gastrosplenic ligament:** connects greater curvature and splenic hilum
2. **Splenorenal ligament:** connects hilum and kidney
3. **Splenophrenic ligament:** suspends posterior aspect from diaphragm
4. **Splenocolic ligament:** attaches inferior pole to the colon

II. **Vasculature**

A. **Splenic artery:** main blood supply (Fig. 15-1)
1. **Origin:** branch of the celiac axis
2. **Course:** travels along the superior border of the pancreas; typically has a tortuous, corkscrew-line course
3. **Branches:** At the hilum, it branches into trabecular arteries, which terminate in small vessels to the splenic pulp.

B. **Short gastric arteries:** arise from the spleen and supply the fundus of the stomach, then course through the gastrosplenic ligament connecting the hilum and the greater curvature

C. **Splenic vein:** crosses at the lower border of the pancreas and joins the superior mesenteric vein to form the portal vein

Histology and Function

I. **Histology:** Capsule comprising dense connective tissue surrounds the spleen. Septations (trabeculae) arising from the capsule subdivides the pulp of the spleen into three discrete zones (red pulp, marginal zone, and white pulp) with distinct architecture and functions.

A. **White pulp:** Contains lymphocytes, macrophages, and plasma cells in a reticular network surrounded by an outer marginal zone; also contains separate areas for T cells and B cells. Its primary function is **immunologic**.

B. **Marginal zone:** Vascular space between the pulps that contains macrophages, which can engulf blood-borne pathogens. It also contains B cells that can generate antibodies.

C. **Red pulp:** Comprises 75% of splenic volume and consists of cords of reticular cells with sinuses in between. Its primary function is to serve as a blood **filter**; it also helps recycle iron.

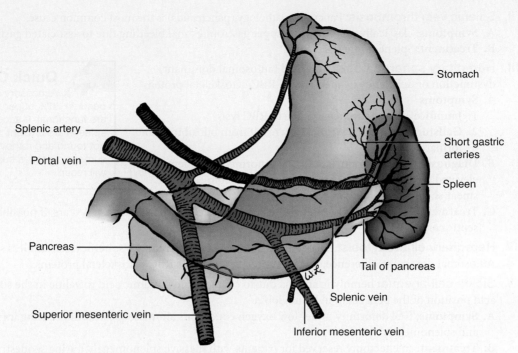

Figure 15-1: Anatomic relationships of the spleen.

II. Functions

A. **Filtration:** removes foreign materials, cellular debris, and damaged erythrocytes from circulation

B. **Immunity:** Removes bacteria from the circulation, including poorly opsonized or encapsulated pathogens. It serves as a site for antigen presentation as well as T-cell and B-cell activation and is the major site of immunoglobulin M (IgM) production.

C. **Reservoir:** In a minor capacity, the spleen serves as a reservoir for platelets and red blood cells (RBCs).

PATHOLOGY

Definitions

I. **Hypersplenism:** functional hyperactivity that results in a loss of one or more hematologic cell populations

A. **Primary hypersplenism:** Functional change in the absence of hematologic disorders or infection. It is rare, more commonly affects women, and is a diagnosis of exclusion.

B. **Secondary hypersplenism:** more common and secondary to another disease process

II. **Splenomegaly:** gross enlargement of the spleen

Symptoms

I. **Anemia:** causes pallor, fatigue, and dyspnea

II. **Leukopenia:** recurrent infections

III. **Thrombocytopenia:** bruising and epistaxis

IV. **Splenomegaly:** If present, may cause pain secondary to capsular distention. Also may present with rupture and hemorrhage.

Causes of Secondary Hypersplenism

I. **Portal hypertension:** most common cause

A. **Symptoms:** often accompanied by congestion and splenomegaly

B. **Treatment:** splenectomy generally not indicated

Quick Cut
Splenomegaly is increased size; *hypersplenism* is increased function. It is possible to have splenomegaly without hypersplenism and vice versa.

Quick Cut
Symptoms of conditions affecting the spleen are chiefly related to underlying cytopenia or splenomegaly.

Quick Cut
Portal hypertension is the most common cause of hypersplenism.

II. **Splenic vein thrombosis:** Pancreatic pathology (pancreatitis) is the most common cause.
   A. **Symptoms:** classically presents with upper gastrointestinal bleeding due to associated gastric varices
   B. **Treatment:** Splenectomy is curative.

III. **Hereditary spherocytosis:** inherited (autosomal dominant) dysfunction or deficiency in **spectrin**, an RBC cytoskeletal protein
   A. **Symptoms**
      1. **Jaundice and splenomegaly:** due to RBC lysis
      2. **Gallstones and biliary colic:** may result from bilirubin stone formation
   B. **Diagnosis:** physical exam, laboratory abnormalities (anemia, elevated serum bilirubin, elevated reticulocyte count), blood smear showing spherocytes
   C. **Treatment:** Splenectomy is curative but should be delayed until after age 4 years, if possible, to avoid septic complications.

> **Quick Cut**
> Accessory spleens occur in 20% of people and are functional. If accessory spleens are present but not found and removed at surgery, diseases such as ITP will recur.

IV. **Hereditary elliptocytosis:** Related to and managed like hereditary spherocytosis but less severe. Autosomal dominant inherence; involves spectrin and other RBC cytoskeletal proteins.

V. **Sickle cell anemia:** hemolytic anemia due to change from glutamic acid to valine in the sixth amino acid position of the beta chain in hemoglobin
   A. **Symptoms:** Cell deformity under low oxygen conditions allows sequestration, causing infarction and splenomegaly.
   B. **Treatment:** splenectomy reserved for patients with massive splenomegaly during sequestration crisis early in life

VI. **Idiopathic autoimmune hemolytic anemia:** caused by autoantibody formation against RBC membrane proteins
   A. **Incidence:** more common in women
   B. **Symptoms:** similar to other hemolytic anemias (jaundice, anemia)
   C. **Diagnosis:** direct Coombs test result is positive; reticulocytosis and increased indirect bilirubin in serum
   D. **Treatment**
      1. **Medical treatment:** Mainstay therapy is high-dose **corticosteroids** (response in 75% of patients).
      2. **Splenectomy:** helpful in some patients refractory to medical therapy (up to 80%)

VII. **Other congenital hemolytic anemias:** splenectomy generally not curative but may be considered for reducing transfusions
   A. **Enzyme deficiencies:** such as glucose-6-phosphate dehydrogenase (G6PD) and pyruvate kinase deficiencies
   B. **Thalassemia major:** Autosomal dominant inheritance characterized by defective hemoglobin synthesis. Causes severe anemia and hepatosplenomegaly.

VIII. **Idiopathic thrombocytopenic purpura (ITP):** autoimmune disorder of unknown etiology, characterized by platelet destruction resulting in low platelet count
   A. **Acute form:** More common in children following a viral upper respiratory illness; 80% recover spontaneously.
   B. **Chronic form:** most common in adults and women
   C. **Symptoms:** Unexplained ecchymoses or petechiae. Splenomegaly is rare.
   D. **Clinical diagnosis:** platelet count less than 100,000; megakaryocytes in bone marrow
   E. **Treatment**
      1. **Medical:** First-line therapy includes platelet transfusion, gamma-Ig, corticosteroids, and Rho(D) Ig.
      2. **After splenectomy failure:** rituximab and romiplostim
      3. **Splenectomy:** indicated in patients refractory to medical therapy or with intracranial hemorrhage; produces sustained remission in 75%–85%

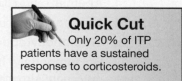

> **Quick Cut**
> Only 20% of ITP patients have a sustained response to corticosteroids.

IX. **Thrombotic thrombocytopenic purpura (TTP):** rapidly progressive and usually fatal; characterized by thrombocytopenia, microangiopathic hemolytic anemia, and neurologic complications
   A. **Clinical presentation:** fever, petechiae, hemolytic anemia, neurologic symptoms, and renal failure
   B. **Diagnosis:** confirmed by **peripheral blood smear**, with schistocytes, nucleated RBCs, and basophilic stippling

C. **Treatment: Plasma exchange (plasmapheresis)** is first-line therapy. Splenectomy reserved for patients with relapse or requiring multiple plasma exchanges.

D. **Prognosis:** poor long-term survival rate (<10%)

X. **Felty syndrome:** complication of long-standing rheumatoid arthritis, characterized by rheumatoid arthritis, splenomegaly, and neutropenia

A. **Symptoms:** recurrent infections and chronic leg ulcers

B. **Treatment:** splenectomy performed for symptomatic neutropenia, anemia requiring transfusions, and severe thrombocytopenia

XI. **Enzyme deficiencies and metabolic diseases (unusual)**

A. **Enzyme deficiencies:** G6PD and pyruvate kinase deficiencies

B. **Gaucher disease:** lysosomal storage disease

> **Quick Cut**
> Felty syndrome is the classic triad of rheumatoid arthritis, splenomegaly, and neutropenia.

Evaluation of Hypersplenism

I. **Peripheral blood smear:** Decreased number of RBCs, white blood cells (WBCs), or platelets or abnormal RBC morphology. **Reticulocytosis** is seen secondary to increased RBC turnovers.

II. **Bone marrow biopsy:** may allow detection of increased hematopoetic progenitor cell populations to compensate for hypersplenism and cytopenia

III. **Radiologic imaging**

A. **Ultrasound:** can help assess the size and texture of the spleen and perisplenic fluid such as blood

B. **Computed tomography (CT) scan:** useful in assessing the size of the spleen as well as determining any structural abnormalities; also helps with guidance of percutaneous procedures and may show other pathology such as lymphadenopathy or varices

C. **Nuclear imaging:** may be useful in locating accessory splenic tissue causing ongoing cytopenia after unsuccessful splenectomy for ITP

> **Quick Cut**
> Ultrasound is usually the first choice in trauma scenarios.

Splenic Cysts

I. **Etiology:** may be idiopathic or induced by trauma

II. **Treatment:** Partial splenectomy or cyst marsupialization should be performed whenever possible to preserve splenic function.

> **Quick Cut**
> Surgery is only indicated with splenic cysts for symptoms such as pain or mass effect (such as early satiety from gastric compression).

Sarcoidosis

I. **Etiology:** multisystem inflammatory disease of unknown etiology characterized by noncaseating granulomas in multiple tissues (especially lungs and lymph nodes)

II. **Treatment:** splenectomy typically only indicated to rule out cancer

Infection

I. **Splenic abscess:** uncommon but has a high mortality rate (40%–100%)

A. **Causes:** Most common organisms are *Staphylococcus aureus* or *Streptococcus.*

1. **Infarction:** resulting in necrosis and suprainfection

2. **Intra-abdominal infection from other source.**

3. **Hematogenous seeding:** in intravenous drug users or during overwhelming bacteremia (e.g., in endocarditis)

B. **Diagnosis:** clinical evidence of sepsis (fever, elevated WBC, etc.), in conjunction with CT findings suggestive of splenic abscess

C. **Treatment:** Initiate broad-spectrum antibiotics. Splenectomy has been considered the gold standard for refractory cases, but percutaneous drainage is increasingly a viable option.

> **Quick Cut**
> Treatment for splenic infection is generally medical, although surgery may be indicated for abscess or disease localized to the spleen.

II. **Viral infections:** Mononucleosis, HIV, and hepatitis may cause transient splenomegaly and hypersplenism.

III. **Parasitic infections:** Malaria, leishmaniasis, or trypanosomiasis may cause splenomegaly. An echinococcal cyst may develop in the spleen. Partial or total splenectomy is curative.

IV. **Fungal infection:** Histoplasmosis produces characteristic areas of calcification within the spleen.

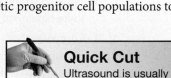

Neoplastic Diseases

I. Primary splenic tumors (sarcoma, hemangioma, and hamartoma): rare

   A. Symptoms: often asymptomatic but may cause symptoms if large enough to cause capsular stretch and pain

   B. Treatment: Splenectomy indicated for indeterminate or suspicious lesions (to confirm or exclude malignancy). Benign, stable hemangiomas (as determined by arterial and venous phase contrast CT) do not necessarily require splenectomy.

II. Metastatic disease: Isolated splenic metastases are rare.

III. Hematologic malignancies

   A. Hodgkin disease: Treatment includes radiation therapy alone, chemotherapy alone, or a combination of both. Overall, there is a good long-term survival rate.

   B. Staging laparotomy: Splenectomy used to be part of the staging but is now rarely indicated because the additional information does not alter therapy.

IV. Non-Hodgkin lymphoma

   A. Staging: uses the same classification as for Hodgkin disease

   B. Splenectomy: may be indicated in select patients to treat hypersplenism or to relieve symptoms of massive splenomegaly

Quick Cut
Splenectomy is no longer required to stage Hodgkin lymphoma.

V. Leukemias

   A. Symptoms: Patients with **chronic lymphocytic leukemia (CLL)**, **chronic myelogenous leukemia (CML)**, and **hairy cell leukemia** may develop hypersplenism and thrombocytopenia.

   B. Treatment: Splenectomy may benefit in cases that are refractory to medical therapy.

Other Lesions

I. Splenic rupture: traumatic cause or spontaneous because of massive splenomegaly due to an associated disease

II. Splenosis: May occur spontaneously after rupture; shed splenic tissue can engraft in the body and can maintain pathologic hypersplenic state after therapeutic splenectomy.

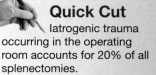

Quick Cut
Iatrogenic trauma occurring in the operating room accounts for 20% of all splenectomies.

III. Splenic artery aneurysms

IV. Ectopic spleen: Results from a long splenic pedicle; splenic location can vary within the abdomen.

V. Accessory spleens: present in 20% of population; greater than 80% located near the splenic hilum and vascular pedicle and less frequently in the tail of the pancreas and in the mesentery

Quick Cut
Blunt trauma is the leading cause of splenectomy. Many cases of traumatic splenic injury can be managed nonoperatively.

Treatment

I. Treatment: depends on the underlying condition

II. Table 15-1: summarizes the role of surgery in various pathologic conditions

TECHNICAL ASPECTS OF SPLENECTOMY

Open Splenectomy

I. Step 1: Mobilize the spleen to midline by dividing the splenic attachments (splenophrenic, splenocolic, splenorenal ligaments) either sharply or bluntly.

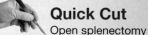

Quick Cut
Open splenectomy may be performed through midline laparotomy or a left subcostal incision.

II. Step 2: Careful dissection of the hilum and application of vascular clamps should be performed to avoid injury to the tail of the pancreas.

III. Step 3: Once the splenic hilum is controlled, identification and ligation of the short gastrics should be performed.

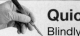

Quick Cut
Blindly applying a clamp to the splenic hilum may injure the pancreatic tail.

Table 15-1: Absolute and Relative Indications for Splenectomy

Type of Pathology	Absolute Indications	Relative Indications
Primary splenic disorders	Symptomatic splenic cyst	Primary hypersplenism
Disorders of splenic blood flow	Bleeding esophagogastric varices associated with splenic vein thrombosis	Portal hypertension with severe hypersplenism
Hematopoietic disorders	Hereditary spherocytosis	Hereditary elliptocytosis Thalassemia major Sickle cell anemia Congenital erythropoietic porphyria
Immune disorders	None	Idiopathic autoimmune hemolytic anemia Idiopathic thrombocytopenic purpura Thrombotic thrombocytopenic purpura Felty syndrome Systemic lupus erythematosus
Infiltrative disorders	None	Myeloid metaplasia Sarcoidosis
Infectious diseases	Splenic abscess Echinococcal cyst	Gaucher disease
Neoplastic diseases	Primary splenic tumors	Staging laparotomy for Hodgkin disease or non-Hodgkin lymphoma Chronic lymphocytic leukemia Chronic myelogenous leukemia Hairy cell leukemia
Miscellaneous	Massive splenic trauma Spontaneous rupture	

Laparoscopy

I. **Operative steps:** similar to a laparotomy, but care must be taken to avoid rupture and consequent splenosis

II. **Technique:** Because splenosis can lead to recurrence of the underlying disease, surgeons must avoid spillage of any part of the splenic specimen; tear-resistant nylon bags are available.

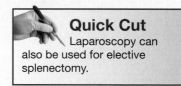

Quick Cut
Laparoscopy can also be used for elective splenectomy.

 ## COMPLICATIONS AFTER SPLENECTOMY

Injury to Surrounding Structures

I. **Gastric wall:** Injury occurs in course of controlling the short gastric vessels. Gastric wall necrosis with delayed perforation with overzealous short gastric ligation may occur.

II. **Tail of the pancreas:** Injury can occur during clamping or stapling of the artery and vein at the hilum, resulting in postoperative pancreatic leak, pancreatitis, abscess, or phlegmon formation. If recognized, a drain should be left postoperatively.

III. **Colonic injury**

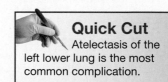

Quick Cut
Atelectasis of the left lower lung is the most common complication.

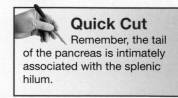

Quick Cut
Remember, the tail of the pancreas is intimately associated with the splenic hilum.

Overwhelming Postsplenectomy Infection/Sepsis

I. **Etiology and incidence:** Occurs because spleen is no longer able to opsonize encapsulated bacteria; incidence is very rare (<1%).

   A. **Causative organisms:** encapsulated bacteria, including *Streptococcus pneumoniae*, *Neisseria meningitidis*, and *Haemophilus influenzae*

B. **Timing:** Most septic episodes occur within 2 years after splenectomy.

C. **Risk:** greatest if splenectomy occurs during the first 2–4 years of life

II. **Clinical presentation:** nonspecific, mild, influenza-like symptoms, which can rapidly progress to high fever, shock, and death

III. **Prevention and treatment**

A. **Vaccines:** should be administered 2 weeks prior to elective splenectomies or anytime following an unplanned splenectomy and include polyvalent pneumococcal vaccine and vaccines for *N. meningitidis* and *H. influenzae*

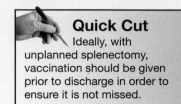

Quick Cut
Ideally, with unplanned splenectomy, vaccination should be given prior to discharge in order to ensure it is not missed.

B. **Prophylactic penicillin:** Daily doses are commonly recommended for children until age 5 years or at least 5 years post splenectomy.

C. **If symptoms begin:** Initiate penicillin therapy immediately.

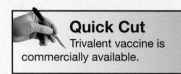

Quick Cut
Trivalent vaccine is commercially available.

Other

I. **Postoperative hemorrhage:** may result from inadequate hemostasis of the splenic pedicle or the short gastric vessels

II. **Subphrenic abscess:** usually accompanied by a left pleural effusion

III. **Thrombocytosis:** Common; if the platelet count is greater than 1 million, **antiplatelet therapy** may be considered to prevent spontaneous thrombosis.

Study Questions for Part IV

Directions: *Each of the numbered items in this section is followed by several possible answers. Select the ONE lettered answer that is BEST in each case.*

1. A 47-year-old woman presents with dysphagia to both solids and liquids equally. She has experienced a 10-kg weight loss over the last several months. A barium swallow reveals a bird's beak narrowing in the distal esophagus. What is the underlying cause of her symptoms?

   A. Disorganized, strong nonperistaltic contractions in the esophagus
   B. Failure of the lower esophageal sphincter to relax
   C. Hiatal hernia
   D. Barrett esophagus
   E. Esophageal stricture secondary to untreated gastroesophageal reflux

2. A 45-year-old male executive is seen because he is vomiting bright red blood. There are no previous symptoms. The man admits to one drink a week and has no other significant history. In the hospital, he bleeds five units of blood before endoscopy. What is the most likely diagnosis?

   A. Gastritis
   B. Duodenal ulcer
   C. Esophagitis
   D. Mallory-Weiss tear
   E. Esophageal varices

3. An 80-year-old male patient is referred for dysphagia with reflux of undigested food. The patient occasionally notices a bulging in his left neck. Which of the following is the most appropriate definitive treatment?

   A. Barium swallow
   B. Upper endoscopy
   C. Cricopharyngeal myotomy
   D. CT scan of the chest
   E. Liquid diet

4. A 42-year-old female patient is diagnosed with gastroesophageal reflux and is started on medical therapy. Which of the following would be an indication for surgical antireflux procedure?

   A. Development of esophageal stricture
   B. Barrett esophagus with severe dysplasia
   C. Esophagitis by biopsy
   D. High lower esophageal sphincter pressure demonstrated by esophageal manometry
   E. Slow and uncoordinated swallowing by barium study

5. A 75-year-old male patient presents to the emergency room 2 hours after developing severe chest pain with repeated episodes of vomiting. He is tachycardic and febrile. A chest radiograph demonstrates a left pleural effusion. Emergent barium swallow reveals extravasation of contrast into the left chest. Proper definitive treatment of this patient would include which of the following?

   A. Observation
   B. Emergent surgical intervention
   C. Placement of left chest tube
   D. Intravenous antibiotics and admission to the hospital
   E. Upper endoscopy

Questions 6–7

A 65-year-old patient has been treated with pharmacologic therapy for an antral gastric ulcer for 12 weeks. A repeat upper gastrointestinal series shows approximately 50% shrinkage of the ulcer.

6. What further management should the patient undergo at this time?

   A. Continued pharmacologic therapy with a repeat upper gastrointestinal series in 8–12 weeks
   B. A change in pharmacologic therapy with a repeat upper gastrointestinal series in 12 weeks
   C. An upper endoscopy with multiple biopsies
   D. Total gastrectomy
   E. Surgery with limited excision of the ulcer

After further diagnostic workup, the patient is found to have a gastric adenocarcinoma. Metastatic workup is negative.

7. Therapy with curative intent would involve which of the following?

   A. Radiation therapy followed by chemotherapy alone
   B. Distal gastrectomy followed by adjuvant chemoradiotherapy
   C. Total gastrectomy
   D. Total gastrectomy and splenectomy
   E. Local excision of the ulcer with clear margins followed by radiotherapy

8. Which of the following statements is true about the performance of a parietal cell vagotomy?

   A. It divides the vagus nerve at the gastroesophageal junction.
   B. It maintains innervation of the pylorus so that a drainage procedure is not required.
   C. The recurrence rate is less than 5%.
   D. It cannot be performed laparoscopically.
   E. It is contraindicated for bleeding or perforated ulcers.

9. What innervates the stomach resulting in parietal cell secretion and gastrin release?

   A. Phrenic nerve
   B. Vagus nerve
   C. Greater splanchnic nerves
   D. Celiac ganglion
   E. T4 root

10. Which of the following is true regarding intestinal absorption of nutrients?

   A. Bile or bile salts are essential for absorption of vitamin B_{12}.
   B. An iron-deficient individual can absorb up to 80% of dietary iron.
   C. Parathormone increases the intestinal absorption of dietary calcium.
   D. Intestinal epithelial cells resynthesize triglycerides before their release into the portal circulation.
   E. Triglycerides are absorbed intact in a bile salt micelle–dependent process.

Questions 11–12

A previously healthy 43-year-old man presents with a 6-month history of nonbloody diarrhea, fever, and 10-lb weight loss and now develops urosepsis. On evaluation, an enterovesical fistula (from the ileum to the bladder) is found. At laparotomy, findings include inflammation and "fat wrapping" of three separate segments of ileum. Each segment is approximately 20 cm in length and is separated by less than 20-cm segments of normal-appearing bowel (skip areas). The distal most of the three segments is more severely inflamed than the others and involves the terminal ileum all the way to the cecum. This segment of ileum is densely adherent to the right superior aspect of the bladder.

11. Which of the following is true?

  A. All of the abnormal-appearing bowel should be resected.
  B. This patient has complications of Meckel diverticulitis.
  C. All of the bladder wall involved in the inflammatory process must be removed.
  D. Extensive resection can reduce the potential for a recurrence to less than 10%.
  E. Closure of the fistula and resection of the involved bowel are preferred.

12. The patient returns to the office 3 years later complaining of abdominal pain, abdominal distention, bloating after meals, and intermittent constipation interspersed with diarrhea. He has lost 20 pounds during the last 3 months, which he ascribes to the aforementioned abdominal symptoms. An upper gastrointestinal series with a small bowel follow-through reveals one area of tight stricture in the distal small bowel. The stricture appears to be 10 cm in length. Which of the following is true?

  A. All strictures require resection; bypass of the involved segment is not an option.
  B. Postoperatively, this patient's chance of another recurrence requiring surgery is 50%.
  C. Because this patient requires surgery for the second time, his risk of cancer is extremely high, and he should have an extensive small bowel resection.
  D. Postoperative anastomotic strictures typically cause symptoms years later.
  E. Because of the patient's prior surgery, folate replacement is essential.

Questions 13–15

A 32-year-old male with long-standing Crohn disease presents with a complete obstruction of the small bowel. At laparotomy, scarring of the distal ileum and cecum cause an obstruction. A 10-cm segment of mid small bowel shows moderate nonobstructive Crohn disease.

13. Which operative procedure should be performed at this time?

  A. Radical resection of the involved segment of mid small bowel, all of the ileum, the cecum, and the right colon
  B. Resection of the distal ileum and right colon with the involved mesentery and lymph nodes
  C. Bypass of the obstructing segment with a side-to-side anastomosis between the ileum and the right colon and no resection
  D. Stricturoplasty of the obstruction plus resection of the short involved segment of mid small bowel
  E. Resection of the distal ileum and cecum

14. Postoperatively, the patient requires an indwelling bladder catheter for 5 days to treat urinary retention. He does well until the 10th postoperative day, at which point he develops a fever of 103°F, right lower quadrant (RLQ) pain, and an ileus. The midline wound is not inflamed. Which of the following is most likely to have developed?

  A. Blind loop syndrome
  B. Pyelonephritis
  C. Recurrent Crohn disease
  D. Intra-abdominal abscess
  E. Pseudomembranous enterocolitis

15. After successful surgery and discharge from the hospital, which of the following is true?

   A. If the diseased bowel is removed, therapy with prednisone and metronidazole can best prevent
   a recurrence.
   B. The chance of a cure is greater than 60%.
   C. The recurrence rate is higher than 50% during the next 5–10 years.
   D. If the terminal ileum is removed, the risk of recurrence is decreased.
   E. If the terminal ileum is removed, the patient will require long-term therapy with oral iron to
   prevent anemia.

Questions 16–17

A 63-year-old man presents with a 3-day history of increasing cramping abdominal pain, constipation,
and intermittent vomiting. He continues to pass gas. Other than the present complaints, he has been
healthy. Examination reveals a distended abdomen with high-pitched bowel sounds. No localized
tenderness is found and no rectal masses are present. The stool is heme positive.

16. Diagnostically, the first step should be to perform which of the following?

   A. Total colonoscopy
   B. Mesenteric angiography
   C. Flat plate and erect abdominal radiographs
   D. Upper gastrointestinal radiographs with small bowel follow-through
   E. Barium enema

17. Therapeutically, the first step should be which of the following?

   A. A Fleet enema, clear liquids by mouth, and careful observation
   B. Emergency colonoscopy for colonic decompression
   C. Intravenous fluids, nasogastric suction, and careful observation
   D. Colonoscopic decompression with use of a rectal tube, if necessary
   E. Immediate exploratory laparotomy

Questions 18–19

A 60-year-old patient who is finishing a course of antibiotic therapy for bacterial pneumonia develops
cramping abdominal pain and profuse watery diarrhea. A diagnosis of pseudomembranous or
antibiotic-associated colitis is suspected.

18. Which of the following is the quickest way to establish the diagnosis?

   A. Stool culture
   B. Barium enema
   C. Stool titer for *Clostridium difficile* toxin
   D. Proctoscopy
   E. Blood culture

19. What would the initial treatment involve?

   A. Metronidazole
   B. Vancomycin
   C. Imodium
   D. Cephalexin
   E. Total abdominal colectomy

20. During exploration for a transverse colon tumor, a surgeon incidentally notices a 2-cm diverticulum of the small bowel located 2 ft proximal to the ileocecal valve. Which of the following statements is **not** true?

   A. This diverticulum should be resected when found due to an associated increased risk of malignancy.
   B. This is an example of the most common type of diverticulum of the gastrointestinal tract, present in 2% of the population.
   C. It is more commonly found in men than women.
   D. When symptomatic in children, it presents as a source of bleeding.
   E. It can cause obstruction via intussusception.

21. A 55-year-old man presents with a 24-hour history of increasingly severe left lower quadrant abdominal pain. On examination, he has tenderness localized in the left lower quadrant with rebound. Fever and leukocytosis are present. The clinical suspicion of diverticulitis would best be confirmed by which of the following?

   A. Barium enema
   B. Colonoscopy
   C. CT scan of the abdomen and pelvis
   D. Magnetic resonance imaging of the abdomen and pelvis
   E. Chest radiograph

22. A 45-year-old woman with diabetes presents with a 2-day history of acute perirectal pain. On examination, a tender fluctuant mass is present to the left of the anus. What treatment should be administered at this time?

   A. Broad-spectrum antibiotic therapy
   B. Abscess drainage and excision of the fistulous tract
   C. Incision and drainage of the abscess
   D. Continued observation
   E. Treatment of Crohn disease

Questions 23–24

A 34-year-old female patient in previous good health presents in the emergency department with spontaneous intraperitoneal hemorrhage. Her only medication is an oral contraceptive that she has been taking for the past 5 years. During resuscitation, a bedside ultrasound reveals a large amount of intraperitoneal blood and a 3-cm mass in the right lobe of the liver.

23. What is the likely cause of her hemorrhage?

   A. Hepatoma
   B. Hemangioma
   C. Focal nodular hyperplasia
   D. Hepatic cell adenoma
   E. Metastatic neoplasm

The patient continues to bleed and requires transfusion.

24. What further treatment should be undertaken?

   A. Observation in the intensive care unit
   B. Right hepatic artery ligation
   C. Right hepatic lobectomy
   D. Angiographic embolization of hepatic artery
   E. CT portogram

25. A 45-year-old man presents to the emergency room with 24 hours of left lower quadrant abdominal pain. Examination reveals fever and focal tenderness in the left lower quadrant but no generalized peritoneal signs. CT scan reveals a collection containing air and fluid. Optimal management of this patient includes which of the following?

   A. Admission for intravenous antibiotics and serial abdominal exams
   B. Urgent operation with resection of diseased bowel and primary anastomosis
   C. Urgent operation with resection of diseased bowel and diverting colostomy
   D. Colonoscopy to rule out the possibility of a perforated cancer followed by CT-guided drainage
   E. CT-guided drainage followed by bowel resection once the patient has fully recovered

Questions 26–28

A 52-year-old alcoholic man with known cirrhosis presents to the emergency department with hematemesis.

26. After resuscitation and stabilization, which procedure should take place?

   A. Arteriography
   B. Upper gastrointestinal series
   C. Endoscopy
   D. Tagged red cell scan
   E. Liver biopsy

Workup reveals acutely bleeding esophageal varices.

27. What should the next treatment be?

   A. Transjugular intrahepatic portosystemic shunt
   B. Emergency portacaval shunt
   C. Splenectomy
   D. Sclerotherapy
   E. Gastroesophageal devascularization

After appropriate therapy, the bleeding ceases and the patient stabilizes. He is found to be a Child's C alcoholic cirrhotic who has been abstinent for 1 year. Evaluation for an orthotopic liver transplant has begun.

28. If his variceal bleeding recurs, it could be managed by all *except* which of the following?

   A. Portacaval shunt
   B. Mesocaval shunt
   C. Sclerotherapy
   D. Transjugular intrahepatic portosystemic shunt
   E. Selective Warren shunt

29. A 73-year-old previously healthy man presents to the emergency room with several days of jaundice followed by 12 hours of right upper quadrant pain and fever. He is mildly hypotensive. CT scan of the abdomen reveals dilatation of the biliary tree. The next step in management includes which of the following?

   A. Laparoscopic cholecystectomy
   B. Open cholecystectomy and T tube placement
   C. Open cholecystectomy and choledochojejunostomy
   D. Fluid resuscitation, antibiotics, and endoscopic retrograde cholangiopancreatography (ERCP)
   E. Fluid resuscitation and hepatitis serologies

Questions 30-31

A 33-year-old man with no significant past medical history presents to the emergency room with abdominal pain and nausea. He is afebrile, and laboratory studies reveal a serum amylase level of 1,200 U/L.

30. Which of the following would not be part of initial management?

    A. Intravenous hydration
    B. Nasogastric decompression
    C. Abdominal imaging with ultrasound and/or CT scan
    D. ERCP to evaluate pancreatic duct anatomy
    E. Intravenous narcotic pain medicine

31. Ten days into his course of pancreatitis, this patient is found to have a fluid collection measuring 4 cm in diameter near the tail of his pancreas. He had a recurrence of his abdominal pain when he was restarted on a diet 2 days prior but is otherwise asymptomatic. He remains on total parenteral nutrition. Appropriate management of this collection would include which of the following?

    A. CT-guided aspiration to assess for infection
    B. Endoscopic drainage via an ultrasound-guided cystogastrostomy
    C. Operative debridement and external drainage
    D. CT-guided percutaneous drainage
    E. Observation alone

32. A 59-year-old patient undergoes exploration for a 4-cm mass in the head of the pancreas that has caused obstructive jaundice. The patient had a biliary stent endoscopically placed prior to the procedure with complete resolution of jaundice. At the time of surgery, two small liver metastases are noted. Which of the following is not part of appropriate management at this point?

    A. Transduodenal pancreatic biopsy
    B. Hepaticojejunostomy
    C. Gastrojejunostomy
    D. Cholecystectomy
    E. Celiac ganglion nerve block

33. A 65-year-old patient presents with a history significant for obstructive jaundice and weight loss. A workup reveals a 2.5-cm mass in the head of the pancreas; needle aspiration reveals adenocarcinoma. Which of the following findings on preoperative CT scan would preclude operative exploration for curative resection?

    A. Presence of replaced right hepatic artery
    B. Loss of fat plane between tumor and portal vein
    C. Loss of fat plane between tumor and superior mesenteric artery
    D. Occlusion of gastroduodenal artery
    E. Occlusion of superior mesenteric vein

Directions: *The group of items in this section consists of lettered options followed by a set of numbered items. For each item, select the lettered option(s) that is(are) most closely associated with it. Each lettered option may be selected once, more than once, or not at all. Match the portion of the stomach, duodenum, or pancreas to the appropriate arterial supply.*

34. Body and tail of pancreas

A. Left gastric artery

35. Duodenum and head of pancreas

B. Right gastroepiploic artery

36. Proximal lesser curvature of stomach

C. Splenic artery

37. Distal greater curvature of stomach

D. Vasa brevia (short gastric arteries)

38. Fundus of stomach

E. Superior mesenteric artery

39. A 35-year-old man complains of severe heartburn. He has been on acid suppression over the counter for 5 years without relief. Endoscopy demonstrates esophagitis, and a pH study documents pathologic reflux. The best treatment for this patient is:

A. Heller myotomy
B. Proton pump inhibitor
C. Nissen fundoplication
D. Repeat endoscopy in 3 months
E. Elevation of head of bed

40. A 20-year-old healthy woman undergoes outpatient endoscopy for abdominal pain. The stomach is unremarkable on endoscopic examination. In the recovery area, she has normal vital signs and oxygen saturation levels, but she complains of severe chest pain, and there is a crunching sound on cardiac auscultation. The most likely etiology for the patient's pain is:

A. Esophageal perforation
B. Acute myocardial infarction
C. Pulmonary embolism
D. Missed peptic ulcer
E. Pneumonia

41. A 59-year-old man has upper abdominal pain, fatigue, and a 20-lb weight loss over 6 months despite eating a regular diet. Esophagogastroduodenoscopy (EGD) is performed, revealing a 4-cm proximal gastric adenocarcinoma. Positron emission tomography (PET) scan suggests bilateral lung nodules in addition to the gastric mass. The best treatment for this patient is:

A. Gastrojejunostomy
B. Gastrectomy with Roux-en-Y reconstruction
C. Palliative chemotherapy
D. Radiation to the abdomen
E. Pulmonary resection followed by total gastrectomy

42. A 60-year-old woman with infrequent medical care presents to the emergency department with diaphoresis, tachycardia, and abdominal pain. Abdominal x-ray reveals free air, and the patient is taken to the operating room. Despite fluid resuscitation, the patient remains tachycardic. A 1.5-cm ulceration with perforation is found in the distal stomach. What is the best course of action?

    A. Close the patient, and begin cyclophosphamide, hydroxydaunomycin, vincristine, and prednisone (CHOP) chemotherapy.

    B. Primary repair

    C. Selective vagotomy and antrectomy

    D. Local excision (wedge resection)

    E. Distal gastrectomy with Roux-en-Y reconstruction

43. A 49-year-old man presents with abdominal pain over the past year. He describes a burning, epigastric pain that is partially alleviated by eating. As a result, he has gained 12 lb. He has taken over-the-counter antacids with significant relief, but he reports that his symptoms are worsening. What is the best initial study for diagnosis?

    A. EGD

    B. Computerized tomography

    C. Abdominal x-ray

    D. Small bowel follow-through

    E. Magnetic resonance cholangiopancreatography

44. A 64-year-old woman presents with abdominal pain. The patient had a previous laparotomy for trauma one decade ago. She now has dull, diffuse pain, nausea, one episode of emesis, and ongoing flatus. She appears distended, with no hernias, and in no distress. Abdominal x-ray shows multiple air-fluid levels. The best treatment for this patient is:

    A. Intravenous fluids and nasogastric decompression

    B. EGD

    C. Capsule endoscopy

    D. Urgent laparotomy

    E. PET

45. A 64-year-old woman presents with abdominal pain. The patient had a previous laparotomy for Crohn disease one decade ago. She now has dull, diffuse pain, nausea, one episode of emesis, and ongoing flatus with multiple loose stools. She has a heart rate of 100 beats per minute, a systolic blood pressure of 120 mm Hg, RLQ tenderness on exam, and no distension. The best treatment for this patient is:

    A. Intravenous fluids and nasogastric decompression

    B. EGD

    C. Computerized tomography

    D. Urgent laparotomy

    E. PET

46. Small intestinal fat absorption is best characterized by:

    A. Passive absorption in the distal duodenum

    B. Active absorption in the distal duodenum

    C. Absorption by micelles in the jejunum

    D. Digestion by amylase and directly absorbed in jejunum

    E. Active transport across distal ileum as a complex

47. A 67-year-old woman undergoes screening colonoscopy and is found to have a sessile adenocarcinoma in the sigmoid colon. There is no evidence of metastatic disease on CT of the chest and abdomen. The most appropriate next step is:

A. Annual colonoscopy
B. Endoscopic polypectomy
C. FOLFOX chemotherapy
D. Segmental colectomy with lymphadenectomy
E. Abdominoperineal resection (APR)

48. A 23-year-old woman has crampy abdominal pain and a new perianal fistula. Workup should include all of the following *except*:

A. WBC count and C-reactive protein (CRP level)
B. Colonoscopy
C. Exam under anesthesia
D. Antineutrophil cytoplasmic antibody (ANCA)/anti–*Saccharomyces cerevisiae* antibody (ASCA)
E. Capsule endoscopy

49. A 45-year-old man with a penicillin allergy undergoes elective ventral hernia repair with mesh and receives clindamycin. Two days later, he develops severe stool frequency with some left-sided abdominal pain but no fever or tachycardia. The best initial treatment is:

A. Loperamide
B. Intravenous vancomycin
C. Oral metronidazole
D. Oral rifampin
E. Colectomy

50. A 34-year-old woman is involved in a minor motor vehicle collision and undergoes CT scan. There is no visceral injury, but a 1-cm mass is noted in the periphery of the right lobe of the liver. The radiologist notes that there is a central scar visible. A sulfur colloid scan shows only the appearance of normal parenchyma. The most appropriate treatment for this lesion is:

A. Observation only
B. Oral contraceptive therapy
C. Hepatic artery ligation
D. Open liver biopsy
E. Surgical excision

51. A 55-year-old woman is referred for cholecystectomy. Three years previously, she had some pain and was diagnosed with gallstones on an outpatient ultrasound but deferred operation. She now has had a history of 1 month of jaundice and right upper quadrant pain. On exam, she has normal vital signs, obvious scleral icterus, and a firm liver palpable four fingerbreadths below the costal margin. The best next step in her management is:

A. Laparoscopic cholecystectomy
B. Right upper quadrant ultrasound
C. Open cholecystectomy
D. CT scan
E. Hepatobiliary iminodiacetic acid (HIDA) scanning

52. A 40-year-old woman presents with a history of gallstones and a recent history of right upper quadrant pain after eating fatty meals. She has had dark-colored urine and some pruritus. Liver function tests demonstrate an elevated total bilirubin level of 4 mg/dL and transaminitis. The next appropriate step in her management is:

A. Laparoscopic cholecystectomy
B. ERCP
C. HIDA scanning
D. Cholecystostomy tube
E. Hepaticojejunostomy

53. A 34-year-old man without previous medical history presents with acute abdominal pain of 2 days' duration radiating to the back. On exam, he has epigastric tenderness. Laboratory exam is most significant for an elevated WBC count of 15,000/mm^3 and an amylase of 1,100 U/L. The most likely reason for his pancreatitis is:

A. Alcohol ingestion
B. Steroid use
C. Gallstones
D. Viral infection
E. Pancreas divisum

54. The same patient from question number 53 is admitted and started on intravenous fluids and antibiotics. After 24 hours, he becomes tachycardic, hypotensive, and has minimal urine output. His pain increases dramatically, with rebound tenderness on exam, and a repeat WBC count is 24,000/mm^3. The most appropriate intervention is:

A. Upper gastrointestinal series
B. EGD
C. ERCP
D. Surgical debridement
E. CT-guided biopsy

55. The most direct connection between the spleen and the stomach is via:

A. The pancreaticosplenic ligament
B. The short gastric arteries
C. The greater omentum
D. The celiac axis
E. The gastroepiploic artery

56. A 68-year-old patient has a history of splenectomy 2 years prior to presentation. The most likely indication for elective splenectomy in an adult is:

A. Primary hypersplenism
B. Hereditary spherocytosis
C. Hereditary elliptocytosis
D. Sickle cell trait
E. ITP

Answers and Explanations

1. **The answer is B** (Chapter 9, Esophageal Motility Disorders, Achalasia, II–III). This patient is presenting with classic symptoms of achalasia. The dysphagia to both solids and liquids is classic, as is the bird-beak narrowing on radiographs. The underlying defect is failure of the lower esophageal sphincter to relax, causing increased pressure in the esophagus and dysfunctional swallowing. Disorganized, strong nonperistaltic contractions in the esophagus are characteristic of diffuse esophageal spasm. Strictures typically have dysphagia to solids well before liquids cause symptoms.

2. **The answer is B** (Chapter 10, Peptic Ulcer Disease, Duodenal Ulcers, IV C 2). Massive upper gastrointestinal bleeding is usually due to a bleeding source proximal to the ligament of Treitz. The cause is most likely to be a posterior duodenal ulcer that is eroding into the gastroduodenal artery. Gastritis, esophagitis, a Mallory-Weiss tear, and esophageal varices are less likely causes of massive upper gastrointestinal bleeding.

3. **The answer is C** (Chapter 9, Esophageal Motility Disorders, Cricopharyngeal Dysfunction and Zenker Diverticulum, I B 4 a). This patient's symptoms are consistent with a Zenker diverticulum. A barium swallow would be diagnostic but not therapeutic. Endoscopy is contraindicated secondary to the risk of diverticular perforation by the endoscope. Surgical myotomy of the cricopharyngeus muscle with resection or suspension of the diverticulum is the treatment of choice. CT scan of the chest is not necessary. Changing the diet would not alter the underlying pathology.

4. **The answer is A** (Chapter 9, Esophageal Motility Disorders, Esophageal Reflux, IV C 1). Development of esophageal strictures is an indication for surgical antireflux procedures. Uncomplicated Barrett esophagus is a controversial indication for an antireflux procedure, as available studies do not agree as to whether or not surgery reverses the mucosal changes associated with Barrett esophagus. Confirmed severe dysplasia is an indication for esophagectomy, not antireflux surgery. Gastroesophageal reflux is associated with a lower esophageal sphincter pressure. Esophageal dysmotility is a contraindication to reflux surgery. Esophagitis should heal with appropriate medical management.

5. **The answer is B** (Chapter 9, Esophageal Perforation, Treatment, I–II). This patient's history, physical examination, and diagnostic studies are consistent with an acute esophageal perforation, and the situation represents a surgical emergency. Whenever possible, primary surgical repair is indicated regardless of the time since perforation. If sepsis and regional inflammation preclude primary repair, resection with cervical esophagostomy and gastrostomy and jejunostomy tube insertion should be performed. Restoration of alimentary continuity with stomach or colon can then be performed in 2–3 months.

6–7. **The answers are 6-C** (Chapter 10, Peptic Ulcer Disease, Gastric Ulcers, III C), **7-B** (Chapter 10, Gastric Cancer, Gastric Adenocarcinoma, VI B). Benign gastric ulcers should heal in 8–12 weeks with maximal medical therapy. If the ulcer does not heal completely during this time period, repeat endoscopy should be performed with biopsy. If gastric adenocarcinoma is diagnosed in this location, the optimal surgical therapy for this condition would be a distal gastrectomy with D1 (regional) lymph node dissection. More extensive surgery, such as total gastrectomy or splenectomy, would be reserved for more proximal gastric lesions. Neither radiation therapy followed by chemotherapy alone without surgery or limited surgery followed by radiotherapy is a treatment plan with curative intent.

8. **The answer is B** (Chapter 10, Peptic Ulcer Disease, Duodenal Ulcers, IV B 3). Parietal cell vagotomy, also termed *highly selective vagotomy*, maintains the nerves of Latarjet that innervate the pylorus. By dividing only the branches that innervate the parietal cells, pyloric function is preserved and outflow of the stomach is maintained. It is a technically demanding operation, in that failure to adequately sever the appropriate nerves will result in recurrences of more than 10%. However, parietal cell vagotomy can be performed for bleeding or perforated ulcers.

9. **The answer is B** (Chapter 10, Stomach, Surgical Anatomy, VI A). The vagal nerves are one of the principal stimulants of gastric acid secretion through direct stimulation of the parietal cells and via gastrin release from antral cells. Although the splanchnic and celiac ganglions are important in gastric motility and sensation, they do not stimulate acid secretion. The T4 root and phrenic nerve are not involved in gastric nervous supply.

10. **The answer is C** (Chapter 11, Introduction, Physiology, III). Both parathormone and vitamin D increase intestinal absorption of dietary calcium. Bile salts are essential for absorption of fats and fat-soluble vitamins. Vitamin B_{12} is a water-soluble vitamin that complexes with intrinsic factor, which is a protein produced by the stomach, and the protein–vitamin B_{12} complex is absorbed in the terminal ileum. The range of iron absorption is only 10%–26% of dietary iron. Triglycerides are not absorbed intact but must first be broken down into free fatty acids and monoglycerides. Once absorbed, they are resynthesized into triglycerides, but they are not released into the portal circulation. Rather, the triglycerides are packaged as chylomicrons and released into the lymphatic circulation.

11. **The answer is E** (Chapter 11, Diseases, Crohn Disease, III–IV). The diagnosis of Crohn disease is supported by the enterovesical fistula, the presence of "fat wrapping" of the bowel, inflammation, and the clinical history. To prevent ongoing contamination of the urinary tract, the fistula must be closed, and resection of the involved segment of bowel would be the standard approach. Regarding the extent of resection, the 50% risk of recurrence is not decreased by more extensive resections; thus, the less bowel removed, the better. In this case, with three widely separated segments of ileum involved, removal of all involved bowel could result in loss of more than half of the ileum and would not be advisable. Crohn disease does not directly involve the bladder and thus resection of the bladder wall is unnecessary except when needed to close the opening of the fistula. Meckel diverticulum occurs proximal to the terminal ileum; it would not affect multiple bowel segments and does not cause "fat wrapping."

12. **The answer is B** (Chapter 11, Diseases, Crohn Disease, VII). This patient presents with recurrent Crohn disease in the form of an obstruction from stricture, which is the most common manifestation that requires surgery. After surgery, the risk of recurrent manifestations of Crohn disease requiring reoperation is 50%, and the risk remains 50% after each surgical procedure. Strictures, unlike fistulas and perforations, can be treated via bypass of the involved segment of bowel, although resection is preferred except when the risk is too great. The risk of cancer is related to the chronicity of the disease and would almost never require extensive small bowel resection, which may leave the patient with short bowel syndrome (a difficult disorder to treat in this population). Postoperative anastomotic strictures cause symptoms very early postoperatively, not years later. If this patient had previously had a resection of the terminal ileum, he would develop a deficiency of vitamin B_{12}, not folate.

13–15. **The answers are 13-E** (Chapter 11, Diseases, Crohn Disease, VI), **14-D** (Chapter 11, Diseases, Crohn Disease, VI C), **15-C** (Chapter 11, Diseases, Crohn Disease, VII). When surgery is necessary to treat complications of Crohn disease, the operations are "conservative," as defined by the length of the resection. Therefore, when an obstructive lesion is present, only a short length of bowel needs to be resected. In the case described, the distal ileum and cecum should be removed. Radical resections are not necessary, as they do not reduce the risk of recurrence and may ultimately contribute to short bowel syndrome if several resections are required over long periods. In addition, resection of mesentery and lymph nodes (e.g., for a cancer operation) is unnecessary. Bypass procedures without resection are reserved for only the most difficult cases where resection cannot be undertaken safely. A stricturoplasty is appropriate occasionally for short symptomatic strictures in the small bowel only.

    The second postoperative week is the usual time for the development of serious complications, such as abdominal wound dehiscence, intestinal anastomotic breakdown, and intraperitoneal abscess. Blind loop syndrome occurs rarely, and although it does cause pain and diarrhea, it does not cause fever and ileus. Pyelonephritis usually causes flank pain and pyuria. Crohn disease does not recur immediately or cause the signs unless complications have occurred. Pseudomembranous enterocolitis causes tenderness over the transverse colon and occasionally over the descending colon, with diarrhea. Of the choices listed, an intra-abdominal abscess is the most likely diagnosis.

The prognosis of Crohn disease, which requires surgery, is not good because 50% of patients require additional surgical procedures within 5 years of the first operation. Therefore, the chance of cure is less than 50%. Medical therapy (including anti-inflammatory agents and antibiotic drugs) has not proved effective for preventing recurrence of the disease. Removal of the terminal ileum has no effect on disease recurrence or iron absorption; however, the absorption of vitamin B_{12} is significantly impaired.

16–17. The answers are 16-C (Chapter 11, Diseases, Small Bowel Obstruction, III B), **17-C** (Chapter 11, Diseases, Small Bowel Obstruction, IV). Flat plate and erect radiographs of the abdomen should be performed first. Further studies may be needed based on the results of this initial survey. As with all bowel obstructions, the initial treatment involves nasogastric suction, intravenous fluids, and resuscitation with careful attention to correcting metabolic and electrolyte abnormalities. Once a patient has been adequately resuscitated, the decision to either observe carefully or intervene operatively can be made.

18–19. The answers are 18-D (Chapter 12, Pseudomembranous Colitis [Antibiotic-Assisted Colitis], Diagnosis, II–III), **19-A** (Chapter 12, Pseudomembranous Colitis [Antibiotic-Assisted Colitis], Treatment, II). Crampy abdominal pain and diarrhea after a course of antibiotic therapy is highly suggestive of antibiotic-associated or pseudomembranous colitis. Diagnosis can be made either by proctoscopy, which demonstrates pseudomembranes, or by stool titer for *Clostridium difficile* toxin. Proctoscopy establishes the diagnosis immediately. Barium enema is contraindicated. The antibiotics should be stopped, and the patient should be started on metronidazole. Oral vancomycin is also effective, but it is more expensive. Colectomy is rarely required only in severe cases.

20. The answer is A (Chapter 11, Diseases, Diverticular Disease, III E). Meckel diverticulum is the most common diverticulum of the gastrointestinal tract and goes by the rule of 2's: 2 ft from ileocecal valve, 2% incidence, 2 cm long, and 2:1 male to female ratio. They can cause bleeding due to heterotropic gastric mucosa as well as intussusception and obstruction. An asymptomatic Meckel diverticulum should not be resected.

21. The answer is C (Chapter 12, Diverticular Disease, Diverticulitis, III). CT scan of the abdomen and pelvis is the most helpful test to confirm the suspected diagnosis of diverticulitis. Free air is detected on the chest radiograph in less than 3% of patients with diverticulitis. Contrast enema should generally be avoided in the initial stages of diverticulitis. Colonoscopy to exclude a sigmoid cancer may be of value after the condition of the patient has stabilized.

22. The answer is C (Chapter 12, Benign Anorectal Disease, Anorectal Abscess and Fistula, III). This patient presents with a classic history and physical findings of perirectal abscess. Antibiotic therapy will not cure an abscess. Definitive drainage is required. This therapy will be curative in approximately 50% of the patients, and the remainder will develop a fistula. However, the physician should deal with the abscess itself at the initial presentation. Attempts to definitely address any fistula tract at initial presentation is not recommended due to potential complications such as injury to the sphincter muscles and difficulties with continence.

23–24. The answers are 23-D (Chapter 13, Hepatic Tumors, Benign Tumors, II A), **24-D** (Chapter 13, Hepatic Tumors, Benign Tumors, II C). Although many liver tumors undergo spontaneous hemorrhage, this condition occurs most frequently with hepatic cell adenomas. Up to 30% of patients present with spontaneous rupture into the peritoneal cavity as their initial finding.

When the patient continues to bleed, emergency liver resection after an acute rupture would be associated with high morbidity and mortality. Although hepatic artery ligation may control the bleeding, this can probably be accomplished less invasively by radiologic embolization. Once the bleeding is controlled and the patient recovers, elective resection should be undertaken to avoid future hemorrhage.

25. The answer is E (Chapter 12, Diverticular Disease, Diverticulitis, V B 2). Cases of diverticulitis complicated by perforation and abscess formation are best managed by percutaneous drainage in the absence of evidence of diffuse peritonitis. Young patients (typically considered as being younger than 50 years of age) with a single severe case such as this should be considered for an interval resection of the diseased section of bowel because of the very high risk of subsequent severe episodes. Older patients are often referred after a second episode. Colonoscopy should not be routinely performed during the acute phase of an episode of diverticulitis but should be performed prior on an interval basis. Operative intervention during the acute phase is reserved for cases that either present with diffuse peritonitis, perforation, or continued worsening of the clinical picture in spite of appropriate nonoperative therapy. Primary anastomosis is typically avoided in the setting of severe infection and contamination.

26–28. **The answers are 26-C** (Chapter 13, Hepatic Abscesses and Cysts, Portal Hypertension, VI A), **27-D** (Chapter 13, Hepatic Abscesses and Cysts, Portal Hypertension, VI B), **28-A** (Chapter 13, Hepatic Abscesses and Cysts, Portal Hypertension, VII). Acute variceal bleeding commonly occurs because of portal hypertension from underlying cirrhosis. Other causes of upper gastrointestinal bleeding that must also be considered in these patients include gastritis and peptic ulcer disease. Upper gastrointestinal endoscopy is the most rapid way of making the diagnosis of the site and identifying the cause of upper gastrointestinal bleeding. Once the diagnosis has been made, sclerotherapy is the preferred method of managing acute variceal bleeding. It is successful in 90% of patients.

Portacaval shunt, mesocaval shunt, sclerotherapy, transjugular intrahepatic portosystemic shunt, and selective Warren shunt for recurrent bleeding would potentially be successful in preventing long-term hemorrhage. However, portacaval shunt would make a subsequent liver transplant extremely difficult and hazardous.

29. **The answer is D** (Chapter 13, Biliary Tree Pathology, Cholangitis, II). Cholangitis is a potentially life-threatening disease. This patient is present with Charcot triad of pain, fever, and jaundice.

30–31. **The answers are 30-D** (Chapter 14, Pancreatitis, Acute Pancreatitis, III D 8), **31-E** (Chapter 14, Pseudocyst, II A, IV). Uncomplicated acute pancreatitis is best managed conservatively with nasogastric decompression, intravenous hydration, bowel rest, and pain medicine. Imaging with ultrasound, CT scan, magnetic resonance imaging, or magnetic resonance cholangiopancreatography can be useful in establishing a possible etiology (gallstones) or detecting complications. ERCP should not be used routinely during the acute presentation due to the risk of ERCP-associated pancreatitis complicating the acute situation. ERCP should be reserved for specific cases where there is evidence of biliary obstruction. Evaluation of pancreatic duct anatomy can be helpful on an interval basis to help assess causes of chronic or recurrent pancreatitis.

32. **The answer is A** (Chapter 14, Pancreatic Malignancies, Pancreatic Adenocarcinoma, IV D, E). When patients are unresectable due to distant metastases at the time of surgery, a surgeon must accomplish several things. A biliary bypass (hepaticojejunostomy) palliates the obstructive jaundice, and a cholecystectomy is performed in conjunction with this. A gastric bypass (gastrojejunostomy) prevents the gastric outlet obstruction observed in 19% of unresected periampullary cancer patients. A celiac axis nerve block has been shown to significantly reduce cancer-related pain. A surgeon must also make a tissue diagnosis, in this case by taking a biopsy of one of the liver metastases. An additional pancreatic biopsy is unnecessary and adds additional risks.

33. **The answer is E** (Chapter 14, Pancreatic Malignancies, Pancreatic Adenocarcinoma, IV A 1). Findings that determine unresectability on preoperative CT scan include encasement of the superior mesenteric artery or proximal celiac axis and occlusion of the superior mesenteric vein or portal vein. Tumor abutting these vessels but not encasing or occluding them is not a contraindication to resection. The gastroduodenal artery is ligated during a pancreaticoduodenectomy, thus its occlusion does not preclude resection. A replaced right hepatic artery is not uncommon and must be preserved. This does not, however, preclude resection.

34–38. **The answers are 34-C, 35-E, 36-A, 37-B, and 38-D** (Chapter 10, Stomach, Surgical Anatomy, IV, and Chapter 14, Anatomy and Physiology, Vasculature, II, III). The blood supply of the viscera is important in gastrointestinal surgery. Three of the four main arteries can be sacrificed, and blood flow to the stomach will still be preserved through collateral circulation. The proximal lesser curvature is supplied by the left gastric artery (arising from the celiac axis). The right gastric artery (arising from the common hepatic artery) supplies the distal lesser curvature. The left and right gastroepiploic arteries supply the proximal and distal greater curvature, respectively. The duodenum and head of the pancreas are supplied by the superior and inferior pancreaticoduodenal arteries that arise from the gastroduodenal and superior mesenteric arteries, respectively. The body and tail of the pancreas are supplied by branches of the splenic artery.

39. **The answer is C** (Chapter 9, Esophageal Motility Disorders, Esophageal Reflux, IV C 2 a). The patient is a candidate for surgical antireflux therapy, having documented reflux and having failed a trial of medical therapy. Heller myotomy is the appropriate surgery for achalasia. Elevating the head of bed is an antireflux measure but unlikely to provide the patient with significant relief.

40. **The answer is A** (Chapter 9, Esophageal Perforation, Etiology, Diagnosis). The most common cause of esophageal perforation is instrumentation (endoscopy). The crunching sound is the result of mediastinal air. Myocardial infarction is unlikely in a young patient, and pulmonary embolism is not consistent with her normal saturation. Peptic ulcer does not typically cause acute chest pain, and pneumonia, although possible, should be more evident by other physical signs.

41. **The answer is C** (Chapter 10, Gastric Cancer, Gastric Adenocarcinoma, VI C). The patient presents with metastatic disease, and the best option is palliative chemotherapy. Bypass, such as gastrojejunostomy, may be used in cases of unresectable obstruction. Gastrectomy may be used for earlier stage tumors, and aggressive therapy such as total gastrectomy has not increased survival. Radiation therapy is not effective in the treatment of gastric cancer.

42. **The answer is D** (Chapter 10, Peptic Ulcer Disease, Gastric Ulcers, VI C). The patient remains hemodynamically compromised, so the procedure of choice is wedge resection and not definitive ulcer procedures involving formal resection. The ulcer specimen can be examined for evidence of malignancy. CHOP chemotherapy is reserved for cases of gastric lymphoma and not used in the setting of acute perforation. Primary repair, or suture closure, does not address the question of malignancy.

43. **The answer is A** (Chapter 10, Peptic Ulcer Disease, Gastric Ulcers, III). The patient has signs and symptoms of ulcer disease. The most sensitive test for ulcer symptoms is EGD. CT is unlikely to provide information on luminal disease. Abdominal x-ray is useful for perforation but unlikely to have findings in uncomplicated cases. Small bowel follow-through assesses the small bowel, although an upper gastrointestinal series with barium may identify stomach ulceration. Magnetic resonance cholangiopancreatography is a reasonable test for hepatobiliary disease but has no role in ulcer patients.

44. **The answer is A** (Chapter 11, Diseases, Small Bowel Obstruction, IV B). The patient has signs and symptoms of a partial small bowel obstruction, likely due to adhesions from his previous surgery. Initial management consists of supportive care, with intravenous fluids for volume resuscitation, correction of electrolyte imbalances, and placement of a nasogastric tube for decompression. EGD will be nondiagnostic for most of the small bowel. Capsule endoscopy provides a glimpse of the mucosa and is most useful in identifying mass lesions. Laparotomy may be indicated if the patient progresses to a complete bowel obstruction. PET scans identify areas of increased metabolic uptake (tumor).

45. **The answer is C** (Chapter 11, Diseases, Crohn Disease, III). The patient has the hallmarks of a flare of Crohn disease. The most appropriate means of diagnosis would be CT scanning, then treatment with anti-inflammatory medicines. Intravenous fluids are rarely contra-indicated, but the patient does not have obstruction or ileus that would warrant nasogastric tube placement. EGD would not be useful in small bowel diagnosis in this instance. Laparotomy would be overly aggressive and may not help the patient. PET is most useful in detecting malignancy, which is not a primary concern in this case.

46. **The answer is C** (Chapter 11, Introduction, Physiology, III C). Fat is processed in micelles to be absorbed in the intestine. Carbohydrate is digested by amylase and absorbed directly. B12 is actively transported in the terminal ileum as a complex with intrinsic factor.

47. **The answer is D** (Chapter 12, Benign and Malignant Colorectal Tumors, Colorectal Carcinoma, VII). The patient has a known malignancy, and in this case, the primary treatment is surgical. Annual surveillance may be employed in the postoperative setting. Chemotherapy may be used for advanced-stage disease. APR is the technique of choice for low rectal tumors only.

48. **The answer is E** (Chapter 12, Inflammatory Bowel Disease, Ulcerative Colitis, VII). The patient may have inflammatory bowel disease, worked up with markers of inflammation (WBC, CRP, erythrocyte sedimentation rate), antibodies (ANCA/ASCA), and colonoscopy. Capsule endoscopy is used to assess the lumen of the small bowel and may be indicated but not as part of the initial workup.

49. **The answer is C** (Chapter 12, Pseudomembranous Colitis [Antibiotic-Assisted Colitis], Pathogenesis and Presentation, II). The patient has antibiotic-associated colitis. The most likely offending organism is *Clostridium difficile*. Antidiarrheal agents such as loperamide (Imodium) are contraindicated. Intravenous vancomycin is not effective, and rifampin may be used only rarely in some refractory cases. Colectomy is reasonable in cases of megacolon, but antibiotic therapy should be attempted first.

50. **The answer is A** (Chapter 13, Hepatic Tumors, Benign Tumors, III). The patient presents with the characteristic findings of focal nodular hyperplasia. It is an incidental finding, with no specific treatment required for small lesions, as spontaneous rupture is rare. There is an association with oral contraceptives, so they should be avoided. Hepatic artery ligation is a useful technique in cases of rupture only. Surgical excision is reserved for larger or symptomatic lesions.

51. **The answer is D** (Chapter 13, Biliary Tree Pathology, III). The patient requires more diagnostic workup prior to undertaking operation. The jaundice, palpable liver, and pain is suggestive of an obstructed biliary tree. CT scan is the most appropriate among the listed choices, as it would demonstrate an anatomic cause, although MRI or ERCP would be appropriate as well. Right upper quadrant ultrasound may demonstrate ductal dilatation but will not provide sufficient information for definitive diagnosis. HIDA is most useful for cholecystitis. Cholecystectomy may be indicated, but a mass lesion should be ruled out first.

52. **The answer is B** (Chapter 13, Biliary Tree Pathology, Choledocholithiasis, IV). The patient is demonstrating evidence of choledocholithiasis. ERCP offers the best anatomic information confirming the presence of stones and the ability to alleviate the obstruction through sphincterotomy. Laparoscopic cholecystectomy is an option but unlikely to address her main symptoms and relatively contraindicated without further intervention. HIDA scanning is unlikely to offer any relevant information beyond confirming obstruction of the biliary tree. A cholecystostomy tube will also alleviate obstruction but is generally reserved for those with cholangitis who are too ill to tolerate more invasive procedures. The hepaticojejunostomy is an effective means of biliary bypass but only in the circumstance of benign biliary stricture rather than stone disease.

53. **The answer is C** (Chapter 14, Pancreatitis, Etiology, I). Gallstones represent the single most important cause of pancreatitis. Alcohol use is another prime etiology but is less likely given the rise in amylase. Steroids cause pancreatitis uncommonly, and this patient has not report its use. Viral infection is less likely without a prodrome. Pancreas divisum is a rare, congenital cause.

54. **The answer is D** (Chapter 14, Pancreatitis, Acute Pancreatitis, V F). This patient presents as shock, likely due to infected pancreatitis or pancreatic necrosis. The patient is likely to deteriorate without prompt debridement. Upper gastrointestinal would be nondiagnostic as would EGD. ERCP is contraindicated, as it is likely to worsen the acute process. Biopsy is reasonable, but given the acute decompensation, surgical debridement is preferred.

55. **The answer is B** (Chapter 15, Introduction, Anatomy, II B). The short gastric arteries arise from the spleen. They serve an important anastomotic network in cases of portal vein thrombosis when they may lead to gastric varices. The gastrosplenic ligament is an important contributor to splenic stabilization; there is no pancreaticosplenic ligament.

56. **The answer is E** (Chapter 15, Pathology, Causes of Secondary Hypersplenism, VIII). Hereditary spherocytosis and hereditary elliptocytosis are indications for splenectomy but very uncommon. Sickle cell disease, not trait, may be an indication if splenomegaly is present. Primary hypersplenism is an indication for splenectomy but exceedingly rare.

Part V

Breast and Endocrine Disorders

Chapter Cuts and Caveats

CHAPTER 16

Breast:

◆ Because breast cancer is so common, self-examinations and screening mammography are important elements for early detection. Screening mammography reduces breast cancer mortality.

◆ A strong family history of breast cancer (multiple family members) or diagnosis at a young age may be associated with genetic mutations including BRCA1 and BRCA2. The presence of these mutations may affect the treatment choices made by the patient.

◆ If a breast biopsy is negative, it is imperative to confirm that the correct lesion was biopsied. This can be accomplished by physical exam, specimen radiography, intraoperative US, or postoperative radiologic evaluation if necessary.

◆ In lesions diagnosed as ductal carcinoma in situ, 10%–20% have an infiltrative component at excision.

◆ Lobular carcinoma in situ confers an increased risk of breast cancer in both breasts.

◆ Survival rates are the same for patients treated with aggressive resection (mastectomy) versus breast conservation (lumpectomy and radiation).

◆ Tumors often drain to particular nodes first, called the *sentinel nodes*. In breast cancer, this is most commonly in the axilla and can be detected by the injection of dye or radiotracer into the lymphatics. If this node is negative for tumor, then the remaining axillary nodes are negative. This technique has saved many patients the morbidity of an axillary lymph node dissection.

◆ Local advanced breast cancer and inflammatory breast cancer requires multimodal therapy including induction chemotherapy, surgical resection, and postoperative radiation therapy.

◆ Nipple discharge is considered concerning if unilateral, bloody, or spontaneous. The most common cause is intraductal papilloma, and the treatment is excision.

CHAPTER 17

Thyroid, Parathyroid, Adrenal Glands, and Thymus:

◆ The first steps of diagnosis of a thyroid nodule include a thorough history, exam for nodes and vocal cord function, FNA, and neck ultrasound.

◆ FNA is the diagnostic method of choice for most thyroid nodules.

◆ The most feared complication of thyroid surgery is injury to the recurrent laryngeal nerve. Compromise of bilateral recurrent laryngeal nerves leads to a loss of the airway.

- Follicular thyroid carcinoma spreads through vessels, is associated with systemic metastasis, and is often treated with lobectomy and isthmusectomy.
- Papillary carcinoma is the most common thyroid cancer and has a high cure rate.
- Papillary and medullary carcinomas are multicentric, spread to regional lymph nodes, and are treated with total thyroidectomy.
- PTH is a major regulator of calcium.
- Primary hyperparathyroidism is due to adenoma and should be treated for symptomatic patients and asymptomatic patients with a serum calcium greater than 11.5 mg/dL.
- Secondary hyperparathyroidism is associated with renal failure, is due to four-gland hyperplasia, and is associated with a low serum calcium.
- Adrenal masses should be removed when large (>5 cm) or when biologically active.
- Pheochromocytoma is the major tumor of the adrenal medulla; always treat with alpha blockade before surgical intervention.
- MEN syndromes arise from a genetic defect and produce lesions in the thyroid, parathyroid, pancreas, or pituitary.
- Thymectomy may improve symptoms in patients with myasthenia gravis.

Chapter 16

Breast

Emily Bellavance, Steven Feigenberg, and Jessica Joines

INTRODUCTION

Anatomy

I. **Borders:** Figure 16-1
   A. **Superior border:** clavicle
   B. **Medial border:** lateral border of the sternum
   C. **Inferior border:** inframammary fold/sixth rib
   D. **Lateral border:** latissimus dorsi
   E. **Posterior border:** pectoralis major

II. **Vasculature:** Because the breast is well-vascularized, the breast surgeon needs to be aware of a number of important vessels.
   A. **Arterial supply**
      1. **Axillary artery**
         a. **Thoracoacromial artery**
         b. **Lateral thoracic artery**
      2. **Internal mammary artery**
         a. **Anterior intercostal perforators**
   B. **Venous return**
      1. **Axillary vein (primary)**
      2. **Posterior intercostal veins**
      3. **Internal mammary veins**
   C. **Lymphatic drainage:** follows venous drainage (Fig. 16-2)
      1. **Axillary chain:** divided into three levels in relation to the pectoralis minor muscle
      2. **Rotter nodes:** between pectoralis major and minor muscles
      3. **Internal mammary chain:** follows the internal mammary vessels and provides medial drainage

BREAST EVALUATION

Physical Examination

I. **Visual inspection:** Patient sits, raises arms upward, and then presses on hips to contract the pectoralis major muscle.
   A. **Symmetry and nipple retraction:** should be seen
   B. **Skin changes:** Observe color, texture, dimpling, edema (peau d'orange), and ulceration (visible tumor).

II. **Palpation:** With patient in supine position with ipsilateral arm above head, palpate for masses or asymmetric densities.
   A. **Nipple discharge:** elicited with pressure on the offending duct; may also be spontaneous
   B. **Nodes:** Examine axillary, cervical, internal mammary, and supraclavicular nodal basins.

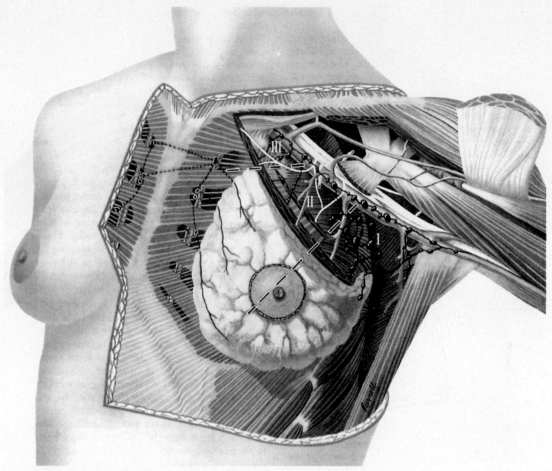

Figure 16-1: Anatomy of the breast. The dashed line represents the pectoralis minor muscle. I, II, and III represent the levels of lymph nodes. (Modified from Harris JR, Lippman ME, Morrow M, et al. *Diseases of the Breast*, 2nd ed. Philadelphia: Lippincott Williams & Wilkins; 2000.)

Radiologic Exam

I. **Mammogram:** Table 16-1

   A. **Baseline mammogram:** starting at age 40 years

   B. **High-risk patients:** start screening at earlier age

   C. **Mammography:** shows breast architecture, asymmetry, skin thickening, irregular masses, and microcalcifications

II. **Ultrasound:** Not recommended for routine screening; axillary ultrasound is useful in assessing lymph nodes.

III. **Magnetic resonance imaging (MRI):** very sensitive but not a specific evaluation of the breast; can detect the extent of tumor within the breast or lymph node basins and residual tumor after lumpectomy or systemic therapy

Biopsy

I. **Needle biopsy**

   A. **Fine-needle aspiration (FNA):** limited use for breast lesions detected on exam or imaging; axillary node biopsy in cancer patients

   B. **Core-needle biopsy:** preferable for breast lesions (Table 16-2)

      1. **Stereotactic biopsy:** uses mammographic equipment to deploy a core needle into mammographic abnormalities

      2. **Ultrasound-guided biopsy:** uses ultrasound to identify lesion and deploy core needle in ultrasound-detected abnormalities

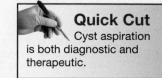
Quick Cut
Breast biopsy is necessary for diagnosis of palpable or image-detected abnormalities.

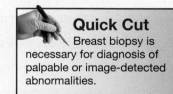
Quick Cut
Cyst aspiration is both diagnostic and therapeutic.

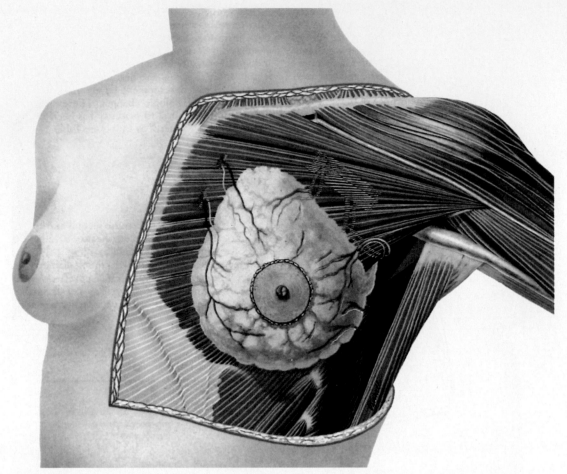

Figure 16-2: The arterial supply may arise from axillay, subclavian, and internal mammary origin. Veins also drain into both axillary and internal mammary systems. Lymphatics (not shown) loosely follow the venous pathways. (Modified from Harris JR, Lippman ME, Morrow M, et al. *Diseases of the Breast*, 2nd ed. Philadelphia: Lippincott Williams & Wilkins; 2000.)

II. **Surgical biopsy (excisional biopsy):** completely removes the lesion
   A. **Excisional biopsy after benign needle biopsy:** See Table 16-2.
   B. **Needle-localized excisional biopsy:** excisional biopsy after the radiologist places a localizing wire in the breast to identify the site

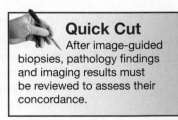

Quick Cut
After image-guided biopsies, pathology findings and imaging results must be reviewed to assess their concordance.

Table 16-1: Indications for Excision Following Core Needle Biopsy

Failure to sample calcifications
Diagnosis of atypical ductal hyperplasia
Diagnosis of atypical lobular hyperplasia or lobular carcinoma in situ*
Lack of concordance between imaging findings and histologic diagnosis
Radial scar (a proliferative breast lesion not related to surgery)
Papillary lesions
Flat epithelial atypia

*Surgical excision for atypical lobular hyperplasia and lobular carcinoma in situ is controversial.
From DeVita VT, Lawrence TS, Rosenberg SA. *Cancer: Principles and Practice of Oncology*, Vol 1. 8th ed. Philadelphia: Lippincott Williams & Wilkins; 2005.

Table 16-2: Indications for Surgical Biopsy after Core-Needle Biopsy

Woman's Risk Level	Mammography	MRI*
Normal	Annual starting at age 40 years	
LCIS, ADH, ALH	Annual after diagnosis	
Personal history of breast cancer	Annual after diagnosis	
BRCA+; multiple first-degree, second-degree relatives; bilateral in first-degree premenopausal relative; breast/ovarian cancer family history	Annual starting at 10 years younger than youngest relative but not younger than age 25 years	Annual
Hodgkin lymphoma treated with mantle radiation	Annual starting 8 years after treatment	Annual

*MRI and mammogram should be scheduled 6 months apart to screen patients twice yearly because cancers in these patients may be rapidly growing.
MRI, magnetic resonance imaging, LCIS, lobular carcinoma in situ; ADH, atypical ductal hyperplasia; ALH, atypical lobular hyperplasia.
From DeVita VT, Lawrence TS, Rosenberg SA. *Cancer: Principles and Practice of Oncology*, Vol 1. 8th ed. Philadelphia, PA: Lippincott Williams & Wilkins; 2005.

BENIGN BREAST DISEASE

Infectious and Inflammatory Breast Diseases
I. **Cellulitis and mastitis:** Infection of the breast is usually associated with lactation.
   A. **Bacteria (*Staphylococcus* or *Streptococcus*):** enter via the nipple
   B. **Treatment:** 10–14-day course of antibiotics and improvements of breastfeeding technique. Lesions that do not resolve require further workup for abscess or inflammatory malignancy.

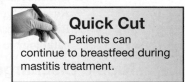
Quick Cut
Patients can continue to breastfeed during mastitis treatment.

II. **Abscess:** collection of purulent fluid within breast parenchyma treated by surgical drainage or aspiration with a course of antibiotics

III. **Chronic subareolar abscess:** A sinus tract develops from the lactiferous duct to the areola.
   A. **Treatment:** requires complete excision of the sinus tract
   B. **Recurrence:** common

IV. **Mondor disease:** phlebitis of the thoracoepigastric vein
   A. **Etiology:** Palpable, tender cord runs along the upper quadrants of the breast along the course of the vein.
   B. **Treatment:** self-limited course, so treatment is nonsteroidal anti-inflammatory drugs (NSAIDs) and warm compresses

Benign Lesions
I. **Fibrocystic changes:** Benign nodularity with or without pain. Any dominant masses should be evaluated with imaging.

II. **Fibroadenoma:** benign tumor of the breast with fibrous stromal tissue with an epithelial component; most common in younger women

III. **Phyllodes tumors:** fibroepithelial breast tumors with more connective tissue abnormalities than fibroadenoma
   A. **Malignancy:** rare; related to number of mitoses per high-power field
   B. **Treatment:** wide local excision or mastectomy
   C. **Sclerosing adenosis:** proliferation of acini in the lobules, which may appear to have invaded the surrounding breast stroma
   D. **Fat necrosis:** associated with trauma or radiation therapy to the breast but may simulate cancer with a mass or skin retraction
   E. **Mammary duct ectasia:** dilatation of the subareolar ducts, which may fill with cellular debris; may present as palpable retroareolar mass or nipple discharge

Quick Cut
Needle aspiration is performed for large symptomatic cysts.

F. **Cysts:** diagnosis made by ultrasound
1. **Color**
a. **Simple cyst:** clear or green fluid and is benign
b. **Galactocele:** milk-filled, benign cyst
c. **Bloody cyst:** may represent atypia or malignancy
2. **Cyst resolution**
a. **Complete resolution:** Perform follow-up ultrasound.
b. **Incomplete resolution:** Treat as a breast mass and excise.
G. **High-risk lesions:** confer an increased risk of breast cancer
1. **Atypical ductal hyperplasia (ADH):** epithelial proliferative lesion of duct
2. **Lobular neoplasia**
a. **Atypical lobular hyperplasia (ALH)**
(1) **Extent:** epithelial proliferative lesion in less than one half of lobular acini
(2) **Risk of upgraded pathology on excision:** 1%–20%
b. **Lobular carcinoma in situ (LCIS)**
(1) **Extent:** epithelial proliferative lesion in greater than or equal to one half of lobular acini
(2) **Risk of upgraded pathology on excision:** 4%–25%
(3) **Prevention:** Tamoxifen can reduce risk of breast cancer by ~50%. Postmenopausal women with LCIS can decrease risk of breast cancer with raloxifene.
3. **Flat epithelial atypia:** Columnar cell lesion in terminal duct lobular units; risk of cancer on excision is **10%–15%**.
4. **Intraductal papilloma:** Polyp of the breast duct; risk of adjacent atypia or malignancy on excision is **10%**.
5. **Radial scar:** Complex sclerosing lesion; risk of upgraded pathology to cancer on excision is **8%–30%**.

 Quick Cut
Tamoxifen for 5 years can reduce the risk of developing breast cancer by 86% in patients with ADH.

Nipple Discharge

I. **Features:** Usually a benign condition secondary to fibrocystic change or papilloma; benign discharge is bilateral with clear, green, or white fluid that occurs with breast stimulation/palpation.

II. **Evaluation and treatment:** Mammogram and ultrasound rule out an associated mass; drainage from an isolated nipple duct should be excised.

Quick Cut
Surgical excision is recommended for ADH, flat epithelial atypia, intraductal papilloma, and radial scar.

Quick Cut
Discharge is suspicious for intraductal papilloma if it is unilateral, bloody, or spontaneous.

Mastalgia

I. **Cyclic pain:** Correlates with the menstrual cycle; treatment includes supportive bra and analgesics.

II. **Noncyclic pain**
A. **Treatment:** Restrict caffeine intake; wear a supportive bra; and take NSAIDs, vitamin E (400 IU/day), and tamoxifen or danazol (for severe cases).
B. **Cancer:** Must be excluded as a cause of pain. All patients should have a thorough exam and mammogram. Ultrasound is indicated for focal pain.

 # MALIGNANT DISEASES

Epidemiology and Risk Factors

I. **Epidemiology:** A woman has a one in eight chance of developing breast cancer.
A. **Incidence:** In 2013, ~240,000 women were diagnosed with breast cancer in the US, and ~40,000 women died of breast cancer.
B. **Mortality rate:** decreased significantly in the last two decades due to earlier detection and improvements in treatment

II. **Risk factors:** Table 16-3
A. **Family history:** produces a threefold higher risk
1. **First-degree relatives (i.e., mother, daughter, sister):** Are affected. Risk is higher if the relative is premenopausal.

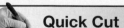 **Quick Cut**
Female gender and increased age are the strongest risk factors for breast cancer.

Table 16-3: Risk Factors for the Development of Breast Cancer

Nonmodifiable Risk Factor	Modifiable Risk Factor
Female sex	Obesity
Age	Alcohol consumption
Family history	Age of parity
High-risk breast lesions	Sedentary life style
Chest wall radiation	Exogenous estrogen
Early menarche	Smoking
High breast density	
Inherited mutation	

2. **Hereditary breast and ovarian cancer:** Breast cancer gene (BRCA) has two forms.
   a. **BRCA-1:** 60%–80% lifetime risk of breast cancer; 40% risk of ovarian cancer
   b. **BRCA-2:** 40%–80% lifetime risk of breast cancer; 10%–20% risk of ovarian cancer

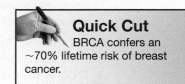

Quick Cut
BRCA confers an ~70% lifetime risk of breast cancer.

B. **Reproductive factors:** early menarche, nulliparity, age of first childbirth older than 30 years, late menopause
C. **Exogenous estrogen:** has been shown to increase the risk of breast cancer in postmenopausal women
D. **Risk estimation: Modified Gail model** is the most commonly used statistical model to estimate breast cancer risk; it accounts for risk related to age, age of menarche, age of parity, history of prior breast biopsies, family history in a first-degree relative, and ethnicity. Other models may be used based on patient's personal and family history.

Risk Reduction with Medication (Chemoprophylaxis)

I. **Selective estrogen receptor modulators (SERMs)**
   A. **Tamoxifen:** estrogen receptor agonist/antagonist that blocks estrogen receptors in the breast and stimulates receptors in uterus, liver, and vagina
      1. **Risk reduction:** ~50% in eligible patients; greater than 80% in ADH patients
      2. **Side effects:** vasomotor symptoms (hot flashes, night sweats), increased risk of endometrial cancer, and thromboembolic events
   B. **Raloxifene:** reduces risk in eligible **postmenopausal** women, similar to tamoxifen but with fewer side effects

Quick Cut
SERMs or AIs can be used to reduce a woman's risk of breast cancer. Eligible women have a greater than 1.7% 5-year risk of breast cancer by Gail model; or history of LCIS.

II. **Aromatase inhibitors (AIs):** block the enzyme that converts androgens to estrogen and are therefore effective in **postmenopausal women** in whom estrogen is derived from androgen conversion rather than from ovaries
   A. **Exemestane:** can decrease risk in eligible postmenopausal women by ~60%
   B. **Adverse effects:** osteoporosis, arthralgia, hot flashes, and night sweats

Breast Cancer Symptoms

I. **Early cancers:** often asymptomatic
II. **Breast mass**
III. **Pain:** rarely a symptom but should be completely evaluated to eliminate the possibility of a malignancy
IV. **Metastatic disease:** may also be the initial symptom
   A. **Axillary nodes:** Two percent of patients present with axillary nodes but no identifiable primary breast tumor. If the results of

Quick Cut
A breast mass is one of the more common presenting symptoms of breast cancer, but it is a late finding.

all studies are negative, treatment is modified radical mastectomy or whole breast radiation with axillary dissection.
B. **Distant organ metastasis:** to the bone, brain, liver, or lungs may cause presenting symptoms

Noninvasive Breast Cancers

I. **Ductal carcinoma in situ (DCIS):** Confined to ductal cells; no invasion of the underlying basement membrane occurs. Treatment options follow.

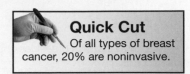

Quick Cut
Of all types of breast cancer, 20% are noninvasive.

A. **Partial mastectomy:** excision with clear margins
   1. **Local recurrence:** varies and is related to grade, tumor size, and margin width
   2. **Fifty percent of recurrences are invasive.**
B. **Lumpectomy and radiation:** Radiation reduces risk of recurrence by 50%.
C. **Total (simple) mastectomy:** Removal of breast tissue and areola/nipple; reconstruction can be done at the time of mastectomy.

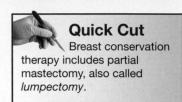

Quick Cut
Breast conservation therapy includes partial mastectomy, also called *lumpectomy*.

D. **Tamoxifen:** taken for 5 years; reduces risk of invasive and noninvasive in-breast recurrence and risk of contralateral breast cancer by ~50%

II. **Paget disease:** Histologically vacuolated cells (Paget cells) are seen in the epidermis of the nipple and result in an eczematous dermatitis.
A. **DCIS or invasive carcinoma:** present in the underlying ducts
B. **Evaluation:** mammography and ultrasound to assess for a subareolar mass
C. **Treatment:** lumpectomy to include nipple areolar complex with adjuvant radiation or mastectomy

Invasive Breast Cancer

I. **Favorable histologic types:** tubular carcinoma, mucinous carcinoma, and papillary carcinoma

II. **Less favorable lesions**
A. **Medullary cancer:** involves lymphocytic infiltration and a well-circumscribed lesion
B. **Inflammatory breast cancer:** Histology shows tumor-plugged subdermal lymphatics. Diagnosis is clinically based on inflammatory signs on exam (e.g., warmth, swelling, and pain).

Staging

I. **Clinical staging**
A. **Diagnostic mammogram:** to define primary tumor, identify additional foci, and evaluate contralateral breast
B. **Breast ultrasound:** to define primary tumor ± axillary node
C. **Chest radiograph:** to detect pulmonary or bone metastasis
D. **Computed tomography (CT) scan of the chest:** may be obtained for node-positive or higher than or equal to stage III patients
E. **Alkaline phosphatase:** sensitive for hepatic metastasis
F. **Bone scan:** if nodes are clinically positive or if nodes are clinically negative but the patient has symptoms of bone pain and stage III or higher
G. **Head CT scan:** if neurologic signs or symptoms are present

II. **Clinical/pathologic staging:** Tables 16-4 and 16-5

Treatment

I. **Surgery:** recurrence risk varies and is related to many factors including age, nodal status, tumor size, margin status, and lumpectomy with radiation; typically reduces risk of recurrence by 60%–75%

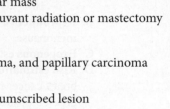

Quick Cut
Treatment for invasive breast cancer includes surgery, chemotherapy, radiation, and/or hormonal therapy.

A. **Mastectomy:** Removal of the breast tissue and nipple/areolar complex. Patients with a large tumor in relation to breast size may have superior cosmetic results with mastectomy.
   1. **Modified radical mastectomy:** includes removal of breast and levels I and II axillary lymph nodes (see Table 16-1)

Quick Cut
There is *no* survival difference between breast conservation and mastectomy.

Table 16-4: American Joint Committee on Cancer Tumor-Node-Metastasis Staging of Breast Cancer

T	Tumor Size	N	Node Metastasis	M	Distant Metastasis
T0	In situ	**N0**	None	**M0**	None
T1	≤2 cm	**Nmi**	Microscopic <2 mm	**M1**	Any
T2	>2cm to ≥5 cm	**N1**	Mobile in level I, II axilla		
T3	>5 cm	**N2**	Fixed in level I, II axilla		
T4	Direct extension to chest wall/skin	**N3**	Level III axillary, internal mammary, supraclavicular		

2. **Skin-sparing mastectomy:** Nonareolar breast skin is preserved; with immediate reconstruction provides more cosmetic result and does not increase recurrence risk.
3. **Radical mastectomy:** includes the pectoralis major and minor muscles and levels I–III axillary nodes

B. **Axillary sampling:** must accompany surgery to accurately stage patient
   1. **Sentinel node biopsy:** for clinically negative nodes; radiotracer and/or vital blue dye is used to identify the first nodes drained by the breast
      a. **Advantages:** allows minimal dissection with a substantial decrease in morbidity (lymphedema)
      b. **Node(s) examined for cancer:** If negative for metastatic disease, no further lymphadenectomy performed. If positive, axillary dissection is performed.
   2. **Axillary dissection:** for patients with clinically positive nodes or with positive sentinel nodes
      a. **Level I and II nodes:** removed in relation to the axillary vein (see Figure 16-2)
      b. **Skip metastasis (i.e., involved level III nodes with negative levels I and II nodes):** occurs in less than 5% of cases
      c. **Long thoracic nerve:** Preserved to prevent denervation of the **serratus anterior** muscle, which results in a **winged scapula**. **Thoracodorsal nerve** and blood supply to the **latissimus** muscle are also preserved.

II. **Adjuvant radiation:** whole breast radiation involves 45–50 Gy; used in breast conservation to decrease recurrence rates
   A. **Advantages:** reduces local recurrences and improves survival following a mastectomy in patients with large tumors (>5 cm), positive nodes, or with chest wall involvement
   B. **Postmastectomy setting:** Nodal radiation is uniformly administered to the axilla, supraclavicular fossa with or without the internal mammary nodes, and the chest wall.

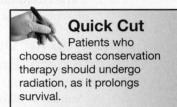

Quick Cut
Patients who choose breast conservation therapy should undergo radiation, as it prolongs survival.

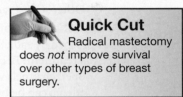

Quick Cut
Radical mastectomy does *not* improve survival over other types of breast surgery.

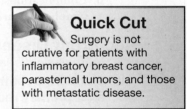

Quick Cut
Surgery is not curative for patients with inflammatory breast cancer, parasternal tumors, and those with metastatic disease.

Table 16-5: Anatomic Stage and Prognostic Groups

Stage 0	In situ disease	M0
Stage 1	T1N0, T0–1Nmi	M0
Stage 2	**T2**N0, T3N0, T1**N1**, T2N1	M0
Stage 3	**T3N1**, any **T4**, any **N2**, any **N3**	M0
Stage 4	Any T, any N	**M1**

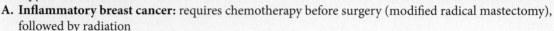

III. **Adjuvant chemotherapy:** Candidates have node-positive, tumor larger than 1 cm, estrogen receptor/progesterone receptor (ER/PR)–negative, HER2/neu receptor–positive pathology.
  A. **Common chemotherapy drugs:** cyclophosphamide, doxorubicin, docetaxel, and paclitaxel for 3–6 months
  B. **Trastuzumab:** used to treat HER2/neu (epidermal growth factor receptor 2)–positive cancers
  C. **Side effects:** myelosuppression, alopecia, and cardiomyopathy (doxorubicin and trastuzumab)
IV. **Adjuvant hormonal therapy:** for ER/PR+ patients
  A. **Premenopausal:** tamoxifen ± ovarian suppression or ablation
  B. **Postmenopausal:** AIs
V. **Neoadjuvant therapy:** systemic therapy given before surgical therapy for local disease
  A. **Inflammatory breast cancer:** requires chemotherapy before surgery (modified radical mastectomy), followed by radiation
  B. **Large, fixed tumors or large nodal disease:** can downstage disease and enable resectability or decrease tumor size and allow breast conservation

> **Quick Cut**
> Hormonal therapy is used in ER+ or PR+ patients.

Follow-up for Operable Breast Cancer (Ipsilateral and Contralateral Breasts)

I. **Observation:** for tumor recurrence and complications
  A. **Annual or biannual breast examination:** by a physician
  B. **Annual mammogram**
  C. **Other:** Chest radiographs, CT scans, and tumor markers are not needed unless clinical suspicion arises.
II. **Lymphedema of the arm:** Ten percent to 30% develop arm edema after axillary dissection, which is worsened by radiation if greater than 10 lymph nodes are removed.
  A. **Treatment:** Because each infection increases lymphatic obstruction by obliterating the remaining open channels with fibrosis, even minor skin infections should be evaluated by a physician; chronic edema can be treated with an elastic sleeve.
  B. **Complications:** Chronic edema lasting 10 years or longer can rarely lead to the development of **lymphangiosarcoma** in the affected arm.

Recurrent Disease

I. **Metastatic disease:** present in 10% of patients with recurrence
II. **Standard treatment (of an isolated breast recurrence after primary radiation therapy):** mastectomy
III. **Chest wall recurrences**
  A. **After mastectomy:** Isolated chest wall recurrences are treated with radiation therapy and resection.
  B. **Ipsilateral recurrences (after breast conservation with adjuvant radiation):** mastectomy
IV. **Distant metastasis**
  A. **Hormone therapy:** Patients with hormone-positive breast cancer who respond to one hormone treatment modality generally continue to respond to sequential hormone therapy.
  B. **Chemotherapy:** for patients with recurrent disease who are ER− or who do not respond to hormone therapy
    1. **Common drugs:** anthracyclines (doxorubicin), taxanes (paclitaxel), and antimetabolites (capecitabine)
    2. **Temporary favorable responses (e.g., decrease in tumor size or pain relief):** occur in 70% of patients with stage IV disease

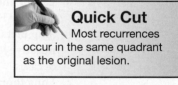

> **Quick Cut**
> Most recurrences occur in the same quadrant as the original lesion.

Special Cases

I. **Breast cancer in pregnancy**
  A. **Incidence:** occurs in 1.5% of women during childbearing years
  B. **Diagnosis:** usually delayed secondary to normal nodularity that forms in breasts during pregnancy
    1. **Suspicious mass:** should have ultrasound, then core biopsy
    2. **Vital blue dye for sentinel node:** contraindicated
    3. **Radiotracer:** appears to be safe

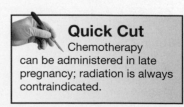

> **Quick Cut**
> Chemotherapy can be administered in late pregnancy; radiation is always contraindicated.

II. Male breast

A. Gynecomastia: unilateral or bilateral enlargement of the breast tissue directly behind the nipple

1. **Types (three)**
   a. **Prepubertal gynecomastia:** rare; caused by adrenal and testicular carcinoma
   b. **Pubertal gynecomastia:** 60%–70% of prepubertal boys
   c. **Senescent gynecomastia:** due to decreased testosterone and increased estradiol and luteinizing hormones

2. **Causes**
   a. **Idiopathic**
   b. **Drug therapies:** thiazide diuretics, digoxin, theophylline, antidepressants, and hormones
   c. **Alcohol and marijuana abuse**
   d. **Disease conditions:** cirrhosis, renal failure, and malnutrition

3. **Evaluation and treatment:** Evaluate for mass with mammography and physical exam; biopsy any dominant mass.
   a. **Negative biopsy:** Treat underlying medical condition; provide reassurance.
   b. **Testicular tumor:** Rarely, gynecomastia can be secondary to testicular tumor. Check serum estrogen, beta-human chorionic gonadotropin, estrogen, and dehydroepiandrosterone; perform testicular exam.

> **Quick Cut**
> Breast enlargement in the healthy male adolescent does not require treatment and will regress with age.

B. Cancer: Accounts for 1% of all breast cancers; average age is 63–70 years and most are ER+.

1. **Klinefelter syndrome:** associated with male breast cancer (testicular hormone factors)
2. **Symptoms:** Most patients present with a painless unilateral mass.
3. **Workup:** identical to that for female breast cancer
4. **Treatment**
   a. **Simple mastectomy:** most common
   b. **Breast conservation with radiation:** an option
   c. **Sentinel node biopsy:** ± axillary dissection
   d. **Tamoxifen:** for ER/PR+ cancers
5. **Survival:** similar to female breast cancer stage for stage

Chapter 17

Thyroid, Parathyroid, Adrenal Glands, and Thymus

John A. Olson Jr.

 THYROID GLAND

Vasculature

I. **Arterial supply:** Figure 17-1
   A. **Superior thyroid artery:** First branch of the external carotid artery supplies the upper pole of the thyroid.
   B. **Inferior thyroid artery:** arises from the thyrocervical trunk of the subclavian artery and supplies the lower pole
   C. **Thyroidea ima artery:** occasionally arises from the aortic arch and connects to the thyroid isthmus inferiorly

II. **Venous drainage:** interconnecting series of veins without valves
   A. **Superior thyroid veins:** drain along the course of the superior thyroid arteries into the internal jugular vein
   B. **Middle thyroid vein:** drains directly into the internal jugular
   C. **Inferior thyroid veins:** drain from the lower pole and isthmus either directly into the internal jugular or the innominate vein

III. **Lymphatic drainage:** to cervical nodes located in the central neck between the carotids and trachea (level 6), along the course of the internal jugular vein (levels 2A, 2B, 3, 4), in the posterior triangle (level 5), or to the paratracheal nodes in the mediastinum (formerly level 7) (Fig. 17-2)

Nerves

I. **Recurrent laryngeal nerve (RLN):** branch of the vagus (cranial nerve [CN] X) that runs in the tracheoesophageal (TE) groove at the posteromedial aspect of the thyroid
   A. **On the right:** RLN recurs around the subclavian artery and runs an oblique course, crossing the inferior thyroid artery before entering the TE groove.
   B. **On the left:** RLN recurs around the ligamentum arteriosum in the mediastinum and runs a course parallel to the TE groove.
   C. **Divisions:** RLN divides at variable locations into an anterior branch and posterior branch.
   D. **Function:** Anterior branch innervates the adductor muscles (thyroarytenoid, interarytenoid, and lateral cricoarytenoid), and posterior branch innervates the abductor muscles (posterior cricoarytenoid).

 Quick Cut
Surgery remains the mainstay of treatment for suspected or proven thyroid cancer and compressive goiters.

 Quick Cut
The nodes in the tracheoesophageal groove (level 6) are most important in the spread of thyroid malignancies because involved nodes may signal tumor extension into the recurrent laryngeal nerve.

 Quick Cut
In ~1% of individuals, the laryngeal nerve is nonrecurrent and enters the larynx by crossing the TE groove at the midpole of the thyroid.

 Quick Cut
The RLN provides motor function and sensory innervation of the glottis and trachea.

Anterior view

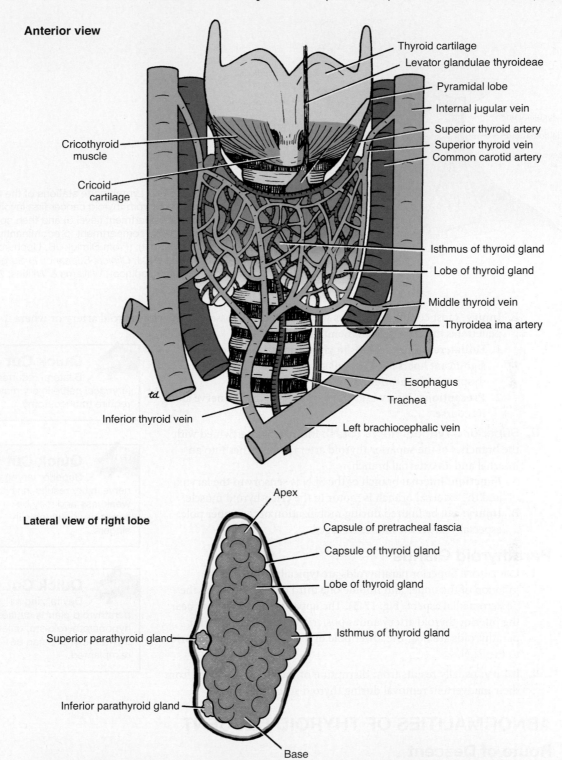

- Thyroid cartilage
- Levator glandulae thyroideae
- Pyramidal lobe
- Internal jugular vein
- Superior thyroid artery
- Superior thyroid vein
- Common carotid artery
- Isthmus of thyroid gland
- Lobe of thyroid gland
- Middle thyroid vein
- Thyroidea ima artery
- Esophagus
- Trachea
- Left brachiocephalic vein

- Cricothyroid muscle
- Cricoid cartilage
- Inferior thyroid vein

td

Lateral view of right lobe

- Apex
- Capsule of pretracheal fascia
- Capsule of thyroid gland
- Lobe of thyroid gland
- Isthmus of thyroid gland
- Superior parathyroid gland
- Inferior parathyroid gland
- Base

Figure 17-1: Blood supply of the thyroid gland. Each lobe of the thyroid has two main arteries and three veins. (From Snell RS. *Clinical Anatomy by Regions*, 9th ed. Baltimore: Lippincott Williams & Wilkins; 2011).

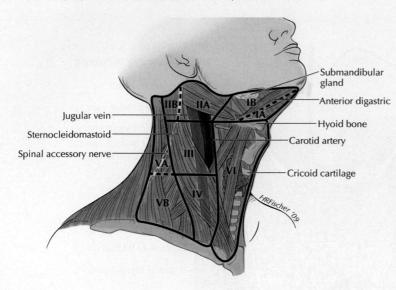

Figure 17-2: Lymph node stations of the neck. Metastases from thyroid cancer first involve the central compartment (level 6) and then spread to the lateral compartment (predominantly levels 3 and 4). (From Dimick JB, Upchurch GR, Sonnenday CJ. *Clinical Scenarios in Surgery*. Baltimore: Lippincott Williams & Wilkins; 2012).

E. Injury: most commonly occurs where the nerve crosses the inferior thyroid artery or where it penetrates the cricothyroid membrane
   1. **Unilateral injury:** results in vocal cord paralysis causing significant hoarseness as well as sensory loss resulting in dysphagia and aspiration
   2. **Precautions:** Injury is avoided by identifying the nerve along its course.

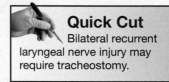

Quick Cut
Bilateral recurrent laryngeal nerve injury may require tracheostomy.

II. Superior laryngeal nerve (SLN): Intimately intertwined with the branches of the superior thyroid artery; it branches into an internal and an external branch.
   A. Function: Internal branch of the SLN is sensory to the larynx, and the external branch is motor to the cricothyroid muscle.
   B. Injury: can be injured during mobilization of the upper pole, especially when the lobe is enlarged

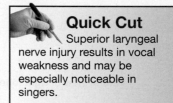

Quick Cut
Superior laryngeal nerve injury results in vocal weakness and may be especially noticeable in singers.

Parathyroid Glands

I. Location: Superior parathyroids are typically located at the junction of the upper and middle one third of the thyroid on the posteromedial aspect (Fig. 17-3). The upper gland is typically near the inferior thyroid artery and is posterior to the RLN. Inferior parathyroids are near the lower pole of the thyroid, usually anterior to the RLN.

II. Injury: usually results from disruption of the blood supply or from their inadvertent removal during thyroid surgery

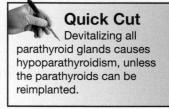

Quick Cut
Devitalizing all parathyroid glands causes hypoparathyroidism, unless the parathyroids can be reimplanted.

◆ ABNORMALITIES OF THYROID DESCENT

Route of Descent

I. Normal descent: Thyroid migrates downward from its point of origin at the foramen cecum at the base of the tongue through the hyoid bone and the thyroglossal duct.

II. Abnormal descent: may result in ectopic placement of thyroid tissue in the tongue, midline of the neck, or mediastinum
   A. Glottic (lingual) thyroid: occurs when the thyroid does not descend into the neck and remains at the base of the tongue
      1. **Symptoms:** Obstruction or difficulty with speech is usually related to goiter formation in the lingual mass.
      2. **Diagnosis:** By inspection or indirect laryngoscopy. A radioiodine (^{131}I) scan should be performed to identify the mass as thyroid tissue.

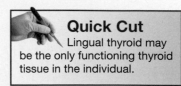

Quick Cut
Lingual thyroid may be the only functioning thyroid tissue in the individual.

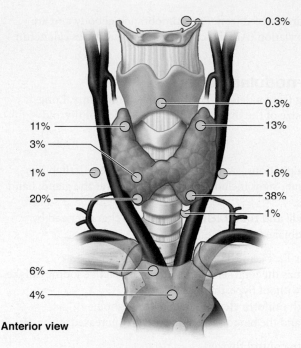

0.3%

0.3%

11% — 13%

3% —

1% — 1.6%

20% — 38%

1%

6%

4%

Anterior view

Figure 17-3: Normal locations of the parathyroid glands. The superior glands are almost always located on the dorsal aspect of the thyroid at the level of the cricoid cartilage. The inferior glands are more variable but are most commonly found on the lateral aspect of the lower pole of the thyroid. (From Moore KL, Agur AMR, Dalley AF. *Clinically Oriented Anatomy*, 7th ed. Baltimore: Lippincott Williams & Wilkins; 2013.)

3. **Management:** Thyroxine (T_4) should be the first step because glottic thyroid tissue is usually hypofunctioning. Surgical removal should be considered when there are obstructive symptoms.

B. **Mediastinal thyroid (substernal goiter):** Most are located in the anterosuperior mediastinum and may represent substernal extensions from an enlarged thyroid or normal thyroid tissue, resulting from aberrant embryologic descent of the thyroid into the mediastinum.

  1. **Evaluation:** Usually, computed tomography (CT) scans are best.
  2. **Substernal extensions:** may be caused by adenomatous hyperplasia and are not usually malignant; usually occur in older age groups
    a. **Symptoms:** TE compression and dysphagia or dyspnea
    b. **Management:** In general, they do not respond to medical therapy. Operation is usually advised to relieve pressure symptoms.

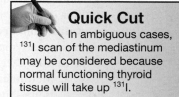

Quick Cut
In ambiguous cases, ^{131}I scan of the mediastinum may be considered because normal functioning thyroid tissue will take up ^{131}I.

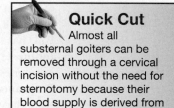

Quick Cut
Almost all substernal goiters can be removed through a cervical incision without the need for sternotomy because their blood supply is derived from the neck.

THYROID DYSFUNCTION REQUIRING SURGERY

Thyroid Hormones

I. **Triiodothyronine (T_3) and T_4: Follicular cells** of the thyroid are derived primarily from the floor of the foregut and produce T_3 and T_4.

  A. **Hormone synthesis and release:** Iodine and tyrosine combine to form T_3 and T_4; both of these hormones bind to thyroglobulin and are stored in the gland.
    1. **Release:** Under the control of thyroid-stimulating hormone (TSH) from the pituitary. TSH is released upon stimulation by thyrotropin-releasing hormone (TRH) from the hypothalamus.
    2. **Feedback regulating TRH and TSH release:** mediated by circulating levels of T_3 and T_4

  B. **Action:** increase metabolic rate and oxygen consumption, increase glycogenolysis (elevated blood sugar), and enhance actions of catecholamines
    1. **Result:** increased pulse rate, cardiac output, and blood flow
    2. **Symptoms:** Nervousness, irritability, muscular tremors, and muscle wasting can also occur.

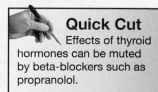

Quick Cut
Effects of thyroid hormones can be muted by beta-blockers such as propranolol.

II. Thyrocalcitonin: Parafollicular cells (C cells) are derived from the ultimobranchial body and are part of the amine precursor uptake and decarboxylation (APUD) cell system that produces calcitonin (whose function is unknown).

Graves Disease (Diffuse Toxic Non-nodular Goiter)

I. Pathogenesis: Autoimmune disease resulting from a defect in cell-mediated immunity. Long-acting thyroid stimulator (LATS) increases the size of the thyroid and its production of thyroid hormone.

II. Clinical presentation

    A. Hypermetabolic state: Symptoms include palpitations, sweating, intolerance to heat, irritability, insomnia, nervousness, weight loss, and fatigue. Signs include an audible bruit over the gland, hand and tongue tremors, and cardiac arrhythmias.

    B. Abnormal deposition of mucopolysaccharide and round cell infiltration: is characterized by exophthalmos, chemosis, and eyelid and pretibial edema

III. Diagnosis: confirmed by increased total serum T_4, T_3, and T_3 resin uptake (T_3RU)

    A. Free T_4 index: Increase of the T_3RU value times the total serum T_4 and of radioactive iodine uptake (RAIU) distinguish this from thyrotoxicosis without hyperthyroidism.

    B. ^{131}I thyroid scan: shows enlarged thyroid with uniform elevated uptake throughout

    C. Other: Serum cholesterol level is decreased, and the blood sugar and ALP are increased.

IV. Medical treatment: Initially, antithyroidals to control thyroid hormone release and block the systemic effects of elevated T_4 and T_3. This is usually followed by thyroid ablation with ^{131}I or surgery.

Quick Cut
Antithyroid drugs are rapidly effective and can reverse symptoms in a short time.

    A. Antithyroid drugs: effective in ~50% of patients, especially those with symptoms of short duration and with a small gland

        1. Action: alter various stages of iodine metabolism

            a. Methimazole and Propylthiouracil (PTU): Methimazole is first-line treatment to control high serum thyroid levels, except in pregnancy because it is teratogenic. Both it and PTU act through competitive inhibition of peroxidase, blocking the oxidation of iodide to thyroid hormone. PTU is reserved for pregnancy and thyroid storm because it also blocks the peripheral conversion of T_4 to T_3, which provides a rapid response. PTU has the potential for serious liver toxicity.

            b. Iodine: High concentrations block the release of thyroid hormones, but the effect only lasts 10–14 days.

            c. Propranolol: Beta-adrenergic blocker reduces the secondary effects of hypermetabolism.

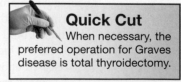

Quick Cut
Methimazole is first line treatment for Graves Disease. PTU is not recommended due to the risk of liver toxicity.

        2. Recurrence: high if the drugs are stopped

        3. Toxicity: Drugs must be discontinued if fever, rash, arthralgia, a lupus-like syndrome, or agranulocytosis occurs.

    B. Ablative doses of ^{131}I: Oral administration is effective and usually preferred in Graves disease.

        1. Advantages: ^{131}I ablation obviates the need for surgery and does not appreciably increase the risk of carcinoma.

        2. Contraindications: pregnancy or planned pregnancy; large, symptomatic goiters; concurrent thyroid nodules at risk for malignancy; Graves ophthalmopathy (relative); and patients in need of rapid resolution of their hyperthyroidism

V. Surgical treatment: usually the second-line ablative option for Graves disease

    A. Indications: Thyroidectomy is indicated when ^{131}I treatment is contraindicated.

    B. Objectives: Remove thyroid tissue to correct the hyperthyroidism. Currently, most experts recommend performing either a near-total thyroidectomy (total lobectomy on one side and a subtotal lobectomy on the other) or total thyroidectomy.

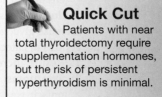

Quick Cut
When necessary, the preferred operation for Graves disease is total thyroidectomy.

Quick Cut
Patients with near total thyroidectomy require supplementation hormones, but the risk of persistent hyperthyroidism is minimal.

C. **Preoperative preparation:** To minimize the risk of thyroid storm, the patient should be euthyroid before operation.
  1. **Antithyroid drugs:** Given until the patient is clinically and biochemically euthyroid (free T_3 <5 pM/L). Lugol solution or saturated potassium iodide (SSKI) is given for 7–10 days before surgery to decrease gland vascularity.
  2. **Beta blockade:** used if there is tachycardia or hypertension despite antithyroid medications
D. **Propranolol:** effective in rapidly restoring the euthyroid state and in reducing vascularity; must be given for 4–5 days postoperatively to prevent thyroid storm because the half-life of circulating thyroid hormone is 5–10 days
E. **Complications**
  1. **Thyroid storm:** severe hypermetabolic state that causes hyperpyrexia and tachyarrhythmias due to uncontrolled hyperthyroidism
    a. **Incidence:** rarely found, unless a patient has undiagnosed hyperthyroidism and has surgery for some unrelated emergency
    b. **Treatment:** large doses of antithyroid drugs, hydrocortisone, iodine, and propranolol
  2. **Hemorrhage:** possible due to increased vascularity in a hyperactive thyroid gland
    a. **Airway obstruction:** caused by hemorrhage resulting in tracheal compression and laryngeal edema
    b. **Treatment:** Secure the airway, evacuate the clot, and control the bleeding.
  3. **Hypoparathyroidism:** usually develops within the first 24 hours after surgery and results in a subnormal serum calcium concentration
    a. **Symptoms of hypocalcemia:** Numbness and tingling periorally or in the fingers and toes, nervousness, and anxiety. Evidenced by a positive Chvostek sign (facial twitch with tapping on the facial nerve) or Trousseau sign (carpopedal spasm with blood pressure cuff insufflation).
    b. **Treatment of hypocalcemia:** Intravenous (IV) oral calcium salts. Activated vitamin D (calcitriol) therapy may be required if the serum intact parathyroid hormone (PTH) level is low. IV calcium should be avoided unless severe hypocalcemia (Ca <7.5 mg/dL) and symptoms are present.

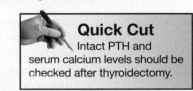

Quick Cut
Intact PTH and serum calcium levels should be checked after thyroidectomy.

  4. **RLN injury:** produces vocal cord paralysis
    a. **Unilateral injury:** Usually manifested by hoarseness. If the nerve is intact (paresis), the patient usually recovers a normal voice within 3 months. If the injury is permanent, therapy to medialize the true vocal cord is necessary.
    b. **Bilateral:** Airway obstruction results due to paralysis of the vocal cords in the midline adducted position, requiring emergency intubation or tracheostomy. If the nerves are intact, recovery usually occurs in 3–6 months.
  5. **Injury to the external branch of the SLN:** This nerve is motor to the cricothyroid muscle and can be injured during ligation of the branches of the superior thyroid artery, causing voice fatigue and a loss of timbre and projection.

Plummer Disease (Toxic Multinodular Goiter)

I. **Characteristics:** Hyperthyroid state caused by several hyperfunctioning nodules in a multinodular gland. Most commonly found in women older than age 50 years and is usually associated with a history of pre-existing nontoxic multinodular goiter.

II. **Clinical presentation:** Hypermetabolic symptoms tend to be subtler than in Graves disease; however, cardiovascular manifestations of hyperthyroidism, such as tachycardia, palpitations, and arrhythmias (atrial fibrillation) are more common. Signs are arrhythmias, occasional muscle wasting, and the presence of a multinodular goiter.

III. **Laboratory studies:** T_3 and T_4 levels are increased, and RAIU is increased in the nodules, which will not be suppressed by exogenously administered T_4.

IV. **Treatment:** Options for treatment are as outlined for Graves disease. [131]I tends to be less effective for toxic multinodular goiter than for Graves disease.
  A. **Preoperative preparation and perioperative management:** same as for Graves disease except for the use of iodides, which may worsen the hyperthyroidism
  B. **Total thyroidectomy:** preferred treatment, especially if the goiter is large or there are compressive symptoms

Toxic Adenoma

I. **Clinical presentation:** hyperthyroidism due to an autonomously hyperfunctioning solitary nodule in an otherwise normal gland

  A. **Symptoms:** Initially, the patient may be asymptomatic because hormone production by the rest of the gland will be suppressed. Eventually, symptoms of hyperthyroidism can occur as the nodule continues to secrete thyroid hormone.

  B. **Signs:** Solitary thyroid nodule may be palpable in an otherwise normal gland.

II. **Laboratory studies:** T_3 and T_4 levels are increased, RAIU is increased in the nodule (hot nodule), and hormone secretion will not be suppressed by exogenous T_4.

III. **Treatment:** Surgical excision of the nodule (lobectomy) is the safest and most expeditious treatment. ^{131}I ablation is also a good option. Preparation for surgery is as outlined for Graves disease.

Thyroid Goiter

I. **Overview:** Enlargement of the thyroid gland are collectively referred to as **goiters**, which may be **diffuse** or **focal** and may be either smooth or nodular. Thyroid function may be normal or abnormal.

II. **Causes:** Diffuse goiters with normal or decreased function have benign causes. Focal or nodular goiters with normal function may be due to neoplasms.

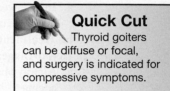

Quick Cut
Thyroid goiters can be diffuse or focal, and surgery is indicated for compressive symptoms.

III. **Colloid and iodine-deficiency goiters:** occur infrequently in the United States

  A. **Clinical presentation:** bulky, soft enlargements

  B. **Treatment:** Surgery is indicated for compressive symptoms, coexistent nodules concerning for malignancy, or occasionally, cosmetic concerns. Thyroid hormone suppression is generally not effective and should be discouraged.

IV. **Thyroiditis:** Inflammation can be acute, subacute, or chronic.

  A. **Acute suppurative thyroiditis:** uncommon disorder caused by the hematogenous spread of microorganisms into the thyroid gland

    1. **Clinical presentation:** pain and tenderness

    2. **Diagnosis:** fine-needle aspiration (FNA)

    3. **Treatment:** open drainage or localized resection with antibiotics

  B. **Subacute thyroiditis (giant cell, granulomatous, or de Quervain thyroiditis):** Thought to be viral and is often preceded by an upper respiratory infection. Course is self-limited, lasting 2–6 months. Nonsteroidal anti-inflammatory drugs (NSAIDs) are used.

  C. **Chronic thyroiditis:** occurs in two major forms, Hashimoto and Riedel

    1. **Hashimoto thyroiditis (struma lymphomatosa):** Relatively common autoimmune disorder that occurs predominantly in women. Thyroid function is normal or hypothyroid. Treatment is usually long-term T_4 supplementation.

Quick Cut
Reidel thyroiditis is usually stony hard on physical exam and difficult to distinguish from thyroid malignancy. Reidel thyroiditis is the only chronic thyroiditis treated surgically.

    2. **Riedel (fibrous) thyroiditis:** Relatively rare form in which the parenchyma is replaced with dense fibrous tissue. Treatment is surgical.

V. **Nodular thyroid enlargements:** Diffuse multinodular goiter is the most common form and is the cause of a palpable nodule in the thyroid in as much as 10% of the adult population.

  A. **Clinical presentation:** These goiters are caused by adenomatous hyperplasia of the thyroid gland, thought to be due to long-standing stimulation of the thyroid by TSH. Thyroid function studies are normal, as are thyroid antibodies.

  B. **Treatment:** If there are no clinical signs of malignancy and the gland is not symptomatic, no treatment is necessary. Surgery is indicated for compressive symptoms.

Thyroid Neoplasms

I. **Overview:** Frequently, a solitary or prominent thyroid nodule is detected on physical examination in an asymptomatic patient. Although most solitary thyroid nodules are benign, the primary concern is thyroid cancer.

Quick Cut
The most common reason for thyroid surgery today is to diagnose or treat a suspected thyroid neoplasm that cannot be diagnosed by other means.

Table 17-1: Indications for Fine-Needle Aspiration of Thyroid Nodules

Patient Risk Category	Ultrasound Feature	Size
High*	Any	>5 mm
Average	Any	>1.5 cm
Average	Microcalcifications Hypoechoic Irregular margin Taller than wide Abnormal lymph nodes	>1 cm†
Average	Spongiform Mixed solid-cystic Cystic	>2cm >1.5–2.0 cm NR‡

*Patients with a family history of thyroid cancer, prior exposure to head and neck radiation, prior history of thyroid cancer status post thyroid lobectomy, or multiple endocrine neoplasia type 2 kindred member.
†Consider biopsy for smaller lesions depending on clinical suspicion.
‡May be done for relief of compressive symptoms.
NR, not reported.

II. **Assessment of thyroid nodules:** Table 17-1
   A. **Patient's age:** In children, 10%–15% of thyroid nodules are malignant; during the childbearing years, most nodules are benign; incidence of cancer in nodules increases by ~10% per decade after age 40 years.
   B. **Patient's sex:** Thyroid cancer is more common in women than in men, but benign thyroid nodules are also more common in women, and the likelihood that a nodule will prove to be malignant is greater in men than in women.
   C. **Other risk factors:** family history of thyroid malignancy and history of exposure to therapeutic radiation, which increases incidence 5–10-fold

III. **Characteristics of the nodule**
   A. **Consistency:** Firmness suggests malignancy.
   B. **Infiltration (into the surrounding thyroid or overlying structures, such as the strap muscles):** suggests malignancy
   C. **Nodulation: Solitary nodules** have a 5% chance of being malignant. **Multiple nodules** are present in as many as 40% of proven cases of thyroid malignancy.
   D. **Growth patterns:** Nodules that suddenly increase in size should be suspected of being thyroid neoplasms.

IV. **Ipsilateral lymph node enlargement:** Suggests thyroid malignancy. In children, as many as 50% of thyroid cancers are first detected because of cervical lymph node enlargement.

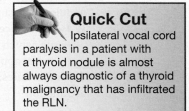

Quick Cut
Ipsilateral vocal cord paralysis in a patient with a thyroid nodule is almost always diagnostic of a thyroid malignancy that has infiltrated the RLN.

V. **Mobility of the vocal cords:** Because vocal cord paralysis may not be associated with voice changes, the cords should be assessed preoperatively by either indirect or direct laryngoscopy in all patients undergoing thyroid operations. Examination should be repeated postoperatively if voice abnormalities occur.

VI. **Diagnostic studies:** Thyroid nodules are common; workup must efficiently seek to determine whether a nodule is functional or likely to be malignant (Fig. 17-4).
   A. **Blood work:** Serum TSH is the first test for thyroid nodules.
      1. **Suppressed TSH:** Patient should be evaluated for hyperthyroidism and then be scheduled for a technetium-99m (^{99m}Tc) pertechnetate/^{131}I thyroid scan.
      2. **Serum calcitonin:** specific biomarker for medullary carcinoma of the thyroid (MTC)
   B. **US:** Using a high-frequency linear transducer (7.5–14 Hz), nodules can be identified as cystic, solid, or complex. Features

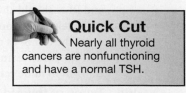

Quick Cut
Nearly all thyroid cancers are nonfunctioning and have a normal TSH.

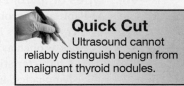

Quick Cut
Ultrasound cannot reliably distinguish benign from malignant thyroid nodules.

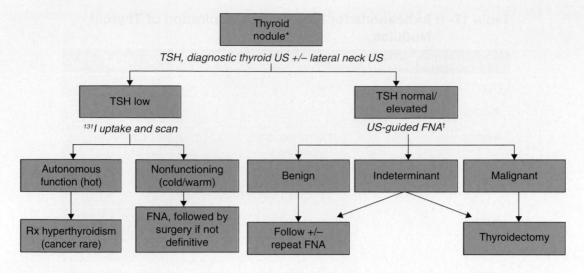

Figure 17-4: Algorithm for the evaluation and management of the asymptomatic thyroid nodule. TSH, thyroid-stimulating hormone; US, ultrasound; FNA, fine-needle aspiration.

* Detected clinically or incidentally on imaging.
† Criteria for FNA listed in Table 16-2.

that may be suggestive of malignancy include the presence of calcifications, solid echo-texture, indistinct borders, local invasion, or increased vascularity.

C. **Needle biopsy (of the thyroid):** allows for the histopathologic or cytopathologic examination of cells as an aid in the diagnosis of thyroid nodules and in planning therapy

> **Quick Cut**
> Needle biopsy is the most useful diagnostic tool for distinguishing benign from malignant thyroid nodules.

1. **FNA and cytology:** Cells are aspirated by applying suction to a syringe attached to a 21- to 25-gauge needle. Technique requires interpretation by a well-trained thyroid cytopathologist but has a good degree of accuracy and specificity (false-negative rate <3%) in diagnosing malignant lesions and is associated with few complications.
2. **Core biopsy and histology:** Using a 14- or 18-gauge especially designed needle (Tru-Cut), a cylinder of tissue is obtained then fixed and stained for histopathologic analysis. Due to a relatively high incidence of bleeding complications, the technique is rarely performed.

D. **Radioisotope scanning (of the thyroid):** Indicated in patients with nodules and a suppressed TSH. May be done with ^{131}I or with ^{99m}Tc.

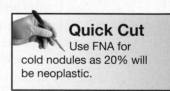

> **Quick Cut**
> Use FNA for cold nodules as 20% will be neoplastic.

1. **Isotope tracers:** Taken up by normally functioning thyroid tissue, which appears as a "hot" area; nodules that do not take up tracer appear as "cold" areas.
2. **Hot nodules:** should be scanned with ^{131}I to determine their function

VII. **Operative approach:** Surgical removal is the mainstay of treatment for nodules at high risk for harboring malignancy. Parathyroid glands and RLN should always be identified and preserved.

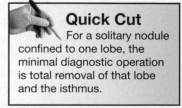

> **Quick Cut**
> For a solitary nodule confined to one lobe, the minimal diagnostic operation is total removal of that lobe and the isthmus.

A. **Extent of the operation:** depends on the histologic type, extent of the tumor as determined from the preoperative assessment and the operative findings, and the tumor's biologic aggressiveness

B. **Lymph node resection:** indicated when nodes are grossly involved

VIII. **Types of thyroid malignancy:** Table 17-2

A. **Papillary thyroid carcinoma (PTC):** accounts for 80% of all thyroid cancers in children and 60% in adults; affects women twice as often as men

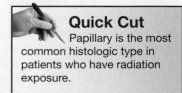

> **Quick Cut**
> Papillary is the most common histologic type in patients who have radiation exposure.

1. **Characteristics:** Slow rate of growth; 50% spread to regional lymphatics; 40% of tumors are multicentric in origin.

Table 17-2: Types of Thyroid Cancer and Treatment

Cancer Type	% Thyroid Cancer	Prognosis	Treatment
Papillary	80%–85%	Excellent	Thyroidectomy, TSH suppression, +/− ^{131}I ablation
Follicular	10%–15%	Good	Thyroidectomy, TSH suppression, +/− ^{131}I ablation
Medullary	5%	Intermediate	Thyroidectomy + LND
Anaplastic	<2%	Poor	Multimodality therapy

TSH, thyroid-stimulating hormone; LND, lymph node dissection.

2. **Treatment: Total thyroidectomy** is the treatment of choice for most PTC >1 cm.
    a. **Cervical lymphadenectomy:** indicated for gross lymph node metastasis
    b. **^{131}I therapy:** to ablate the thyroid remnant and treat microscopic node disease; indicated for intermediate and high-risk patients (e.g., age >45 years, tumors >2 cm, lymph node metastasis)
3. **Prognosis:** excellent with occult or well-encapsulated intrathyroidal carcinoma; poor when there is extrathyroidal invasion or if the patient is older than age 45 years

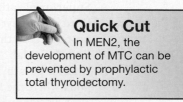

Quick Cut
Patients with well-encapsulated papillary tumors have a 20-year survival rate greater than 90%.

B. **Follicular thyroid carcinoma (FTC):** accounts for 10%–15% of all thyroid malignancies; more common in areas where iodine-deficiency goiter is prevalent
    1. **Incidence:** Affects women twice as often as men; relative frequency increases after age 40 years.
    2. **Characteristics:** slow-growing and usually unifocal tumor spreads primarily through the bloodstream and uncommonly (<10%) to regional lymph nodes
    3. **Treatment: Total thyroidectomy** is the treatment of choice for most FTC >1 cm.
        a. **Lymph node metastasis:** Occurs in 10%; lymphadenectomy is indicated for gross lymph node metastasis.
        b. **^{131}I therapy:** to ablate the thyroid remnant and treat microscopic node disease; indicated for intermediate- and high-risk patients who also benefit from TSH suppressions
    4. **Prognosis:** good with minimal vascular invasion (80% 20-year survival rate); poor with gross invasion (20-year survival rate <20%)
C. **MTC:** accounts for less than 5% of all thyroid cancers and most commonly occurs sporadically but also can be familial as a part of multiple endocrine neoplasia (MEN) syndrome type II
    1. **Characteristics:** Early spread to the lymph nodes is characteristic and spread to liver and bone is also common. Arises from the C cells of the thyroid and produces calcitonin.
    2. **Treatment: Total thyroidectomy and central compartment** (bilateral level 6) is indicated for all MTC patients; **lateral compartment-oriented cervical lymphadenectomy** is indicated for patients with gross adenopathy.
    3. **Prognosis:** poorer than for PTC or FTC and is related to stage
        a. **Overall survival:** ~86% at 5 years and ~65% at 10 years
        b. **Poor prognostic factors:** advanced age, TNM stage III or IV, reoperation, and having MEN2B

Quick Cut
Calcitonin is a useful tumor marker to detect recurrence of MTC.

Quick Cut
In MEN2, the development of MTC can be prevented by prophylactic total thyroidectomy.

D. **Anaplastic thyroid carcinoma (ATC):** accounts for less than 2% of all thyroid cancers but is the most common cause of thyroid cancer–specific death
    1. **Incidence:** most common between ages 50 and 70 years and is three times more common in women than men
    2. **Characteristics:** can be reliably diagnosed by FNA or core biopsy, which shows small cells, giant cells, or spindle cells; may arise from a pre-existing, well-differentiated thyroid neoplasm
    3. **Growth:** Usually rapid, involving the trachea and esophagus; they metastasize early, so they are usually unresectable.

4. **Treatment:** Small ATC (<5 cm) limited to the thyroid have the greatest chance of prolonged survival with **total thyroidectomy** followed by adjuvant chemotherapy and radiation therapy.
   a. **Patients with locally advanced disease:** may benefit from up-front chemoradiation
   b. **Secure airway:** Often the immediate need for ATC patients. Tracheostomy may be performed, but endotracheal stenting is preferred.
5. **Prognosis:** Poor, with a fatal outcome in almost all, regardless of treatment. Palliation is aimed at maintaining patency of the esophagus and the airway.

E. **Thyroid lymphoma:** Two percent of all thyroid malignancies, affecting mostly women 50–70 years of age. Chronic Hashimoto thyroiditis is the principal risk factor.

1. **Characteristics:** Rapidly enlarging goiter with neck pain, dysphagia, hoarseness, dyspnea, and cough. Physical findings include a firm thyroid goiter with fixation to surrounding structures.

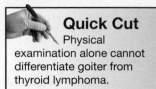

Quick Cut
Physical examination alone cannot differentiate goiter from thyroid lymphoma.

2. **Diagnosis:** FNA and core biopsy are the mainstays. Patients should undergo CT scan of the neck, chest, and abdomen to evaluate the extent of disease.
3. **Type:** almost exclusively of the non-Hodgkin type and of B-cell origin

Quick Cut
Unless the tumor is small and confined to the thyroid lobe, surgical excision of lymphoma is generally not indicated.

4. **Treatment:** Combination of chemotherapy and radiation. Surgery has a limited role. Tracheostomy should be considered in any patient with actual or impending airway compromise.
5. **Prognosis:** Outcome is dependent on stage and grade of lymphoma. Overall 5-year survival has been estimated to be 35%.

PARATHYROID GLANDS

Overview

I. **Embryology:** Most individuals have two superior and two inferior parathyroid glands that differ in their embryologic origin.

A. **Superior parathyroid glands:** Arise from the fourth branchial pouch in close proximity to the origin of the thyroid and descend into the neck. Because of the embryologic origin, abnormal parathyroid locations may be either intrathyroidal or within the posterior mediastinum near the TE groove.

Quick Cut
There is no current satisfactory replacement for PTH, and the patient with hypoparathyroidism is doomed to a lifetime of episodic, symptomatic hypocalcemia.

B. **Inferior parathyroid glands:** Arise from the third branchial pouch in relationship to the thymic anlage and cross the superior glands in their descent into the neck. They are frequently associated with the thymus gland in the anterosuperior mediastinum.

II. **Anatomy:** Most people have four parathyroid glands, but as few as three glands and as many as five have been identified. The average parathyroid gland weighs from 40 to 70 mg.

A. **Superior parathyroid glands:** Usually lie at the junction of the upper and middle one third of the thyroid gland on its posteromedial surface or in the TE groove; they usually lie posteriorly to the RLN and are in close proximity to the thyroid. Occasionally, they may even be intrathyroidal.

B. **Inferior parathyroid glands:** Lie within a circle with a 3-cm diameter, the center of which is the point where the RLN crosses the inferior thyroid artery; usually anterior to the RLN. They may be in close proximity to or within the cervical limb of the thymus gland.

C. **Arterial supply:** Derived mainly from the inferior thyroid artery. Superior parathyroid glands receive their blood supply from the superior thyroid artery in 10%.

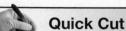

Quick Cut
Both parathyroid adenomas and hyperplasia primarily involve chief cells, making the pathologic distinction difficult.

D. **Venous drainage:** is into the superior, middle, and inferior thyroid veins

E. **Histopathology:** Normal parathyroid gland has a significant amount of fat interspersed with chief and oxyphil cells.

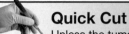

Parathyroid Hormone

I. **Calcium metabolism:** PTH is a major regulator of calcium metabolism.

   A. **Action:** PTH acts in conjunction with activated vitamin D_3 to regulate the plasma concentration of the ionized form of calcium. There is a reciprocal relationship between the serum calcium and PTH secretion—as serum calcium levels decrease, the secretion of PTH increases.

   B. **Affected organs:** PTH exerts its biologic effect on bone (mobilizes calcium from bone), intestine (increases intestinal absorption of calcium), and kidney (active reabsorption of calcium in the distal nephron).

II. **Increased, unopposed PTH secretion:** Clinical effects include hypercalcemia, altered calcium excretion (initially, hypocalciuria occurs due to increased reabsorption, which reverts to hypercalciuria in chronic hyperparathyroid states when the hypercalcemia exceeds the renal threshold), hypophosphatemia, and hyperphosphaturia.

III. **Laboratory tests:** Serum PTH levels can be measured by radioimmunoassay.

Hyperparathyroidism

I. **Primary hyperparathyroidism (PHPT):** relatively common disorder that most commonly occurs sporadically

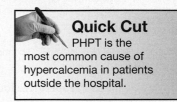

Quick Cut
PHPT is the most common cause of hypercalcemia in patients outside the hospital.

   A. **Etiology and pathology:** Most PHPT cases are due to a solitary adenoma; 10%–15% are due to four-gland hyperplasia; PTC accounts for less than 1% of PHPT; 0.4% of cases are due to multiple adenomas involving more than one gland.

   B. **Clinical presentation:** Most patients are clinically asymptomatic.

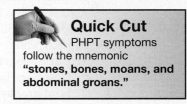

Quick Cut
PHPT symptoms follow the mnemonic **"stones, bones, moans, and abdominal groans."**

     1. **Kidney stones:** Nephrolithiasis occurs in 50%.

     2. **Bones:** Osteitis fibrosa cystica (von Recklinghausen disease of bone) is found mostly in secondary and tertiary hyperparathyroidism.

     3. **Moans:** Psychiatric manifestations—personality disorders or frank psychosis—are uncommon.

     4. **Abdominal groans:** Peptic ulcer disease may occur, usually associated with hypergastrinemia; cholelithiasis or pancreatitis may also occur. Many patients have nonspecific symptoms, such as weakness, easy fatigability, lethargy, constipation, and arthralgia.

   C. **Diagnosis**

     1. **Laboratory studies:** Increased serum calcium is the cornerstone of diagnosis, which should be shown on at least two blood specimens drawn on different occasions.

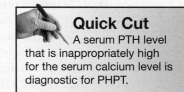

Quick Cut
A serum PTH level that is inappropriately high for the serum calcium level is diagnostic for PHPT.

       a. **Other causes of high serum calcium:** include metastatic bone disease, myeloma, sarcoidosis, the use of thiazide diuretics, milk-alkali syndrome, hypervitaminosis, thyrotoxicosis, and Addison disease

       b. **Serum 25-hydroxy vitamin D:** should be measured to exclude secondary hypoparathyroidism

       c. **Other:** Serum phosphorus level is decreased, and the serum chloride-to-phosphorus ratio usually exceeds 33:1.

     2. **Radiographic studies:** Plain radiographs are rarely indicated. Historically, in x-rays, the proximal ends of the long bones may show bony reabsorption or brown tumors. Ultrasound, CT, or scintigraphy may be used to assess the parathyroid glands.

   D. **Indications for surgery:** Table 17-3

     1. **Symptomatic patients:** All should be considered for surgery.

     2. **Asymptomatic patients:** if younger than age 50 years, serum calcium levels greater than 1 mg/dL above the normal range; decrease in bone density (T score < -2.5 at any site), hypercalciuria; decrease in creatinine clearance less than 60 mL/min or patients who are unable to have close medical follow-up

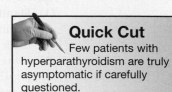

Quick Cut
Few patients with hyperparathyroidism are truly asymptomatic if carefully questioned.

Table 17-3: Indications for Surgery in Hyperparathyroidism

HPT Type	Symptom Status	Patients Eligible	Treatment
Primary	Symptomatic "Vaguely" symptomatic Asymptomatic	All Most[†] NIH guidelines[‡] met NIH guidelines not met	Parathyroidectomy* Parathyroidectomy* Parathyroidectomy* Observation
Secondary	Symptomatic** Asymptomatic	All PTH >300–500 pg/mL despite maximal medical therapy	Subtotal parathyroidectomy or total parathyroidectomy with autotransplantation
Tertiary	Asymptomatic Symptomatic	Ca^{+2} >12 mg/dL All	Parathyroidectomy[††] Parathyroidectomy[††]

*Directed parathyroidectomy with intraoperative parathyroid hormone monitoring or four-gland exploration.
[†]Symptoms improve 30%–50% of the time.
[‡](Any) Ca^{+2} 1 mg/dL elevation, age younger than 50 years, T score less than 2.5 any site, glomerular filtration rate less than 60 mL/min, or follow-up unlikely.
**Symptoms in secondary hyperparathyroidism (SHPT) that warrant parathyroidectomy include calciphylaxis, bone pain, osteodystrophy, and severe pruritus.
[††]Four-gland exploration.
HPT, hyperparathyroidism; "vaguely symptomatic," patient with musculoskeletal, neuropsychiatric, and abdominal complaints; NIH, National Institutes of Health; PTH, parathyroid hormone.

E. **Preoperative localization of the parathyroid glands:** helpful to permit a minimal access approach, define the anatomy in patients who have had prior surgery, and aid in defining the pathology in patients who have persistent or recurrent hypercalcemia

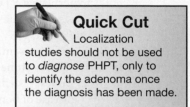

Quick Cut
Localization studies should not be used to *diagnose* PHPT, only to identify the adenoma once the diagnosis has been made.

1. **Ultrasonography (US):** will define an enlarged parathyroid in most cases; least expensive first test for parathyroid localization
2. **Scintigraphy:** Using ^{99m}Tc sestamibi can localize 75% of parathyroid adenomas.
   a. **Delayed images:** show persistent uptake by enlarged parathyroid glands
   b. **Sestamibi scanning:** useful in demonstrating ectopic glands, such as the mediastinum
   c. **Single positron emission computerized tomography (SPECT):** may reveal what traditional planar imaging does not
3. **CT:** particularly successful in localizing enlarged parathyroids in the mediastinum
4. **Magnetic resonance imaging (MRI):** Seems to be as successful as CT in localizing parathyroids on the T_2-weighted image. Cost is high.
5. **Selective venous sampling and PTH assay:** Because the study is costly and time consuming, it is reserved only for patients with negative noninvasive imaging. Retrograde injection of the thyroid veins is performed.
   a. **High PTH level:** Disproportionately high PTH in one or more of the venous samples helps to localize the lesion to one side of the neck.
   b. **Four-gland hyperplasia:** suggested by significant increase in samples obtained from veins on both sides of the neck
F. **Surgical treatment:** Parathyroid surgeon must be able to reliably identify all four parathyroid glands.
1. **Solitary adenoma:** Should be completely excised. Currently, localization techniques and intraoperative assay of PTH levels allow for a minimal access approach to parathyroid adenomas in most patients.
   a. **PTH levels:** Drawn at the beginning of the operation, and then a limited dissection is performed to excise the adenoma. Following excision, additional PTH levels are drawn at specific intervals.
      (1) **Significant drop:** Due to the short half-life of PTH (5 minutes), a drop occurs if all abnormal parathyroid tissue has been removed.
      (2) **If the levels do not drop sufficiently:** Abnormal tissue remains.
   b. **If tumor cannot be found in the normal locations:** Exploration should continue in regions where ectopic parathyroids may be found, including the deep thymus,

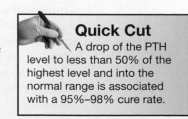

Quick Cut
A drop of the PTH level to less than 50% of the highest level and into the normal range is associated with a 95%–98% cure rate.

the prevertebral space behind the esophagus, behind the upper pole of the thyroid, and intrathyroidal.

    2. **Four-gland hyperplasia:** managed as follows

        a. **Subtotal parathyroidectomy (leaving a well-vascularized remnant [50–100 mg of parathyroid tissue] to provide for normal parathyroid function):** Intraoperative PTH levels are obtained to ensure that an adequate excision of parathyroid tissue has been performed. There is a 5% recurrence rate.

        b. **Total parathyroidectomy (with autotransplantation of minced parathyroid tissue):** There is a real danger of permanent hypoparathyroidism.

  G. **Postoperative management:** Hypocalcemia usually develops after successful therapy. Asymptomatic hypocalcemia greater than 8 mg/dL requires no treatment.

    1. **Symptomatic hypocalcemia:** Calcium less than 8.0 mg/dL always requires treatment.

        a. **Treatment:** should begin with IV calcium gluconate

        b. **Mildly symptomatic patients:** May be given oral calcium. The gastrointestinal (GI) tract is able to absorb a maximum of 30% of ingested oral calcium daily, which corresponds to doses of calcium salts ranging from 3–4 g/day.

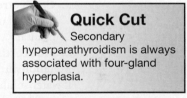

Quick Cut
Patients with significant bone disease require prolonged calcium supplementation to permit skeletal remineralization.

    2. **Vitamin D:** may be needed if hypocalcemia remains symptomatic despite calcium supplementation

II. Secondary hyperparathyroidism (SHPT): Found in chronic renal failure. These patients are unable to synthesize the active form of vitamin D and develop chronic hypocalcemia and hyperphosphatemia.

  A. **Multiple gland enlargement:** results from chronic hypocalcemia sensed by the parathyroid

  B. **Unresponsiveness to calcium and vitamin D:** Calcium-sensing and vitamin D receptors are frequently downregulated.

  C. **Clinical presentation:** Symptoms include fatigue, muscle weakness, pruritus, bone pain, joint pain, and metastatic soft tissue calcifications causing tissue necrosis (calciphylaxis). Untreated SHPT may result in symptomatic renal osteodystrophy (adynamic bone, osteomalacia, and osteitis) with risk of fracture.

  D. **Diagnosis:** increased serum intact PTH level, hypocalcemia, vitamin D deficiency, hyperphosphatemia, and elevated alkaline phosphatase (ALP)

  E. **Imaging studies:** US, ^{99m}Tc sestamibi, or CT scan

  F. **Medical treatment:** indicated in most patients and includes phosphate binders, vitamin D analogues, and calcimimetics such as cinacalcet

Quick Cut
Secondary hyperparathyroidism is always associated with four-gland hyperplasia.

  G. **Surgical treatment:** Subtotal parathyroidectomy or total parathyroidectomy with autotransplantation of parathyroid tissue is indicated for patients who are refractory to medical therapy or who have intractable symptoms.

III. Tertiary hyperparathyroidism (THPT): Hyperparathyroidism that persists in patients who have chronic renal disease despite a successful renal transplant; it produces the same symptoms as PHPT.

Quick Cut
Tertiary hyperparathyroidism occasionally occurs after transplantation, resulting in hypercalcemia.

  A. **Etiology:** Autonomous clones of unresponsive, hypersecretory parathyroid cells develop from the parathyroid hyperplasia of long-standing renal disease.

  B. **Diagnosis:** Serum PTH is elevated; hypercalcemia, hypophosphatemia, and elevated ALP are common.

  C. **Imaging studies:** may include ultrasound, ^{99m}Tc sestamibi, or 4D CT scan

  D. **Surgical treatment:** When persistent longer than 12 months following transplantation, THPT is treated by subtotal parathyroidectomy or total parathyroidectomy with autotransplantation.

ADRENAL GLAND

Overview

  I. **Embryology:** consists of two distinct parts, the **cortex** and the **medulla**, each of which has a different embryologic origin

  A. **Medulla:** From ectodermal cells of neural crest origin; other **extra-adrenal medullary tissue** can be found in the paraganglia,

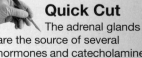

Quick Cut
The adrenal glands are the source of several hormones and catecholamines and play a key role in blood pressure regulation.

in the organ of Zuckerkandl just below the origin of the inferior mesenteric artery, and in the mediastinum.

   B. Adrenal cortex: derived from mesodermal cells, which can occasionally become separated and form **adrenocortical rests** and are most commonly found in the ovary or testis

II. **Anatomy:** Two adrenal glands, each lying on the medial aspect of the superior pole of a kidney; their normal combined weight is ~10 g.

   A. Histology: Three distinct areas can be recognized in the cortex.
      1. **Zona glomerulosa:** outer zone that produces mineralocorticoids (e.g., aldosterone)
      2. **Zona fasciculata:** produces cortisol and glucocorticoids
      3. **Zona reticularis:** inner zone where **androgens** and **estrogens** are made

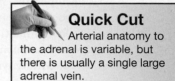

Quick Cut
Arterial anatomy to the adrenal is variable, but there is usually a single large adrenal vein.

   B. Arterial supply: from three primary sources—the phrenic artery, aorta, and renal arteries
   C. Venous drainage: Short (~1 cm) right adrenal vein drains into the vena cava, and the left adrenal vein joins the phrenic vein to empty into the left renal vein.
   D. Adrenal portal system: Venous blood from the cortex, containing high levels of glucocorticoids, drains into the medulla, helping to induce the enzyme phenylethanolamine-N-methyltransferase, which methylates norepinephrine to form epinephrine.

Adrenal Hormones and Catecholamines

I. **Steroid hormones (three classes):** glucocorticoids, mineralocorticoids, and sex steroids (androgens and estrogens)

   A. Glucocorticoids: Most important physiologically is **cortisol**, which has a diurnal variation, with the highest serum levels occurring around 6:00 A.M.

Quick Cut
Cortisol exerts a negative feedback on ACTH at the hypothalamic-pituitary level.

      1. **Regulation:** Adrenocorticotropic hormone (ACTH; corticotropin) is produced by the anterior pituitary gland. ACTH stimulates the production of cortisol by the adrenal.
         a. **Corticotropin-releasing factor (CRF):** produced by the hypothalamus and stimulates release of ACTH from the pituitary
         b. **Free cortisol:** is the active hormone
      2. **Metabolism:** Cortisol is metabolized in the liver by conjugation with glucuronide, which renders it water soluble for urinary excretion. The level of urinary 17-hydroxycorticosteroids reflects glucocorticoid production and metabolism.
   B. Mineralocorticoids: Major hormone produced is **aldosterone**.
      1. **Regulation:** Aldosterone production is regulated by the renin-angiotensin system and changes in plasma concentrations of sodium and potassium.
         a. **Renin:** released by the juxtaglomerular cells of the kidney in response to decreased blood pressure; converts **angiotensinogen** (made in the liver) to **angiotensin I**
         b. **Angiotensin I:** is converted to **angiotensin II** by **angiotensin-converting enzyme**, which is produced by endothelial cells
         c. **Angiotensin II:** stimulates the adrenal cortex to release **aldosterone**
         d. **Sympathetic nervous system (SNS):** can also stimulate release of aldosterone
      2. **Metabolism:** Aldosterone is metabolized in a similar manner to cortisol. It is excreted in the urine in small quantities and can be measured by radioimmunoassay.
   C. Sex steroids: Androgens and **estrogens** are produced in the **zona reticularis** of the adrenal cortex. The urinary level of 17-ketosteroids reflects androgen production. Estrogens can be measured directly in the urine.

II. **Catecholamines: Adrenal medulla** is the site of catecholamine production, including dopamine, norepinephrine, and epinephrine.

   A. Regulation: Catecholamine production is under the control of the SNS.
   B. Metabolism (Fig. 17-5): Levels of metanephrine, normetanephrine, vanillylmandelic acid (VMA), and catecholamines can be measured in the urine. Fractionated catecholamine metabolites may be measured in plasma.

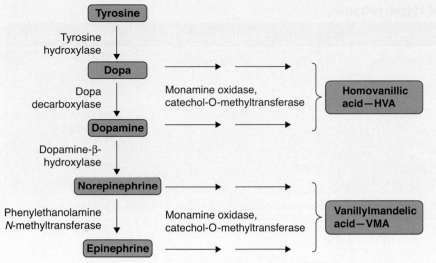

Figure 17-5: Schematic for catecholamine production. HVA, homovanillic acid. (From Philip PA, David PG. *Principles and Practice of Pediatric Oncology*, 6th ed. Baltimore: Lippincott Williams & Wilkins; 2010.)

Adrenocortical Insufficiency (Addison Disease)

I. **Primary disease:** results in diminished or absent function of the adrenal cortex caused by autoimmune disease, bilateral adrenal tuberculosis, adrenal fungal infections, or bilateral adrenal hemorrhage (secondary to meningococcal septicemia, postpartum, or in patients on anticoagulant therapy)

II. **Secondary disease:** atrophy of the adrenal cortex secondary to a decreased pituitary ACTH (Cushing syndrome) caused by ACTH suppression by corticosteroid drugs or primary pituitary pathology (Cushing disease)
    A. **Clinical presentation:** Symptoms include anorexia, malaise, weight loss, poor tolerance of stress, hypoglycemia, hypotension, and occasionally, skin hyperpigmentation.
    B. **Aldosterone deficiency:** results in volume depletion, hyponatremia, hyperkalemia, azotemia, and acidosis
    C. **Perioperative steroid replacement:** Handled on an individual basis and depends on the length of steroid therapy, the dosage taken, and the magnitude of the planned procedure. In general, the target is 100–150 mg of hydrocortisone IV daily for 2–3 days; preoperative oral dosage is resumed after 3 days.

Hypercortisolism

I. **Cushing syndrome:** results from chronically increased cortisol levels
    A. **ACTH dependent**
        1. **Pituitary source (Cushing disease):** accounts for 70% of the cases of endogenous Cushing syndrome and is more common in middle-aged women. Overproduction of ACTH by the pituitary results in bilateral adrenal hyperplasia; most come from a pituitary adenoma.
        2. **Ectopic Cushing syndrome:** accounts for 15% of the cases and is more common in older men
            a. **Cause:** ACTH is produced by an extra-adrenal, extrapituitary neoplasm, most commonly small cell carcinoma of the lung but can also occur with bronchial carcinoids, thymomas, and pancreas or liver tumors.
            b. **ACTH level:** quite high (>500 ng/mL)
    B. **ACTH independent:** Adrenal Cushing syndrome accounts for 15% of the cases.
        1. **Cause:** Excess cortisol produced autonomously by the adrenal cortex due to an adenoma, a carcinoma, or bilateral nodular dysplasia and ectopic cortisol-producing tumors; remaining

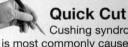

Quick Cut
Patients with Addison disease cannot tolerate the stress of surgery without receiving corticosteroid support.

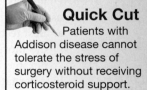

Quick Cut
Cushing syndrome is most commonly caused by suppression of the cortex secondary to exogenous corticosteroids.

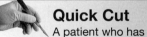

Quick Cut
A patient who has taken steroids regularly for any period during the past year is assumed to have inadequate adrenal reserve.

Table 17-4: Adrenal Causes of Hypertension

Name(s)	Hormone(s)	Adrenal Source	Diagnostic Test(s)
Aldosteronoma (Conn syndrome)	Aldosterone	Cortex: zona glomerulosa	Aldo/PRA Aldo suppression AVS
Cortisol-producing adenoma (Cushing syndrome)	Cortisol	Cortex: zona fasciculata	1 mg dexamethasone suppression test ACTH
Pheochromocytoma	Epinephrine Norepinephrine	Medulla	PFMs 24-hr catecholamines

Aldo, serum aldosterone; PRA, plasma renin activity; aldo suppression, aldosterone response to salt loading; AVS, adrenal vein sampling for aldosterone/cortisol; ACTH, adrenocorticotropic hormone; PFMs, plasma fractionated metanephrines.

adrenocortical tissue atrophies, and ACTH levels are low because of suppression by the excess cortisol.

2. **Clinical presentation:** Most common manifestations are listed in Table 17-4.
3. **Diagnosis:** Normal **diurnal rhythm** of cortisol secretion is usually lost. Cushing syndrome is a state of cortisol excess.
   a. **Best test for hypercortisolism:** elevated (>2 μg/dL) morning sample after a suppressing dose of 1 mg dexamethasone the night before
   b. **Alternative test:** Measure salivary cortisol at midnight, which is normally less than 1.6 ng/mL.
   c. **Elevated (>55 μg/day) 24-hour urinary free cortisol:** reliable index of hypercortisolism due to the increased renal clearance of unmetabolized cortisol

> **Quick Cut**
> No one test is conclusive for Cushing syndrome: Laboratory test results and clinical presentation must be considered together to make an accurate diagnosis.

4. **Pathogenesis:** Plasma ACTH level gives a good indication if Cushing syndrome is ACTH-dependent or independent.
   a. **Extremely low values:** found with adrenal Cushing syndrome due to the suppressive effects of cortisol
   b. **Very high levels:** occur with ectopic Cushing syndrome due to the autonomous ACTH production
   c. **Normal values:** Present in 50% of pituitary Cushing syndrome
   d. **Intermediate range:** Differentiating ectopic from pituitary Cushing syndrome can be difficult.
      (1) **High-dose dexamethasone suppression test:** Patient is given dexamethasone, 8 mg/day for 2 days, and the urine is collected for measurement of 17-hydroxycorticosteroids. In pituitary disease, the 17-hydroxycorticosteroid levels will usually decrease to less than 50% of normal, whereas they will show no suppression in the ectopic syndrome.
      (2) **Also helpful:** Corticotropin-releasing hormone (CRH) stimulation, jugular and peripheral ACTH levels, and plasma lipotrophic hormone may also be helpful.
5. **Localization of pituitary and ectopic tumors:** MRI and CT are the best tests to identify small pituitary adenomas; chest film usually shows an ectopic neoplasm; however, CT or MRI may be necessary.
6. **Localization of adrenal tumors:** CT or MRI can correctly identify greater than 90%, including adenomas less than 1 cm in diameter, carcinomas, and bilateral hyperplasia.
      (1) **Radioisotope scanning:** Radiocholesterol analogue **NP-59** (iodomethylnorcholesterol) can localize functioning adrenocortical tumors. This test is rarely used.
      (2) **Adrenal vein sampling for cortisol:** can also localize the source of cortisol production
7. **Curative therapy for pituitary Cushing syndrome**
   a. **Trans-sphenoidal resection of the tumor:** procedure of choice
   b. **Pituitary irradiation from an external source:** Has been effective in up to 80% of children. However, the cure rate is only about 15%–20% for adults.

   c. **Bilateral total adrenalectomy:** now reserved for cases in which no pituitary adenoma is found, radiation has failed, or when the patient cannot tolerate the prolonged radiation process

     (1) **Advantage:** immediate and complete control of the cushingoid state

     (2) **Disadvantages:** Increased morbidity and mortality. In 15% of the cases, an ACTH-secreting pituitary tumor develops (**Nelson syndrome**).

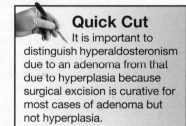

Quick Cut
Bilateral adrenalectomy produces a permanent Addisonian state.

  8. **Ectopic Cushing syndrome treatment:** Directed to the underlying neoplasm. Removal of the tumor is curative; however, because of the diffuse nature of small cell lung cancers, often only palliative therapy can be offered.

  9. **Adrenal Cushing syndrome treatment:** total adrenalectomy via laparoscopic or open techniques

   a. **Approach:** transabdominally or retroperitoneally via the flank or back

   b. **Large or aggressive lesions:** Open adrenalectomy via an anterior or flank approach is advisable for significant heterogeneity, nodal involvement, and local soft tissue or vascular invasion.

Quick Cut
Laparoscopic adrenalectomy has become the preferred approach for adrenal lesions less than 6 cm in size.

   c. **Partial resection:** If all of the malignant tissue cannot be removed, palliative therapy is improved.

  10. **Palliative chemotherapy: offered to those patients who have unresectable malignancies and to those undergoing radiation treatments**

   a. **Remission:** obtained in ~60% of the cases, but relapse is rapid after drug cessation

   b. **Agents:** may include bromocriptine and cyproheptadine or mitotane

Primary Hyperaldosteronism (Conn Syndrome)

  I. **Overview:** excess secretion of aldosterone by the adrenal as a result of a unilateral adenoma (85%), bilateral adenomas (5%), and hyperplasia (10%)

  II. **Types:** In primary hyperaldosteronism, plasma renin levels are normal or low. In the secondary form, the aldosterone increase is secondary to increased plasma renin from a decrease in pressure on the renal juxtaglomerular cells. Common causes include renal artery stenosis, malignant hypertension, and edematous states, such as congestive heart failure, cirrhosis, and the nephrotic syndrome.

Quick Cut
It is important to distinguish hyperaldosteronism due to an adenoma from that due to hyperplasia because surgical excision is curative for most cases of adenoma but not hyperplasia.

  III. **Signs and symptoms:** Increased aldosterone leads to hypertension, muscle weakness, fatigue, polyuria and polydipsia, and headaches.

  IV. **Diagnosis:** Spironolactone should be discontinued 6 weeks before testing, as it can affect laboratory values.

   A. **Plasma electrolytes:** Serum potassium value less than 3.5 mEq/L and urinary potassium excretion greater than 30 mEq/day supports a diagnosis of primary hyperaldosteronism.

   B. **Screening:** Concurrent serum aldosterone and plasma renin. Plasma aldosterone concentration (PAC) of greater than 20 ng/dL and a PAC/plasma renin activity (PRA) ratio of greater than 30 are diagnostic for aldosteronoma with ~90% sensitivity.

   C. **Confirmation:** Achieved by demonstrating inappropriate aldosterone secretion with salt loading, which involves a 24-hour urine collection for sodium and aldosterone after 3 days of a high-sodium diet. IV saline infusion test or captopril challenge test is also a reliable method but are not usually required.

  V. **Localization of adenomas**

   A. **High-resolution adrenal CT:** best test for localization of an adrenal tumor

   B. **Adrenal vein sampling (to lateralize the source of aldosterone production):** useful in patients when there is no adrenal abnormality on CT but technically difficult

    1. **Technique:** Percutaneous transfemoral cannulation of both adrenal veins is performed and IV ACTH (50 μg/hr) is administered. Simultaneous adrenal vein blood samples

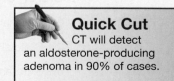

Quick Cut
CT will detect an aldosterone-producing adenoma in 90% of cases.

for aldosterone and cortisol are taken before and after ACTH injection, and their ratios are determined.

2. **Results:** PAC is markedly higher (at least four-fold) on the side of an adenoma, whereas there is little or no left–right gradient present in cases of bilateral adrenal hyperplasia.

VI. Surgical treatment: For patients who have primary hyperaldosteronism due to an adrenocortical adenoma, the treatment of choice is laparoscopic adrenalectomy; it is important to restore potassium levels before surgery.

VII. Medical management with spironolactone: Direct antagonism to aldosterone at the kidney tubule gradually leads to a reduction in blood pressure and a return to normal potassium levels; used in primary hyperaldosteronism caused by adrenal hyperplasia and in the preoperative restoration of normal serum potassium levels in patients who have adenomas.

> **Quick Cut**
> Favorable response to spironolactone in potassium and blood pressure may predict successful improvement after adrenalectomy.

Pheochromocytoma

I. Overview: Functionally active tumors that develop from the neural crest–derived chromaffin tissue; "10% rule" has been applied to these tumors (Table 17-5).

A. Characteristics: produce excess amounts of catecholamines; can occur as part of MEN2 and are usually bilateral in these patients

B. Malignancy: most of these tumors (90%) are benign; higher incidence of malignancy with extra-adrenal tumors

1. **Determination:** Histologic examination is not an accurate means; presence of metastases or direct invasion by the tumor determines malignancy.

2. **Cause:** Pheochromocytomas may be due to mutations in succinate dehydrogenase genes

II. Location: Ninety percent are found in the adrenal medulla; 10% of these are bilateral. Of the extra-adrenal tumors, most are found in the organs of Zuckerkandl, the extra-adrenal paraganglia, the urinary bladder, and the mediastinum.

III. Signs and symptoms: Hypertension results from the excess production of catecholamines. Other findings include attacks of headaches, sweating, palpitations, tremor, nervousness, weight loss, fatigue, abdominal or chest pains, polydipsia and polyuria, and convulsions.

> **Quick Cut**
> Hypertension from pheochromocytoma is intermittent in half of cases.

IV. Diagnosis: Urinary levels of metanephrine and VMA are the most reliable diagnostic screening tests.

A. Fractionated plasma and urinary catecholamine levels: can increase the accuracy of the diagnosis to virtually 100%

B. Provocative tests: Using histamine, tyramine, or glucagon is potentially hazardous and seldom used.

V. Localization of the tumor: CT and MRI have emerged as the most accurate localizing tools. Scintigraphy with ^{131}I-labeled *m*-iodobenzylguanidine (MIBG), which structurally resembles norepinephrine, has been helpful for small extra-adrenal tumors. Selective venous sampling is rarely necessary.

VI. Preparation for surgery: should include adrenergic blockade with both alpha- and beta-blockers

A. Adrenergic blockade: helpful to provide preoperative control of hypertension, reduce the risk of dramatic swings in blood pressure during surgery, and provide vasodilation, allowing restoration of a normal blood volume

> **Quick Cut**
> Alpha blockade should precede beta blockade in pheochromocytoma patients.

1. **Alpha blockade:** Achieved first; phenoxybenzamine therapy is begun 2 weeks before surgery, starting with 40 mg/day and adjusting the dose until hypertension is controlled.

Table 17-5: Ten-Percent Rule of Pheochromocytoma

10% Malignant	10% Multiple
10% Bilateral	10% Familial
10% Extra-adrenal	10% Children

    2. Beta blockade: Propranolol is started about 3 days before surgery, to control tachycardia, at a dose of 40 mg/day.

   B. Newer drug regimens to manage hypertension: selective alpha-1-adrenergic antagonists (terazosin and doxazosin) and calcium channel blockers (nifedipine and nicardipine)

VII. Operation: Patient should be monitored with an arterial and a central venous pressure line because of the potential for wide blood pressure changes; laparoscopic, transabdominal approach is preferred.

   A. Sporadic pheochromocytomas: Adrenalectomy is the procedure of choice.

   B. Malignant pheochromocytomas: Surgical excision of the tumor. Chemotherapy or therapeutic MIBG ^{131}I can be used for extensive metastatic disease.

   C. Component of MEN: Bilateral cortex adrenalectomy should be considered.

Adrenal Cysts and Other Adrenal Tumors

I. Incidental adrenal masses: Discovered at autopsy in up to 9% of patients. With the growing use of CT and MRI scanning, an increased number of these "incidentalomas" are being discovered during life.

   A. Routine screening: includes tests for pheochromocytoma (plasma fractionated metanephrines), hypercortisolism (low-dose overnight dexamethasone suppression test), and hyperaldosteronism (PAC/PRA ratio)

Quick Cut
Incidental adrenal masses must be assessed for hormonal production and malignancy.

   B. Imaging: Characteristics on CT indicate the likelihood of malignancy. Tumors greater than 5 cm are at risk of cancer and should be removed.

   C. Routine biopsy: should be avoided unless a patient has a prior risk of malignancy (e.g., lung or melanoma) and pheochromocytoma has been ruled out biochemically

II. Adrenocortical carcinoma: rare (incidence of 0.5–2 cases per million per year), very aggressive (most patients present with advanced disease), and produce frequent hormone overproduction syndromes (hypercortisolism, hyperaldosteronism, or virilization)

   A. Diagnosis: Contrast-enhanced CT of the abdomen and chest is important to diagnose local tumor invasion and metastatic lesions as well as to confirm a functioning contralateral kidney.

Quick Cut
Complete resection of locally confined tumor is the only chance for cure from adrenocortical carcinoma.

   B. Treatment: Surgical resection is the mainstay for all stages; however, distant or local spread is evident in 65% of cases at presentation.

   C. Prognosis: Poor; median survival following diagnosis for all patients is 18 months.

III. Adrenal cysts: occur infrequently

   A. Types: Most are either endothelial cysts (lymphangiomatous or angiomatous) or pseudocysts, resulting from hemorrhage into normal adrenal tissue or into an adrenal neoplasm. Rarely are they retention cysts or cystic adenomas.

   B. Symptoms: Large cyst can present as a palpable mass and can cause dull aching or GI symptoms due to pressure.

   C. Diagnosis: CT and MRI are the best methods available.

   D. Treatment: Because a neoplasm cannot be excluded, these cysts should be surgically excised.

TUMORS OF THE ENDOCRINE PANCREAS

Pathophysiology

I. Pancreatic neuroendocrine tumors (PNETs): Arise from normal neuroendocrine cells located in the pancreatic islets. Most are sporadic, but they can be hereditary.

II. Classification: according to their clinical virulence

   A. Well-differentiated tumors: have a slow-growing, indolent course

   B. Poorly differentiated tumors: high grade and may be very aggressive

III. Functionality: Most PNETs are nonfunctional; however, they may secrete a variety of hormones including insulin, gastrin, glucagon, and vasoactive intestinal peptide (VIP).

Insulinoma

I. **Pathogenesis:** Tumor originating from the beta cells of the pancreatic islets that releases abnormally high amounts of insulin. Most are solitary and benign adenomas; ~10% are malignant with the potential to metastasize.

II. **Clinical presentation:** Hypoglycemia may result in bizarre behavior, unconscious episodes, palpitations, nervousness, and other symptoms of sympathetic discharge.

III. **Diagnosis:** Have the patient fast for 72 hours then measure the insulin and glucose levels. Measurement of elevated insulin C peptide and sulfonylurea in blood is used to identify iatrogenic insulin and oral hypoglycemic overdose, respectively.

IV. **Surgical treatment:** based on preoperative localization of the tumor, which may be detectable on CT or MRI
   A. **Endoscopic US:** best imaging test because most are less than 1.5 cm
   B. **Percutaneous catheterization (of the portal vein with serial insulin measurements):** can localize the tumor to the head, body, and tail
   C. **Surgical resection:** Only curative treatment; options are enucleation or distal pancreatectomy.
   D. **Surgical exploration (of the entire pancreas):** Often needed to identify a small radiographically occult insulinoma. Intraoperative US is helpful.
   E. **Extent:** When islet cell hyperplasia is present, an 80%–90% subtotal pancreatectomy will usually control the symptoms; if the tumor is not localized, blind pancreatectomy should be avoided.

> **Quick Cut**
> The Whipple triad includes (1) episodes of neuroglycopenic symptoms (abnormal mentation, anxiety, irritability, diaphoresis, tremulousness, fatigue) precipitated by fasting; (2) hypoglycemia during the episodes, usually with blood glucose levels less than 60 mg/dL; and (3) relief of symptoms by glucose administration.

> **Quick Cut**
> An increased insulin level in the presence of a low glucose level (insulin-to-glucose ratio greater than 0.25) effectively confirms an insulinoma.

Gastrinoma (Zollinger-Ellison Syndrome)

I. **Pathogenesis:** Neuroendocrine tumors that arise from enteroendocrine cells of the pancreas or intestine (duodenum); most gastrinomas are sporadic but may be a component of MEN type I and can precede development of hyperparathyroidism.

II. **Clinical presentation:** Symptoms result from oversecretion of gastrin, the consequence of which is peptic ulceration due to high gastric acid secretion, which may cause abdominal pain, GI bleeding, perforation, or gastric outlet obstruction.

III. **Inhibition of pancreatic enzymes:** Leads to diarrhea, steatorrhea, and increased intestinal motility. Profound dehydration and malnutrition may be present.

IV. **Diagnosis:** Made based on the presence of the clinical syndrome, not whether the tumor stains for gastrin. Zollinger-Ellison syndrome (ZES) should be considered in any patient with an ulcer that is refractory to intensive treatment with antacids, H_2-receptor blockers, or proton pump inhibitors (PPIs); recurrent peptic ulcer after a standard surgical procedure for peptic ulcer disease; and peptic ulcer disease and refractory diarrhea.
   A. **Laboratory findings:** provide the diagnosis
      1. **Fasting gastrin level:** Greater than 1,000 pg/mL (normal <110 pg/mL) in the presence of gastric acid (gastric pH <2.0) makes a diagnosis of ZES.
      2. **Secretin stimulation testing:** May clarify the cause of modest elevations in gastrin. In ZES, an infusion of secretin will increase gastrin by 120–200 pg/mL or more.
   B. **Localization of the tumor:** Endoscopic US is the best test to identify small gastrinomas in the duodenal wall and pancreas.
      1. **CT scan and MRI:** best cross-sectional imaging studies
      2. **Somatostatin receptor scintigraphy (SRS) with 111-indium-penetreotide with SPECT:** less accurate than CT but used to determine metastatic sites

V. **Treatment:** must control gastric hyperacidity and should remove all gross tumor
   A. **Gastrinoma triangle:** defined by the junction of the cystic and common bile ducts superiorly, the junction of the second and

> **Quick Cut**
> Most (80%) gastrinomas are located in the **"gastrinoma triangle."**

third portions of the duodenum inferiorly, and the junction of the neck and body of the pancreas medially

    B. Standard surgical approach: Remove all identifiable tumors (frequently multifocal), transilluminate the duodenum, open the duodenum and resect submucosal tumors, and remove surrounding lymph nodes.

    C. ZES in the setting of MEN1: Uncommonly cured surgically; medical therapy is preferred until tumors reach 2 cm in size.

    D. Total gastrectomy: Previously the classic treatment for refractory ZES. It should be performed rarely.

VI. Prognosis: Good if the GI hyperacidity can be controlled; although two thirds of the causative tumors are malignant, they are very slow growing.

VIPoma (Pancreatic Cholera)

I. Overview: syndrome of severe secretory diarrhea (low [<50 mOSm/kg] osmotic gap in stool sample) due to hypersecretion of VIP

II. Clinical presentation: also known as **WDHA syndrome** because of **w**atery **d**iarrhea; **h**ypokalemia (with resultant profound muscular weakness due to the high potassium content in the stool), and **a**chlorhydria

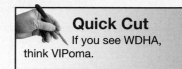
Quick Cut If you see WDHA, think VIPoma.

III. Pathogenesis: PNET is solitary in 80% of cases and is usually localized to the body or tail of the pancreas; 50% are malignant.

IV. Diagnosis: Most VIPomas are greater than 3 cm in size at diagnosis and may be effectively localized with CT scanning.

V. Treatment: Somatostatin receptor analogues (octreotide or lanreotide) are usually very effective in controlling the secretory diarrhea. Surgical excision of the primary tumor is indicated for localized disease.

VI. Prognosis: stage dependent and often poor due to the presence of metastasis at the time of diagnosis

Glucagonomas

I. Overview: rare PNETs that produce glucagonoma syndrome

II. Clinical presentation: Symptoms of glucagonoma syndrome include necrolytic migratory erythema (NME) (erythematous plaques on the face, perineum, and extremities), weight loss, diabetes mellitus, anemia, diarrhea, venous thrombosis, and neuropsychiatric symptoms.

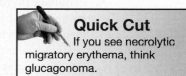
Quick Cut If you see necrolytic migratory erythema, think glucagonoma.

III. Pathogenesis: Due to tumors of the pancreatic alpha islet cells; most glucagonomas originate in the pancreatic tail and are malignant.

IV. Diagnosis: made by measurement of serum glucagon, which usually exceeds 500–1,000 pg/mL

    A. CT or MRI: used to localize the tumor

    B. Endoscopic US: useful to guide biopsy and evaluate for suspicious adenopathy

V. Treatment: Surgical resection of all localized gross disease, including liver metastases. As most patients (50%–100%) have metastatic disease, treatment is most often palliative. For patients with widespread disease, octreotide may be helpful.

MULTIPLE ENDOCRINE NEOPLASIA

Types (Three)

I. MEN type 1 (Table 17-6): rare autosomal dominant condition predisposing affected individuals to tumors of the parathyroid glands, anterior pituitary gland, and enteropancreatic endocrine cells

    A. Clinical definition: two or more primary MEN1 tumor types or the occurrence of a single tumor type in a member of a MEN1 kindred

    B. Cause: Inheritance of a mutated menin gene on chromosome 11q13. The exact function of this gene is unknown but it is thought to act as a tumor suppressor.

    C. Hyperparathyroidism: present in 90% or more of the patients usually before age 50 years, with most having multiple parathyroid gland adenomas

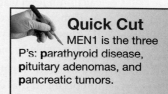
Quick Cut MEN1 is the three P's: parathyroid disease, pituitary adenomas, and pancreatic tumors.

    D. Pituitary adenomas: present in ~20%–60% of cases and are usually lactotroph adenomas

Table 17-6: Multiple Endocrine Neoplasia Syndromes

Syndrome	Clinical Presentation	Treatment	Gene/Test
MEN1	Primary hyperparathyroidism Prolactinoma Gastrinoma/insulinoma/PPoma/VIPoma/glucagonoma/ nonfunctional enteropancreatic tumor	Parathyroidectomy Bromocriptine Pancreatectomy/duodenal tumor enucleation	Menin
MEN2A	Medullary thyroid cancer Pheochromocytoma Primary hyperparathyroidism	Thyroidectomy/CLND Adrenalectomy Parathyroidectomy	RET
MEN2B	Medullary thyroid cancer Pheochromocytoma Ganglioneuroma	Thyroidectomy/CLND Adrenalectomy None	RET

MEN, multiple endocrine neoplasia; PP, pancreatic polypeptide; VIP, vasoactive intestinal peptide; CLND, central cervical lymph node dissection; RET, rearranged during transfection tyrosine kinase proto-oncogene.

- E. **Enteropancreatic tumors (PNET):** present in up to 80% of patients
    1. **Common:** Gastrinoma is the most common symptomatic tumor and occurs in up to 60% of MEN1 patients. Image-detected nonfunctioning tumors of the pancreas are as common.
    2. **Less common:** Symptomatic insulinoma, glucagonoma, and VIPoma can occur.
    3. **Metastasis:** Both functioning and nonfunctioning PNET may metastasize to liver; malignant PNET is the most common cause of MEN1-specific mortality.
- II. **MEN type 2A:** Comprises MTC, pheochromocytoma, and, in MEN 2A, parathyroid hyperplasia. MEN2 syndromes are caused by mutation of the RET gene, which maps to 10q11.2 and acts as a dominant oncogene.
    - A. **Medullary thyroid carcinoma:** Occurs in all patients; it is usually multifocal and preceded by nonmalignant hyperplasia of the C cells. Serum calcitonin levels are increased.
    - B. **Pheochromocytomas:** ~40% of patients; often bilateral, asynchronous, and usually benign; often presenting later than medullary thyroid cancer
    - C. **Parathyroid hyperplasia (with consequent hyperparathyroidism):** develops in 60% of patients with MEN 2A and is often milder than the parathyroid hyperplasia of MEN 1
- III. **MEN type 2B:** as in MEN 2A, medullary thyroid carcinoma and pheochromocytoma
    - A. **Features:** marfanoid body habitus and the development of multiple neuromatous mucosal nodules
    - B. **Presentation:** first or second decade of life with a much more aggressive course

Diagnosis

- I. **MEN1:** Hyperparathyroidism in MEN1 is typically asymptomatic and is usually detected by laboratory abnormalities (calcium and PTH).
    - A. **Clinical presentation:** Patients with MEN1 may present with symptoms of peptic ulceration related to the pancreatic gastrinoma or with symptoms related to the pituitary tumor.
    - B. **Genetic testing:** Mutations in menin testing is available to any index patient with clinical MEN1 and all first-degree relatives of known MEN1 mutation carriers.
    - C. **Asymptomatic biochemical screening:** involves calcium and may include other more detailed hormonal screening for gastrin, fasting glucose, insulin, insulinlike growth factor 1, prolactin, and chromogranin A
- II. **MEN2A:** Should be suspected in any patient with MTC; patient should be referred for genetic counseling and testing for mutation of the RET proto-oncogene. Finding of an increased serum calcitonin level leads to the diagnosis.
    - A. **Hyperparathyroidism:** usually detected by increases in the serum calcium and PTH levels
    - B. **Pheochromocytomas or adrenal medullary hyperplasia:** may be asymptomatic but should be detectable by biochemical screening
- III. **MEN2B:** Most patients are diagnosed in early childhood; because it is aggressive, early diagnosis is important so that effective treatment can begin promptly. Diagnosis is similar to that for MEN2A. The early appearance of mucosal neuromas and the marfanoid body habitus aids diagnosis.

Treatment

I. **MEN1:** PHPT in MEN1 involves all glands, usually asymmetrically. Surgery is not curative but parathyroidectomy may reduce circulating PTH. Choice of approach is largely based on surgeon training and experience.

    A. **Subtotal (3.5 gland) parathyroidectomy:** Leaving a normal-sized well-vascularized remnant of parathyroid tissue is a common approach.

    B. **Total parathyroidectomy (with nondominant forearm parathyroid autotransplantation):** may also be performed

    C. **PNETs (located within the pancreas and duodenum):** Resection is performed to reduce threat of malignant spread and to reduce hormonal symptoms. Resection of nonfunctioning PNETs should be considered with greater than 2 cm lesion.

> **Quick Cut**
> Autotransplantation of parathyroid tissue to the forearm has the advantage of avoiding repeat neck surgery if recurrence develops.

        1. **ZES:** enucleation of the tumor located in the gastrinoma triangle

        2. **Insulinoma:** enucleation of tumors in the pancreatic head and may include distal subtotal pancreatectomy

    D. **Pituitary tumors:** Usually treated medically with bromocriptine. Trans-sphenoidal hypophysectomy may be needed in some cases.

II. **MEN2A:** Patients with known MEN2A–associated RET mutations should receive prophylactic total thyroidectomy, which is curative.

    A. **Pheochromocytoma or adrenal medullary hyperplasia:** Adrenalectomy (preferable laparoscopic) before thyroidectomy because these hormone-producing disorders can lead to hypertensive crises during thyroidectomy.

    B. **Hyperparathyroidism:** can be treated at the time of total thyroidectomy by either subtotal parathyroidectomy or total parathyroidectomy and forearm parathyroid autotransplantation

III. **MEN2B:** Treated similarly with MEN2A. Because MEN2B assumes such an aggressive course, prompt and effective treatment is important.

THYMUS GLAND

Overview

I. **Introduction:** Thymus is the origin of a variety of tumors and is significantly involved in the development of cellular immunity.

    A. **Cortex:** consists primarily of lymphocytes, which appear to migrate to the medulla and then emigrate from the thymus

    B. **Two limbs:** extend into the neck and are often associated with the inferior parathyroid glands

II. **Functions:** Essential for the development of cellular immunity, which controls delayed hypersensitivity reactions and transplant rejection. Histologic abnormalities in the thymus (e.g., lymphoid hyperplasia or thymic tumors) are frequently found in association with autoimmune diseases.

Myasthenia Gravis

I. **Overview:** Autoimmune disease of neuromuscular transmission that causes skeletal muscle weakness. The most common symptoms are ptosis, double vision, dysarthria, dysphagia, nasal speech, and weakness of the arms and legs.

> **Quick Cut**
> Myasthenia gravis exacerbations may be precipitated by upper respiratory infections.

II. **Normal neuromuscular transmission:** Acetylcholine (ACh) is produced at the nerve terminal of the myoneural junction and binds to receptor sites on the muscle endplates, which triggers muscle contraction.

III. **Neuromuscular transmission in myasthenia gravis:** ACh receptor antibodies develop, resulting in reduced muscle contraction.

IV. **Treatment:** Sustained improvement is achieved with medication in only 33% of patients without surgery and in 85% of patients after thymectomy.

    A. **Medical treatment:** Patients respond to drugs that stimulate the neuromuscular junction, such as neostigmine and pyridostigmine.

    B. **Surgical treatment:** Removal of the thymoma is advised, although the effect on the myasthenia is unpredictable. However, even in patients without thymic tumors, thymectomy appears to be the treatment of choice.

Study Questions for Part V

Directions: *Each of the numbered items in this section is followed by several possible answers. Select the ONE lettered answer that is BEST in each case.*

1. A 40-year-old man has a subtotal thyroidectomy performed for Graves disease. Several hours later, he complains of difficulty breathing. On examination, he has stridor and a markedly swollen, tense neck wound. What should be one of the first steps in the management of this patient?

   A. Intubate with an endotracheal tube.
   B. Perform a tracheostomy.
   C. Control the bleeding site in the operating room.
   D. Open the wound to evacuate the hematoma.
   E. Aspirate the hematoma.

2. A 50-year-old hypertensive man has definitive biochemical evidence of a pheochromocytoma. CT scan and MRI do not reveal any abnormalities, and MIBG scanning is not readily available. What should be the next step in the management of this patient?

   A. Abdominal exploration
   B. Continued clinical observation
   C. Mediastinoscopy
   D. Selective venous sampling
   E. Mediastinal exploration

3. A 55-year-old woman with progressive but episodic muscle weakness is diagnosed as having myasthenia gravis. Her chest radiograph is normal and reveals no evidence of mediastinal mass or tumor. What is the most definitive treatment that can be offered to this patient?

   A. Prednisone
   B. Neostigmine
   C. Thymectomy
   D. Plasmapheresis
   E. Atropine

4. A first-degree relative of a patient found to have advanced MTC is referred for further evaluation. Which screening measure is the choice for detection of medullary thyroid pathology?

   A. Careful physical examination
   B. Serum calcitonin level
   C. Stimulated serum calcitonin level (calcium and pentagastrin)
   D. Gastrin level
   E. Carcinoembryonic antigen (CEA) level

5. If a first-degree relative of a patient with MEN2A syndrome is found to have medullary pathology requiring surgical exploration of the thyroid gland, what should the preoperative screening include?

   A. Serum cortisol level
   B. Fasting glucose and insulin
   C. CT scan of the head
   D. Urinary aldosterone and renin
   E. Urinary VMA and metanephrines

6. A 60-year-old female patient has a workup for episodic symptoms of palpitations, nervousness, and bizarre behavior, all of which tend to occur during fasting states. Biochemically, she is diagnosed as having an insulinoma. What is the best choice for localizing this tumor?

   A. CT scan
   B. MRI
   C. Selective arteriography
   D. Percutaneous catheterization of the portal vein with selective venous sampling
   E. Surgical exploration and intraoperative ultrasound

7. A 55-year-old female patient is evaluated for new onset of diabetes mellitus. Her medical history is largely unremarkable. Her physical examination is unrevealing except for the presence of an erythematous skin rash. Her further evaluation should include an investigation of the possibility of which of the following?

   A. Insulinoma
   B. Glucagonoma
   C. Gastrinoma
   D. Carcinoid tumor
   E. Pancreatic cholera

8. A 23-year-old woman has a palpable mass in her left breast. Ultrasound suggests a cystic lesion. On aspiration, some dark fluid is retrieved, but the mass does not completely resolve. What is the next step in treatment?

   A. Observation
   B. NSAIDs
   C. Repeat aspiration
   D. Excision
   E. Simple mastectomy

9. The best treatment for ductal carcinoma in situ is:

   A. Observation and reassurance
   B. Lumpectomy
   C. Partial mastectomy with radiation
   D. Simple mastectomy
   E. Modified radical mastectomy

10. The nerve that supplies the latissimus dorsi muscle and may be injured during axillary node dissection is:

    A. Long thoracic
    B. Thoracodorsal
    C. C7
    D. Intercostal brachial
    E. Lateral brachial

11. A 30-year-old man has hypertension and has complaints of weakness and fatigue. His physical examination is unremarkable. Routine labs are normal except for a potassium of 3.0 mEq/L. He undergoes abdominal CT scan, which demonstrates a 3-cm left adrenal mass. The best next step in management is:

    A. MRI of the abdomen with T2 imaging
    B. Urinary cortisol monitoring
    C. Beta blockade
    D. Adrenocorticotropic hormone stimulation
    E. Laparoscopic adrenalectomy

12. A 56-year-old woman is undergoing surgery for a left-sided parathyroid adenoma. The initial parathyroid level is 100 pg/mL. After incision, the inferior gland is identified and removed, and the parathyroid level at 10 minutes falls to 90 pg/mL. The next step is:

    A. Closure of incision
    B. Monitoring of 20-minute PTH levels
    C. Exploration of the left superior gland
    D. Total parathyroidectomy with autotransplantation
    E. Stat calcium measurement

13. Which of the following is not associated with an increased incidence of invasive ductal carcinoma of the breast?

    A. Sclerosing adenosis
    B. Lobular carcinoma in situ
    C. Atypical ductal hyperplasia
    D. Epithelial hyperplasia
    E. Papillomatosis

Questions 14–17

Match the correct treatment with each inflammatory or infectious process of the breast.

14. Mastitis   A. Surgical drainage

15. Abscess   B. Excision of sinus tract

16. Chronic subareolar abscess   C. Antibiotics

17. Mondor disease   D. NSAIDs

18. The preferred treatment for new-onset pubertal gynecomastia is:

    A. Radical excision with latissimus dorsi flap
    B. Observation
    C. Suction lipectomy
    D. Tamoxifen therapy
    E. Simple mastectomy

Questions 19–20

A 65-year-old woman with no other significant past medical history presents with a large mass in the right breast. The mass measures approximately 6 cm in diameter and appears to be fixed to the chest wall. In addition, bulky adenopathy is present in the right axillary region. The patient states that the mass has been enlarging for the last several years.

19. Following mammography, what should be the next step in this patient's evaluation?

    A. FNA
    B. Incisional or core biopsy
    C. Excisional biopsy
    D. Modified radical mastectomy
    E. Radical mastectomy

The diagnosis for this patient is invasive ductal carcinoma. A mammogram reveals no other lesions in the right breast and no abnormalities in the left breast. A chest radiograph, bone scan, and liver function tests are normal.

20. What should the next step in the management of this patient involve?

    A. Neoadjuvant chemotherapy

    B. Radiation therapy to the breast and axilla

    C. Radical mastectomy

    D. Modified radical mastectomy

    E. Simple mastectomy

Answers and Explanations

1. **The answer is D** (Chapter 17, Thyroid Dysfunction Requiring Surgery, Graves Disease, V E 2). Postoperative bleeding after thyroidectomy can cause airway compromise due to tracheal compression. The first step should be to open the wound to evacuate the hematoma, followed by a return to the operating room to control the bleeding site. Attempts to perform either endotracheal intubation or tracheostomy may be difficult until the external compression of the hematoma is relieved.

2. **The answer is D** (Chapter 17, Adrenal Gland, Pheochromocytoma, V). Although 90% of pheochromocytomas are located in the adrenal glands, they can occur in any tissue that is derived from neuroectoderm. When CT scan and MRI do not identify a tumor, MIBG scanning can be helpful; however, this is not always available. Selective measurements of catecholamines drawn at various levels from the vena cava and its major branches should be obtained before surgical exploration.

3. **The answer is C** (Chapter17, Thymus Gland, Myasthenia Gravis, IV B). Myasthenia gravis is an autoimmune disease of neuromuscular transmission that causes skeletal muscle weakness. Parasympathomimetic drugs have been found to improve muscle strength in these patients. Prednisone has also been used with some success because of the autoimmune nature of this disease. Plasmapheresis may be effective in preparing the patient preoperatively. The treatment of choice for all forms of myasthenia, except purely ocular, appears to be thymectomy. An increased percentage of patients have permanent remission. The response to medication is improved in patients who do not achieve a complete remission.

4. **The answer is B** (Chapter 17, Thyroid Dysfunction Requiring Surgery, Thyroid Neoplasms, VI A 2). All first-degree relatives of patients with MTC should be screened for this disorder because it can occur in a familial pattern. Physical examination of the thyroid gland should be performed for the detection of any nodules. An increased serum calcitonin or an increased stimulated serum calcitonin test will also indicate underlying medullary pathology, either hyperplasia or carcinoma. The stimulated tests will detect disease at an earlier, more curable stage. Increased gastrin levels are associated with ZES and are not part of this MEN type 2 syndrome. CEA is elevated in some GI malignancies.

5. **The answer is E** (Chapter17, Adrenal Gland, Pheochromocytoma, IV). MTC may present as a sporadic or familial form associated with MEN type 2A or 2B. Both are associated with pheochromocytomas. If a pheochromocytoma is present, it should be diagnosed and treated first to avoid the morbidity of cervical exploration in a patient with untreated pheochromocytoma. Urinary VMA and metanephrines should be evaluated preoperatively.

6. **The answer is E** (Chapter 17, Tumors of the Endocrine Pancreas, Insulinoma, IV). The patient has had a definitive biochemical diagnosis of insulinoma. These tumors can be present anywhere in the pancreas. Because they are usually small in size, arteriography, CT, and MRI are less sensitive than they would be for larger tumors. With careful surgical exploration and intraoperative ultrasound, approximately 90% of these tumors can be localized at the time of surgery.

7. **The answer is B** (Chapter 17, Tumors of the Endocrine Pancreas, Glucagonomas, II). Glucagon-producing tumors of the pancreas secrete glucagon in large amounts. Patients tend to present with new onset of diabetes mellitus (hyperglycemia). Affected individuals also characteristically have a migratory erythematous skin rash.

8. **The answer is D** (Chapter 16, Breast Evaluation, Biopsy, II). Cysts that do not resolve completely on aspiration should be treated as solid lesions and excised. NSAIDs are useful in Mondor disease (thrombophlebitis). Repeat aspiration may be attempted, but a cyst that recurs once is likely to recur again. Mastectomy is too radical a therapy.

9. **The answer is C** (Chapter 16, Malignant Diseases, Noninvasive Breast Cancer, I A). Excision with clear margins is the standard of care, and radiation reduces the risk of recurrence by 50%.

10. **The answer is B** (Chapter 16, Malignant Diseases, Treatment, I B 2 c). The thoracodorsal supplies the latissimus. The long thoracic supplies serratus anterior, and injury produces a winged scapula.

11. **The answer is E** (Chapter 17, Adrenal Gland, Primary Hyperaldosteronism [Conn Syndrome], VI). The patient has signs and symptoms of aldosteronoma and imaging consistent with a left adrenal adenoma. Further cross-sectional imaging is unnecessary. Cortisol testing is used for suspicion of adrenal hyperfunction or insufficiency but is not needed in this case. Beta blockade may be useful for management of hypertension but would not be indicated in the initial management of pheochromocytoma. In practice, an aldosterone level could be checked preoperatively to confirm the diagnosis, then laparoscopic left adrenalectomy.

12. **The answer is C** (Chapter 17, Parathyroid Glands, Hyperparathyroidism, I F 1). The patient has evidence of loss of parathyroid tissue but not a sufficient response to consider the abnormal gland removed. It is expected that there is both a 50% reduction in the PTH level as well as a movement into the normal range. Given that this did not occur, exploration of the remaining glands is the next step. Total parathyroidectomy is overly aggressive, and monitoring of additional lab values of PTH or calcium does not alter the decision-making process.

13. **The answer is A** (Chapter 16, Benign Breast Disease, Benign Lesions, III G). Epithelial hyperplasia, atypical ductal hyperplasia, and papillomatosis are proliferative lesions of the breast that carry an increased risk of invasive ductal carcinoma of the breast. Papillomatosis is simply a description of the pattern the cells assume (papillary). Lobular carcinoma in situ of the breast carries an increased risk bilaterally for an invasive breast cancer, which can be ductal or lobular. Sclerosing adenosis is a proliferation of the acini that appear to invade, but it is not a malignant or premalignant lesion.

14–17. **The answers are 14-C, 15-A, 16-B, and 17-D** (Chapter 16, Benign Breast Disease, Infectious and Inflammatory Breast Diseases, I–IV). Cellulitis of the breast (mastitis) requires treatment with antibiotics to cover *Staphylococcus* and *Streptococcus* infection. An acute abscess requires surgical drainage. A chronic recurrent abscess requires excision of the sinus tract to avoid recurrence. Mondor disease is a phlebitis of the superficial veins, and although self-limited, treatment with NSAIDs can alleviate the discomfort.

18. **The answer is B** (Chapter 16, Malignant Diseases, Special Cases, II A 3). Gynecomastia represents breast growth in a male due to hormonal imbalance. The initial presentation during puberty should be observed, as the lesion often regresses. Symptomatic cases can be treated medically with tamoxifen or surgically with suction lipectomy. More aggressive surgery such as mastectomy is not warranted.

19–20. **The answers are 19-B** (Chapter 16, Breast Evaluation, Biopsy, I B) and **20-A** (Chapter 16, Invasive Breast Cancer, Treatment, V B). Although FNA can be performed, it may not be conclusive to warrant further treatment. A core-needle biopsy can easily be performed on a mass of this size. Excision is inappropriate in masses larger than 5 cm. Definitive surgical therapy should not be performed until after neoadjuvant chemotherapy is given.

Part VI

Special Subjects
Chapter Cuts and Caveats

CHAPTER 18

Head and Neck Surgery:

◆ The most common neck lesion is a reactive lymph node. All adults with a persistent neck mass have a malignancy until proven otherwise.
◆ Most head and neck cancers are squamous cell and are treated with surgery, radiation, or chemotherapy. Cosmetic and functional deficits may be frequent.
◆ Congenital lesions are abnormal variants of normal structures. Thyroglossal duct cysts are midline structures that rise and fall with swallowing. They should be resected if symptomatic, after making sure there is adequate residual thyroid tissue.
◆ Tonsillectomy was once an extremely common operation and is now reserved for those with repeated infections, as the risk of surgery outweighs the benefits for most patients.

CHAPTER 19

Bariatric Surgery:

◆ Obesity affects more than one third of Americans and an increasing percentage of children and adolescents. Obesity creates metabolic comorbidities and decreases life span.
◆ BMI is the most useful marker for obesity; people qualify for bariatric surgery with BMI greater than 40 kg/m^2 or 35 kg/m^2 with medical comorbidities.
◆ Bariatric procedures are classified as primarily restrictive or malabsorptive. Roux-en-Y gastric bypass is the most common operation and is a blend of the two. Gastric banding and sleeve gastrectomy are restrictive, and the duodenal switch operation is malabsorptive.
◆ Postoperative bariatric patients are susceptible to a variety of unique complications, including internal hernia, marginal ulceration, and nutritional deficiencies.
◆ Tachycardia in a postoperative patient is a surgical complication until proven otherwise. The patient must be assessed for anastomotic leak and DVT/PE.

CHAPTER 20

Minimal Access Surgery:

◆ Minimally invasive surgery relies on technology to decrease the size of the access incisions; visual cues largely replace tactile ones.
◆ The first steps in minimally invasive procedures are establishment of pneumoperitoneum and diagnostic laparoscopy.
◆ Pneumoperitoneum is an artificial state that has a mechanical (pressure) component that can mimic abdominal compartment syndrome. The use of carbon dioxide gas also creates an acidosis. This does not have a significant clinical impact for brief procedures in patients who have minimal physiologic compromise.

- Most general surgical procedures have minimally invasive options, including surgery on the gallbladder, appendix, intestines, and hernias. Robotic procedures are especially useful in anatomically confined cases, such as low pelvic surgery or prostatectomy.

CHAPTER 21

Surgical Oncology:

- Oncology is increasingly multidisciplinary. *Benign* and *malignant* refer to behavior, not outcomes—benign lesions may be fatal, and malignant processes may be indolent.
- Oncogenes drive the cell cycle; tumor suppressor genes provide a natural checkpoint. Dysregulation of either may lead to cancer.
- Imaging, serum markers, and genomics can all provide diagnosis well in advance of clinical symptoms. Screening can reduce mortality in breast, colon, cervical, and prostate cancer.
- The TNM system provides a common language to group and stage tumors.

CHAPTER 22

Trauma and Burns:

- Primary survey: ABCs. Remember the ABCDE of trauma: airway, breathing, circulation, disability, everything else.
- Hemodynamically unstable patients should not go to the CT scanner. Intubate all patients with a low GCS or those with massive injury.
- Fatal hemorrhage occurs in five major locations: chest, abdomen, retroperitoneum, thigh, and externally.
- Hypovolemia is the most common cause of hypotension in trauma and is treated with fluid resuscitation. However, tension pneumothorax and cardiac tamponade cause hypotension, are not associated with hypovolemia, and are not treated with fluid resuscitation. They should be considered early during resuscitation.
- FAST exam reliably detects free fluid and can provide an early, safe means of diagnosing the need for operation.
- Initial resuscitation of burn victims may be massive: use 4 mL/kg/% BSA over the first 24 hours. Use the rule of 9's to estimate BSA.
- Hypothermia may cause coagulopathy and resultant bleeding after trauma.
- Simple pneumothorax usually presents with dyspnea and is not emergent, whereas a tension pneumothorax presents with hypotension and requires emergent decompression.

CHAPTER 23

Organ Transplantation:

- Calcineurin inhibitors have considerable nephrotoxicity.
- Organ transplantation is considered for irretrievable end-organ dysfunction.
- The main complications of immunosuppression are susceptibility to infections and the development of malignancy.
- Kidney transplants are the most successful solid organ transplants. Although dialysis is a replacement option, patients live longer with kidney transplants than on dialysis; therefore, all end-stage renal patients are considered transplant candidates. Although outcomes are superior with living donors, deceased donors and extended criteria donors have produced acceptable results.
- Because no alternative exists to replace a dysfunctional liver, transplantation remains the only option for severe liver failure but is fraught with complications due to the extent of disease in most of these patients.
- Most acute rejection occurs in the first year after transplant and may be related to infection or inadequate immunosuppression. The cornerstones of immunosuppression are corticosteroids, but immune modulators have been developed that affect all aspects of T-cell function and differentiation.
- Islet cell transplantation may provide the cure of diabetes without the heavy immunosuppression of whole organ transplant. To date, results are promising.

CHAPTER 24

Pediatric Surgery:

◆ Pediatric surgery represents a separate discipline, since the physiology of children differs from that of adults.

◆ Congenital hernias may be associated with other conditions and require careful assessment before repair. In general, umbilical hernias are not repaired, as they may close spontaneously. Inguinal hernias are repaired with high ligation of the sac. Diaphragmatic hernias are repaired but with caution, as pulmonary dysfunction may also be present.

◆ Many specific problems can arise within the neonatal GI tract. Malrotation and necrotizing enterocolitis may require urgent surgery and may result in long-term problems such as short gut syndrome.

◆ Failure to pass meconium in the first 24 hours suggests a diagnosis of Hirschsprung disease, which is confirmed on rectal biopsy.

◆ Projectile vomiting in a 1-month old infant may represent hypertrophic pyloric stenosis. Treatment is a surgical pyloromyotomy after correction of any metabolic derangements.

◆ Wilms tumor and neuroblastoma are the two most common childhood solid tumors.

◆ Gastroschisis is an abdominal wall defect with no sac and has rare associated congenital anomalies.

◆ Omphalocele has a sac and has a high association with congenital anomalies.

◆ Esophageal atresia is most commonly a proximal esophageal pouch and distal tracheoesophageal (TE) fistula and is associated with cardiac and VACTERL anomalies.

◆ Intestinal malrotation usually presents with bilious vomiting.

◆ Duodenal atresia shows an abdominal double-bubble sign, is corrected by duodenoduodenostomy and is commonly associated with other congenital anomalies.

◆ Jejunal and more distal bowel atresia occur from in-utero vascular accidents and have few associated congenital anomalies.

Chapter 18

Head and Neck Surgery

Andrea Hebert and Jeffrey S. Wolf

 COMPONENTS OF THE HEAD AND NECK EXAM

General

I. **Breathing:** Note whether the patient is breathing comfortably and the presence of stridor, stertor, or the use of accessory muscles.

II. **Voice:** Note the quality of the patient's voice (e.g., hoarseness or muffled or breathy qualities) and any dysarthria.

III. **Swallow:** Note if the patient is able to tolerate secretions or if he or she is drooling.

> **Quick Cut**
> *Stridor* is a high-pitched sound produced by turbulent flow through a partially obstructed upper airway. *Stertor* is lower pitched, snoring-type sound.

Head

I. **General**

A. **Trauma:** visible ecchymosis, edema, bony abnormalities, or lacerations

B. **Masses/lesions:** skin lesions, biopsy sites or surgical scars, edema, firmness, induration, fluctuance, or erythema

II. **Eyes**

A. **Examination:** Be sure to note extraocular motion and pupillary response and to report nystagmus.

B. **Tests**

1. **Visual acuity:** if the patient is complaining of any change in vision

2. **Visual field test:** if the patient is complaining of diplopia

III. **Ears:** Standard office assessment of hearing includes the Weber and Rinne tests.

A. **Weber test:** Tuning fork is struck and placed on the midline of the patient's head to determine if the sound lateralizes and identifies unilateral hearing loss.

B. **Rinne test:** involves placing the vibrating tuning fork on the mastoid process and comparing the perception to that of the sound directly adjacent to the ear; also helps discriminate between conductive and sensorineural hearing loss

> **Quick Cut**
> Perform a Weber and Rinne exam if the patient has any otologic complaints.

C. **Auricle:** Note any deformity, tenderness to palpation of the tragus or mastoid, or tenderness with tugging of the pinna.

D. **External auditory canal:** Note any canal stenosis, debris, erythema, or otorrhea.

E. **Tympanic membrane:** Note whether intact, the presence and characteristics of fluid behind the tympanic membrane, presence of middle ear masses, and whether the membrane retracts.

IV. **Nose:** Perform anterior rhinoscopy on all patients.

A. **Septum:** Examine for deviations or lesions.

B. **Nasal cavity:** Note inferior turbinate hypertrophy, nasal masses or polyps, and the presence of rhinorrhea.

V. **Oral cavity/oropharynx:** Note any masses or lesions and specify the color, friability, and tenderness. Note any ulceration and palpate with a gloved finger to determine softness or firmness.

    A. **Teeth:** Note the quality of the dentition and the presence of any tenderness.

    B. **Assess:** Look for any erythema, edema, palatal asymmetry, or tonsillar deviation. Note any uvular deviation and trismus.

VI. **Larynx:** Perform a laryngeal mirror exam if not performing fiberoptic laryngoscopy.

VII. **Neck:** Palpate for lymphadenopathy or thyroid masses. Note surgical scars, crepitus, or decreased range of motion.

VII. **Neurologic:** Perform a complete cranial nerve (CN) exam.

BENIGN LESIONS OF THE HEAD AND NECK

Overview

I. **Reactive lymph node:** most common neck mass and most often secondary to bacterial or viral infections

II. **Malignancy:** Most neck masses in children are benign; in adults, neck masses are more likely to be malignant.

Workup for Acquired Lesions

I. **Detailed history:** Obtain details about the following.

    A. **Family history:** malignancy and personal history of cancer

    B. **Risk factors:** smoking; alcohol consumption; exposure to radiation, sawdust, or other potential carcinogens; and exposure to human papillomavirus (HPV) 16 or 18

    C. **Recent illnesses:** upper respiratory infection (URI), sinusitis, or tonsillitis; otitis or conjunctivitis; and dental problems

II. **Physical examination:** See earlier discussion.

III. **Laboratory tests:** may include tuberculin test for tuberculosis, heterophil titer (monospot test) for mononucleosis, thyroid function tests or thyroid scan, serologic tests for syphilis, and viral titers (especially for Epstein-Barr virus, which is associated with nasopharyngeal carcinoma and Burkitt lymphoma)

IV. **Radiologic studies:** may include soft tissue radiographs of the neck, barium swallow, chest x-ray, or scanning procedures such as computed tomography (CT) and magnetic resonance imaging (MRI)

V. **Endoscopy:** indicated if a primary neoplasm is suspected

VI. **Treatment:** depends on the findings (Fig. 18-1)

    A. **Antibiotics:** if a bacterial infection is suspected

    B. **Consultation:** may be helpful

        1. **Dental consultation:** if the teeth seem to be a source

        2. **Dermatology consultation:** if skin lesions are present

    C. **Surgical biopsy:** may be indicated if a mass does not shrink significantly over 6 weeks and a source of infection is not found

        1. **Fine-needle aspiration (FNA):** used with suspected malignancy

        2. **Excisional biopsy:** indicated for persistent cervical adenopathy

NECK ABSCESSES

Types

I. **Peritonsillar abscesses (quinsy):** most common abscesses in the parapharyngeal space (Table 18-1)

    A. **Cause:** arise as a complication of acute tonsillitis

    B. **Clinical presentation:** Ipsilateral palatal edema, contralateral deviation of the uvula, "hot potato" voice, trismus, and dysphagia. The patient may have only a low-grade fever or be afebrile.

Quick Cut
The most common neck mass is a reactive lymph node.

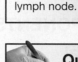
Quick Cut
The "rule of 7's" provides a guide for etiology of neck masses: A mass that has been present for 7 days is inflammatory; 7 months, malignant; 7 years, congenital.

Quick Cut
Scrofula is mycobacterial lymphadenitis in the neck.

Quick Cut
Endoscopic biopsy and radiologic studies should precede any open biopsy of the neck.

Quick Cut
FNA can diagnose carcinoma but is usually inadequate to define lymphoma.

Quick Cut
A patient presenting with fever and an erythematous, painful, fluctuant neck mass most probably has an abscess.

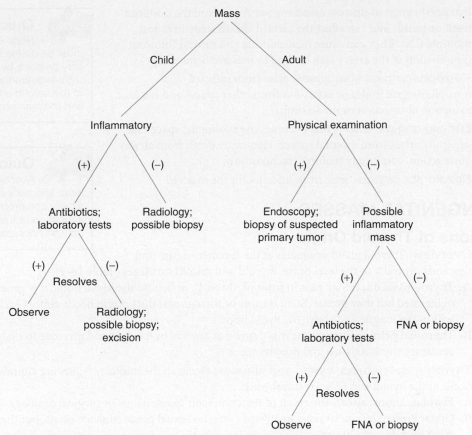

Figure 18-1: Basic algorithm for treatment of head and neck cancer. FNA, fine-needle aspiration.

Table 18-1: Neck Abscesses

Signs and Symptoms
Pain
Swelling
Dysphagia
Dyspnea
Leukocytosis
Fever
Air in soft tissue radiograph
Treatment
Airway protection
Incision and drainage
Antibiotics

II. **Parapharyngeal space abscesses:** Arise from the posterior teeth or tonsils and can affect the carotid sheath structures and multiple CNs. They can cause mediastinitis and carotid "blowout" (i.e., erosion of the artery wall leading to massive hemorrhage).

III. **Retropharyngeal abscesses:** arise from infected retropharyngeal nodes or extension from other spaces and can lead to airway obstruction or mediastinitis

IV. **Ludwig angina:** abscess that occupies the sublingual space that generally arises from a dental source. Can cause death from airway obstruction, commonly requires tracheostomy

V. **Bezold abscesses:** arise from infection in the mastoid

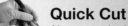

Quick Cut
Neck infections must be drained but should only be done by those familiar with neck anatomy owing to the carotid artery, airway, and the cranial nerves.

Quick Cut
Abscesses in the head and neck can cause airway compromise, and intubation or tracheostomy may be necessary.

CONGENITAL MASSES

Lesions of Thyroid Origin

I. **Overview:** Thyroid gland originates at the foramen cecum and descends centrally to the level of the thyroid and cricoid cartilages (Table 18-2).
  A. **Thyroglossal duct:** May pass in front of, through, or behind the hyoid bone; it is generally obliterated but may persist. Solid tumors of thyroglossal duct origin occur almost exclusively within the tongue and above the hyoid bone.
  B. **Thyroidal primordium:** Some may remain at any site in the duct and give rise to cysts, fistulas, accessory thyroid tissue, and neoplasms.

II. **Thyroglossal fistulas, cysts, and sinuses:** Occur in the midline; ~20% are suprahyoid, 15% occur at the hyoid, and 65% are infrahyoid.
  A. **Fistulas:** almost always the result of infection with spontaneous or surgical drainage
  B. **Cysts:** Present by age 10 years in 50% of cases; no sexual predominance exists, but they are most often found in caucasians.
    1. **Size:** usually measure 2–4 cm in diameter and gradually increase in size, although the size may fluctuate
    2. **Behavior:** rise and fall with the larynx during swallowing
  C. **Sinus tract:** may form as direct connection to the skin and result in persistent drainage
  D. **Treatment:** total surgical excision

Quick Cut
Imaging is important to ensure a normal thyroid gland is present elsewhere before excision of a thyroid rest.

III. **Thyroid rests:** may be lingual or may occur in the neck
  A. **Endotracheal ectopias:** may occur
  B. **Palpation:** of the normal position of the thyroid often reveals no evidence of thyroid tissue
  C. **Treatment:** dictated by the degree of obstruction and by the presence of other thyroid tissue
  D. **Thyroid scan:** Ensures that functional thyroid tissue exists in the usual location; 75% of patients have no other functional thyroid.

Branchial Cleft Anomalies

I. **Embryology:** In week 4, five ridges and grooves appear on the ventrolateral surface of the embryonic head that form the branchial arches and clefts, respectively, and the pharyngeal pouches develop internally at the same level as the external grooves.

Table 18-2: Congenital Neck Masses

Type	Location	Examination	Treatment
Thyroglossal cysts	Midline	Firm, nontender	Surgical excision
Branchial cleft cyst	Preauricular anterior	Firm, nontender	Surgical excision
Teratoma	Anywhere	Firm	Surgical excision
Hemangioma	Anywhere	Diffuse	Observation; laser treatment
Cystic hygroma	Posterior triangle	Diffuse	Partial excision

II. **Types**
   A. **Sinus (incomplete fistula):** has either an internal or an external opening
   B. **Complete fistula:** has both internal and external openings
   C. **Cyst:** has neither internal nor external openings
   D. **Combinations (of any of the preceding types):** can occur

III. **Anatomy:** Anomalies are generally located along the anterior border of the sternocleidomastoid (SCM) muscle or deep to it; they can occur anywhere between the external auditory canal and the clavicle.
   A. **First cleft anomalies:** always superior to the hyoid bone
      1. **Fistula:** if present, courses superiorly and end near the external auditory canal
      2. **Cyst and tract:** may lie in the parotid gland, with a variable relationship to the facial nerve
   B. **Second cleft anomalies:** most common type
      1. **External opening:** approximately two thirds down the SCM muscle anteriorly if present
      2. **Fistula:** if present, ascends with the carotid sheath and ends at the tonsillar fossa
   C. **Third cleft anomalies:** rare
      1. **External opening:** occurs in the same position as in a second cleft fistula
      2. **Tract:** ascends along the carotid sheath and opens in the piriform sinus
   D. **Fourth cleft anomalies:** have never been seen in their entirety

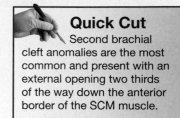

Quick Cut
Second brachial cleft anomalies are the most common and present with an external opening two thirds of the way down the anterior border of the SCM muscle.

IV. **Characteristics:** generally smooth, round, nontender masses
   A. **Size increase:** common during URI
   B. **Infected cyst:** may abscess or rupture spontaneously to form a sinus
   C. **Symptoms:** determined by size and location of the anomaly
      1. **Large cysts:** may cause dysphagia, stridor, and dyspnea
      2. **Small cysts:** often undiscovered until adulthood because of their slow rate of growth and minor symptoms

Quick Cut
Consider a neck mass to be a branchial cleft anomaly if it is located laterally, increases in size with URIs, and has been present since birth.

V. **Treatment:** Complete excision without damage to the surrounding vital structures is the definitive treatment.
   A. **Timing:** Excision is delayed until antibiotic treatment is completed.
   B. **Incision and drainage:** avoided, if possible, because it makes subsequent excision more difficult

Teratomas

I. **Definition and types:** growths that consist of multiple tissues foreign to the part of the body in which they arise
   A. **Epidermoid cysts:** most common type; lined by squamous epithelium and have no adnexa
   B. **Dermoid cysts:** epithelium-lined cavities containing skin appendages (e.g., hair, glandular tissue, and follicles)
   C. **Teratoid cysts (rare in the head and neck):** lined with simple stratified squamous or respiratory epithelium and contain cheesy keratinous material

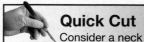

Quick Cut
Epidermoid cysts = ectoderm; *dermoid* cysts = ectoderm and mesoderm; *teratoid* cysts = ectoderm, mesoderm, and endoderm

II. **Cervical teratomas:** most commonly present at birth
   A. **Characteristics:** usually 5–12 cm, semicystic, and unilateral
   B. **Symptoms:** Infants usually have stridor, apnea, or cyanosis because of tracheal compression, and dysphagia may also be present. Some infants are asymptomatic at birth but become symptomatic within weeks or months.
   C. **Associated anomalies:** increased incidence of maternal hydramnios but no increase in associated infant anomalies
   D. **Treatment:** Early excision in infants is *mandatory*.

III. **Malignant teratomas (of the neck):** rare; occur exclusively in adults with a very poor prognosis

IV. **Nasal dermoids:** commonly apparent shortly after birth
   A. **Location:** Nasal dorsum is the most common site, but they may occur in the tip of the nose or the columella (the external end of the nasal septum).

Table 18-3: Congenital Nasal Masses

	Associated Congenital Anomalies	Can Be Midline	Associated with Infections of Skin	Meningitis Risk	Sinus Tract	Compressible
Dermoid	No	Yes	Yes	Yes	Yes	No
Glioma	No	Yes	No	Yes	No	No
Encephalocele	Yes	Yes	No	Yes	No	Yes

  B. **Characteristics (Table 18-3):** male predominance of 2:1; must be differentiated from encephaloceles and gliomas
  C. **Treatment:** Early removal is important; recurrences secondary to incomplete removal are common.

Vascular Tumors

I. **Hemangiomas:** Most common tumors of the head and neck in children. Girls are more often affected, and lesions are usually solitary.
  A. **Capillary hemangiomas:** Include nevus flammeus (port-wine stain) and strawberry nevus and are characteristically found in the dermis. They have an early period of evolution, after which they often regress. They may develop suddenly and grow quite large.
  B. **Cavernous hemangiomas:** More permanent; spontaneous regression is more likely for hemangiomas present at birth than in those appearing later.
  C. **Arteriovenous hemangiomas:** occur almost exclusively in adults and have a predilection for the lips and perioral skin
  D. **Invasive hemangiomas:** occur in the deep subcutaneous tissues, deep fascial layers, and muscles
    1. **Presentation:** Present as neck masses, predominantly in children; masseter and trapezius are the muscles most commonly involved. Intramuscular hemangiomas most commonly present in young adults as palpable, mobile, noncompressible masses.
    2. **Characteristics:** Tend to recur after excision but do not metastasize; they are generally without thrills, pulsations, or bruits; and pain secondary to compression of other structures is usually present.
  E. **Subglottic hemangiomas:** Usually capillary in type. Owing to their location, they often present at birth with stridor and usually with cutaneous involvement.
  F. **Treatment**
    1. **Congenital cutaneous hemangiomas:** Many lesions regress spontaneously, but several treatment options exist for those that do not.
      a. **Medical:** Glucocorticosteroids, interferon alfa, vincristine, and imiquimod have been used for treatment. Propranolol has been shown to induce involution of infantile hemangiomas.
      b. **Excision:** Laser excision is preferred in areas with cosmetic or functional concern (pulsed dye laser is used). Surgical excision can also be performed.
    2. **Subglottic lesions:** may require tracheotomy, steroids, propranolol, and, in some cases, laser excision
    3. **Extensive lesions:** Surgery may be needed.
    4. **Radiation therapy:** Used to suppress tumor growth in areas that are inaccessible surgically; however, the use of radiation alone is controversial and is known to increase risk of thyroid, breast, and skin cancers.

> **Quick Cut**
> When evaluating a newborn with stridor, conducting a thorough skin exam is important.

II. **Cystic hygromas:** found predominantly in the neck and are usually noted at birth
  A. **Location:** They are more common in the posterior triangle and may extend up into the cheek or parotid region and down into the mediastinum or axilla.
    1. **Large masses:** extend past the SCM muscle into the anterior compartment and may cross the midline
    2. **Floor of the mouth and base of the tongue:** may be involved

B. **Signs and symptoms:** difficulty nursing, facial or neck distortion, respiratory distress, brachial plexus compression with pain or hyperesthesia, and a sudden increase in size secondary to spontaneous hemorrhage, *which can be fatal*

C. **Characteristics:** Can be progressive, static, or regressive and generally transilluminate; no gender predilection exists, for right or left side.

1. **Small lesions:** unilocular and firm
2. **Large tumors:** loculated, shiftable, and compressible
3. **Cyst walls:** Usually tense, and because the loculi tend to communicate, rupture of one locule can cause all of them to partially collapse.

D. **Treatment:** Surgery is the mainstay of treatment, but recurrences are common because resection is often incomplete.

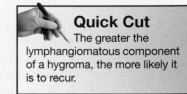

Quick Cut
The greater the lymphangiomatous component of a hygroma, the more likely it is to recur.

III. **Oral and perioral lymphangiomas:** Relatively common lesions usually found at birth or soon after. They behave very much like cystic hygromas.

 ## ACQUIRED LESIONS

Tonsillar and Adenoidal Hypertrophy

I. **Obstructive hypertrophy:** Patients benefiting from tonsillectomy with adenoidectomy are those with airway obstruction, sleep apnea, dysphagia, or failure to thrive.

II. **Adenoidectomy:** performed in children with chronic nasal obstruction, especially when they also demonstrate chronic serous otitis media or orthodontic problems

Leukoplakia, Erythroplakia, and Keratosis

I. **Definition:** Leukoplakia presents as white lesions that occur on the mucosa of the mouth, pharynx, or larynx. **Erythroplakia** is a similar red patch.

II. **Etiology:** These lesions are associated with repeated trauma (e.g., from poorly fitting dentures and decayed teeth), smoking, or use of alcohol.

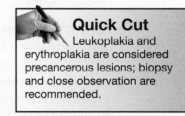

Quick Cut
Leukoplakia and erythroplakia are considered precancerous lesions; biopsy and close observation are recommended.

III. **Transformation:** Leukoplakia is precancerous, with a transformation rate ranging from 11% to 36%. Erythroplakia has a higher transformation rate. Little correlation exists between the clinical appearance and their histology.

IV. **Diagnosis:** Biopsy, to rule out squamous cell carcinoma, should be performed in high-risk patients (smokers and drinkers) and if the lesion persists after the removal of an irritative focus.

V. **Treatment:** Benign leukoplakic lesions require no treatment but do require continued observation.

Papillomas

I. **Squamous papillomas of the oral cavity:** usually occur as one lesion but may be multiple and are common on the palate and faucial arches

A. **Characteristics:** usually pedunculated and cauliflowerlike in appearance

B. **Recurrence:** rare after excision

II. **Nasal (schneiderian) papillomas**

A. **Benign lesions of the sinonasal tract:** from the schneiderian mucosa and classified into three types: fungiform, oncocytic, and inverted

B. **Inverted papillomas:** Typically arise from the lateral nasal wall and can invade the sinuses and orbits. Grossly, the lesions appear bulky and deep red to gray in color and vary in consistency; unlike allergic polyps, they are unilateral.

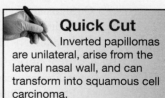

Quick Cut
Inverted papillomas are unilateral, arise from the lateral nasal wall, and can transform into squamous cell carcinoma.

1. **Characteristics:** Patients generally present with nasal obstruction, a postnasal drip, and headaches. These lesions occur mainly in men age 50–70 years.
2. **Malignant transformation:** Incidence is 10%.
3. **Treatment:** Complete excision that includes the lateral nasal wall and ethmoid sinus. Recurrence is common; therefore, lifelong follow-up is usually recommended.

III. **Laryngeal papillomas:** most common laryngeal tumors of childhood and may be found at any age

A. **Juvenile type:** occurs predominantly in childhood and tends to involute at puberty

1. **Etiology:** Viral; HPV 6 and 11 are the most common viral strains.

2. **Characteristics:** Multiple papillomas typically occur and may involve the airway from the epiglottis to the bronchi. The vocal folds are usually involved; hoarseness and obstruction occur late.

3. **Treatment:** Laryngoscopic removal, often by the use of surgical microdebridement, is the mainstay of therapy.

a. **Tracheotomy:** may be necessary but predisposes to papilloma seeding

b. **Recurrence and spread:** common

B. **Adult type:** In this form, the papilloma is generally single.

1. **Recurrence:** As in the juvenile form, the papilloma tends to recur following excision.

2. **Malignant transformation:** in recurrent lesions, particularly in patients exposed to radiation

> **Quick Cut**
> Laryngeal papilloma, or *respiratory papillomatosis*, is associated with HPV6 and 11 and typically presents as hoarseness in a child.

Nasal Polyps

I. **Incidence:** rare before age 5 years and occur more commonly in men

II. **Etiology:** believed to be an allergic response

A. **Samter triad:** They may be associated with asthma and an idiosyncratic reaction to aspirin.

B. **In children:** should prompt a sweat test to rule out cystic fibrosis

III. **Characteristics:** Inflammatory polyps are almost always bilateral and may recur; paranasal sinus involvement is common.

IV. **Treatment:** Polyps are excised if they obstruct the nasal airways or the sinus drainage pathways; patients are placed on a topical steroid medication to prevent recurrence, and management of their allergies is vital.

Peripheral Nerve Tumors

I. **Schwannomas:** solitary, encapsulated tumors surrounded by a nerve that are primarily located centrifugally and are often painful and tender

II. **Acoustic neuromas:** constitute a type of slow-growing schwannoma

A. **Etiology:** arise from CN VIII, usually within the internal auditory canal (IAC)

B. **Signs and symptoms:** may include hearing loss, tinnitus, imbalance, and vertigo

C. **Evaluation:** Testing includes an audiogram and MRI with gadolinium enhancement.

D. **Treatment:** Because these tumors grow slowly, they can be observed in the right clinical context. Other treatment options are surgical resection or radiation therapy.

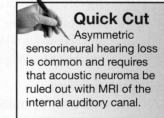

> **Quick Cut**
> Asymmetric sensorineural hearing loss is common and requires that acoustic neuroma be ruled out with MRI of the internal auditory canal.

III. **Von Recklinghausen neurofibromatosis (NF I):** Neurites (axons) pass through the tumor; lesions are usually multiple, unencapsulated, located centripetally, and characteristically asymptomatic.

A. **Etiology:** Caused by a nerve growth factor gene on chromosome 17q11.2; inheritance is autosomal dominant.

B. **Malignant transformation:** 8%

C. **Signs and symptoms:** Café au lait spots, vitiligo, gliomas (especially optic), osseous changes, Lisch nodules (iris hamartomas), meningitis, spina bifida, syndactyly, hemangiomas, axillary or inguinal freckles, NF I in a first-degree relative, or retinal and visceral manifestations may be present.

IV. **Central neurofibromatosis (NF II):** Classically, slow-growing, bilateral acoustic neuromas or neurofibromas cause hearing loss or dizziness and lead to a diagnosis by age 20 years.

A. **Etiology:** Chromosomal abnormality involves encoding of a suppressor protein *schwannomin*. Inheritance is autosomal dominant, but almost 50% of cases are new mutations.

B. **Diagnosis:** may also be established by a unilateral CN VIII mass and a relative with NF II or any two of the following: glioma, juvenile posterior subscapular lenticular opacity, meningioma, neurofibroma, or schwannoma.

C. **Signs and symptoms:** Café au lait spots, hearing loss and balance issues. Lisch nodules, and cutaneous neurofibromas are uncommon.

D. **Wishart type:** early-onset rapid growth and other fibromatous tumors in addition to CN VIII masses

E. **Gardner type:** later onset, slow growth rate; usually bilateral acoustic neuromas only

V. **Treatment:** Most neurogenous tumors of the head and neck can be excised safely without sacrificing nerves.

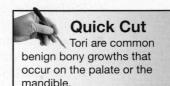

Quick Cut
If an important nerve must be cut at surgery, it should be generally reanastomosed or a nerve graft should be interposed.

Nondental Jaw Lesions

I. **Fibrous dysplasia:** Developmental anomaly of the bone that manifests as a defect in osteoblastic differentiation and maturation. Any bone(s) in the body can be affected, including the craniofacial skeleton.

A. **Characteristics:** active growth in childhood and stabilization in adulthood

B. **Signs and symptoms:** bone enlargement; the maxilla is more commonly involved than the mandible.

C. **Radiographs:** reveal sclerosis, lytic lesions, or unilocular lesions

D. **Treatment:** Obvious deformity, pain, or interference with function suggests the need for surgery; conservative resection appears to be the best treatment.

E. **Malignant transformation:** possible but uncommon

II. **Torus:** Benign bony growth, occurring at the midline of the palate (**maxillary torus**) or bilaterally lingual to the bicuspid (**mandibular torus**). They grow slowly and generally have no significance except that they may interfere with the fitting of dentures.

Quick Cut
Tori are common benign bony growths that occur on the palate or the mandible.

III. **Osteomas:** Slow-growing, benign tumors in the sinuses, jaws, or external ear canals. They may require excision if they produce symptoms.

Laryngeal Lesions

I. **Laryngocele:** Dilatation of the laryngeal saccule, producing an air sac that communicates with the laryngeal ventricle. Pressure increases the size of a laryngocele (e.g., coughing, straining, playing a wind instrument).

A. **Laryngopyocele:** infected laryngocele that can be fatal if it results in asphyxia or if the purulent contents are aspirated

B. **Location:** Laryngoceles may be unilateral or bilateral. They may also be internal (within the larynx), external (presenting in the neck), or both (combined).

1. **Internal laryngocele:** causes bulging of the false cord and aryepiglottic fold

2. **External laryngocele:** appears as a neck swelling at the level of the hyoid and anterior to the SCM muscle

C. **Characteristics**

1. **Internal laryngoceles:** cause hoarseness, breathlessness, and stridor on enlargement

2. **External laryngoceles:** increase in size with coughing or the Valsalva maneuver; are tympanic to percussion and may produce hissing as the laryngocele empties air into the larynx when the air pressure is reduced

D. **Diagnosis:** CT and MRI scans

E. **Treatment**

1. **Symptomatic laryngoceles:** excised

2. **Laryngopyoceles:** Incision, drainage, and subsequent excision. Antibiotics are also appropriate.

II. **Laryngeal webs**

A. **Characteristics:** May be congenital or follow vocal fold trauma. When extensive, they present with stridor, weak phonation, and feeding problems in infants.

B. **Treatment:** Excision or division is generally the preferred treatment, and placement of a stent or keel is often required.

III. **Vocal nodules:** bilateral benign masses that usually occur at the junction of the true vocal folds

A. **Etiology:** associated with vocal abuse

B. **Treatment:** Best treated by modifying the patient's speaking or singing technique through voice therapy. Surgery is rarely necessary

IV. **Vocal polyps**
   A. **Characteristics:** usually unilateral and often do not regress with speech therapy
   B. **Treatment:** Recommended therapy is careful excision with microscopic visualization and avoidance of injury to the underlying lamina propria; in selected cases, the laser may be helpful.

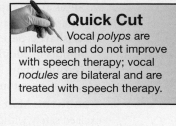

Quick Cut
Vocal *polyps* are unilateral and do not improve with speech therapy; vocal *nodules* are bilateral and are treated with speech therapy.

V. **Laryngeal granulomas (intubation granulomas):** occur over the vocal processes of the arytenoid cartilages
   A. **Etiology:** Generally the result of trauma, usually from an endotracheal tube, and are usually associated with reflux laryngitis. Voice abuse may be a factor.
   B. **Treatment:** Antireflux and speech therapies often help them regress.
      1. **Persistent granulomas:** best treated by excision after a period of voice and medical therapy
      2. **Botulinum toxin:** used for selected, recurrent cases

VI. **Arytenoid dislocation:** generally is the result of endotracheal tube or external trauma
   A. **Characteristics:** Soft, breathy voice after extubation. Flexible fiberoptic exam will reveal an immobile vocal cord.
   B. **Treatment:** Prompt reduction is advisable; otherwise, the arytenoid usually becomes fixed in the dislocated position. However, late reduction (after months or years) can be successful.

VII. **Contact ulcers:** mucosal disruptions usually located posteriorly on the vocal folds
   A. **Etiology:** sometimes result from trauma (e.g., from intubation), occasionally from vocal abuse, and often from gastric reflux laryngitis or heavy coughing
   B. **Treatment:** antireflux medication and behavioral changes such as elevation of the head of the bed; avoidance of caffeine, chocolate, late-night snacks, and fatty foods
      1. **Antacid therapy:** usually results in prompt resolution
      2. **Antibiotics:** may be helpful if infection is present

HEAD AND NECK INFECTIONS

Tonsillitis and Adenotonsillitis

I. **Tonsillectomy with adenoidectomy:** Once the most common operation performed in the United States. It remains quite prevalent but is now performed only for specific indications.
   A. **Obstructive hypertrophy:** See earlier discussion.
   B. **Recurrent infection:** Patients with documented recurrent adenotonsillitis are improved after tonsillectomy with adenoidectomy.

II. **Peritonsillar abscess:** Tonsillectomy is often suggested after treatment for inpatients with a history of previous tonsillitis.

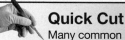

Quick Cut
Many common infections such as ear infections (otitis) can be treated with antibiotics alone.

Quick Cut
A history of three to six episodes of adenotonsillitis annually is a relative indication for tonsillectomy with adenoidectomy.

Atypical Mycobacteria Infection

I. **Characteristics:** Presents as an inflamed mass or draining sinus in the head and neck, commonly associated with the parotid or submandibular glands and is most common in children and adolescents. Pulmonary involvement is rare.
   A. **Results:** Fixation of overlying skin and sinus formation are common.
   B. **Biopsy:** can lead to a chronically draining sinus tract

II. **Treatment:** Surgical excision or curettage and drainage. Antimycobacterial drug therapy is *not* indicated because this is not systemic but a localized problem.

MALIGNANT LESIONS OF THE HEAD AND NECK

Overview

I. **Characteristics:** Table 18-4 shows the basic characteristics of head and neck cancer.

II. **Epidemiology:** Primary malignant neoplasms of the head and neck, excluding skin cancer, account for 5% of new cancers each year in the United States.
   A. **Incidence:** Male to female ratio is 3:1 to 4:1, and most lesions occur in patients older than age 40 years.

Table 18-4: Basic Characteristics of Head and Neck Cancer

Most Prominent		Risk of	
Location	Symptom	Risk Factor	Cervical Metastases
Nose and sinus	Mass	Nickel, wood	Moderate
Nasopharynx	Neck mass; serous otitis media	Epstein-Barr virus	High
Oral cavity	Pain	Tobacco, alcohol	Moderate
Oropharynx	Dysphagia	Tobacco, alcohol, HPV 16 and 18	High
Larynx	Hoarseness	Tobacco	Glottic, low; supraglottic, high
Hypopharynx	Dysphagia	Tobacco, alcohol	High
Salivary glands	Mass	Radiation	High-grade, high; other, low

    B. **Types:** Approximately 80% of primary head and neck malignancies are squamous cell carcinomas; the remainder includes thyroid cancers, salivary neoplasms, lymphoma, and other less common tumors.

III. **Risk factors:** Tobacco use, alcohol consumption, and exposure to radiation are etiologic factors in most squamous cell carcinomas of the head and neck.

    A. **Smoking:** Approximately 85% of patients with head or neck cancer smoke or formerly smoked cigarettes at the time of diagnosis.

    B. **HPV:** associated with some head and neck squamous cell carcinomas, most commonly strains 16 and 18

> **Quick Cut**
> The number of patients with a second primary malignancy of the upper aerodigestive tract at the time of initial presentation has been reported to be as high as 17%.

Evaluation

I. **History:** Evaluation of the patient starts with a careful history, especially head or neck malignancy.

    A. **Exposure to etiologic agents:** such as tobacco, alcohol, sawdust, other toxins, and irradiation

    B. **Associated symptoms:** hoarseness or sore throat of more than 3 weeks' duration, dysphagia, otalgia, dyspnea, nonhealing ulcers, hemoptysis, and neck mass

    C. **Nutritional status**

        1. **Malnourishment:** Either because of alcoholism or an obstructive tumor; some patients may require nutritional supplements.

        2. **Severe malnourishment:** Consider refeeding syndrome.

    D. **Family history:** critical with inherited factors (i.e., medullary thyroid cancer)

> **Quick Cut**
> Otalgia is often a referred pain, secondary to involvement of CNs IX and X.

II. **Physical examination:** must include an inspection of all the skin and mucosal surfaces of the head and neck

    A. **Intranasal examination and indirect mirror examination:** of the nasopharynx and hypopharynx

    B. **Careful palpation:** of the oral cavity, base of the tongue, and oropharynx

    C. **Fiberoptic examination:** of the nose, pharynx, and larynx is indicated in all patients who are being evaluated for cancer

> **Quick Cut**
> Treatment needs to be individualized to the needs of the patient as well as their ability to comply with the treatment plan.

Treatment

I. **Surgery (Fig. 18-2):** Indicated for many patients with head and neck cancer. The effects of radiation are avoided, and radiation can be saved for recurrent disease or other primary cancers. The choice of surgery can be influenced by many factors.

    A. **Malnourishment:** can increase the perioperative risk of morbidity

>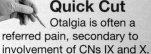
> **Quick Cut**
> Treatment is based on the site and pathology of the primary cancer and the extent of the local, regional, and distant disease.

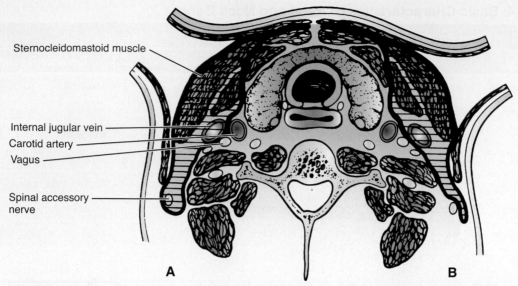

Figure 18-2: Types of neck dissection, including traditional neck dissection and various levels of modification. In a radical neck dissection **(A)**, the sternocleidomastoid muscle, internal jugular vein, and spinal accessory nerve are removed. In the most conservative modification **(B)**, only the fascial compartment with the lymphatic tissue is removed, and all of the structures are spared.

B. Coexistent systemic disease: Diabetes, chronic obstructive pulmonary disease, coronary artery disease, etc. increase the surgical risk.

C. Results: Necessary procedures can be disfiguring and can leave the patient with severe functional deficits and is best performed in institutions that can provide the full range of rehabilitative services.

1. **Resection of the larynx:** alters communication
2. **Surgery on the tongue, oropharynx, hypopharynx, or mandible:** can alter or prevent swallowing

D. Contraindication: Surgery for a cure is generally contraindicated in patients with distant metastases.

II. Radiation therapy: Radiation alone is adequate treatment for many early lesions.

A. Benefits: It can provide a cure without the functional or cosmetic deficits associated with surgery, can treat multiple primary lesions simultaneously, and can prophylactically treat regional nodes that are clinically negative.

B. Planned postoperative radiation: can significantly increase the survival rate for patients with advanced lesions

> **Quick Cut**
> A dental examination and possibly extraction is required before radiotherapy. Dental treatment during and up to 2 years after radiotherapy can be hazardous because of decreased vascularity and consequent delayed healing.

C. Hyperfractionation (more than one daily treatment) and concomitant chemotherapy: Studies show that these techniques can enhance the response to radiation therapy, but they increase the risk and severity of local side effects.

D. Complications: mucositis, xerostomia, loss of taste, dermal and soft tissue fibrosis, dental caries, and bone and soft tissue necrosis

III. Chemotherapy: not curative as a single treatment modality in head and neck squamous cell carcinoma

A. Neoadjuvant treatment: to reduce the tumor burden before radiation or surgery

B. Concomitant radiation therapy: to increase response rates in advanced tumors

C. Palliation: in patients with unresectable tumors or distant metastases

IV. Rehabilitation: should be planned at the same time as treatment

A. Surgical flaps: Cosmetic and functional defects are reconstructed at the time of the cancer resection whenever possible.

1. **Local flaps:** nasolabial, forehead
2. **Distant pedicled skin flaps:** deltopectoral, omocervical
3. **Pedicled myocutaneous flaps:** pectoralis major, latissimus dorsi, trapezius

> **Quick Cut**
> The choice of a surgical flap depends on the size of the defect, history of peripheral vascular disease, prior surgeries, or procedures in the desired donor region and general health and nutritional status of the patient.

B. **Esophagectomy:** Gastric "pull-up" (raising the stomach into the chest to replace the esophagus) or colon interposition are options for reconstruction.

C. **Free microvascular flaps:** have a high rate of complications but can be very effective

D. **Prosthetic rehabilitation:** necessary when portions of the maxilla, orbit mandible, or palate are resected

E. **Voice restoration:** When the larynx is removed, intensive rehabilitation is required to re-establish the voice with an electrolarynx that is applied to the neck surface, regurgitated air (esophageal speech), or with a prosthesis placed in a tracheoesophageal fistula.

F. **Swallowing training:** Many patients who undergo partial laryngectomy, pharyngectomy, or glossectomy need this to avoid aspiration.

 NECK CANCER

Anatomy

I. **Divisions:** anterior and posterior triangles

A. **Anterior triangle:** Bounded by the midline of the neck, the inferior mandible border, and the anterior SCM muscle. It can be subdivided further into submandibular, submental, superior carotid, and inferior carotid triangles.

B. **Posterior triangle:** Bounded by the posterior border of the SCM muscle, the anterior border of the trapezius, and the clavicle. It is divided further into supraclavicular and occipital triangles.

II. **Lymphatic drainage:** Fascial planes of the neck enclose the lymphatic system and are important when discussing spread of infections and malignancy in the head and neck.

A. **Superficial fascia:** subcutaneous and envelops the platysma

B. **Deep fascia:** three parts:

1. **Superficial layer:** invests the SCM and trapezius muscles and the parotid and submandibular glands

2. **Middle layer:** divided into muscular and visceral divisions

a. **Muscular division:** invests the strap muscles and pharyngeal constrictors and buccinators

b. **Visceral division:** also called the *pretracheal fascia*; envelopes the trachea, esophagus, and thyroid

3. **Deep layer:** divided into the alar fascia anteriorly and the prevertebral fascia posteriorly

C. **Retropharyngeal space:** lies anterior to the alar fascia and is an important plane when discussing spread of malignancy and infection

D. **Neck lymph nodes:** Many drain specific areas of the upper aerodigestive tract. These are divided into six levels based on location and drainage patterns.

1. **Deep jugular and spinal accessory chains:** where most lymph nodes lie

2. **Jugular chain divisions:** superior, middle, and inferior groups

Neck Mass Evaluation in Adults with No Primary Cancer Seen on Exam

I. **History and physical examination:** Careful history is taken, and the head and neck are examined for evidence of a possible primary cancer.

II. **Diagnosis:** If the primary cancer is not identified on the initial examination, the subsequent workup should include the following.

A. **Imaging:** Chest x-ray, barium swallow, and CT scan of the neck are indicated in most patients. MRI or ultrasound of the neck is guided by findings on the history and physical examination.

1. **MRI:** particularly useful in defining deeply invasive tongue, pharynx, and larynx tumors

2. **CT of the sinuses:** can be used to search for primary tumors

3. **Staging:** CT or MRI of the chest and abdomen are often used.

B. **FNA:** should be performed to provide a tissue diagnosis

C. **Panendoscopy:** direct laryngoscopy, esophagoscopy, bronchoscopy, and nasopharyngoscopy to identify any obvious lesions for biopsy

1. **Random biopsies:** If the result of the endoscopic survey is negative, biopsy of the nasopharynx (right, middle, and left), piriform sinuses, tongue base, and a tonsillectomy may also be considered.

2. **Next step:** If all biopsies have negative results, proceed with open neck biopsy and frozen section.

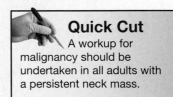
Quick Cut
A workup for malignancy should be undertaken in all adults with a persistent neck mass.

Treatment

I. Types of neck dissection: Figure 18-3

   A. Radical neck dissection: en bloc dissection of the cervical lymphatics that includes removal of the SCM muscle, internal jugular vein, or spinal accessory nerve

   B. Modified (functional, conservative) neck dissection: removes the cervical lymphatics within their fascial compartments that spares the SCM muscle, internal jugular vein, and spinal accessory nerve

   C. Segmental neck dissection: refers to removal of less than five nodal groups on one side of the neck (e.g., submandibular triangle dissection, supraomohyoid dissection)

II. Elective neck dissection: surgical treatment with no known cervical disease; controversial because radiation therapy can provide prophylaxis for metastatic neck disease in many cases

   A. Choice between surgery and radiation: usually depends on the treatment of the primary tumor

   B. In general: performed for a primary cancer that has at least a 20% chance of occult metastasis

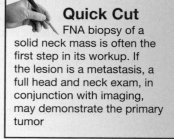

Quick Cut
FNA biopsy of a solid neck mass is often the first step in its workup. If the lesion is a metastasis, a full head and neck exam, in conjunction with imaging, may demonstrate the primary tumor

NASAL CAVITY AND PARANASAL SINUS CANCER

Anatomy and Classification

I. Basic structure: Sinuses are contiguous with the nasal cavity through natural ostia, and the nose and sinuses are lined with a respiratory mucosa, which is pseudostratified columnar with goblet cells and cilia.

II. Lymphatic drainage: to the parapharyngeal or retropharyngeal nodes

III. Location: Most tumors (59%) are in the maxillary sinus, 24% are in the nasal cavity, 16% in the ethmoid, and 1% in the frontal/sphenoid sinuses.

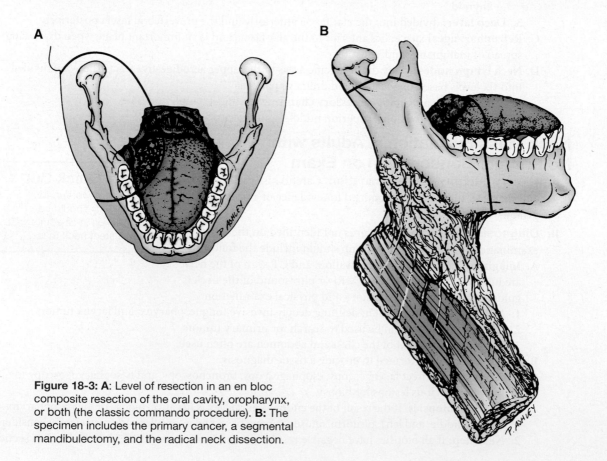

A

B

Figure 18-3: A: Level of resection in an en bloc composite resection of the oral cavity, oropharynx, or both (the classic commando procedure). **B:** The specimen includes the primary cancer, a segmental mandibulectomy, and the radical neck dissection.

IV. **Classification:** Nasal and sinus cancers are locally invasive. Nodal metastases are unusual and tend to occur late, even with extensive local disease.
   A. **Squamous cell carcinoma:** ~80%
   B. **Adenocarcinomas:** including adenoid cystic carcinoma, ~10%–14%

Quick Cut
Squamous cell carcinoma is the most common malignancy of the nasal cavity and paranasal sinuses.

Clinical Evaluation

I. **Presenting symptoms:** can include nasal obstruction; epistaxis; localized pain; tooth pain; CN deficits; mass in the face, palate, or maxillary alveolus; proptosis; and trismus

II. **Diagnosis:** Extent of the disease is determined by physical examination and radiographic studies.
   A. **CT scan:** useful for identifying bony erosions and orbital or intracranial extension
   B. **MRI:** can be used for intraorbital and intracranial invasion

Quick Cut
Be suspicious for a malignancy in a patient who presents with unilateral nasal obstruction, epistaxis, localized facial pain, or CN deficits (III, IV, VI, or VII).

Treatment and Prognosis

I. **Maxillary sinus cancer**
   A. **Less advanced cancers:** Subtotal or radical maxillectomy. Adjuvant radiation may be used.
   B. **Advanced cancers:** Usually receive a combination of surgical resection followed by chemotherapy and/or radiotherapy. Orbital exenteration and skin resection are performed when necessary.

II. **Ethmoid sinus or nasal cavity tumors:** combination of surgical resection and chemotherapy and/or radiation

III. **Extensive cancers:** Combined craniofacial resection for selected patients. Chemotherapy is used for treatment or palliation.

IV. **Cervical lymph node metastases:** treated with radiotherapy or surgery

V. **Prognosis**
   A. **Overall cure rate:** ~30%–35%
   B. **5-year survival rate:** less advanced lesions, 70%; decreases to 15%–20% with more advanced disease

NASOPHARYNX CANCER

Overview

I. **Anatomy:** Nasopharynx is the most cephalad part of the pharynx; its roof is formed by the basioccipital and sphenoid bones, and its posterior wall is formed by the atlas.
   A. **Walls:** Roof and posterior wall are covered by mucosa, and the adenoid tissue is embedded; the lateral wall contains the orifice of the eustachian tube, and, just posterior to that, the fossa of Rosenmüller.
   B. **Limits:** Choanae define the anterior limit, and the free edge of the soft palate provides the inferior limit.
   C. **Lymphatic drainage:** to the lateral retropharyngeal, jugulodigastric (tonsillar), and high spinal accessory nodes

II. **Epidemiology:** High incidence among people living in China. People of Chinese ancestry who live in other countries do not have the same incidence, suggesting an environmental risk factor (i.e., consumption of smoked fish) contributing to the increased incidence.
   A. **Elevated Epstein-Barr virus titer:** high incidence among persons with nasopharyngeal cancer
   B. **Age:** occurs at younger ages than do most solid head and neck tumors

III. **Classification:** Eighty-five percent of nasopharyngeal tumors are epithelial; 7.5% are lymphomas. Epithelial tumors commonly arise in the fossa of Rosenmüller.

Clinical Evaluation

I. **Presenting symptoms:** Epistaxis, cervical adenopathy, serous otitis media, and nasal obstruction (headache, diplopia, facial numbness, trismus, ptosis, and hoarseness may also be present); 70% of patients will have nodal disease, 40% will have CN involvement.

Quick Cut
An adult with a unilateral middle ear effusion should have nasopharyngoscopy to rule out a nasopharyngeal mass.

II. **Diagnosis:** confirmed by biopsy of a metastatic lymph node
   A. **Staging:** CT and MRI
   B. **Elevated Epstein-Barr virus titer:** Monitoring of the titer should show a decrease with successful treatment and an increase with recurrences.

Treatment and Prognosis

I. **Radiation:** Primary treatment for all epithelial nasopharyngeal tumors. The dose is delivered to the nasopharynx and to both sides of the neck. Improved responses are possible with combined chemotherapy and radiation in patients who can tolerate the increased toxicity.

II. **Radical neck dissection:** performed for residual nodes if the primary tumor is controlled

III. **5-year survival rate:** 40% in patients without positive nodes and 20% in patients with positive nodes

◆ ORAL CAVITY CANCER

Overview

I. **Anatomy:** Oral cavity extends from the lip anteriorly to the faucial arches posteriorly and includes the lips, buccal mucosa, gingivae, retromolar trigones, hard palate, anterior two thirds of the tongue (the oral tongue), and floor of the mouth.

II. **Lymphatic drainage:** to the submental, submandibular, and deep jugular nodes

III **Etiology:** Ninety percent of patients are heavy users of tobacco (either smoking or chewing); ~80% of patients are heavy drinkers.

Quick Cut
The seven subsites of the oral cavity are the lips, buccal mucosa, gingivae, retromolar trigone, hard palate, oral tongue, and the floor of the mouth.

Clinical Evaluation

I. **Presenting symptoms:** Can include loose teeth, painful or nonhealing ulcers, odynophagia, otalgia (with posterior lesions), and cervical adenopathy. The lip is the most common site of carcinoma, followed by the oral tongue and floor of the mouth.

II. **Diagnosis:** Pain, which is a late symptom, occurs after ulceration develops.
   A. **Mandibular radiographs:** assess the bony involvement by adjacent tumors
   B. **Nodal metastases:** Common, especially in the floor of mouth and oral tongue with more advanced primary tumors; much are microscopic (occult) disease.
   C. **Metastases:** uncommon; usually occur late in cancer of the lip or the buccal mucosa

Treatment and Prognosis

I. **Small tumors with no lymph node involvement:** can be treated with either local excision or radiotherapy

II. **Larger lesions:** should be treated with combined surgery and radiation
   A. **Surgery:** involves an en bloc resection and neck dissection
   B. **Technique:** Either a partial mandibulectomy is included or the tumor is "pulled through" medially to the mandible into the neck (i.e., the tumor is removed en bloc, leaving the mandible intact).

Quick Cut
Most malignancies of the oral cavity are treated with surgery, with or without radiation.

III. **Tumors attached to the mandible:** May be removed with a partial thickness of mandible (i.e., the lingual plate or alveolar process). The mandibular arch is kept intact when possible.

IV. **Tumors demonstrating bony erosion in the mandible:** removed with a full-thickness portion of bone

V. **5-year survival rate:** overall, for cancer of all oral cavity sites, is ~65%
   A. **Lip cancer:** Rates as high as 90% have been reported.
   B. **Tongue lesions:** Prognosis is worse if the lesion is posterior.
      1. **Anterior (mobile) tongue lesions:** Often diagnosed when they are small; overall 5-year survival rate is more than 65%.
      2. **Posterior lesions:** less than 40%

OROPHARYNX CANCER

Overview

I. **Anatomy**
   A. **Boundaries:** free edge of the soft palate superiorly, the tip of the epiglottis inferiorly, and the anterior tonsillar pillar anteriorly
   B. **Contents:** soft palate, tonsillar fossae and faucial tonsils, lateral and posterior pharyngeal walls, and base of the tongue
   C. **Parapharyngeal space:** directly lateral to the oropharynx; contains the glossopharyngeal, lingual, and inferior alveolar nerves; pterygoid muscles; internal maxillary artery; and carotid sheath and is a site of early extension of an oropharyngeal tumor that also provides a pathway for the tumor to spread to the base of the skull
   D. **Lymphatic drainage:** Primarily to the jugulodigastric (tonsillar) nodes; tumors of the soft palate, lateral wall, and tongue base also spread to the retropharyngeal and parapharyngeal nodes.

>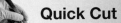
> **Quick Cut**
> Tobacco, alcohol use, and HPV 16 and 18 exposures are risk factors for oropharyngeal squamous cell carcinoma.

II. **Etiology:** Alcohol and tobacco use are commonly found together in patients with oropharyngeal cancer.
   A. **HPV strains 16 and 18:** associated with squamous cell cancer of the oropharynx with increasing incidence
   B. **Local mucosal irritation, malnutrition, and immune defects:** also implicated

> **Quick Cut**
> A synergistic effect seems to exist between alcohol and tobacco in oropharynx cancer, but it has not been defined.

Clinical Evaluation

I. **Presenting symptoms:** Most common is a persistent sore throat, which is frequently accompanied by ipsilateral otalgia (referred pain via the tympanic branch of the glossopharyngeal nerve), vague sensation of throat irritation, restriction of tongue motion ("hot potato voice"), odynophagia, and bleeding.
   A. **Malnourishment:** Most patients are significantly malnourished.
   B. **Cervical adenopathy:** Nodal metastases are found in ~70% of patients with cancer of the base of the tongue and in 60%–80% of patients with tonsillar cancer; most of these nodes are palpable.

II. **Initial examination:** Must include careful palpation of the base of the tongue. Many small tumors are difficult to see but may be palpated easily.

III. **Diagnosis:** Often made late in the course; many patients are asymptomatic until tumors are large; others are treated conservatively for incorrectly diagnosed lesions.
   A. **Endoscopy under general anesthesia:** for all lesions before treatment is chosen
   B. **CT and MRI:** useful in determining tumor extension

Treatment and Prognosis

I. **Small lesions:** most commonly treated with radiotherapy

II. **Large lesions:** Combined therapy offers improved survival rates and is indicated when nodal metastasis is present.

III. **Composite resection (the jaw-neck or commando procedure):** most commonly used to resect large lesions of the oropharynx and involves a neck dissection and a partial mandibulectomy in conjunction with excision of the tumor (Fig. 18-3) and reconstruction (Fig. 18-4).
   A. **Tracheotomy:** routine treatment
   B. **Total glossectomy:** Occasionally, the larynx is spared after in young and otherwise healthy patients.
   C. **Laryngectomy:** performed when either the tumor invades the pre-epiglottic space or the entire tongue base and both hypoglossal nerves are removed

IV. **Transoral robotic surgery (TORS):** now used at some centers for surgical resection of oropharyngeal tumors
   A. **Reduced morbidity:** due to ability to resect the tumor without splitting the mandible
   B. **Decreased need for feeding tubes following resection:** demonstrated by some studies

V. **Prognosis:** Related to the HPV status of the tumor; patients who have HPV+ tumors generally have a better prognosis than those who have HPV− tumors.

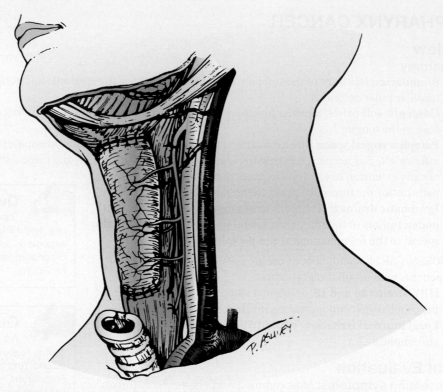

Figure 18-4: Reconstruction of a circumferential pharyngeal defect with a jejunal free graft. The vascular pedicle has been anastomosed to branches of the external carotid artery and internal jugular vein.

HYPOPHARYNX AND CERVICAL ESOPHAGUS CANCER

Overview

I. **Anatomy**
   A. **Boundaries:** Hypopharynx extends from the pharyngoepiglottic fold to the inferior border of the cricoid area, excluding the larynx.
   B. **Contents:** includes the piriform sinuses, the postcricoid area, and the posterior pharyngeal wall
   C. **Lymphatic drainage:** Hypopharynx has a rich lymphatic network.
      1. **Piriform sinuses:** drain to jugulocarotid and midjugular nodes
      2. **Posterior pharyngeal wall:** drains primarily to retropharyngeal nodes
      3. **Lower hypopharyngeal areas:** drain to paratracheal and low jugular nodes
      4. **Cervical esophagus:** drained by mediastinal nodes

II. **Classification:** Ninety-five percent of the tumors in this region are epithelial cancers; ~60%–75% arise in the piriform sinuses and 20%–25% on the posterior pharyngeal wall; tumors rarely arise in the postcricoid area.

III. **Etiology:** as with other head and neck tumors, related to heavy use of alcohol and tobacco

Clinical Evaluation

I. **Presenting symptoms:** Triad of throat pain, referred otalgia, and dysphagia is present in more than 50% of patients.

II. **Hoarseness and airway obstruction:** indicate laryngeal involvement

III. **Small postcricoid tumors:** often present with mild symptoms of sore throat, globus (a "lump in the throat"), and throat clearing

IV. **Cervical lymph node metastases:** found in 75% of patients with piriform sinus cancers (41% occult) and in 83% of patients with pharyngeal wall tumors (66% occult)

V. **Diagnosis:** CT scan of the neck with contrast and endoscopy with biopsy complete the workup.

Treatment and Prognosis

I. **Advanced lesions:** Laryngopharyngectomy and radical neck dissection followed by radiotherapy are necessary for most.

II. **Small tumors that spare the apex of the piriform sinus:** Supraglottic laryngectomy can be considered.

III. **Small tumors:** can be treated by radiation therapy alone or by surgical resection via a lateral pharyngotomy

IV. **Cervical esophagus cancer:** can require removal of the pharynx, esophagus, and larynx

V. **Prognosis:** poor because of extensive submucosal spread and the high incidence of cervical metastasis
   A. **Overall 5-year survival rate:** ~30%
   B. **If eligible for supraglottic laryngectomy:** Five-year survival rate rises to 50%.

VI. **Chemotherapy with radiation therapy:** in organ-sparing protocols

LARYNX CANCER

Overview

I. **Anatomy**
   A. **Divisions:** three regions
      1. **Supraglottis:** extends from the tip of the epiglottis to include the false vocal folds and roof of the ventricle
      2. **Glottis:** extends from the depth of the ventricle to 1 cm below the free edge of the true vocal fold
      3. **Subglottis:** extends from 1 cm below the free edge of the true vocal fold to the inferior border of the cricoid cartilage
   B. **Lymphatic drainage**
      1. **Supraglottis:** rich network that crosses the midline and drains to the deep jugular nodes
      2. **Glottis:** poorly developed sparse lymphatics
      3. **Subglottis:** drains through the cricothyroid membrane to the prelaryngeal (delphian) and pretracheal nodes

II. **Etiology:** More than 90% of patients have a significant history of smoking, and heavy alcohol consumption is a common but not definite etiologic factor.

III. **Classification**
   A. **Squamous cell carcinomas:** account for 95%–98% of the tumors
   B. **Verrucous carcinoma:** variant of squamous cell carcinoma that is locally invasive but almost never metastasizes

Clinical Evaluation

I. **Presenting symptoms:** Most common symptom is hoarseness.
   A. **Other:** Stridor, cough, hemoptysis, odynophagia, otalgia, dysphagia, and aspiration also occur.
   B. **Neck masses:** uncommon at the time of presentation

II. **Diagnosis:** All patients require direct laryngoscopy and biopsy; barium swallow, stroboscopic laryngoscopy, and CT scan may be helpful.

> **Quick Cut**
> Glottic cancers are usually diagnosed relatively early compared to other cancers of the head and neck due to the presenting symptom of hoarseness.

Treatment and Prognosis

I. **Carcinoma in situ:** excision of the involved vocal fold mucosa and close monitoring

II. **Early-stage lesions:** Many are treated with radiation because the resultant voice is usually of better quality than the one after surgical excision (at least initially). However, surgery is still indicated for many patients.
   A. **Removal of the involved vocal fold:** by traditional techniques or by carbon dioxide laser yields equivalent local control
   B. **Hemilaryngectomy (vertical laryngectomy):** for some glottic lesions that involve the anterior commissure because of the increased risk of cartilage involvement
   C. **Limited surgical resection:** for some small lesions of the tip of the epiglottis

III. **Large supraglottic tumors:** Supraglottic (horizontal) laryngectomy spares the true vocal folds but removes the epiglottis, aryepiglottic folds, and false vocal folds.

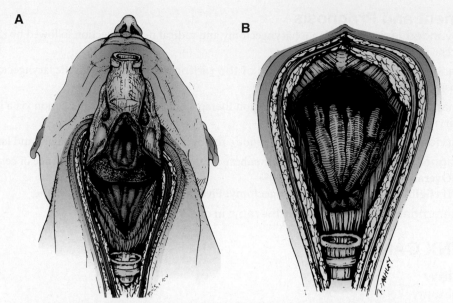

Figure 18-5: **A:** Total laryngectomy specimen ready for removal, attached only to the tongue base. **B:** Pharyngeal defect following total laryngectomy. Closure is usually accomplished in layers in a T fashion.

IV. **Transglottic tumors:** For supraglottic tumors that spread to a true vocal fold, a suprahemilaryngectomy may be considered. Neck dissection, radiation, or both are often necessary.

V. **Advanced tumors:** Usually require a total laryngectomy, often combined with neck dissection (Fig. 18-5). Postoperative radiotherapy is usually indicated.

VI. **Verrucous carcinoma:** Conservation laryngectomy, when possible. There is no need for elective neck dissection, and the use of radiotherapy is controversial.

VII. **Concurrent chemoradiotherapy protocols:** achieve cure rates comparable to those for traditional combined surgical therapy and allow some patients to avoid total laryngectomy (Fig. 18-6)

VIII. **Prognosis:** better than with cancer of other head and neck sites

SKIN CANCER

Basal and Squamous Cell Carcinomas

I. **Etiology:** sunlight, radiation, arsenic, burns, scars, and genetic disorders (xeroderma pigmentosum, basal cell nevus syndrome, albinism)

II. **Clinical evaluation:** Usually present as slowly enlarging cutaneous or subcutaneous lesions; some lesions form nonhealing ulcers. Nodal metastasis is uncommon.

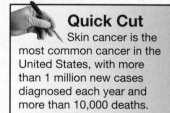

Quick Cut
Skin cancer is the most common cancer in the United States, with more than 1 million new cases diagnosed each year and more than 10,000 deaths.

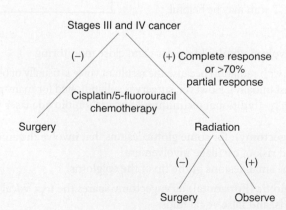

Figure 18-6: Example of organ-sparing neoadjuvant chemotherapy protocol.

III. **Treatment:** Therapy includes electrodesiccation, curettage, cryosurgery, excision, Mohs surgery, radiation, and topical fluorouracil.

A. **Squamous cell carcinoma:** Surgical excision is preferred because it allows removal of a margin.

B. **Basal cell carcinomas:** Of the nasolabial folds, medial and lateral canthi, or postauricular regions are especially aggressive. They can invade multiple tissue planes and, therefore, require an extensive surgical resection.

C. **Mohs surgery:** involves the precise mapping and frozen-section control of the entire resection bed

D. **Radiation therapy:** usually reserved for advanced lesions in areas where surgical excision leaves a cosmetically unacceptable defect (e.g., the nose, eyelid, and lip)

E. **All positive nodes:** should be treated with neck dissection or radiotherapy

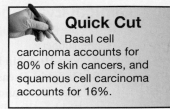
Quick Cut
Basal cell carcinoma accounts for 80% of skin cancers, and squamous cell carcinoma accounts for 16%.

Malignant Melanoma

I. **Epidemiology:** Accounts for 1% of all cancers; incidence is increasing by 5%–7% each year.

II. **Etiology:** Sun exposure and heredity play important roles.

III. **Pathologic variants:** lentigo maligna melanoma, superficial spreading melanoma, and nodular melanoma

IV. **Staging:** depth of primary lesion, see part VII Chapter Cuts and Caveats

V. **Treatment:** wide excision with treatment of nodal basins for deeper melanomas

A. **Sentinel node biopsy:** for intermediate depth of invasion to assess for nodal disease

1. **Lymphoscintigraphy:** Radiotracer is injected intradermally around the melanoma lesion. Lymphatic imaging is then performed after injection to confirm appropriate uptake of the radiotracer.

2. **Technique:** Blue dye and radiotracer are injected intradermally at the site of the lesion. The dye is visible and a gamma probe is used to identify radiotracer activity and an incision is made in the area.

3. **Neck dissection:** performed for positive nodes

4. **Parotidectomy:** added for lesions of the anterior scalp, eyelids, auricles, and cheeks because the first-level lymphatic drainage is to the periparotid nodes

B. **Radiation therapy:** usually reserved for palliative treatment of recurrent disease

C. **Chemotherapy:** used for disseminated melanoma

VI. **Prognosis:** Survival rate is related to the tumor staging; the prognosis in patients with mucosal melanoma is extremely poor.

Quick Cut
Twenty-five percent of all melanomas arise in the head and neck.

Quick Cut
When describing skin lesions concerning for melanoma, use the ABCD system: *a*symmetry, *b*order irregularity, *c*olor (uneven color pattern), and *d*iameter greater than 6 mm.

Quick Cut
A sentinel node is the first node involved in lymphatic spread of a malignancy.

HEAD AND NECK LYMPHOMA

Overview

I. **Epidemiology:** Eighty percent of all malignant lymphomas arise from nodes, many of which are in the head and neck.

A. **Hodgkin lymphoma:** Seventy percent of patients have cervical lymph node involvement.

B. **Extranodal presentation:** rare in Hodgkin disease but occurs in 20% of patients with non-Hodgkin lymphoma

II. **Classification**

A. **Non-Hodgkin lymphoma:** really a group of diseases, which are classified into favorable and unfavorable types on the basis of therapeutic response

B. **Hodgkin lymphoma:** Histology influences the prognosis.

Clinical Evaluation

I. **Presenting symptoms:** Usually a single, enlarged cervical node; most lymphomatous nodes are firm and rubbery.
   A. **Non-Hodgkin lymphoma:** typically presents in upper cervical nodes
   B. **Hodgkin disease:** discovered in nodes throughout the cervical chain
   C. **Sites of extranodal involvement in non-Hodgkin lymphoma:** Head and neck, particularly in Waldeyer tonsillar ring. Other sites include the nasal cavity, paranasal sinuses, orbit, and salivary glands.
   D. **Systemic symptoms:** Approximately 40% of patients with Hodgkin lymphoma have fever, sweats, weight loss, and malaise.

II. **Diagnosis:** Usually made by excisional biopsy of a lymph node; one of the largest nodes should be removed in its entirety.
   A. **FNA of the lymph node and endoscopy:** should be performed to rule out squamous cell carcinoma
   B. **If a possible extranodal source has been discovered:** Biopsy first.
   C. **Frozen-section diagnosis:** of little value except to exclude squamous cell carcinoma
   D. **Additional workup aids in staging:** Chest radiograph, CT scan of the abdomen, and bone marrow biopsy are recommended.

Treatment and Prognosis

I. **Treatment:** Combination of chemotherapy agents and radiation therapy are used depending on the stage and pathology.

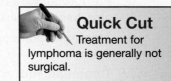

Quick Cut
Treatment for lymphoma is generally not surgical.

II. **Prognosis**
   A. **Hodgkin disease:** Favorable prognostic factors include localized disease, limited number of anatomic sites, absence of massive disease, and a favorable histology.
   B. **Survival rates:** Patients with limited disease have 5-year, relapse-free rates of 80%–90%; the rate falls to 60%–80% in patients with advanced disease treated with combined therapy; and rates as low as 30% occur in advanced disease.
   C. **Non-Hodgkin lymphoma survival:** Radiation therapy for limited disease yields 50%–70% cure rates.
      1. **With more advanced lesions:** Patients with a favorable histology can have a 60%–70% 5-year survival rate and a 30% cure rate.
      2. **Patients with an unfavorable histology:** face a 24%–40% 5-year survival rate with little chance for a cure

UNUSUAL TUMORS

Carotid Body Tumors

I. **Characteristics:** Usually present as slow-growing, painless neck masses; 3% are bilateral (increasing to 26% in patients with a familial tendency for paragangliomas). The mass may be pulsatile and may have a bruit.

II. **Large tumors:** can cause dysphagia, airway obstruction, and CN palsies

III. **Diagnosis:** Angiography shows a tumor blush at the carotid bifurcation that splays the internal and external carotids.

IV. **Treatment:** Surgical excision; large tumors may require carotid bypass.

PAROTID GLAND

Overview

I. **Embryology:** Largest of the salivary glands; average gland weighs 25 g. It appears in the fourth week of gestation and originates from the epithelium of the oropharynx.

II. **Anatomy:** Covers the masseter muscle, extends beyond the vertical ramus of the mandible, and abuts the external auditory meatus.
   A. **Fascial sheath:** Encloses the gland; the tightness of this fascia is responsible for the severe pain that accompanies acute swelling of the gland (acute parotitis).
   B. **Lobes:** Classically, the parotid gland was thought to have two lobes, superficial and deep, which is useful when discussing the surgical treatment of parotid disease.

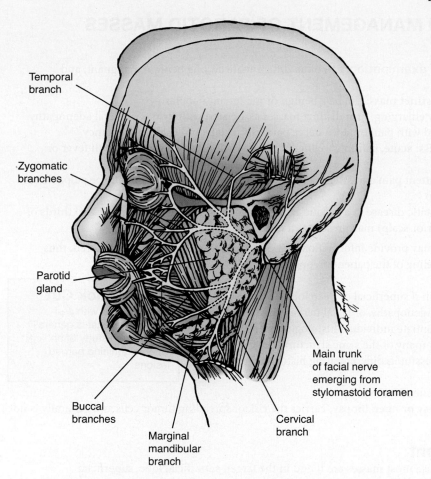

Figure 18-7: Facial nerve branches pass through the parotid gland.

Temporal branch

Zygomatic branches

Parotid gland

Buccal branches

Marginal mandibular branch

Main trunk of facial nerve emerging from stylomastoid foramen

Cervical branch

III. **Stensen duct:** Drains saliva; this duct exits anteriorly, pierces the buccinator muscle, and enters the oral cavity opposite the second upper molar. The opening is marked by the parotid papilla, which may be felt by the tongue or a finger.

IV. **Innervation (Fig. 18-7):** Facial nerve enters the posterior part of the gland immediately after emerging from the stylomastoid foramen.

A. **Divisions (two):** Facial nerve divides within the substance of the gland into two parts (zygomaticofacial and cervicofacial) at the pes anserinus or goose's foot.

B. **Major branches (five):** temporal, zygomatic, buccal, mandibular, and cervical

C. **Facial nerve and its branches:** separate the superficial and deep portions of the gland (Fig. 18-8)

D. **Muscles of expression:** supplied by the facial nerve on the ipsilateral side of the face

> **Quick Cut**
> Generations of students have used the mnemonic "To Zanzibar By Motor Car" to remember the branches of the facial nerve.

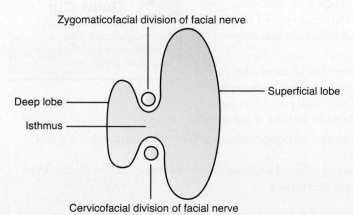

Zygomaticofacial division of facial nerve

Deep lobe

Isthmus

Superficial lobe

Cervicofacial division of facial nerve

Figure 18-8: Frontal cross section of the parotid gland.

EVALUATION AND MANAGEMENT OF PAROTID MASSES

Overview

I. **History and physical examination:** can often differentiate among benign, malignant, and inflammatory processes

    A. **Slowly enlarging, distinct mass:** can be a benign or malignant neoplasm

    B. **Malignancy:** Rapidly enlarging, firm distinct masses associated with firm, ipsilateral adenopathy, and masses associated with pain or facial nerve paralysis usually indicate a malignancy.

    C. **Inflammatory process:** acute, painful swelling in one or both glands, associated with fever or systemic symptoms

    D. **Sialadenitis:** Intermittent pain and swelling in the gland; a stone may occasionally be palpable on intraoral examination.

    E. **Parotid mass:** Metastatic disease in a parotid lymph node (drainage from the upper two thirds of the face and the anterior scalp) may present as a mass.

II. **Diagnostic studies:** may provide information that dictates the extent of surgery required, thus permitting better counseling of the patient preoperatively

    A. **Radiologic studies**

        1. **MRI:** Can establish if superficial or deep lobes are involved, suspicious lymphadenopathy, or facial nerve invasion. It may also help to differentiate individual histologic lesions.

        2. **CT scans:** discern many of the same structural details but are not nearly as successful in differentiating histologic lesions

    B. **Invasive tests**

        1. **FNA:** provides tissue diagnosis

        2. **Core-needle biopsy or open biopsy:** carries the risk of spreading tumor cells and generally is not indicated

>
> **Quick Cut**
> MRI with and without contrast is generally the imaging study of choice when examining parotid lesions.

Surgical Management

I. **Benign lesions:** Because most masses are found in the larger, superficial lobe, superficial parotidectomy is usually sufficient, but complete excision is required. "Shelling out" a mass often leads to recurrence.

II. **Malignant lesions:** If the lesion is small, low grade, and completely confined to the superficial lobe, then resection of only that lobe may be sufficient. Otherwise, total parotidectomy should be performed.

    A. **Facial nerve:** Should be sacrificed if it is involved. Nerve grafting allows restoration of some function in 6–12 months.

    B. **Neck dissection:** indicated for high-grade lesions

    C. **Postoperative radiation therapy:** may be used for unfavorable high-grade lesions or in cases where a limited dissection was performed

PAROTID NEOPLASMS

Benign

I. **General:** Eighty percent of parotid tumors are benign. The most common presenting feature of these tumors is a painless mass, and facial paralysis is rare. Very careful identification and surgical treatment, which consists of excision that includes a margin of normal gland, are required.

>
> **Quick Cut**
> Be highly suspicious for malignancy if there is a parotid mass and the patient has facial weakness.

II. **Pleomorphic adenomas (mixed tumors):** So named because they contain both stromal and epithelial components; they are the most common benign salivary tumors (60% of all parotid tumors and are slow growing but may be quite large at the time of presentation).

III. **Papillary adenocystoma (cystadenoma) lymphomatosum (Warthin tumors):** consist of both epithelial and lymphoid elements

    A. **Presentation:** They are soft (cystic) when palpated and contain mucoid material that may appear purulent. They are neoplastic and noninflammatory.

B. **Incidence:** found in men five times as frequently as in women and usually occurs in people ages 40–60 years

C. **Etiology:** associated with cigarette smoking

III. **Benign lymphoepithelial tumor (Godwin tumor):** Characterized by slowly progressive lymphoid infiltration of the gland; care must be taken not to confuse this lesion with a lymphoma. It is associated with HIV.

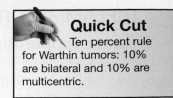

Quick Cut
Ten percent rule for Warthin tumors: 10% are bilateral and 10% are multicentric.

IV. **Oxyphil adenomas:** consist of acidophilic cells called *oncocytes*, occur most frequently in elderly patients, grow slowly, and do not usually grow larger than 5 cm

V. **Miscellaneous lesions:** For example, hemangiomas and lymphangiomas also occur. Hemangiomas that do not regress are treated by resection.

Malignant

I. **Mucoepidermoid carcinoma:** Arises from the ducts of the gland. It is the most common parotid malignancy and constitutes 9% of all parotid tumors.

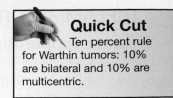

Quick Cut
Malignant tumors constitute 20% of all parotid neoplasms. They are often characterized by pain and facial nerve paralysis.

A. **Types**

1. **Low-grade tumors:** more common form and are the tumors seen most frequently during childhood

   a. **Presentation:** They generally feel soft when palpated and appear encapsulated at surgery.

   b. **Treatment:** excision, with preservation of facial nerve branches that are not directly involved by the lesion

   c. **Prognosis:** When treated properly, 5-year survival rate is ~95%.

2. **High-grade tumors:** extremely aggressive, unencapsulated tumors that invade the gland widely

   a. **Treatment:** Total parotidectomy plus neck dissection (even without palpable nodes); surgery is usually supplemented by postoperative radiation.

   b. **Prognosis:** Five-year survival rate is 42% with optimal treatment.

II. **Malignant mixed tumors (carcinoma ex pleomorphic adenoma, carcinosarcoma):** Second most common type of malignancy and responsible for 8% of all parotid tumors. The treatment is total parotidectomy; a neck dissection is also done for either palpable adenopathy or a high-grade tumor.

III. **Squamous cell carcinoma:** Rare in the parotid gland; it is important to differentiate this lesion from a metastasis arising from a primary tumor elsewhere in the head and neck such as a skin cancer.

A. **Presentation:** hard on palpation and accompanied by pain and nerve paralysis

B. **Prognosis:** Five-year survival rate is ~20%.

IV. **Other lesions:** include adenoid cystic carcinoma (cylindroma), acinic cell adenocarcinoma, and adenocarcinoma

A. **Treatment:** Total parotidectomy; neck dissection is added when obvious nodal disease is present.

B. **High-grade, recurrent, and inoperable tumors:** treated with radiation

V. **Malignant lymphoma:** May arise as a primary tumor in the gland. The treatment is the same as for other lymphomas.

PAROTID TRAUMA

Lacerations and Foreign Bodies

I. **Parenchymal damage:** usually heals spontaneously if Stensen's duct is not injured

II. **Stensen duct:** the conduit for saliva from the parotid to the mouth, near the upper second molar. If lacerated or transected, it should be repaired over a small catheter, which will remain in place until the duct heals.

III. **Facial nerve injuries:** May recover spontaneously if only an anterior aspect of a distal branch is injured. If a main trunk is injured, it requires repair by primary anastomosis or nerve grafting.

IV. **Foreign bodies (e.g., bullets):** should be removed

INFLAMMATORY DISORDERS

Acute Suppurative Parotitis

I. **Etiology:** usually found in patients who are debilitated and dehydrated and who have poor oral hygiene

II. **Causal organism:** usually *Staphylococcus aureus*, which most likely enters the gland from the mouth via Stensen duct
   A. **Dehydration:** Patient whose salivary glands are not secreting actively is susceptible to rapid growth of the organism in this favorable environment.
   B. **Bacterial proliferation:** leads to an intense inflammatory reaction in the gland, with edema and severe pain

III. **Initial treatment:** includes hydration, antibiotics, and measures to promote salivation, such as occasionally sucking on a lemon
   A. **Cultures:** taken from Stensen duct
   B. **Antibiotics:** initially directed against *S. aureus* and are later adjusted as indicated by the results of the cultures

IV. **Surgical drainage:** required if the process is not arrested by the preceding measures

Calculous Sialadenitis

I. **Overview:** Condition caused by stones in the salivary ducts. If obstruction of the duct occurs, inflammation and intermittent painful swelling of the gland follow.

II. **Diagnosis:** Radiographs may show the stones. In the parotid gland, only 60% of stones are radiopaque.

III. **Surgery:** should be postponed if there is an acute infection present
   A. **Location:** When the stone is near the end of the duct, it can be removed transorally; if it is deep in the gland, it can be removed by an external incision.
   B. **Multiple stones and pain recurrence:** Remove the entire gland.
   C. **Sialoendoscopy (endoscopy of the ducts of the salivary glands):** has become an increasingly common way to diagnose and treat non-neoplastic disorders of the salivary gland, including calculi, strictures, and intraductal masses

IV. **Variants:** Sialadenitis can occur without stones. If symptoms persist, surgery may be necessary to remove the gland.

Chapter 19

Bariatric Surgery

Mark D. Kligman

 BACKGROUND

Obesity

I. **Classification and comorbidity**
   A. **Table 19-1:** classifies obesity
   B. **Table 19-2:** shows the risk of obesity-related comorbidities rising with increasing **body mass index (BMI)**

II. **Prevalence**
   A. **Incidence:** In the United States, obesity affects 35% of adults; ~17% of children and adolescents (ages 2–19 years) are also affected.
   B. **Demographics**
      1. **Ethnicity:** Prevalence of obesity is increased in African Americans and Hispanics.
      2. **Socioeconomics:** Poverty and poor education are also associated with an increased risk of obesity.

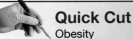 **Quick Cut**
Obesity comorbidities have broad effects on both the affected individual and society by limiting daily function, reducing life expectancy, and increasing health care costs.

Patient Selection

I. **General criteria:** Patients must demonstrate the following to qualify for bariatric surgery.
   A. **BMI:** greater than 40 kg/m² or BMI 35–39.9 kg/m² with a significant obesity-related comorbidity
   B. **Nonsurgical weight management programs:** documented failure
   C. **Surgical:** acceptable operative risk and adequate mental capacity to actively participate in pre- and postoperative care
   D. **Other:** absence of current alcohol or illicit drug abuse and of poorly controlled psychosis or depression

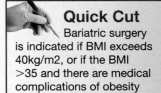 **Quick Cut**
Bariatric surgery is indicated if BMI exceeds 40kg/m2, or if the BMI >35 and there are medical complications of obesity

Table 19-1: Classification of Obesity

	Body Mass Index (BMI) (kg/m²)	Risk of Obesity-Related Comorbidity
Underweight	<18.5	Low
Normal	18.5–24.9	Average
Overweight	25.0–29.9	Mild
Class I obesity	30.0–34.9	Moderate
Class II obesity	35.0–39.9	Severe
Class III obesity	≥40	Very severe

Table 19-2: Obesity-Related Disorders

Cardiovascular	Musculoskeletal
Coronary artery disease	Osteoarthritis
Congestive heart failure	**Genitourinary**
Hypertension	Stress urinary incontinence
Dyslipidemia	**Gynecologic**
Venous stasis disease	Infertility
Pulmonary	**Hematopoietic**
Obstructive sleep apnea	Deep venous thrombosis
Obesity hypoventilation syndrome	Pulmonary embolism
Asthma	**Neurologic**
Endocrine	Pseudotumor cerebri
Insulin resistance	Stroke
Type 2 diabetes mellitus	
Polycystic ovarian syndrome	
Gastrointestinal	
Gastroesophageal reflux disease	
Nonalcoholic fatty liver disease	
Gallstones	

II. **Special populations**

A. **Adolescent patients:** Bariatric surgery has been demonstrated to be both safe and effective in adolescents.

1. Surgery is currently reserved for high-BMI patients (typically, BMI ≥ 50 kg/m^2) with major comorbidities (e.g., diabetes mellitus [DM], obstructive sleep apnea).

2. Patients must reach bone maturity prior to surgery to avoid growth retardation.

3. Family counseling is thought to improve compliance and is mandatory in most programs.

B. **Elderly patients:** Careful consideration of the current health status and desired goals/results must be undertaken in patients age older than 65 years.

C. **Class I obesity:** Early data is very promising for extending the indications for bariatric surgery to class I obesity (especially for DM treatment), but the practice is not yet considered the standard of care.

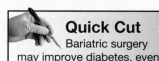

Quick Cut
Bariatric surgery may improve diabetes, even when performed in patients with normal BMI.

III. **Patient evaluation:** done by a multidisciplinary team that typically includes nutritionists, mental health professionals, and exercise physiologists

A. **Medical subspecialists (most commonly endocrinology, cardiology, or pulmonary medicine):** Consultation is based on specific patient needs.

B. **Studies:** Laboratory testing, radiologic evaluation, endoscopy, cardiac evaluation, and other studies are also based on specific needs.

SURGICAL TREATMENT OF OBESITY

Bariatric Operation Classification System

I. **Restrictive operations:** procedures that limit oral intake

A. **Adjustable gastric banding (Fig. 19-1):** Proprietary silastic band is placed around the stomach just below the gastroesophageal junction (GEJ), forming the outlet of a small gastric pouch.

1. **Mechanism:** Balloon attached to the band's inner surface is connected via tubing to a subcutaneous port; when sterile water is injected into the port, the balloon inflates, which narrows the outlet and thus limits food intake.

2. **Advantage:** This operation is easily reversed.

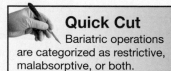

Quick Cut
Bariatric operations are categorized as restrictive, malabsorptive, or both.

Quick Cut
There is a hormonal component to weight management, which is poorly understood. The best studied of these hormones is ghrelin.

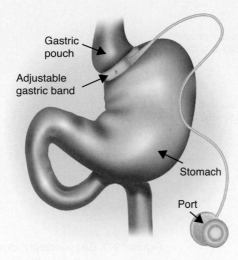

Figure 19-1: Adjustable gastric band.

B. **Sleeve gastrectomy (Fig. 19-2):** creates a narrow tube from the lesser curvature of the stomach by resection of the greater curvature of the gastric body and fundus
   1. **Mechanism:** Sleeve reduces food intake by impeding its transit through the stomach.
   2. **Disadvantage:** This procedure is not reversible.

II. **Malabsorptive operations:** procedures that limit nutrient absorption
   A. **Biliopancreatic diversion (Fig. 19-3):** features a 200–500-mL gastric pouch created from the proximal stomach by resection of the gastric antrum and distal gastric body
      1. **Mechanism:** The small intestine is divided 200–300 cm proximal to the ileocecal valve to form the alimentary limb (a combination of the Roux limb and common channel), which is used to drain the gastric pouch. The biliopancreatic limb is composed of the remaining small intestine and is anastomosed to the alimentary limb 50–150 cm proximal to the ileocecal valve, providing drainage for hepatic and pancreatic secretions.
      2. **Complication:** commonly causes dumping syndrome
   B. **Biliopancreatic diversion with duodenal switch (Fig. 19-4):** Gastric sleeve is used as the gastric pouch, thereby preserving the pylorus and eliminating the risk of dumping syndrome as a complication.

> **Quick Cut**
> Roux-en-Y gastric bypass is the standard weight loss operation, as it balances effective weight loss and risk of complications.

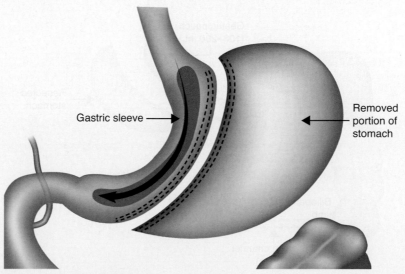

Figure 19-2: Sleeve gastrectomy.

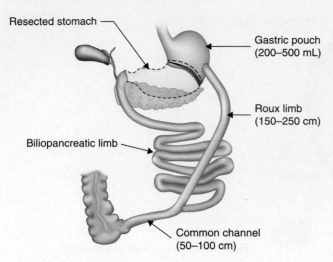

Figure 19-3: Biliopancreatic diversion.

III. Combined restriction and malabsorption (Fig. 19-5):
Gastric bypass is essentially a restrictive operation with limited malabsorption in which the volume of the gastric pouch is reduced to 15–30 mL, and the size of the pouch outlet is also limited.
A. **Mechanism:** Alimentary limb is formed from the entire small intestine except for the 40–75 cm required to provide drainage for hepatic and pancreatic secretions.
B. **Advantages:** Compared to malabsorptive operations, gastric bypass has similar weight loss with fewer nutritional complications.

Postoperative Considerations
I. **Vitamin and mineral supplementation:** Begins preoperatively and continues lifelong. Supplements commonly include multivitamins, vitamin B_{12}, vitamin D, calcium, and iron.

II. **Medical follow-up:** necessary to adjust medications and to assess nutritional status
A. **Frequency:** at least four times in the first postoperative year and annually thereafter
B. **Gastric band patients:** additionally assessed for weight loss rate and the band is adjusted as appropriate

III. **Multidisciplinary follow-up:** includes nutritional, exercise, and mental health counseling and educates patients for optimal results

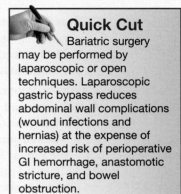

Quick Cut
Bariatric surgery may be performed by laparoscopic or open techniques. Laparoscopic gastric bypass reduces abdominal wall complications (wound infections and hernias) at the expense of increased risk of perioperative GI hemorrhage, anastomotic stricture, and bowel obstruction.

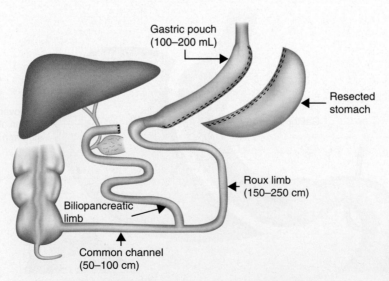

Figure 19-4: Biliopancreatic diversion with duodenal switch.

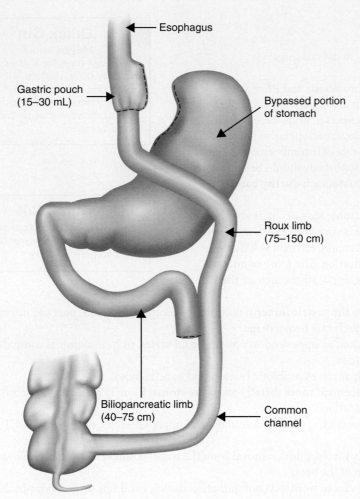

Esophagus

Gastric pouch
(15–30 mL)

Bypassed portion
of stomach

Roux limb
(75–150 cm)

Biliopancreatic limb
(40–75 cm)

Common
channel

Figure 19-5: Roux-en-Y gastric bypass.

Outcomes

I. **Weight loss:** usually reported as percentage of excess weight loss (EWL)

    A. **EWL:** calculated as (current weight − ideal body weight)/ (preoperative weight − ideal body weight) × 100%

    B. **Average weight loss:** influenced by the choice of operation

        1. **Adjustable gastric band:** 40%–50%

        2. **Sleeve gastrectomy:** 50%–65%

        3. **Biliopancreatic diversion (with or without duodenal switch):** 65%–75%

        4. **Gastric bypass:** 60%–75%

II. **Comorbidities (see Table 19-2):** improve or enter remission in 60%–95% of those affected and is directly related to percentage of EWL

III. **Survival:** Bariatric surgery reduces the overall 10-year risk of death from disease by ~50%.

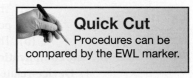

Quick Cut
Procedures can be compared by the EWL marker.

Quick Cut
In the severely obese, weight loss by any means, including surgical, will improve survival.

◆ POSTOPERATIVE MORTALITY AND COMPLICATIONS

Mortality

    I. **Rate:** Overall mortality rate is 0.2%.

    II. **Risk:** varies by type of operation (malabsorptive > combined > restrictive)

    III. **Causes:** Most common are sepsis, cardiac complications, and pulmonary embolism (PE).

Complications

I. Gastric banding

A. Early complications (within 30 days of surgery)

1. **Thromboembolism**
   a. **Incidence:** deep vein thrombosis and PE = 0.15% or less, much lower than for any other bariatric procedure
   b. **Diagnosis and treatment:** as in non-obese patients
   c. **Prevention:** Pharmacologic perioperative prophylaxis is controversial given the rate of thromboembolic events; however, mechanical prophylaxis should be considered in all patients.

2. **Perforation (of esophagus/stomach during band placement):** rare

3. **Device-related complications:** May occur at any time in the patient's postoperative course and commonly require operative repair. Diagnosis and treatment is based on the specific type of complication. The more commonly occurring device-related complications include the following.
   a. **Band penetration (into the gastric lumen):** may present as epigastric pain, port site infection, loss of restriction, or (rarely) GI hemorrhage
      (1) **Diagnosis:** established by upper endoscopy, upper GI series, or by abdominal computed tomography (CT) scan
      (2) **Treatment:** initially involves antibiotic therapy and band removal
   b. **Band slip (band displacement more distally on to the stomach):** may present with vomiting due to pouch outlet distortion
      (1) **Diagnosis:** confirmed using plain abdominal films, upper GI series, or abdominal CT scan
      (2) **Treatment:** initially involves fluid removal from the band to relieve symptoms, followed by surgical revision of the band
   c. **Port infection:** may be caused by direct contamination during band fills or, secondarily, due to band penetration
      (1) **Evaluation:** Abdominal CT scan and upper endoscopy are required to rule out band penetration.
      (2) **Treatment:** initially involves antibiotic therapy and port removal
         (a) The band and its tubing are left in the peritoneal cavity, and the skin overlying the port is left to heal secondarily.
         (b) The tubing is later retrieved and connected to a new port, completing band salvage.

B. Late complications (more than 30 days after surgery)

1. **Device-related complications:** (see above)
2. **Nutritional deficiencies:** rare

II. Sleeve gastrectomy

A. Early complications (within 30 days of surgery)

1. **Bleeding**
   a. **Incidence:** less than 1%
   b. **Site:** Bleeding can be intraluminal from the staple line or from an intraperitoneal source.
   c. **Diagnosis**
      (1) **History:** Intraluminal bleeding often presents with hematemesis.
      (2) **Physical examination:** Often unremarkable; however, significant bleeding can cause hemorrhagic shock.
   d. **Treatment**
      (1) **Initial therapy:** may include resuscitation with fluids and blood products and hemodynamic and urinary output monitoring
      (2) **Definitive treatment**
         (a) **Intraluminal bleeding:** Controlled using endoscopic techniques; surgical exploration is reserved for failed endoscopic therapy.
         (b) **Intraperitoneal bleeding:** requires surgical exploration to control hemorrhage site

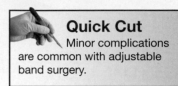

Quick Cut
Malabsorptive operations have the highest mortality rates, restrictive operations have the lowest mortality rates, and combined operations have intermediate mortality rates.

Quick Cut
Minor complications are common with adjustable band surgery.

2. **Staple line leak**
   a. **Incidence:** less than 3%
   b. **Etiology:** Most leaks occur near the GEJ and may be associated with partial obstruction in the more distal sleeve.
   c. **Diagnosis**
      (1) **Physical examination (abdominal):** Unreliable; peritonitis is a late finding.
      (2) **Abdominal CT:** best diagnostic modality for stable patients
      (3) **Surgical exploration:** definitive diagnostic tool and mandatory for diffuse peritonitis
   d. **Treatment:** fluid resuscitation, broad-spectrum antibiotics, and nutritional support
      (1) **Wide peritoneal drainage of the leak site:** surgically or percutaneously with image guidance; first-line treatment
      (2) **Direct repair of the leak site:** occasionally successful and used in conjunction with wide drainage
      (3) **Endoscopic techniques:** used to seal leaks, typically in conjunction with drainage

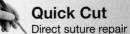

> **Quick Cut**
> The most common presenting signs of leak after bariatric surgery are those of early sepsis—tachycardia and tachypnea.

> **Quick Cut**
> Direct suture repair of a GI leak may sound appealing, but the sutures will not hold in the setting of peritonitis and inflammation.

B. **Late complications** (more than 30 days after surgery)
   1. **Gastric sleeve stricture:** from postoperative scarring or a technical error in sleeve construction
      a. **Incidence:** 0.5%
      b. **Clinical presentation:** Most common symptoms are nausea and vomiting; typically, patients tolerate fluids better than solids.
      c. **Diagnosis**
         (1) **Physical examination:** Usually unremarkable. Epigastric pain, if present, is mild.
         (2) **Radiologic evaluation:** abdominal CT, upper GI series, and upper endoscopy
      d. **Treatment**
         (1) **Endoscopic stenting and surgical stricturoplasty:** successful in some cases
         (2) **Conversion to gastric bypass:** usually the best option

III. **Gastric bypass**
   A. **Early complications** (within 30 days of surgery)
      1. **Bleeding**
         a. **Incidence:** 4%
         b. **Site:** can be intraluminal, from an anastomosis or staple line, or intraperitoneal
         c. **Diagnosis**
            (1) **History:** Hematemesis, hematochezia, or melena suggests an intraluminal source.
            (2) **Physical examination:** Often unremarkable; however, significant bleeding can cause hemorrhagic shock.
         d. **Treatment**
            (1) **Initial therapy:** may include resuscitation with fluids and blood products and hemodynamic and urinary output monitoring
            (1) **Definitive treatment:** determined by hemorrhage site
               (a) **Intraluminal bleeding:** Often controllable endoscopically; surgical exploration is reserved for failed endoscopic therapy, endoscopically inaccessible bleeding sites, or for unstable patients.
               (b) **Intraperitoneal bleeding:** often requires surgical exploration to control hemorrhage site
      2. **Anastomotic leak**
         a. **Incidence:** less than 4%
         b. **Etiology:** Most leaks occur 5–14 days from surgery and are related to tissue ischemia; earlier leaks are usually due to technical error.
         c. **Clinical presentation:** Most common presenting signs are those of early sepsis—tachycardia and tachypnea—and patients may appear anxious.

> **Quick Cut**
> Anastomotic leak is the most feared early complication of bariatric surgery. Reoperation may be the best means of diagnosis.

d. Diagnosis

(1) **Physical examination (abdominal):** Unreliable; peritonitis is a late finding.

(2) **Abdominal CT:** best diagnostic modality for stable patients

(3) **Surgical exploration:** definitive diagnostic tool and mandatory for diffuse peritonitis

e. Treatment: fluid resuscitation, broad-spectrum antibiotics, and nutritional support

(1) **Uncontained leak:** Surgical drainage is often the only necessary intervention; direct repair (or resection) is rarely successful.

(2) **Contained leaks:** can often be drained percutaneously under imaging guidance

2. Venous thromboembolism

a. **Incidence (of DVT and PE):** each less than 1%

b. **Diagnosis and treatment:** beyond chapter scope

c. **Prevention:** Perioperative prophylaxis should follow American College of Chest Physicians (ACCP) recommendations for high-risk general surgery patients.

> **Quick Cut**
> PE accounts for ~50% of all postoperative deaths following gastric bypass.

(1) Pharmacologic agents (unfractionated heparin or low-molecular-weight heparin) may be combined with leg compression devices.

(2) Prophylactic placement of inferior vena cava filters is controversial.

B. Late complications (more than 30 days after surgery)

1. Dumping syndrome

a. **Incidence:** Up to 85% of patients experience dumping syndrome at some point in their postoperative course.

b. **Etiology:** usually related to poor food choices, specifically foods containing refined sugars (e.g., high-fructose corn syrup) or high-fat concentrations (especially fried foods)

c. **Clinical presentation:** follows two patterns

(1) **Early dumping syndrome:** Typically begins 20–30 minutes after meals and is triggered by the rapid passage of food with high osmolality into the small intestine. The hypertonic intraluminal load induces a rapid shift of extracellular fluid into the intestinal lumen, producing either GI symptoms (e.g., nausea and vomiting, epigastric fullness, cramping abdominal pain, and diarrhea) or cardiovascular symptoms (e.g., flushing, dizziness, diaphoresis, palpitations, tachycardia, and syncope).

(2) **Late dumping syndrome:** Begins 1–3 hours after meals and is triggered by rapid passage of carbohydrates into the small intestine, which produces a hyperglycemic spike. The insulin released in response is excessive in relation to the total carbohydrate load, subsequently causing

> **Quick Cut**
> Dumping syndrome may occur after any gastrojejunostomy.

hypoglycemia that leads to catecholamine release from the adrenal gland. Symptoms include tremulousness, diaphoresis, light-headedness, tachycardia, and (rarely) confusion.

d. **Diagnosis:** Careful history is usually diagnostic.

e. **Treatment**

(1) Avoid refined sugars and fatty foods.

(2) Somatostatin analogues or acarbose may be helpful for those patients with persistent symptoms of late dumping syndrome despite dietary changes.

2. Anastomotic stricture: occurs almost exclusively at the gastrojejunostomy and may be associated with marginal ulceration

a. **Incidence:** 1%–15%

b. **Clinical presentation:** Typically involves persistent nausea and vomiting; patients often progressively limit their diet to foods that are able to traverse the stricture (i.e., soft foods or liquids).

c. **Diagnosis**

(1) **Physical examination:** often unremarkable

(2) **Upper endoscopy:** best diagnostic tool

d. **Treatment**

(1) **Endoscopic balloon dilation:** highly effective in providing permanent symptomatic relief

(2) **Surgical revision:** required rarely

3. **Marginal ulcers:** occur near the gastrojejunostomy
   a. **Etiology:** Factors include increased acid secretion, *Helicobacter pylori* infection, nonsteroidal anti-inflammatory drug (NSAID) use, and smoking.
   b. **Incidence:** 3%–10%
   c. **Clinical presentation:** most commonly epigastric pain associated with postprandial nausea and vomiting
   d. **Diagnosis**
      (1) **Physical examination:** Patients usually have focal epigastric tenderness.
      (2) **Upper endoscopy:** best method for patients with the typical pain pattern
      (3) **Upper GI series or abdominal CT scan:** sometimes useful
      (4) *H. pylori* **testing**
   e. **Treatment**
      (1) **Uncomplicated ulcers:** First-line treatment is medical therapy with cytoprotective agents (sucralfate), proton pump inhibitors, and antibiotics (if *H. pylori* present); patients should avoid NSAID use and smoking.
      (2) **Nonhealing ulcers: surgical** revision of the gastrojejunostomy
   f. **Complications:** include upper GI hemorrhage and perforation
4. **Internal hernia (Fig. 19-6):** results from small intestine trapped in mesenteric defects created during gastric bypass construction
   a. **Sites (three):** Petersen space, transverse mesocolic, or small bowel mesenteric defects are possible.
   b. **Incidence:** 3%–13%
   c. **Clinical presentation:** depends on hernia duration and severity
      (1) **Most common symptom:** abdominal pain
      (2) **Intestinal obstruction at the hernia site:** may produce nausea, vomiting, obstipation, and abdominal distension
   d. **Diagnosis**
      (1) **Physical examination:** Patients usually have periumbilical or left upper quadrant tenderness. Peritoneal findings or frank peritonitis suggest intestinal strangulation.
      (2) **Radiologic evaluation:** identifies ~80%
         (a) **Abdominal CT:** test of choice
         (b) **Upper GI series:** sometimes helpful
      (3) **Surgical exploration:** consider for patients with persistent unexplained abdominal pain despite thorough evaluation
   e. **Differential diagnosis:** adhesive bowel obstruction
   f. **Treatment:** requires surgical exploration with reduction of herniated intestine, resection of nonviable intestine, and closure of all potential hernia sites

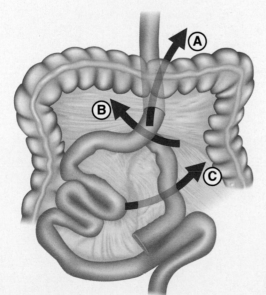

Figure 19-6: Sites for internal hernia following gastric bypass include (*A*) the transverse mesocolic defect, (*B*) Petersen space, and (*C*) the small bowel mesenteric defect.

5. **Cholelithiasis**
   a. **Incidence:** Symptomatic cholelithiasis occurs in up to 30% of patients within 3 years following gastric bypass.
   b. **Prevention:** two approaches
      (1) **All patients undergo prophylactic cholecystectomy (at the time of gastric bypass):** eliminates the possibility of symptomatic gallbladder disease
      (2) **Only patients with symptomatic cholelithiasis have cholecystectomy at the time of gastric bypass:** All other patients receive a 6-month course of ursodiol (300 mg by mouth twice daily). This approach reduces the incidence of subsequent symptomatic gallbladder disease to ~2%.
6. **Nutritional deficiencies:** relatively uncommon in patients who are compliant with postoperative vitamin and mineral supplementation

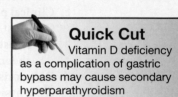

Quick Cut
Nutritional deficiencies are avoidable with routine testing and supplementation.

   a. **Vitamin B$_{12}$ deficiency:** due to both an overall reduction in intrinsic factor production and from bypass of the site of vitamin B$_{12}$ production within the stomach
   b. **Calcium and iron deficiency:** result from bypass of the duodenum and proximal jejunum where divalent cations are most efficiently absorbed
   c. **Fat-soluble vitamin deficiency (especially vitamins D and A):** due to reduced fat absorption in the jejunum and ileum
   d. **Vitamin B$_1$ deficiency (bariatric beriberi):** although uncommon, can occur with prolonged episodes of vomiting; may present with neuropsychiatric abnormalities (Wernicke encephalopathy) composed of confusion, ataxia, ophthalmoplegia, nystagmus, and impaired short-term memory or with cardiac findings including peripheral edema, dyspnea with exertion, paroxysmal nocturnal dyspnea, and tachycardia

Quick Cut
Vitamin D deficiency as a complication of gastric bypass may cause secondary hyperparathyroidism

IV. **Biliopancreatic diversion with or without duodenal switch:** similar to gastric bypass complications

Chapter 20

Minimal Access Surgery

Daniel Medina, Hugo Bonatti, and Stephen M. Kavic

HISTORY

Technical Advances

I. **Celioscopy:** Kelling was the first person to perform peritoneal "celioscopy" in a canine model with a cystoscope and air insufflation in 1901. In 1910, Jacobaeus used the same technique in humans.

II. **Image resolution:** Fiberoptic light sources replaced incandescent lights in the 1960s, and the addition of digital cameras greatly improved resolution of images. More recent developments include high-definition three-dimensional cameras and flexible camera heads.

III. **Stapling and intracorporeal energy device development:** based on ultrasound and electricity; allow more effective division of tissue, hemostasis, and anastomoses

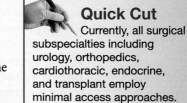

Quick Cut
Minimal access surgery is heavily technology dependent.

IV. **Hand ports:** 5-cm incisions and a gelcap through which one hand can be passed while keeping the abdomen air-sealed

V. **Single access surgery:** relies on a 3-cm incision and an occluding device with multiple ports through which all instruments can be introduced

VI. **Robotic technology:** Independently developed by the National Aeronautics and Space Administration and other institutions; the surgeon remotely and precisely operates various arms that hold modified laparoscopic instruments.

VII. **Hybrid procedures:** performed with cooperation of a minimal access surgeon and an interventionist, such as a radiologist or gastroenterologist

VIII. **Natural orifice access surgery:** Instruments are introduced through the stomach, rectum, or vagina; reduces scars, but is not yet the standard of care for most procedures.

Operative Milestones

I. **Laparoscopic appendectomy:** pioneered by Semm (1982); improved diagnosis of pelvic pathology in female patients.

II. **Laparoscopic cholecystectomy:** First performed by Erich Muhe (1985) in Germany, then by Dubois, Mouret, and Perrisat (1987) in France. The procedure was introduced and popularized in the United States by McKernan and Saye, and Reddick in the late 1980s.

Quick Cut
Currently, all surgical subspecialties including urology, orthopedics, cardiothoracic, endocrine, and transplant employ minimal access approaches.

III. **Other:** By the early 1990s, the technical feasibility of a laparoscopic approach was demonstrated for virtually all major abdominal surgical procedures.

GENERAL PRINCIPLES

Differences between Minimal Access and Open Surgery

I. **Operative field:** Unlike open surgery in which the operative field is exposed through a lengthy skin incision, minimal access surgery depends on accessing a natural or created cavity through small incisions.

II. **Visual control:** Operation is displayed on a video screen, which allows for magnification of structures but results in the loss of three dimensions.

III. **Instruments:** In open surgery, tactile feedback is an essential part of operative control; in minimal access surgery, control is largely visual.

> **Quick Cut**
> Minimally invasive surgeons rely heavily on visual cues to replace the loss of tactile feedback.

Advantages and Disadvantages of Minimal Access Surgery

I. **Advantages:** include improved visualization of anatomy, less tissue trauma and physiologic stress, less postoperative pain, shorter hospital stay, earlier return to normal activity after discharge, improved cosmetic result, and decreased perioperative complication rates (e.g., superficial wound infection, incisional hernia, and atelectasis)

II. **Disadvantages:** decreased tactile sensation, diminished depth perception, reduced degrees of freedom (instrument movement), difficult hemostasis, and resource intensive (cost and training)

III. **Cost-effectiveness:** Uncertain; minimal access procedures use expensive equipment and often disposable supplies, which increases costs. However, this cost increase may be offset by a faster return to normal activity and fewer complications.

Patient Preparation

I. **Preoperative preparation:** Essentially the same as for laparotomy; special attention is paid to the following.
   A. **Underlying medical problems**
   B. **Assessment of coagulation status**
   C. **Cardiopulmonary disease**

II. **General anesthesia:** employed in nearly all advanced minimal access procedures

III. **Intraoperative conduct:** Field is draped widely in case an open exploration is necessary.
   A. **Antithromboembolic pumps:** applied to the lower extremities to minimize the possibility of deep venous thrombosis (DVT)
   B. **Appropriate anesthetic monitoring:** necessary, especially end-tidal CO_2 monitoring

> **Quick Cut**
> Physiologic changes with pneumoperitoneum (elevated pressure and decreased venous return) may increase the risk of postoperative DVT.

General Operative Technique

I. **Room setup:** Patient position, video monitor placement, location of the operating team, and equipment testing are critical.

II. **Establishment of intra-abdominal access:** Filtered CO_2 is used because it is readily available, inexpensive, does not support combustion, and possesses a high diffusion coefficient. CO_2 is insufflated to a maximum pressure of 12–15 mm Hg in adults.
   A. **Safe, airtight entry into the peritoneal cavity:** may be achieved by various techniques
      1. **Closed pneumoperitoneum method:** Spring-loaded obturator needle (Veress needle) is inserted through the abdominal wall into the peritoneal cavity.
         a. **Left upper quadrant:** safe entry point
         b. **Desired pressure:** Once 12–15 mm Hg is achieved, transparent trocar with coupled camera is advanced under direct visualization through the abdominal wall.
      2. **Laparoscopic-assisted method:** Specialized disposable transparent port is necessary.
         a. **Laparoscope:** placed in the operating port while it is advanced directly through the abdominal wall
         b. **Gas:** Once the laparoscope is inside, gas is insufflated through the operating port into the peritoneal cavity.
      3. **Open pneumoperitoneum method:** A 2-cm incision is made, and the abdominal wall is dissected under direct vision. A specialized operating port with a blunt obturator (Hasson cannula) is inserted, and CO_2 is insufflated.
   B. **Exploration:** Thorough visual inspection is made of the surfaces (i.e., peritoneum, liver, omentum, stomach, and exposed bowel). This overview may help to guide the placement of additional ports.

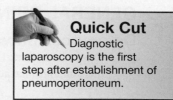

> **Quick Cut**
> Diagnostic laparoscopy is the first step after establishment of pneumoperitoneum.

C. **Insertion of accessory operating ports:** Two to six ports are necessary to accomplish most laparoscopic procedures.

D. **Hand-assisted laparoscopic surgery (HALS):** also known as "handoscopy"; hybrid alternative to conventional laparoscopy

1. **Technique:** Small laparotomy incision (6–8 cm) is made, allowing the surgeon to introduce a hand into the abdomen during laparoscopy for exposure and dissection maneuvers. HALS requires a specialized gel device to provide an air-tight seal between the skin incision and the surgeon's hand.

2. **Advantages:** restores tactile sensation; improves traction, dissection, and tissue exposure; improves control of bleeding; aids handling and extraction of large, bulky specimens

3. **Disadvantages:** requires an additional incision that increases surgical trauma; alters port placement and operative strategy; presence of surgeon's hand minimizes free space in abdomen

Relative Contraindications

I. **Severe cardiopulmonary disease:** Increased abdominal pressure associated with pneumoperitoneum decreases venous return and worsens pulmonary compliance, potentially leading to acidosis, hypotension, and dysrhythmias.

II. **Generalized peritonitis:** usually best treated with laparotomy

III. **Prior abdominal operations and adhesions:** increase the technical difficulty and potential danger of laparoscopy, especially at initial injury

IV. **Severe coagulopathic states:** Associated risk of hemorrhage is a contraindication for laparoscopy.

V. **Morbidly obese patients:** Very thick abdominal wall can hinder operating port placement and movement of laparoscopic instruments.

VI. **Uterine enlargement (during advanced pregnancy):** may preclude sufficient intraperitoneal space to perform laparoscopic procedures

VII. **Portal hypertension:** especially when associated with varices, significantly increases the risk of hemorrhage

> **Quick Cut**
> Critically ill patients and those with significant comorbidities may be best served by open surgery.

> **Quick Cut**
> The second trimester is the optimal time for surgery in pregnant patients.

Physiologic Changes Associated with Pneumoperitoneum

I. **Carbon dioxide:** produces hypercarbia and acidosis, which quickly resolves

II. **Increased intra-abdominal pressure (secondary to pneumoperitoneum):** Decreases venous return via compression of retroperitoneal veins, subsequently reducing cardiac output. Decreased venous return predisposes to stasis and DVT.

III. **Pneumoperitoneum:** may increase systemic vascular resistance and mean arterial pressure

IV. **Respiratory function:** affected by reduced pulmonary compliance (i.e., due to diaphragmatic elevation during pneumoperitoneum)

Complications

I. **Overall mortality and morbidity rates:** Generally similar to those observed in their corresponding open procedures. Surgical site infections should not exceed 2% in "clean" surgical wounds.

> **Quick Cut**
> Minimal access surgery has a decreased risk of wound complications relative to open surgery.

II. **Complications specific to laparoscopy:** include the following:

A. **Complications due to access:** Abdominal wall vessels may be injured in ~2% of cases.

1. **Abdominal wall hernias:** may occur through 10-mm or larger trocar sites, especially at the umbilicus

2. **Organ injury:** May occur, especially with adhesions. Placement of an orogastric tube and urinary catheter may reduce the risk of bowel or bladder perforation.

B. **Complications due to pneumoperitoneum:** Pneumomediastinum, pneumothorax, or subcutaneous emphysema are usually the result of excessive insufflation pressures (>20 mm Hg).

1. **Decreased cardiac output and dysrhythmia:** can occur due to compression of venous return or hypercarbic acidosis

2. **Postoperative shoulder self-limited pain:** Occurs in 10%–20% of patients. It is referred pain believed to be due to either stretching of the diaphragm by the pneumoperitoneum or direct irritation of the diaphragm by CO_2.

3. **Gas embolism:** may occur due to direct placement of an insufflation needle into a vessel or CO_2 flow directly into an open vessel exposed in dissection

Quick Cut
Postoperative shoulder pain is referred pain from the diaphragmatic nerves.

C. **Complications from instrumentation:** Examples include thermal (from electrocautery) or mechanical injury occuring in <1% of cases. These complications almost always require reoperation and may be life threatening if missed.

SELECTED LAPAROSCOPIC PROCEDURES

Laparoscopic Cholecystectomy

I. **Indications:** include biliary colic, symptomatic cholelithiasis, cholecystitis, biliary dyskinesia, or polyps

II. **Contraindications**

A. **Absolute contraindications:** suspicion of malignancy; uncontrolled coagulopathy

B. **Relative contraindications:** severe gallbladder inflammation (acute or chronic), hepatic cirrhosis, portal hypertension, and biliary fistula

III. **Complications**

A. **Common bile duct injuries:** occur more commonly (~0.25%) with laparoscopy than with the open technique (0.1%); requires laparotomy and major biliary reconstruction (Fig. 20-1)

B. **Bile leak:** bile may leak from the gallbladder bed or cystic duct stump (latter most commonly due to a clip coming off the duct)

1. **If suspected:** Patient should undergo either an abdominal ultrasound or computed tomography (CT) scan.

2. **If present:** usually amenable to percutaneous drainage, typically followed by endoscopic retrograde cholangiopancreatography (ERCP) to diagnose and treat the leak

C. **Retained common bile duct stone:** Occurs in ~10% of patients with common bile duct stones found during cholecystectomy. ERCP is usually diagnostic and therapeutic (e.g., sphincterotomy, stent, etc.).

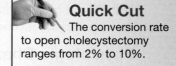
Quick Cut
The conversion rate to open cholecystectomy ranges from 2% to 10%.

IV. **Summary:** Laparoscopic cholecystectomy has been demonstrated to be safe and cost-effective when compared with open cholecystectomy and is the procedure of choice for most biliary disease.

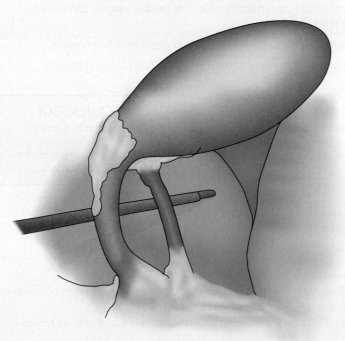

Figure 20-1: The "critical view" of safety during laparoscopic cholecystectomy after dissection of the neck of the gallbladder away from its bed. The cystic duct is seen on the left, and the cystic artery is on the right. This dissection should prevent bile duct injuries during laparoscopic cholecystectomy. (From Yamada T, Alpers DH, Laine L, et al. *Textbook of Gastroenterology*, 4th ed. Philadelphia: Lippincott Williams & Wilkins; 2003.)

V. **Intraoperative cholangiography (IOC):** indicated for the detection of common bile duct stones and the identification of biliary anatomy

Laparoscopic Appendectomy

I. **Indications:** Technically possible in nearly all patients with suspected appendicitis, including many with perforation. It is also useful when the diagnosis is uncertain or the patient is female.

II. **Relative contraindications**

    A. Appendiceal abscess: best treated by percutaneous drainage and appendectomy several weeks later or with open appendectomy and drainage

    B. Known or suspected appendiceal tumors

III. **Complications:** Same as with open appendectomies; the conversion rate to the open technique ranges from 3% to 10% and is usually caused by bleeding, abscesses, extensive abdominal contamination, difficulty in localization, poor exposure, or appendiceal dissection. (Fig. 20-2)

IV. **Controversies and conclusions:** Laparoscopic appendectomy is safe and effective.

    A. Advantages: slightly shorter hospital stay, lower incidence of wound infection, and less postoperative pain

    B. Disadvantages: More expensive and takes longer to perform than open appendectomy. The risk of postoperative intra-abdominal abscess also appears to be greater.

Laparoscopic Inguinal–Femoral Hernia Repair

I. **Indications:** Laparoscopic inguinal repair is used for reducible, recurrent, and bilateral hernias.

II. **Contraindications**

    A. Absolute: inability to tolerate general anesthesia; infarcted bowel in the hernia sac

    B. Relative: prior bladder or prostate surgery; hernia repair in children

III. **Technique:** can be performed from an intraperitoneal or preperitoneal approach (Fig. 20-3)

    A. General anesthesia: Required; dissection in the peritoneal cavity increases the risk of bowel injury, adhesion formation, and postoperative small bowel obstruction.

    B. Intraperitoneal procedure: can be performed with spinal or epidural anesthesia in some patients

        1. Step 1: After diagnostic laparoscopy, the peritoneum is incised above the level of the hernia sac. Blunt dissection is used to created peritoneal flaps and to reduce the hernia sac from the spermatic cord structures.

        2. Step 2: Cooper's ligament is identified and mesh secured with tacks.

        3. Step 3:.The peritoneum is closed over the mesh

IV. **Complications:** Risk of recurrent hernia after laparoscopic hernia repair is 1%–5% within the first 5 years of surgery.

    A. Genitofemoral and lateral femoral cutaneous nerve injuries: can result in significant postoperative groin and thigh pain and are usually caused by inadvertent staple placement too close to the nerves

    B. Injury to bowel, bladder, or major blood vessels: Although rare, these injuries occur more commonly after laparoscopic than open repair.

V. **Advantages:** earlier return to normal activity; less postoperative pain and numbness

VI. **Disadvantages:** longer operative times; higher risk of rare serious injuries (viscera and vessels)

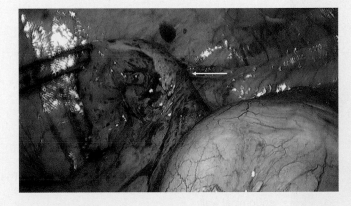

Figure 20-2: Laparoscopic appendectomy. The *arrow* points to the appendix. (From Shirkhoda A. *Variants and Pitfalls in Body Imaging*, 2nd ed. Philadelphia: Lippincott Williams & Wilkins; 2010.)

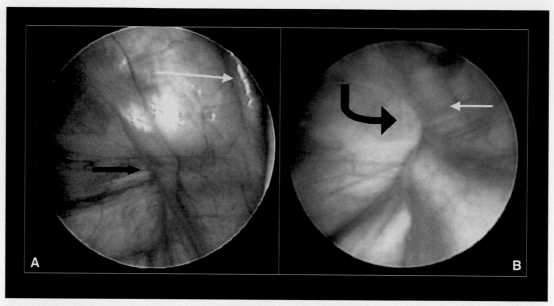

Figure 20-3: Inguinal canal anatomy as viewed during laparoscopic exploration of the peritoneal cavity. **A:** The normal anatomy of the inguinal region from within the peritoneal cavity. *Black arrow* indicates the closed deep inguinal ring; *white arrow*, the inferior epigastric vessels. **B:** An indirect inguinal hernia. *Curved black arrow* indicates the mouth of the hernial sac; *white arrow*, the inferior epigastric vessels. (Courtesy of N.S. Adzick.)

Laparoscopic Ventral Hernia Repair

I. **Indications:** Any symptomatic abdominal wall fascial defect, asymptomatic defects, or "Swiss cheese" abdomen (Fig. 20-4). Commonly, abdominal wall hernias are ventral, incisional, periumbilical, or a combination thereof.

II. **Contraindications**
   A. **Absolute:** loss of abdominal domain
   B. **Relative:** Incarcerated incisional hernias, patients with cirrhosis or portal hypertension, and patients with a history of long-term peritoneal dialysis (may develop a thick, inflammatory peel in the abdomen). Hernias of the lateral abdominal wall and lumbar region are technically more difficult than anterior hernias.

III. **Technique:** Abdomen is usually entered laterally, away from the hernia.
   A. **Step 1:** Three operating ports are placed laterally on one or both sides of the hernia (additional hernia defects are commonly seen during laparoscopy that were not appreciated on physical exam).
   B. **Step 2:** Size of the hernia defect(s) is measured, and an appropriate-sized piece of prosthetic mesh is chosen (should be sufficiently large to overlap the edges of the hernia defect by 5 cm in all directions).
   C. **Step 3:** Mesh is placed over the defect and is secured using sutures, tacks, or both.

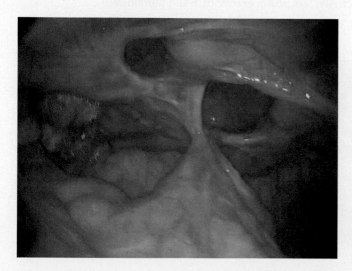

Figure 20-4: Laparoscopic umbilical hernia repair. The hernia defects are easily visualized as "holes" in the abdominal wall.

IV. **Complications**
   A. **Recurrent hernia:** Initial data show 5%–10% recurrence rates at 1–2 years after surgery.
   B. **Seroma:** At least 20% of patients develop a fluid collection between the mesh and the skin that resolves spontaneously in most cases, although aspiration is occasionally necessary.
   C. **Bowel or bladder injury:** occurs in ~2% of cases
   D. **Infection:** Wound infection occurs in ~1.5%–2% of patients; a few cases require mesh removal.

> **Quick Cut**
> Laparoscopic ventral hernia repair has a lower recurrence rates than open ventral hernia repair.

Fundoplication for Gastroesophageal Reflux Disease

I. **Indications:** severe gastroesophageal reflux disease (GERD), characterized by the following:
   A. **Failure of medical therapy:** with proton pump inhibitors
   B. **Severe nonhealing esophagitis:** despite aggressive medical therapy
   C. **Complications of GERD:** esophageal stricture, recurrent pneumonia or aspiration, and severe asthma

> **Quick Cut**
> Minimal access techniques can be applied to all foregut procedures, such as antireflux procedures performed either through the chest or the abdomen.

III. **Contraindications**
   A. **Shortened esophagus:** Severe, long-standing GERD causes fibrosis and shortening of the esophagus.
   B. **Prior laparoscopic fundoplication:** considered a relative contraindication

IV. **Technique:** All antireflux procedures have two common features—repair of a hiatal hernia, when present, and augmentation of lower esophageal sphincter pressure.
   A. **Full (360 degrees) fundoplication (Nissen):** primarily used for patients with GERD (Fig. 20-5) It is important to assess esophageal motility with manometry or UGI prior to operation.
   B. **Partial 270 degrees fundoplication (Toupet):** used in patients with poor esophageal motility

V. **Complications:** Esophageal perforation (<1%), pneumothorax or pneumomediastinum; splenic injury; complications fall into two general categories.
   A. **Mechanical failure:** results from either dehiscence of the suture line or, more commonly, herniation of an intact fundoplication through the diaphragm into the chest (recurrent hiatal hernia)
   B. **Fundoplication dysfunction:** Due to improper construction and resulting in significant dysphagia. Vagal nerve injury may also result in poor gastric emptying.

> **Quick Cut**
> The symptom complex of dysphagia and poor gastric emptying is known as "gas bloat syndrome" or "post-Nissen syndrome."

VI. **Controversies and conclusions:** Laparoscopic fundoplication is considered the procedure of choice in patients requiring surgical therapy for GERD.

Diagnostic Laparoscopy

I. **Indications:** Used to diagnose abdominal or pelvic pathology. It is the first step in any advanced laparoscopic procedure, and may find unrecognized conditions.

II. **Other indications**
   A. **Acute pelvic or lower abdominal pain:** differentiate acute appendicitis from other problems (e.g., pelvic inflammatory disease, ovarian torsion, or hemorrhagic cyst of ovary)
   B. **Tubal ectopic pregnancy:** fallopian tube excision or incision with evacuation of the tubal pregnancy
   C. **Ovarian torsion or infarction:** Treatment options include detorsion or resection of the ovary.
   D. **Infertility:** invaluable in establishing some causes of infertility, including adhesions, endometriosis, and tubal stricture
   E. **Staging of gynecologic malignancy:** Intra-abdominal disease can be staged with aortic and iliac lymph node sampling.
   F. **Ovarian masses:** differentiate benign from malignant ovarian lesions

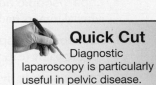

> **Quick Cut**
> Diagnostic laparoscopy is particularly useful in pelvic disease.

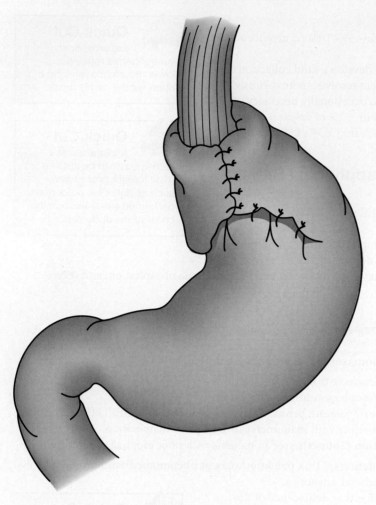

Figure 20-5: Nissen fundoplication.

Laparoscopic Staging of Malignancy

I. **"Formal" staging procedures:** Usually include exploration, lymph node sampling or dissection, liver biopsy, and other interventions as needed for the particular disease process, such as gastrointestinal cancers (esophagus, lung, stomach), genitourinary cancers (testicular, bladder, prostate), lymphoma, and gynecologic cancers. Results may guide treatment prior to definitive surgery.

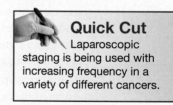

Quick Cut
Laparoscopic staging is being used with increasing frequency in a variety of different cancers.

II. **Directed staging to assess resectability with curative intent:** Such as for pancreatic cancer. The abdomen is inspected for occult metastases not found by imaging.

III. **Biopsy:** of specific abnormalities detected on imaging studies or screening exams

Other Laparoscopic Procedures

I. **Laparoscopic adrenalectomy:** regarded as the procedure of choice for most patients with benign adrenal tumors under 10 cm diameter

II. **Laparoscopic splenectomy:** ideal in patients without severe splenomegaly or uncorrectable coagulopathy (e.g., well-controlled idiopathic thrombocytopenic purpura [ITP])

III. **Laparoscopic liver resection:** All types of resection, from wedge resection to true anatomic resection, have been reported.

IV. **Laparoscopic donor nephrectomy:** Considered the procedure of choice for harvest of renal allografts in appropriate patients. Allograft function from laparoscopic donors is equivalent to that of kidneys from open donors.

V. **Laparoscopic surgery for morbid obesity:** See Chapter 19.

VI. **Laparoscopic colectomy:** See Chapter 12.

 # ROBOTIC TECHNOLOGY

History and Approach

I. **History:** The technology for robotic surgery was first implemented in the late 1980s. By the late 1990s, general surgery, gynecology, urology, and cardiothoracic surgery fields were employing robotic surgery in major surgical centers.

   A. **Procedures:** Generally, procedures amenable to minimal access surgery (e.g., laparoscopy, thoracoscopy) may be performed robotically; a few procedures, such as prostatectomy, may be best performed robotically.

   B. **Robot types:** During the past two decades, numerous types have been developed that rely on the remote control of the surgeon over the robotic arms, which hold the surgical instruments (Fig. 20-6). This property of robotic surgery allows remote surgery where the surgeon and the patient are geographically separated.

II. **Approach:** Placement of ports through which the robotic arms manipulate instruments is essentially the same as those of laparoscopic surgery.

Advantages, Disadvantages, and Conclusions

I. **Advantages:** relative to standard laparoscopic surgery, provides improved precision and recovery of three-dimensional vision, ambidexterity, and degrees of freedom

II. **Disadvantages:** lack of cost-effectiveness, requires expensive machinery and a well-trained staff, steep learning curve for the surgeon, and lack of tactile feedback

III. **Conclusions:** allows for the performance of complex procedures in experienced hands, for example, in cardiothoracic surgery (robotic coronary artery bypass), general surgery (Whipple procedure, transplant), bariatric surgery (gastric bypasses), orthopedics (joint surgery), neurosurgery (stereotactic procedures), gynecology (hysterectomy), and urology (prostatectomy)

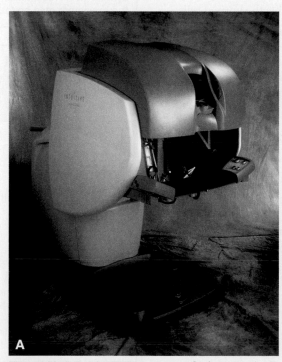 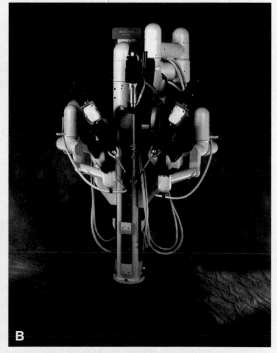

Figure 20-6: DaVinci robot system. **A:** the console. **B:** "the robot." (From Ballantyne GH, Marescaux J, Giulianotti PC. *Primer of Robotic and Telerobotic Surgery*. Philadelphia: Lippincott Williams & Wilkins; 2004.)

Chapter 21

Surgical Oncology

Keli Turner, Natalie A. O'Neill, and Stephen M. Kavic

CANCER

Definitions

I. **Tumor:** abnormal mass of tissue

II. **Neoplasia:** new growth or the development of tumors

III. **Dysplasia:** abnormal growth

IV. **Malignant:** harmful or having the tendency to displace normal function

V. **Benign:** does not tend to spread to other anatomic areas

Grade

I. **Overview:** Tumor grade is assessed on a microscopic level and represents how much divergence there is between normal cells and the cells of the tumor.
   A. **Well-differentiated cells:** similar in appearance to normal cells
   B. **Poorly differentiated cells:** do not resemble the normal cells

II. **Prognosis:** Tumor grade can indicate prognosis.

Subtypes

I. **Carcinoma:** malignant tumor that arises from epithelium
   A. **Adenocarcinoma:** arises from epithelium and has a glandular component
   B. **Squamous cell carcinoma:** arises from squamous epithelium and has keratinization or other characteristics peculiar to this cell

II. **Sarcoma:** arises from mesodermal tissue (mesenchymal cells)

III. **Lymphoma:** arises from the cellular component of lymph nodes (LNs), typically B cells or T cells

CANCER ETIOLOGY AND EPIDEMIOLOGY

Genetic Basis

I. **Oncogenes:** genes that have the potential to cause cancer, usually by thwarting the normal process of apoptosis
   A. **"Proto-oncogenes":** Become activated to form oncogenes; mutation in only one gene is required for a gain of function.
   B. *ras*: signal oncogene that encodes a signal transduction protein; commonly mutated in colon cancer

Quick Cut
Cancer is the general term for disease caused by unregulated growth and spread of cells.

Quick Cut
Malignant tumors infiltrate and metastasize.

Quick Cut
Benign lesions can still cause significant symptoms: A focal lesion near the brainstem may be fatal.

Quick Cut
In general, the less differentiated the tumor, the worse the prognosis.

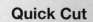
Quick Cut
Proto-oncogenes are expressed during cellular proliferation (embryonic development or the healing response).

C. HER-2/*neu*: membrane receptor that codes for a protein similar to the receptor for epidermal growth factor; commonly mutated in breast and ovarian cancer

D. *C-myc*: nuclear transcription factor; often mutated in solid tumors

II. **Tumor suppression genes:** function to suppress or regulate cellular proliferation

A. **Loss of function:** Mutation or deletion in both genes is required.

B. **p53:** best known of these genes

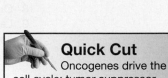

> **Quick Cut**
> Loss of p53 is the single most common genetic defect in human malignancy.

III. **DNA repair genes:** Encode proteins that correct errors in replicated DNA. DNA mismatch repair mutations (MSH2 and MLH1) are associated with hereditary nonpolyposis colon cancer (HNPCC).

Cellular Mechanisms

I. **Cell cycle:** Tightly regulated under normal conditions; cancer cells are characterized by a breakdown in normal regulation of proliferation.

II. **Metastasis:** may require additional elements, such as modification of the extracellular matrix, altered expression of cellular adhesion molecules, and angiogenic factors

> **Quick Cut**
> Oncogenes drive the cell cycle; tumor suppressor genes provide a natural checkpoint.

III. **Adenoma–carcinoma sequence:** See Figure 21-1

IV. **Colorectal cancer:** may develop as a result of a number of mutations

A. **Alterations in the APC gene:** This early change may permit adenoma formation.

B. **Mutations in kRas:** may lead to adenomatous polyps

C. **Further mutations in p53:** may allow the formation of adenocarcinoma

> **Quick Cut**
> Carcinogens are substances that are known to be causative agents in cancer development.

Carcinogens

I. **Chemical**

A. **Tobacco smoke:** squamous cell carcinoma of the lung

B. **Asbestos:** mesothelioma of the pleura

II. **Physical**

A. **Neck irradiation:** papillary thyroid cancer

B. **Ultraviolet (UV) light:** basal cell skin carcinoma

> **Quick Cut**
> No single etiology causes cancer: multiple factors lead to neoplastic transformation.

III. **Infection**

A. **Epstein-Barr virus:** Burkitt lymphoma

B. **Hepatitis B or C:** hepatocellular carcinoma

IV. **Geographic/epidemiologic**

A. **Japan:** gastric cancer

B. **China:** esophageal cancer

Epidemiology

I. **Incidence:** Number of new cases of a particular disease that appear in a given time period. Table 21-1 lists the top 10 cancers by diagnosis.

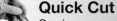

> **Quick Cut**
> Prevalence is the overall proportion of cases within a given population.

II. **Mortality:** Parallels cancer incidence but not directly—some tumors are more aggressive biologically (Table 21-2).

A. **Men:** Prostate cancer is the most common malignancy in men.

B. **Women:** Breast cancer is the most common malignancy in women.

C. **Overall:** Lung cancer is the most common cause of cancer death for both sexes.

> **Quick Cut**
> One in four Americans will develop some type of cancer.

Gene alteration	Loss of APC		Activation of Ras		Loss of a tumor suppressor gene	Loss of p53 activity	Other alterations	
Cell type	Normal epithelium	→ Hyperproliferative epithelium	→ Early adenoma	→ Intermediate adenoma	→ Late adenoma	→ Carcinoma	→ Metastasis

Figure 21-1: The adenoma–carcinoma sequence for colon cancer. Multiple mutations are required to progress from normal epithelium to overt cancer. APC, adenomatous polyposis coli gene. (From Swanson TA, Kim SI, Glucksman MJ. *BRS Biochemistry, Molecular Biology, and Genetics*, 5th ed. Baltimore: Lippincott Williams & Wilkins; 2009.)

Table 21-1: Incidence of Cancer by Site and Gender

Male	Female
1. Prostate	1. Breast
2. Lung	2. Lung
3. Colon	3. Colon
4. Bladder	4. Uterus
5. Melanoma	5. Thyroid
6. Kidney	6. Lymphoma
7. Lymphoma	7. Melanoma
8. Oral cavity	8. Kidney
9. Leukemia	9. Pancreas
10. Liver	10. Leukemia

SCREENING AND DIAGNOSIS

Overview

I. **Screening:** Used when a disease process may be detected early enough in its course to allow for optimal management, which relies on a sufficiently sensitive test as well as a disease process with significant prevalence for a given population. Although a detailed discussion of screening is beyond the scope of this chapter, the American Cancer Society (ACS) recommends screening for the following processes.

   A. **Colorectal cancer:** Current guidelines recommend endoscopy (colonoscopy, sigmoidoscopy, or computed tomography [CT]–based virtual colonoscopy) or barium enema starting at age 50 years. Other screening tests may include fecal occult blood testing or stool DNA.

   B. **Breast cancer:** Current recommendation remains for annual mammography starting at age 40 years, combined with clinical breast exam every 3 years and routine surveillance with breast self-examination.

   C. **Cervical cancer:** Starting at age 21 years, it is recommended that women have Pap smears every 3 years until age 30 years, then every 5 years in conjunction with a human papilloma virus (HPV) test until age 65 years.

   D. **Prostate cancer:** Men older than age 50 years are eligible for prostate-specific antigen (PSA), but it is not routinely recommended for all men, as there is no proven survival benefit.

II. **Diagnosis:** It may take years before a tumor is clinically detectable; symptoms may be a late appearance of malignancy.

   A. **Mass effect:** obstruction or impairment of an adjacent structure due to compression

   B. **Bleeding:** may be related to neovascularization and angiogenesis related to a tumor

   C. **Systemic signs of malignancy:** include fever, malaise, and cachexia

> **Quick Cut**
> A single malignant cell that undergoes 30 doublings results in 1 billion cells and a 1-cm diameter tumor.

Table 21-2: Cancer Mortality

Male	Female
1. Lung	1. Lung
2. Prostate	2. Breast
3. Colon	3. Colon
4. Pancreas	4. Pancreas
5. Liver	5. Ovary
6. Leukemia	6. Leukemia
7. Esophagus	7. Uterus
8. Bladder	8. Lymphoma
9. Lymphoma	9. Liver
10. Kidney	10. Brain

Table 21-3: **Common Tumor Markers**

Marker	Malignancy
Alpha-fetoprotein	Germ cell tumors, hepatocellular carcinoma
Beta-human chorionic gonadotropin	Choriocarcinoma, testicular cancer
BCR-ABL gene	Chronic myeloid leukemia
CA 19-9	Pancreas, bile duct, stomach
CA 125	Ovarian
Calcitonin	Medullary thyroid
Carcinoembryonic antigen	Colorectal
Chromogranin A	Neuroendocrine tumors
Lactate dehydrogenase	Germ cell tumors
Prostate-specific antigen	Prostate
Thyroglobulin	Thyroid

D. Tumor markers (Table 21-3): substances typically made by normal cells (but in lower quantities than in cancer cells) that are detectable on laboratory tests and indicate the presence of tumors or tumor-specific products such as hormones or enzymes
    1. Screening: Tumor markers may be used such as PSA for prostate cancer.
    2. Disease recurrence: Some markers may be useful in the early identification of recurrence, such as carcinoembryonic antigen (CEA) in colon cancer.

Imaging

  I. **Cross-sectional imaging:** Dominant role in the diagnosis and follow-up of solid tumors. CT and magnetic resonance imaging (MRI) both have applications for particular tumor types. Many tumors are initially diagnosed incidentally on imaging obtained for other purposes.

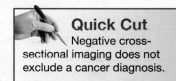

Quick Cut
Negative cross-sectional imaging does not exclude a cancer diagnosis.

  II. **Functional imaging:** Positron emission tomography (PET) is a means of assessing the functional status of metabolically active tissue.
    A. Complementary test: Although the images do not provide precise anatomic information, PET describes regions of high metabolic activity, such as rapidly dividing cancer cells.
    B. Fluorodeoxyglucose (FDG): most commonly used tracer for PET scans
    C. Combination: PET may be combined with CT to produce images at the same time in the same machine. Lesions less than 1 cm may not be easily visible on PET scans.

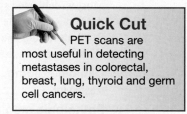

Quick Cut
PET scans are most useful in detecting metastases in colorectal, breast, lung, thyroid and germ cell cancers.

◆ DIAGNOSTIC PROCEDURES

Biopsy

  I. **Fine-needle aspiration (FNA):** Performed by pushing a small-gauge needle, typically 20 gauge or smaller, into the lesion of interest and sending material contained in the lumen for analysis to determine the basic cell type. However, FNA cannot reliably diagnose invasive disease, as architecture may not be revealed on a small specimen.

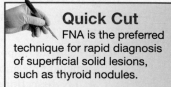

Quick Cut
FNA is the preferred technique for rapid diagnosis of superficial solid lesions, such as thyroid nodules.

  II. **Core-needle biopsy:** Larger needle is used, typically 14 gauge, and passed multiple times through the same lesion, which decreases sampling error, but it is slightly more invasive than FNA. The sample may incorporate some of the tissue around the lesion and provide clues to tumor invasiveness.

III. **Image-guided biopsy:** Percutaneous needle biopsy may be performed using imaging guidance when the lesion is not superficial or palpable. Techniques include ultrasound-guided, CT- or MRI-guided, or stereotactic biopsy.

IV. **Incisional biopsy:** Such as surgical biopsy with a portion of a lesion removed. This technique is usually reserved for larger lesions.

V. **Excisional biopsy:** complete removal of a lesion for diagnostic purposes

Molecular Diagnostics

I. **Receptor status:** Certain cancers may carry prognostic and treatment implications. Perhaps best known is the estrogen receptor (ER) and progesterone receptor (PR) status of breast cancer, determined by direct analysis of tumor specimens.

II. **Genomic studies:** Analyze the structure and function of a DNA sequence. The promise of genomics is that specific genetic sequences may yield prognostic information on tumor behavior or response to therapy. Gene arrays are now available but have not yet been incorporated into common clinical practice.

III. **Proteomics:** Study of protein structure and their functions. An increasing body of information is being generated on cancer gene products and their specific protein signatures that may aid in cancer diagnosis and treatment.

Operation

I. **Operative intervention:** may be necessary to determine the diagnosis or the extent of the disease process

II. **Laparoscopy:** has become a standard diagnostic tool for upper abdominal malignancies, as it is more sensitive than cross-sectional imaging for the detection of metastatic disease and less invasive than laparotomy

STAGING

Overview

I. **Prognosis:** By standardizing malignancies into groups that have similar behavior, accurate prognostic information can be obtained.

II. **Treatment:** Algorithms can be developed for a particular stage of cancer, and these can be rigorously studied, as cancers are grouped into comparable stages.

III. **Tumor, nodes, and metastasis (TNM) system (Table 21-4):** Most widely used system is based on tumor, nodes, and metastases.
   A. **T:** describes the extent of tumor
   B. **N:** describes the presence of local or distant LN involvement
   C. **M:** describes the presence of distant metastatic disease

IV. **Clinical staging:** made based on biopsy and imaging before treatment

V. **Pathologic staging:** determined after definitive intervention

Quick Cut
Staging is the process of grouping cancers based on type and extent of disease.

Quick Cut
TNM is the dominant staging system used for most forms of cancer, and staging is specific to each cancer type.

SURGICAL TREATMENT

Diagnostic

I. **Tissue diagnosis:** Surgical intervention may yield a cancer diagnosis through incisional or excisional biopsy.

II. **LN status:** important for staging any malignancy, but it is particularly used in breast cancer and malignant melanoma
   A. **LN dissection:** Lymphadenectomy involves removing the lymphatic tissue in a known anatomic distribution from the site of a tumor.
   B. **Sentinel LNs:** first LN in a chain that drains the area of interest
      1. **Identification:** Sentinel node can be identified through the use of dye (isosulfan blue) or radioactive tracer (technetium-99–labeled sulfur colloid) and use of an intraoperative gamma probe.

Table 21-4: Tumor, Nodes, and Metastasis Classification System and Stage Grouping for Gastric Adenocarcinoma

Tumor (T)	
T0	No evidence of primary tumor
Tis (in situ)	Tumor limited to mucosa
T1	Tumor limited to mucosa or submucosa
T2	Tumor to but not through the serosa
T3	Tumor through the serosa but not into adjacent organs
T4	Tumor into adjacent organs (direct extension)
Nodes (N)	
N0	No metastases to lymph nodes
N1	Only perigastric lymph nodes within 3 cm of the primary tumor
N2	Only regional lymph nodes more than 3 cm from tumor but removable at operation
N3	Other intra-abdominal lymph nodes involved
Metastases (M)	
M0	No distant metastases
M1	Distant metastases
Stage grouping	
Stage 0	Tis, N0, M0
Stage 1	T1, N0, M0
Stage 2	T2 or T3, N0, M0
Stage 3	T1–T3, N1 or N2, M0
Stage 4	Any T4, any T3, any N3, any M1

2. **Surgical technique:** Identified sentinel node can be excised and undergo analysis, providing diagnostic information without the morbidity of a full lymphadenectomy (such as lymphedema). False-negative rate is less than 5%; may be complicated by previous surgery or biopsies that alter the native patterns of lymph drainage.

> **Quick Cut**
> Sentinel node techniques were developed to avoid the potentially substantial morbidity of LN dissection.

Prophylactic

I. **Breast:** Prophylactic mastectomy may be indicated when the risk of breast cancer approaches 100%; it reduces the risk of breast cancer by more than 90% but not completely, as some breast tissue may remain on the chest wall or in the axilla. Candidates include:
   A. **Bilateral:** BRCA-1– or BRCA-2–positive women
   B. **Contralateral:** women with invasive breast cancer in one breast

> **Quick Cut**
> Prophylactic surgery may be offered when the risk of developing malignancy seems certain.

II. **Ovary:** Prophylactic oophorectomy is offered in women who are BRCA-1 or BRCA-2 positive; it decreases the risk of ovarian cancer by 90% and the risk of breast cancer by 50% in premenopausal women.

III. **Thyroid:** Thyroidectomy is recommended for cases of RET mutation in families with multiple endocrine neoplasia (MEN) that causes medullary thyroid carcinoma; typically performed in childhood and requires lifelong thyroid hormone supplementation.

IV. **Colon:** Colectomy is reserved for cases of genetic conditions where the risk of colon cancer is high (familial adenomatous polyposis or HNPCC); patients may opt for permanent end ileostomy or internal reconstruction with an ileoanal pouch anastomosis.

> **Quick Cut**
> Whenever possible, oncologic surgery is performed with curative intent.

Curative

I. **Excision:** May be adequate for small or low-grade lesions; wide local excision is the preferred treatment for basal cell skin carcinoma.

II. **Radical resection:** Involves the removal of the tumor and its surrounding tissues and may involve removal of multiple LN basins; en bloc resections involve portions of adjacent organs or viscera in direct contact with the tumor.

Palliative

I. **Debulking:** Removal of the majority of a tumor, leaving known residual disease, is performed when complete resection would be excessively debilitating; it may increase efficacy of adjuvant therapies due to decreased tumor burden. Most commonly employed in treatment of ovarian cancer.

II. **Metastasectomy:** may alleviate symptoms when control of the primary tumor is obtained; commonly used in resection of liver metastases from colon cancer

III. **Symptomatic treatment:** used to alleviate a specific symptom from metastatic disease (e.g., decompression of an obstructing colon mass may prolong life and minimize suffering in a patient with known metastases)

Quick Cut
There are several common principles in surgical oncology, including minimal manipulation of the tumor and early ligation of vessels to avoid vascular dissemination, gentle tissue handling and dissection to minimize local recurrence, and excision of lymphatic channels to minimize the risk of lymphatic spread.

Follow-up

I. **Surveillance:** After surgical resection, patients are monitored closely in order to detect any recurrence of cancer with a combination of history and physical examination, laboratory tests including tumor markers, and imaging.

II. **Frequency and timing of visits:** Based on the type and stage of the cancer. If a tumor is detected, patients should undergo restaging to determine the most appropriate treatment.

MULTIDISCIPLINARY TREATMENT

Adjuvant/Neoadjuvant Therapy

I. **Adjuvant therapy:** systemic treatment in a patient with primary control with the goal to minimize the risk of recurrence or metastasis

II. **Neoadjuvant therapy:** adjuvant therapy given before there is control of the primary tumor (i.e., preoperatively)

Quick Cut
A hallmark of modern care of the cancer patient is the involvement of many disciplines to optimize patient outcomes.

Chemotherapy

I. **Definition:** systemic use of chemical agent to impede or destroy rapidly dividing cancer cells

Quick Cut
Adjuvant therapy is not a substitute for good surgical technique.

II. **High dose:** Certain medications may be given in higher local doses through regional techniques, such as use of a hepatic artery catheter for liver lesions, isolated limb perfusion for lesions of the extremities, or intraperitoneal chemotherapy for peritoneal malignancies.

III. **Side effects:** include toxicity to normal cells that undergo division, such as hair and the mucosal surface of the gastrointestinal (GI) tract

Radiation Therapy

I. **Definition:** involves the use of energy delivered through external beams or internal implants (i.e., brachytherapy) to damage the DNA of target cells

II. **Goal:** may be curative or palliative

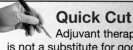

Quick Cut
The precise regimen of primary and adjuvant treatments depends on the tumor type, location, grade, and stage as well as patient factors such as age, comorbid conditions, and patient preferences.

Other

I. **Immunotherapy:** also called *biotherapy*; systemic modulation of the immune system to combat cancer

    A. Monoclonal antibodies: More than 12 have been approved by the U.S. Food and Drug Administration (FDA) for use against specific cancer cells.

    B. Cancer vaccines: Currently, only one agent is FDA approved—sipuleucel-T—for the treatment of prostate cancer.

II. **Hormonal therapy:** Some malignancies are potentiated by hormones, and hormonal blockade may provide some anticancer benefit.
   A. **Breast cancer:** Most are ER positive; tamoxifen blocks the receptor itself, and aromatase inhibitors block estrogen production. Both have demonstrated a survival benefit.
   B. **Prostate cancer:** Androgen inhibitors may be of benefit.

III. **Genetic therapy:** In principle, missing or defective genes could be replaced through transfection; current genetic therapy remains experimental.

RESEARCH AND TRAINING

Clinical Trials

I. **Trial design:** Surgical oncologists are frequently involved in the development and assessment of new treatments and should be familiar with the basic concepts of trial design.

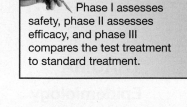

Quick Cut
Phase I assesses safety, phase II assesses efficacy, and phase III compares the test treatment to standard treatment.

   A. **Phase I:** Studies test safety; these are often small studies that establish side effects as well as a safe dosage range.
   B. **Phase II:** Studies test efficacy; these studies involve more participants and look for a clinical effect of the treatment.
   C. **Phase III:** Studies are comparative to a standard treatment.

II. **Institutional review board (IRB):** independent review committee that oversees human subject research
   A. **Mandate:** Code of Federal Regulations, Part 46
   B. **Ethical research:** guided by three principles (the Belmont report):
      1. **Beneficence:** Research should maximize possible benefits and minimize possible harms.
      2. **Justice:** There should be fairness in selection, and those groups that bear the risks of research should benefit from its conclusions.
      3. **Respect for persons:** Autonomy is the guiding principle, with protection for vulnerable populations.

Training

I. **Surgical oncologists:** should pursue advanced training for their particular field

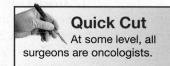

Quick Cut
At some level, all surgeons are oncologists.

II. **Fellowships:** currently available beyond surgical residency in general oncologic surgery, hepatobiliary surgery, breast surgery, and complex surgical oncology

Trauma and Burns

Brandon Bruns and Thomas Scalea

Chapter 22

TRAUMA

Epidemiology

   I. **Incidence:** leading cause of death for individuals ages 1–44 years

   II. **Cause:** More than 50% of these deaths are caused by motor vehicle collisions (MVCs).

Patient Evaluation

   I. **Prehospital:** Network of prehospital providers and transport is paramount for optimal trauma patient outcomes.

   II. **Initial evaluation:** The American College of Surgeons (ACS), through the advanced trauma life support course (ATLS), teaches a systematic approach to the initial evaluation of trauma patients.

     A. Primary survey: ABCDE

       1. **Airway:** Ensure the patient is capable of protecting his or her airway; inspect the oropharynx for any potential for obstruction (e.g., blood, teeth); if necessary, establish an airway via tracheal intubation (most guidelines suggest for a depressed neurologic status with a Glasgow Coma Scale [GCS] score <8).

       2. **Breathing:** Auscultate the bilateral lung fields for breath sounds; decreased breath sounds may indicate the presence of a pneumothorax.

       3. **Circulation:** Check for femoral and distal pulses, and check the patient's blood pressure (BP) and heart rate (HR); tachycardia may precede a drop in BP as the first indication of hypovolemia.

       4. **Disability (Fig. 22-1):** Rapidly assess the patient's GCS (15 is the maximum); if an endotracheal tube is present, add "T" to the end (e.g., GCS 11T).

       5. **Exposure:** Patient is fully disrobed for complete physical evaluation.

     B. Adjuncts: to the primary survey

       1. **Chest radiograph:** Evaluate the chest x-ray systematically, starting with ensuring the correct patient.

         a. **Airway:** Inspect the trachea to ensure it is midline; deviation to either side could indicate pneumothorax, hemothorax, or aortic injury.

         b. **Breathing:** Ensure lung markings are present; absence indicates the presence of a pneumothorax, and opacification of a lung field may indicate a hemothorax.

         c. **Cardiac silhouette:** Inspect the borders of the heart and mediastinum; classically, a mediastinum greater than 8 cm is suggestive of thoracic aortic injury.

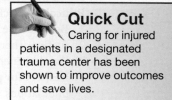

Quick Cut
Caring for injured patients in a designated trauma center has been shown to improve outcomes and save lives.

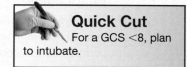

Quick Cut
For a GCS <8, plan to intubate.

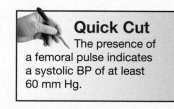

Quick Cut
The presence of a femoral pulse indicates a systolic BP of at least 60 mm Hg.

Eye Opening	
Spontaneous	4
To speech	3
To pain	2
None	1
Verbal Response	
Oriented	5
Confused	4
Inappropriate words	3
Moans	2
None	1
Motor Response	
Follows commands	6
Localizes pain	5
Withdrawals	4
Decorticate (Flexion)	3
Decerebrate (Extension)	2
None	1

Figure 22-1: The Glasgow Coma Scale. Score = E + V + M; minimum score is 3, maximum is 15. (From Zaslau S. *Step-Up to Surgery*. Baltimore: Lippincott Williams & Wilkins; 2014.)

    d. Diaphragm: Injury to a diaphragm may be suggested by diaphragmatic contour irregularity or the presence of a hollow viscus in the chest.

    e. Everything else: Examine the bones for fracture or misalignment; look for subcutaneous air, which could indicate an occult pneumothorax.

  2. Pelvic radiograph: commonly obtained to evaluate for fracture, which, in combination with hypotension, may lead the evaluating surgeon to suspect pelvic bleeding as the cause of hypotension

  3. Ultrasound: Surgeon-performed ultrasound at the bedside enables a rapid assessment of the peritoneal cavity for the presence of fluid, which may indicate blood (hemoperitoneum).

    a. Pericardium: also inspected for the presence of fluid, which may indicate blood within the pericardium

    b. Thorax: may be scanned to examine for the presence of pneumothorax or hemothorax

C. Secondary survey

  1. Physical examination: Full head-to-toe physical examination is done.

  2. History: AMPLE

    a. A: allergies

    b. M: medications

    c. P: previous illnesses

    d. L: last meal

    e. E: events surrounding injury

D. Tertiary survey: Once removed from the chaotic nature of the initial trauma evaluation, the patient undergoes another complete head-to-toe examination 12-24 hours after arrival.

Shock

I. Initial treatment: Obtain venous access.

A. Options: large-bore (18 gauge or greater) needle in the antecubital fossa, central venous access (subclavian or femoral line), or saphenous vein cutdown

B. If unable to obtain venous access: Use intraosseous access.

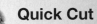

Quick Cut
Chest radiograph interpretation is done the same way every time: patient identification, airway, bilateral lung fields, cardiac silhouette, diaphragm, and everything else (bones, subcutaneous air, foreign bodies).

Quick Cut
Ultrasound is a very useful diagnostic tool because it is rapid, available, and inexpensive and may provide an early indication of bleeding.

Quick Cut
The tertiary survey often leads to the identification of distal extremity fractures and other injuries missed initially.

Quick Cut
The ultimate goal of the trauma evaluation is to identify and control sources of bleeding that lead to shock.

II. **Next steps:** Rapid control of bleeding is essential to ensuring patient survival.
  A. **Infusion:** isotonic crystalloid (lactated Ringer, normal saline, Plasma-Lyte) or blood and blood products
  B. **Identify bleeding source:** Physical examination, chest and pelvic x-rays, and ultrasound all help.
  C. **With uncontrolled blood loss from an injured extremity:** Apply a tourniquet, which may decrease blood loss.

Resuscitative Thoracotomy

I. **Overview:** previously called *emergency department thoracotomy*; performed in an emergent setting when the patient loses vital signs to relieve pericardial tamponade (blood within the pericardium causing shock)

II. **Technique:** An incision is made in the pericardium, any blood is evacuated, and the aorta is clamped.

III. **Results:** increases blood flow to the brain and coronary arteries and may help stop uncontrolled intra-abdominal or extremity bleeding

IV. **Manual compression of the heart:** may be more effective than chest compressions when the patient is in hypovolemic shock

V. **Indications:** controversial and will most likely remain so, but commonly used criteria are the following:
  A. **Penetrating trauma:** cardiac arrest and trauma to the chest or abdomen within 15 minutes of arrival to the trauma center (much higher chance of survival if chest injury)
  B. **Blunt trauma:** cardiac arrest if the arrest occurs while in front of the trauma team's eyes
  C. **Devastating neurologic injury (e.g., transcranial gunshot wound):** Many surgeons would not proceed with thoracotomy, although reports of survival and organ donation do exist.

 # SPECIFIC INJURIES

Head and Neck

I. **Brain:** Identification of a decreased GCS during the primary survey may warn of potential brain injury.
  A. **Pupil examination:** Imperative; a dilated and nonreactive pupil may indicate increased pressure secondary to intracranial bleeding.
  B. **Rapid assessment with computed tomography (CT):** often necessary to better characterize the injury
  C. **Initial treatment for intracranial hemorrhage:** aimed at decreasing the ICP while preserving cerebral blood flow
  D. **Rapid neurosurgical consultation:** will decrease time to definitive management of injuries

II. **Cervical spine:** Immobilization with a cervical collar should be maintained in all blunt trauma patients until they are able to be fully evaluated and "cleared," including during rolling and any procedures (e.g., oral–tracheal intubation).
  A. **During secondary survey:** Cervical spine is palpated to identify tenderness or bony deformity (step-off).
  B. **Physical examination:** can be used to "clear" the cervical spine if the patient is not intoxicated, does not have a "distracting" injury, and does not have a decreased GCS
  C. **CT imaging:** evaluates for the presence of fracture with cervical spine pain or the conditions listed earlier

Quick Cut
Patients can bleed to death in five locations: chest, peritoneal cavity, retroperitoneum/pelvis, extremities (mainly the thigh), and *the street* (i.e., massive blood loss at the scene).

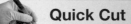
Quick Cut
Although it is important to establish the full extent of injury in trauma patients, unstable patients belong in the OR, not undergoing a lengthy radiographic evaluation.

Quick Cut
Resuscitative thoracotomy is a high-risk procedure that is reserved for patients with some expectation of survival.

Quick Cut
Monro-Kellie doctrine: The brain is enclosed in the skull vault; the addition of blood or any space-occupying lesion greatly increases intracranial pressure (ICP).

Quick Cut
Avoiding hypotension and hypoxia is paramount to prevent brain ischemia, as these contribute to worse outcomes after brain injury.

Quick Cut
First-line maneuvers to help decrease the ICP: analgesia and sedation, head of bed elevation, mannitol (avoid in hypotension), hypertonic saline, and loosening the cervical collar.

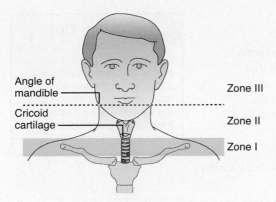

Angle of mandible

Cricoid cartilage

Zone III

Zone II

Zone I

Figure 22-2: Schematic drawing of the zones of the neck. The junction of zones 1 and 2 is variously described as being at the cricoid cartilage or at the top of the clavicles. The important implication of a zone 1 injury is the greater potential for intrathoracic great vessel injury. (From Fiser SM. *ABSITE Review*, 3rd ed. Baltimore: Lippincott Williams & Wilkins; 2010.)

III. **Penetrating cerebrovascular:** Treatment of vessel injury in the neck is mainly surgical, but interventional radiologic approaches are increasing in frequency. The neck is divided into three zones (Fig. 22-2).
   A. **Zone 1:** thoracic inlet to hyoid bone
   B. **Zone 2:** Hyoid bone to angle of mandible; classically, injuries here are treated with operative exploration because of the relatively easy surgical access (i.e., not hidden in the thorax [zone 1] or base of skull [zone 3]).
   C. **Zone 3:** angle of mandible to cranium

IV. **Blunt cerebrovascular injury (BCVI):** Principally carotid artery injury. Risk factors require additional screening for injury identification and include cervical spine injury, displaced midface fracture (Le Fort II and III), pulsatile epistaxis, hanging or clothesline mechanism, basal skull fracture, significant neck hematoma, and neurologic exam not explained by CT of the head.
   A. **Grades of carotid artery injury**
      1. **I:** luminal irregularity or dissection, less than 25% narrowing
      2. **II:** luminal irregularity or dissection, 25% or greater narrowing
      3. **III:** pseudoaneurysm
      4. **IV:** occlusion
      5. **V:** transection
   B. **Diagnosis:** CT neck scans with intravenous (IV) contrast or angiography
   C. **Treatment:** anticoagulation or antiplatelet therapy

Spinal Cord and Spinal Column

I. **Primary survey:** During the disability assessment, attention should be paid to the patient's ability/inability to move all four extremities; the patient should also be rolled and the full spinal column assessed for the presence of pain or bony deformity (step-off).

II. **Spinal immobilization (in the prehospital and in-hospital phases):** maintain with a backboard and during rolling until determination has been made that a spinal fracture does not exist

III. **Diagnosis:** Definitive identification of spinal fracture is most frequently made with CT imaging.
   A. **MRI:** often employed to better define and visualize injury to the spinal cord itself
   B. **Steroids:** *not* indicated; shown to increase infectious complications without decreasing spinal cord edema

Quick Cut
All blunt trauma patients are treated as if they have a cervical spine injury until proven otherwise.

Quick Cut
Remember, CT of the C-spine rules out bony injury, not ligamentous injury. Magnetic resonance imaging (MRI) is the preferred test to evaluate for ligamentous injury.

Quick Cut
Classic teaching: zone 1 and zone 3 penetrating neck injuries require additional imaging (computed tomography angiography/angiography). Zone 2 penetrating neck injuries are treated with surgical exploration.

Quick Cut
Excessive blunt force leads to stretching of the neck vessels.

Quick Cut
Carotid artery injuries lead to an increased risk of stroke if left untreated.

Pneumothorax and Hemothorax

I. **Definitions**

A. **Pneumothorax:** presence of air in the pleural space (outside of the lung), which causes increased pressure within that hemithorax and difficulty with ventilation

B. **Tension pneumothorax:** Increased pressure pushes the mediastinum to the contralateral side and causes decreased venous return and decreased BP.

C. **Hemothorax:** presence of blood in the pleural space

II. **Auscultation:** Decreased breath sounds during the primary survey may alert the physician to his or her potential.

III. **Diagnosis:** Chest x-ray assists. CT may better evaluate the pathology and can identify occult pneumothoraces (not visible on x-ray).

IV. **Treatment:** Chest tubes drain air or blood and should be placed into the pleural space under sterile conditions during initial trauma evaluation.

A. **Incomplete drainage of a hemothorax:** leads to a retained hemothorax and possible an empyema if not addressed and drained early

B. **Thoracotomy:** used to treat massive hemothorax

C. **Excessive bleeding into the chest:** requires surgical evacuation of bleeding and identification and control of the bleeding vessel or repair of bleeding structure

Quick Cut
Tension pneumothorax is a clinical (not radiographic) diagnosis and is an *emergency* that requires decompression of the air in the pleural space (needle decompression or chest tube placement).

Quick Cut
Massive hemothorax is often defined as greater than 1 liter of blood from the chest tube initially or greater than 200–250 mL of blood per hour, for 4 hours or more, managed with emergent thoracotomy.

Cardiac Injury

I. **Blunt:** Forceful blow to the chest can cause injury to the heart (e.g., steering wheel to chest); these patients should get an electrocardiogram (ECG) during initial trauma evaluation.

A. **Diagnosis:** suggested by an arrhythmia (most frequently sinus tachycardia) on ECG

B. **Echocardiogram:** for further characterization of the injury if the patient's ECG is abnormal or the patient is hemodynamically abnormal

C. **Treatment:** typically nonoperative and consists of inpatient cardiac monitoring for arrhythmia

D. **Effects:** Patients can develop structural lesions (cardiac aneurysms, septal wall ruptures, valvular problems).

II. **Penetrating:** Initial evaluation is made during the primary survey adjuncts with ultrasound evaluation of the heart (Fig. 22-3).

A. **Diagnosis:** Presence of fluid within the pericardium may indicate blood, which is highly suggestive of a cardiac injury and may cause cardiac tamponade leading to shock; further diagnostic techniques include a "pericardial window" performed in the operating room.

B. **Treatment:** Operative; the preferred approach is median sternotomy.

Quick Cut
Any penetrating injury to the "cardiac box" should raise the suspicion of a cardiac injury.

Blunt Thoracic Aortic Injury

I. **Diagnosis:** Initial chest x-ray may suggest the injury.

A. **Other:** widened mediastinum (>8 cm), pleural cap from bleeding into the pleural space near the apex; loss of aortopulmonary window, left mainstem bronchus depressions, and nasogastric tube displacement to the right

B. **Definitive diagnosis:** contrast-enhanced chest CT in most cases today

II. **Treatment:** Initial treatment is focused around decreasing the HR and BP; definitive treatment may include endovascular treatment, open surgical treatment, or nonoperative management and observation.

Quick Cut
Most patients with blunt injury to the thoracic aorta die at the scene.

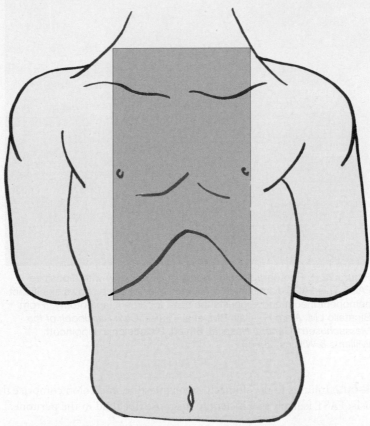

Figure 22-3: Schematic drawing of the "cardiac box." *Shaded area* represents the danger zone for transmediastinal injury. (From Peitzman AB, Rhodes M, Schwab CW, et al. *The Trauma Manual: Trauma and Acute Care Surgery*, 3rd ed. Philadelphia: Lippincott Williams & Wilkins; 2006.)

Esophageal and Tracheal Injury

I. **Diagnosis:** physical examination (bubbling in a wound, presence of food particles), endoscopy (bronchoscopy/esophagoscopy; predominant diagnostic tool in the chest), or swallow study (contrasted x-ray for identification of esophageal injury)

II. **Treatment:** operative repair

III. **Effects:** Tracheal injury may lead to excessive subcutaneous emphysema; missed tracheal and esophageal injury can lead to mediastinitis and death.

Abdominal Injury

I. **Solid organs (liver and spleen):** Initial evaluation begins with the focused abdominal sonography for trauma (FAST) to assess for free fluid (likely blood) within the peritoneum (Fig. 22-4).

A. **Hemodynamically normal patient:** Further evaluation with abdominal/pelvic CT may be pursued.

B. **Grading:** Splenic and liver injuries are graded I–V (with V being the most severe), with more severe injuries likely requiring operative exploration for definitive treatment.

C. **Treatment:** Interventional radiology with embolization may be available in specific situations.

> **Quick Cut**
> Patients with a positive FAST (fluid in the peritoneal space) and a low BP or significant tachycardia (*shock*) belong in the operating room, *not* the CT scanner.

> **Quick Cut**
> The presence of a "blush" on CT scan with IV contrast indicates extraluminal contrast extravasation (active bleeding) and may require interventional radiographic embolization or surgical intervention.

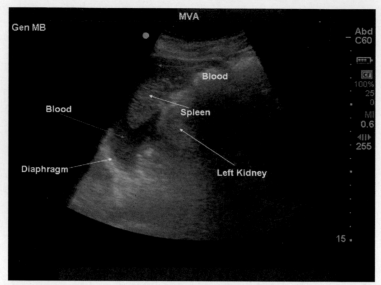

Figure 22-4: Photograph of left upper quadrant view with a positive FAST. This FAST examination of the perisplenic space shows significant hemoperitoneum and suggests the need for urgent laparotomy. (From Bigatello LM, Alam H, Allain RM, et al. *Critical Care Handbook of the Massachusetts General Hospital*, 5th ed. Philadelphia: Lippincott Williams & Wilkins; 2009.)

II. **Hollow viscus:** Injuries to the stomach, small intestine, and colon comprise this group of injuries.
   A. **Diagnosis:** FAST is likely insufficient to diagnose free fluid in the peritoneal cavity in this type of injury.
      1. **Physical examination:** Blunt hollow viscus injury may present with frank peritonitis, which mandates operative exploration.
      2. **Other presentations:** Free fluid on abdominal/pelvic CT in the *absence* of solid organ injury requires either operative exploration with exploratory laparotomy; diagnostic peritoneal lavage (DPL); serial abdominal exams; or, in some centers, diagnostic laparoscopy.
   B. **Treatment:** operative repair of injury or resection

> **Quick Cut**
> The presence of a "seatbelt sign" (significant abdominal wall hematoma caused by seatbelt strap) should raise the suspicion of a hollow viscus injury.

III. **Abdominal vascular injuries:** include aortic, mesenteric, iliac, and cava injuries that most frequently occur as a result of penetrating injury (gunshot and stab wounds)
   A. **Presentation:** shock (hypotension, tachycardia, depressed mental status, pallor, cool extremities) and a positive FAST
   B. **Diagnosis:** In blunt or penetrating injury, a positive FAST exam in the face of shock requires no further evaluation and mandates an emergent trip to the operating room for exploration via midline incision (exploratory laparotomy).
   C. **Treatment:** ligation of the bleeding vessel, repair, or bypass

> **Quick Cut**
> Patients with abdominal vascular injury commonly feel cold, are very thirsty, and say "I'm going to die"—*believe them; they might be right.*

IV. **Genitourinary:** include injuries to the kidneys, ureters, bladder, and urethra
   A. **Kidney:** Most injuries can be managed nonoperatively; operative identification of a kidney injury should prompt the surgeon to examine the contralateral kidney to ensure the patient has two kidneys.
   B. **Ureters:** Injuries are most often repaired surgically.
   C. **Bladder:** Injuries are further placed into two categories.
      1. **Intraperitoneal:** Rupture into the peritoneal cavity is repaired surgically.
      2. **Preperitoneal:** Ruptures into the preperitoneal space are most often managed without an operation and with a urinary catheter for 10-14 days of drainage.

Pelvic Fracture

I. **Initial evaluation:** plain film radiograph (pelvic x-ray)

II. **Pelvic binder:** In a patient with a suspected or verified pelvic fracture *and* hypotension, a binder placed around the greater trochanters bilaterally decreases the pelvic volume and minimizes ongoing hemorrhage.

III. **Treatment for ongoing hemorrhage and shock:** may include angioembolization, preperitoneal packing in the operating room, and endovascular aortic occlusion.

IV. **Treatment for orthopedic injuries:** may include definitive or external fixation

V. **Special consideration:** Urethral injury is suggested by blood at the urethral meatus, a high-riding "ballotable" prostate, and/or significant perineal ecchymosis.

Quick Cut
Pelvic fracture must be recognized quickly, as life-threatening hemorrhage can occur.

Quick Cut
Suspected urethral injury should be further evaluated with a retrograde urethrogram (RUG). Do *not* place a Foley catheter, which could convert a partial urethral injury into a full transection.

Extremities

I. **Fractures:** Fractured long bones (femurs) have the potential to bleed vigorously and lead to shock.

   A. **Diagnosis:** Plain film x-rays are the mainstay.

   B. **Reduction:** Reducing a femur fracture (pulling to length) and stabilizing will decrease patient pain and potentially decrease bleeding, but the act of reduction is very painful to the patient.

   C. **Arterial injury:** Calculation of the ankle-brachial index (ABI) or ankle-ankle index (AAI) can help detect arterial injury (1.0 is normal, <0.9 needs further evaluation).

   D. **Antibiotic prophylaxis:** paramount for open fractures to treat infection

Quick Cut
Distal pulse and neurologic exam are *essential* in the evaluation of any extremity fracture.

Compartment Syndrome

I. **Definition:** most commonly found in the lower leg and forearm but can be found in any extremity and buttock

   A. **Forearm:** classically described as having three compartments—dorsal, ventral, and mobile wad

   B. **Lower leg:** classically described as having four compartments—anterior, lateral, superficial posterior, and deep posterior

II. **Diagnosis:** most typically made on physical examination by the presence of a tense compartment and the sensation of numbness/paresthesias/pain

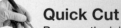

Quick Cut
The "6 P's of arterial insufficiency" are *p*ulselessness, *p*aresthesias, *p*oikilothermia, *p*allor, and *p*aralysis pain.

Quick Cut
Pulselessness is the *last* physical exam finding to occur in compartment syndrome. Treatment for compartment syndrome consists of a fasciotomy performed in the operating room.

 BURNS

Burn Injury

I. **Initial treatment:** Based on the same principles of initial trauma evaluation (airway/breathing/circulation). The patient must be removed from the source of thermal injury, and all burning clothes and/or chemicals should be removed.

   A. **Avoid hypothermia:** Burn wounds can be placed under running room-temperature water (in an effort to stop the burning process) but should not be placed under cold water so as not to exacerbate the injury. Burn wounds should then be covered with a sterile sheet to avoid evaporative heat loss and protect the wound.

   B. **Early pain control:** IV opioids are warranted, as burn wounds are exceedingly painful.

   C. **Other early steps:** Give tetanus toxoid and place a nasogastric tube to decompress the stomach (in anticipation of paralytic ileus) and as a means to provide early enteral nutrition, which is vital in the hypercatabolic response to burn injury.

Quick Cut
Because the initial presentation of a major burn can be quite dramatic, having an orderly approach to management is essential.

II. Intubation: Extensive burns to the face along with singed nasal hairs and carbonaceous sputum should alert the physician to the possibility of airway injury—early intubation is key.

III. Resuscitation: Two large-bore (18 gauge or larger) IV lines should be placed into the bilateral antecubital fossae; lactated Ringer is the classical fluid of choice.

A. Adults: Parkland formula for second and third degree burns

B. Fluid resuscitation: Should be tailored to urine output; calculated requirement of fluid is from the time of burn.

1. **Timing:** First 50% of fluid is given in the initial 8 hours, with the rest in the remaining 16 hours.

2. **Urinary catheter:** placed to monitor urine output

> **Quick Cut**
> Parkland formula for burn resuscitation: 4 mL × total body surface area burned (TBSA) × weight (kg) = estimated fluid requirements in the first 24 hours

Evaluation and Treatment

I. Types

A. Superficial burns: confined to the epidermis, blister, are painful, and do not require surgery

B. Partial-thickness burns: involve the dermis, are mottled and pale in areas with some preserved epidermal appendages, are painful, and require surgery if deep partial-thickness burns

C. Full-thickness burns (to the bone or fascia): are leathery or white in appearance, are insensate, and require surgery

II. Burn size estimation: "Rule of 9's" is used to calculate IV fluid requirements (Fig. 22-5).

III. Topical antimicrobials: should be applied after the full evaluation of the burn injury to prevent localized bacterial growth. Common agents include the following.

A. Silver sulfadiazine (Silvadene): painless; may cause neutropenia (*rare*)

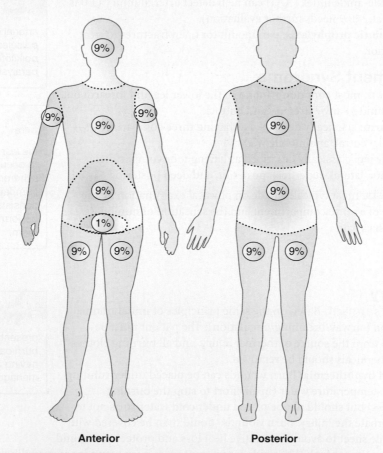

Anterior **Posterior**

Figure 22-5: Rule of 9's in estimating body surface area in burn victims. Remember that for this calculation, burns are scored as second degree and above. (From Van Kleunen JP. *Step-Up to USMLE Step 2*. Baltimore: Lippincott Williams & Wilkins; 2005.)

B. **Mafenide acetate (Sulfamylon):** painful application; penetrates eschar; may cause metabolic acidosis (it is a carbonic anhydrase inhibitor)

C. **Silver nitrate:** used for face burns; may cause electrolyte imbalances and stains everything black

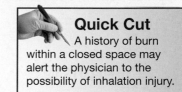

Quick Cut
Systemic antibiotics *should not* be administered in the absence of a specific infection.

IV. **Operative treatment:** "Early" excision and grafting of burn wounds is the current standard of care.

V. **Escharotomy (eschar [*Greek:* "scar"]):** may need to be performed during initial evaluation in the presence of circumferential wounds because burn eschar can impede perfusion or ventilation

Inhalation Injury

I. **Treatment:** Early intubation may be warranted to protect the patient's airway from edema.

A. **Carboxyhemoglobin level:** should be obtained and elevated levels treated with 100% oxygen by facemask

B. **Bronchoscopy:** may be warranted to remove particulate matter

Quick Cut
A history of burn within a closed space may alert the physician to the possibility of inhalation injury.

II. **IV fluid requirement:** Inhalation injury typically requires more than expected to maintain adequate urine output.

Electrical Burns

I. **Muscle damage:** Excessive muscle damage may lead to compartment syndrome of an extremity, warranting emergent fasciotomy in the operating room.

A. **High-voltage (>1,000 volts) injuries:** should raise the suspicion of extensive muscle destruction and cardiac conduction abnormalities

B. **Myoglobinuria:** may be caused by products of muscle breakdown and may lead to a red tint to the urine and places the patient at greater risk of acute kidney injury

Quick Cut
The visible contact burn will vastly underestimate the degree of muscular damage that an electrical burn has caused.

II. **Treatment:** Myoglobinuria should be treated with titration of resuscitation to a urine output of 100 mL/hr. Diuretics may be indicated to maintain urine output.

III. **Rehabilitation:** Trauma and burn injuries are chronic conditions which require lifelong care; rehabilitation can take years and leads to a significant loss of productivity.

Chapter 23

Organ Transplantation

Joseph R. Scalea, Max Seaton, Silke Niederhaus, and Jonathan Bromberg

OVERVIEW

Reasons for Transplantation

I. **End-organ dysfunction:** Transplantation of solid organs is reserved for patients with end-organ dysfunction to prolong life (heart, lung, liver, kidney) and improve quality of life (all organs).

II. **Limitations:** shortage of donor organs and the comorbidities of chronic immunosuppression

Transplant Candidate Evaluation

I. **Recipients:** are evaluated, including all disease-related problems

II. **Other potentially involved organ systems must be evaluated:** Evaluation of a liver transplant candidate includes evaluation for coronary artery disease (CAD) and pulmonary hypertension. A patient with renal failure from diabetes may also have significant CAD, aortoiliac vascular disease, or unidentified carotid stenosis.

III. **General health issues:** Are evaluated; age, body mass index (BMI), and adequate social support are relevant factors in determining candidacy for transplant.

> **Quick Cut**
> Patients with certain cancers that are controlled or eradicated are candidates for organ transplantation.

   A. **Cancers and infections:** must be ruled out or addressed
   B. **Cardiac evaluation:** is a must for all transplant recipients

IV. **Typical studies:** The following workup is needed for each organ system
   A. **Pulmonary:** chest radiograph. If indicated: pulmonary function tests, right heart catheterization
   B. **Cardiac:** electrocardiogram (ECG) and transthoracic echocardiogram. If indicated, stress test or cardiac catheterization
   C. **Gastrointestinal (GI):** Liver function tests (LFTs); computed tomography (CT), ultrasound (US), or magnetic resonance imaging (MRI) of abdomen/pelvis to evaluate vessels and exclude liver masses. In liver patients, esophagogastroduodenoscopy (EGD). In pancreas patients, fasting C-peptide.
   D. **Renal/urologic:** creatinine. If there is a concern that disease may recur, kidney biopsy (eg, glomerulonephritis)
   E. **Immunologic:** tuberculosis (purified protein derivative [PPD]); rapid plasmin reagin (RPR) test; serology for hepatitis B and C, cytomegalovirus (CMV), Epstein-Barr virus (EBV), and HIV; and calculated panel reactive antibody (cPRA) to assess sensitization to human leukocyte antigens (HLAs)
   F. **Cancer screening:** Colonoscopy if age >50 years. In women, mammography and Papanicolaou (Pap) test as indicated. In men, prostate-specific antigen as indicated. For liver transplants, alpha-fetoprotein (AFP).

Terminology

I. **Genetic relationships:** between the donor and the recipient
   A. **Autograft:** tissue transfer within the same individual (e.g., skin graft)
   B. **Isograft:** between genetically identical individuals (e.g., identical twins)

C. **Allograft:** between genetically nonidentical members of the same species; includes living related and unrelated donors and deceased donor human transplants

D. **Xenograft:** Between different species; xenografts are experimental.

II. **Surgical terms**

A. **Orthotopic graft:** Old organ is removed, and the new one is placed in the same position (liver, lung, heart).

B. **Heterotopic graft:** New organ is placed in a different position (kidney, pancreas, some hearts).

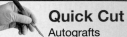

Quick Cut
Autografts and xenografts require immunosuppression to prevent rejection.

Donors and Donor Selection

I. **Deceased donors:** have brain injury resulting in irreversible neurologic injury *or* brain death

A. **Donors after brain death (DBD):** irreversible cessation of brain function, as shown on neurologic exam, revealing unresponsiveness and absence of both spontaneous movement and reflexes from the brainstem and higher

B. **Donors after cardiac death (DCD):** Patients with irreversible neurologic injury who are not brain dead may donate their organs if the family wishes to withdraw support and donate. Organs are not recovered until cessation of cardiac function has persisted for 5 minutes, which, depending on the declaring physician, is absence of either a palpable pulse or electrical activity.

C. **Causes:** most often cerebrovascular disease or trauma

D. **Exclusions:** cancer, infection, and poor donor organ function

II. **Living donors:** are individuals motivated by altruism

A. **Living unrelated donors (e.g., a spouse):** share no more genes with a recipient than deceased donors

B. **Living related donors:** share a substantial portion of their genes with the recipient

C. **Requirements:** Living donors must be in good health, have normal function of the organ under consideration, and be good candidates for anesthesia and the operative procedure.

D. **Full transplant workup:** See "III. General health issues" earlier.

E. **Risks:** Risk of death varies by organ (e.g., 1 in 3,000 for kidneys; 1 in 150 for livers).

1. **Kidney:** Perioperative mortality for living kidney donors is 0.03%. A living donor provides one kidney; the remaining kidney hypertrophies and achieves 80% of pre-donation creatinine clearance

2. **Liver:** Donation of the left lateral segment or either lobe of the liver uses open technique, with 0.5%–1% mortality risk.

3. **Lung:** Live donor lobar lung transplantation is very rare and mostly performed to help a waiting child. The operation is done with an open procedure and involves removal of a lower lobe. For adult recipients, two donors are necessary.

III. **Donor operation:** Donor organ is removed, wherein the blood supply of the organ is controlled and then the organ is rapidly flushed with a cold (4°C) preservation solution to minimize ischemic injury.

IV. **Cold ischemia:** The practical limit with current preservation methods is 4 hours for the heart, 6 hours for a lung, 12 hours for the liver, 20 hours for the pancreas, and 36 hours for a kidney.

Quick Cut
Organ selection is crucial because infections or cancer from the donor may be transmitted to the immunosuppressed recipient.

Quick Cut
Strict criteria for brain death must be met before consideration of organ donation. Brain death criteria include: comatose, apneic, no response to pain, without cranial nerve reflexes or brain stem reflexes

Quick Cut
Sepsis with positive cultures is an absolute contraindication for organ donation.

Quick Cut
The mortality for living kidney donation is very low but not zero.

Quick Cut
Organs are more sensitive to warm ischemia than to cold ischemia.

Quick Cut
As cold ischemic time increases, so does the risk of permanent damage and delayed or loss of function of the organ.

Immunologic Considerations

I. **ABO blood group compatibility:** Same rules apply as those for red blood cell (RBC) transfusions.

II. **HLAs:** histocompatibility antigens
A. **HLA-A, HLA-B, HLA-C, HLA-DR, HLA-DP, and HLA-DQ (six):** Standard tissue typing includes HLA-A, HLA-B, and HLA-DR only.
B. **HLAs are encoded on chromosome 6:** Transplant candidates have six HLAs, defined by tissue typing (i.e., two each for HLA-A, HLA-B, and HLA-DR).
C. **Cross-match compatibility:** Recipient's serum is tested for the presence of cytotoxic antibodies directed against surface antigens (anti-HLA) on the donor lymphocytes.
1. **Positive cross match:** implies the presence of preformed antidonor antibodies in the serum of the recipient and generally precludes transplantation
2. **Panel reactive antibody (PRA):** High-PRA patients have preformed anti-HLA antibodies against a high proportion (>80%) of a **panel of random human cells**, which is used to screen for reactivity. Therefore, good donors for high-PRA patients are difficult to find, resulting in longer waiting times.
3. **Donor-specific antibody (DSA):** Anti-HLA antibody in the recipient directed at one or multiple donor alleles, either major histocompatibility complex (MHC) class I or II. DSA is part of the diagnosis of antibody-mediated rejection (AMR).

Rejection

I. **Hyperacute rejection:** occurs when the serum of the recipient has pre-formed antidonor antibodies, which adhere to the endothelium, resulting in immediate graft infarction

II. **Acute cellular rejection (ACR):** Cell-mediated immune response initiated by helper T cells (Fig. 23-1). The pace of proliferation of alloreactive T cell clones dictates that acute rejection occurs after the sixth post-transplant day; a memory immune response can trigger ACR sooner.
A. **Diagnosis:** by graft dysfunction and biopsy
B. **Treatment:** ACR is usually reversible by a short course of high-dose immunosuppressive drugs.
C. **Timing:** ACR usually occurs between weeks 1 and 12 post-transplant and rarely after the first year, unless triggered by infection or inadequate immunosuppression.

III. **Antibody mediated rejection (AMR):** results from pre-formed antibody or from plasma cell production of antibody to the transplanted organ
A. **Diagnosis:** made by the triad of graft dysfunction, presence of DSA in the serum, and complement (C4d) staining on biopsy
B. **Treatment:** No good treatment exists, but steroids, plasmapheresis, and intravenous immunoglobulin (IVIG) are commonly used.
C. **Timing:** 1-12 weeks post transplant

IV. **Chronic rejection:** Usually happens after 1 year or later. It has an insidious onset and is multifactorial, involving the cell-mediated and humoral arms of the immune system.

V. **Immunologic tolerance:** Tolerance is a state in which the recipient's immune system responds normally to all antigens except those of the donor (i.e., the donor antigens are "tolerated"). Small human trials have demonstrated that tolerance is possible.

Quick Cut
Immunologic compatibility of the donor and recipient influences the outcome for any type of organ transplant.

Quick Cut
Cross-match compatibility must be present for kidney, pancreas, and some heart transplants.

Quick Cut
If donor-specific antibodies are present in the recipient, the donor organ is unacceptable due to risk of hyperacute rejection and destruction of the organ.

Quick Cut
A positive preoperative cross match between donor and recipient is highly predictive of hyperacute rejection. If hyperacute rejection occurs, it cannot be treated.

Quick Cut
Antibody mediated rejection leads to graft failure much sooner than acute cellular rejection.

Quick Cut
Chronic rejection is poorly understood and considered neither treatable nor reversible.

Quick Cut
The ultimate goal in transplantation is tolerance, where this is no need for immunosuppression.

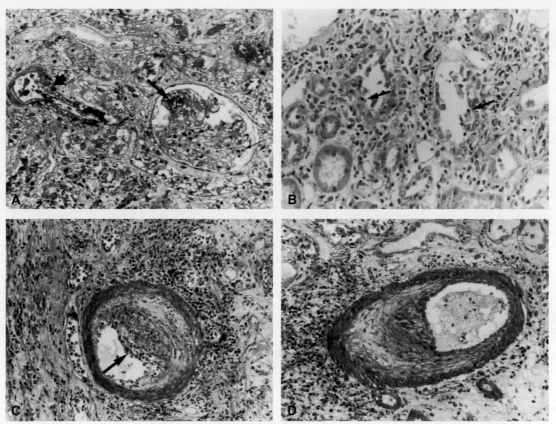

Figure 23-1: Kidney rejection. **A:** Hyperacute rejection characterized by microthrombi in the glomerular capillaries (*large arrow*), infiltration with neutrophils (*small thin arrow*), and endothelial destruction (*thick arrow*). **B:** Acute tubulointerstitial rejection showing an interstitial lymphocytic infiltrate, interstitial edema, and infiltration of lymphocytes into the epithelium of the tubules (tubulitis; *arrows*). **C:** Acute vascular rejection with a subendothelial lymphocytic infiltrate (*arrow*), along with some evidence of chronic vascular rejection. **D:** Chronic rejection with severe proliferative endarteritis. (Courtesy of Roger D. Smith, MD.)

Immunosuppression

I. **General characteristics:** Most allografts require indefinite suppression of the recipient's immune system to prevent rejection.

    A. **Purpose:** to disable components of the immune response (typically lymphocytes)

    B. **Multiple drug therapy:** standard; aims for synergistic immunosuppression while minimizing the side effects

II. **Classification (three types):** Induction regimens, maintenance therapy, and antirejection regimens. Specific immunosuppression medications are described in detail in Table 23-1.

    A. **Induction regimens:** Aim to avoid rejection within the first few post-transplant weeks. They consist of a high-dose steroid taper and an antilymphocyte drug, which can be either lymphocyte depleting (e.g., antithymocyte globulin or alemtuzumab) or nonlymphocyte depleting (e.g., basiliximab).

    B. **Maintenance therapy:** provides long-term immunosuppression to prevent rejection and usually include two to three drugs from separate classes

    C. **Antirejection regimens:** high-dose, short-term (<3 weeks) treatments aimed at reversing acute rejection episodes

Complications of Immunosuppression

I. **Infections:** Nonspecificity of current immunosuppression also impairs host defenses against a diverse group of pathogens and causes opportunistic infections.

    A. **CMV:** common in the early (3–6) months after a transplant and presents with fever and leukopenia

        1. **Risk:** Varies by prior exposure (serostatus). CMV seronegative recipients of seropositive donors are at the highest risk.

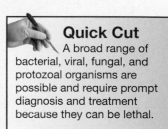

Quick Cut
A broad range of bacterial, viral, fungal, and protozoal organisms are possible and require prompt diagnosis and treatment because they can be lethal.

Table 23-1: Immunosuppressive Medications

Drug	Class	Effect	Side Effects	Comments
Induction Agents and Antirejection Therapy				
Methylprednisolone, dexamethasone, hydrocortisone	Glucocorticoid (IV)	Anti-inflammatory; inhibits all leukocytes	Obesity, cushingoid facies, poor healing, skin atrophy, striae, acne, diabetes, hypertension, osteoporosis, aseptic necrosis of the hips, cataracts, peptic ulcers, psychosis	
Antithymocyte globulin (thymoglobulin, ATGAM)	Depleting polyclonal antibody	Depletes T lymphocytes	Fevers, chills, pulmonary edema, cytokine release syndrome, thrombocytopenia	Requires premedication with steroids, diphenhydramine, and acetaminophen, up to 21 days/doses
Induction Agents				
Alemtuzumab (Campath)	Depleting monoclonal antibody (anti-CD52)	Depletes both T and B lymphocytes	Leukopenia	Single dose
Basiliximab (Simulect)	Nondepleting monoclonal antibody (anti-CD25)	Inhibits costimulation by blocking the IL-2 receptor	Rare anaphylaxis	Two doses
Maintenance Therapy				
Tacrolimus (Prograf, FK506)	Calcineurin inhibitor	Inhibits T-cell function by decreasing IL-2 production	Nephrotoxicity, hypertension, neurotoxicity, tremor, alopecia, diabetes	Vasoconstricts the preglomerular arterioles
Cyclosporine A (Sandimmune, Neoral)	Calcineurin inhibitor	Inhibits T-cell function by decreasing IL-2 production	Nephrotoxicity, hypertension, hirsutism, diabetes, gingival hyperplasia	Vasoconstricts the preglomerular arterioles
Mycophenolate mofetil (CellCept, Myfortic)	Antimetabolite	Inhibits clonal T-cell proliferation by inhibiting purine salvage	Bone marrow suppression; GI disturbances (nausea, diarrhea)	
Azathioprine	Antimetabolite	Inhibits clonal T-cell proliferation by inhibiting purine metabolism	Bone marrow suppression; skin cancer	
Prednisone, prednisolone	Glucocorticoid (oral)	Anti-inflammatory; inhibits all leukocytes	Obesity, cushingoid facies, poor healing, skin atrophy, striae, acne, diabetes, hypertension, osteoporosis, aseptic necrosis of the hips, cataracts, peptic ulcers, psychosis	

(continued)

Table 23-1: Immunosuppressive Medications *(continued)*

Drug	Class	Effect	Side Effects	Comments
Sirolimus (Rapamycin)	Mammalian target of rapamycin inhibitor	Inhibits T-cell activation	Poor wound healing, hernias, proteinuria, hypercholesterolemia, hypertriglyceridemia, mild bone marrow suppression	Should be stopped perioperatively in all patients due to hernia risk
Everolimus	Mammalian target of rapamycin inhibitor	Inhibits T-cell activation	Poor wound healing, hernias, proteinuria, hypercholesterolemia, hypertriglyceridemia, mild bone marrow suppression	
Belatacept	CTLA-4-Ig fusion protein, costimulatory blockade	Blocks costimulation of T-cells by binding to CTLA-4	PTLD, PML	IV only; contraindicated in EBV-mismatched recipients

IV, intravenous; IL-2, interleukin-2; GI, gastrointestinal; CTLA-4-Ig, cytotoxic T-lymphocyte antigen 4 immunoglobulin; PTLD, post-transplant lymphoproliferative disorder; PML, progressive multifocal leukoencephalopathy; EBV, Epstein-Barr virus.

2. **Prophylaxis:** valganciclovir
3. **Treatment:** intravenous (IV) ganciclovir or foscarnet if it is resistant
  B. **BK polyoma virus:** urothelial virus that can invade a kidney transplant and cause allograft failure
   1. **Prophylaxis:** does not exist, so monitoring of BK viremia/viruria is performed selectively
   2. **Treatment:** minimizing immunosuppression
  C. *Pneumocystis carinii* **pneumonia (PCP):** Prophylaxis is given for 1 year with Bactrim, dapsone, or pentamidine. Bactrim also prevents *Nocardia* infections.
  D. **Fungal infections**
   1. **Common:** Candidal overgrowth can cause thrush, esophagitis, and yeast infections. Prophylaxis is 3 months of clotrimazole troches or nystatin swish and swallow.
   2. **Rare:** *Aspergillus*, *Nocardia*, histoplasmosis, cryptococcosis, and coccidioidomycosis occur occasionally and must be treated promptly.
  E. **Toxoplasmosis:** Kittens should be vaccinated and fresh transplant patients should not change cat litter.
  F. **Tuberculosis:** can become reactivated after transplant, so all patients are screened for prior exposure or disease

II. **Neoplasia:** Risks are skin cancer, post-transplant lymphoproliferative disorders (PTLDs), and oral squamous cell or female genital tract cancers.
  A. **Skin cancer:** Squamous and basal cell cancers of sun-exposed skin are very common post transplant. Daily sunscreen and annual dermatologic exams are recommended.
  B. **PTLD:** form of lymphoma, commonly arising from B cells and usually associated with EBV
   1. **Early stages:** may respond to acyclovir
   2. **Later stages:** require CHOP chemotherapy (*c*yclophosphamide, *h*ydroxydaunorubicin, *O*ncovin, and *p*rednisone) and rituximab, but the prognosis is poor
   3. **Oral squamous cell cancers/female genital tract cancers:** occur frequently in post-transplant patients
   4. **Other:** All other cancer screening (such as mammograms or colonoscopy) should follow current guidelines for all patients.

III. **Parenthood after transplantation:** Organ failure is associated with endocrine abnormalities that result in fertility problems. These abnormalities are reversed after transplantation.
  A. **Immunosuppression:** Pregnancy results in metabolic changes that can result in allograft rejection (and sometimes loss) if not carefully managed. Recipients must be transitioned to

> **Quick Cut**
> Papillomavirus is implicated in cancers of the skin, oral cavity, and female genital tract.

a mycophenolate-free regimen at least 2 months prior to conception because this drug is highly teratogenic.

    B. Outcomes: Premature deliveries and low birth weight infants are common. Mycophenolate is contraindicated; associated with early miscarriage and craniofacial, limb, cardiac, esophageal, and renal malformations.

Quick Cut
As drug metabolism increases, as in pregnancy, higher doses of immunosuppression are necessary to prevent rejection.

 # ORGAN-SPECIFIC CONSIDERATIONS

Heart Transplantation

  I. Preoperative assessment: heart failure survival score (HFSS) calculated for risk stratification

    A. Indications: End-stage heart failure (New York Heart Association class III and IV). Most common causes are dilated and ischemic cardiomyopathies, recurrent life-threatening arrhythmias, congenital heart disease, and severe valvular disease.

    B. Contraindications: severe nonreversible pulmonary hypertension; peak oxygen consumption (VO_2) <12 mL/kg/min

Quick Cut
Most immunosuppressive regimens have little increased risk of fetal malformation except mycophenolate.

  II. Operative strategy

    A. Dissection and cardiectomy: Heart transplantation is mostly orthotopic via a median sternotomy. Patients are placed on cardiopulmonary bypass.

    B. Order of reanastomosis: variations exist; left atrium, right atrium, pulmonary artery, then aorta

Quick Cut
The major limitation of cardiac transplant is chronic rejection, producing symptoms of heart failure and accelerated atherosclerosis.

  III. Postoperative management and complications

    A. Location: cardiac surgery intensive care unit (ICU)

    B. Cardiac output (CO): Monitored and heart rate is maintained at 90–110 beats per minute; epicardial pacing or isoproterenol can be useful because the heart is no longer innervated.

    C. Fluid status and volume: Swan-Ganz catheters assess the patient's physiology and guide volume resuscitation. Urine output and ABGs are also useful.

    D. Cardiac tamponade: should be suspected with hypotension, decreased chest tube output, and elevated central venous pressure (CVP)

    E. Severe rejection: may manifest as ventricular failure

  IV. Outcomes: Post-transplant mortality is somewhat dependent on etiology; 1-, 2-, and 5-year patient survivals are 87%, 84%, and 75%, respectively.

  V. Immunosuppression

    A. Induction: Patients age younger than 40 years, those with prior ventricular assist devices (VADs), African Americans, and sensitized patients generally require induction. Polyclonal (thymoglobulin) and monoclonal (anti-CD25, anti-CD52) have been described.

    B. Maintenance: generally tacrolimus, steroids, and antimetabolites

Quick Cut
African American recipients have lower survival possibly due to higher rates of hypertension post orthotopic heart transplant (OHT).

  VI. Rejection: May manifest as graft dysfunction; African Americans, those age younger than 40 years, and patients with prior VAD are at higher risk. Endomyocardial biopsy confirms diagnosis.

  VII. Alternatives to transplantation: Efficacy of VADs (for both left and right ventricles) is constantly improving. OHT is currently the best option for patients with heart failure.

Pulmonary Transplantation

  I. Preoperative assessment

    A. Indications: single lung, bilateral lung, or combined heart-lung

      1. Single lung transplant: chronic obstructive pulmonary disease; idiopathic pulmonary fibrosis

      2. Bilateral lung transplant: cystic fibrosis; pulmonary hypertension without right-sided heart failure

      3. Heart/lung transplant: pulmonary hypertension with associated heart failure (typically right sided); Eisenmenger syndrome

    B. Contraindications: specific to pulmonary transplant, nonreversible pulmonary hypertension, and significant cardiac disease

II. **Operative strategy**

A. **Single-lung transplantation:** Can be done through a posterolateral thoracotomy. The bronchial anastomosis is performed first (which is "telescoped"), then the pulmonary arterial and left atrial anastomoses. An omental wrap may be used to prevent leak around the bronchial anastomosis.

B. **Double-lung transplantation:** can be done in two ways: via sequential lung transplant technique, as described for single-lung transplantation, or via a single tracheal, arterial, and venous anastomosis, requiring cardiopulmonary bypass (clamshell incision or midline sternotomy)

C. **Heart/lung transplantation:** Typically performed through a median sternotomy. These organs are transplanted en bloc.

III. **Postoperative management and complications**

A. **Location:** cardiac surgery ICU

B. **Graft dysfunction:** manifests as hypoxemia, infiltrative pattern on chest x-ray, and heavy secretions from the endotracheal tube

C. **Volume status and physiology:** Aggressive diuresis may be required. Urine output, ABGs, and CO measurements help guide volume resuscitation.

D. **Ventilation:** High levels of positive end-expiratory pressure (PEEP) may be used to maintain patency of the small airways; patients may remain on extracorporeal membrane oxygenation (ECMO) until the lungs are functional.

E. **Airway complications:** Although reduced with surgical experience and improved technique, 10%–15% of lung recipients experience airway complications (leaks, fungal infections, stenosis) because of poor blood supply to the anastomosis. These complications are less likely with heart/lung transplant.

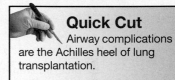

Quick Cut
Airway complications are the Achilles heel of lung transplantation.

F. **Infection:** *Candida* and *aspergillus* infections are more serious than bacterial; mostly seen in the first 3 months post transplant. *Pseudomonas aeruginosa* and CMV infections are common.

IV. **Outcomes:** Both donation after brain death and cardiac death are suitable in lung transplantation. Overall 1-, 2-, and 10-year graft survivals are ~80%, 70%, and 50%, respectively.

V. **Immunosuppression**

A. **Induction:** Approximately 50% of patients receiving lung transplants get induction.

B. **Maintenance:** calcineurin inhibitor–based triple therapy

VI. **Rejection**

A. **Diagnosis:** Confirmation of suspected rejection is performed via transbronchial biopsy and bronchoalveolar lavage.

B. **Acute:** associated with lymphocytic infiltrate and typically seen early post transplant

C. **Chronic:** characterized by fibrosis and obliteration of the small airways and vessels, designated as *obliterative bronchiolitis*

Quick Cut
In heart/lung transplant recipients, rejection of lung transplants may occur without rejection of the heart.

VII. **Alternatives to transplantation:** There are few options for end-stage pulmonary disease. Patients who are not candidates for organ transplants are generally referred to hospice.

Hepatic Transplantation

I. **Preoperative assessment**

A. **Indications**

1. **Adult:** cirrhosis (hepatitis C virus [HCV], nonalcoholic steatohepatitis [NASH], alcohol, etc.), fulminant hepatic failure, hepatocellular carcinoma (HCC), and metabolic disorders

2. **Pediatric:** biliary atresia, Alagille syndrome, and metabolic disease

B. **Contraindications:** Recent or continued alcohol or substance use and poor neurologic status. Complete thrombosis of the entire portal and mesenteric venous system may anatomically preclude liver transplant.

II. **Operative strategy:** Figure 23-2

A. **Piggyback:** Recipient liver is dissected, leaving a short recipient hepatic vein cuff that can be anastomosed to the inferior vena cava.

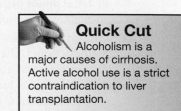

Quick Cut
Alcoholism is a major causes of cirrhosis. Active alcohol use is a strict contraindication to liver transplantation.

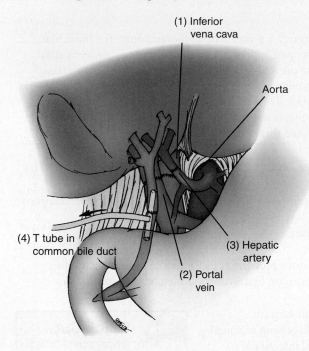

(1) Inferior
vena cava

Aorta

(4) T tube in
common bile duct

(3) Hepatic
artery

(2) Portal
vein

Figure 23-2: Standard anastomoses used for orthotopic liver transplant: (*1*) suprahepatic inferior vena cava (IVC) and infrahepatic IVC anastomoses, (*2*) portal vein anastomoses, (*3*) hepatic (splenic) artery anastomosis, (*4*) anastomosis for biliary drainage. (From Blackbourne LH. *Advanced Surgical Recall*, 2nd ed. Baltimore: Lippincott Williams & Wilkins; 2004.)

B. **Bicaval:** Donor's supra- and infrahepatic venae cavae are anastomosed to the recipient's. This procedure sometimes uses venovenous bypass.

C. **Living donor:** involves transplant of the right liver (adult to adult) or left lateral segment (adult to child)

D. **Pediatric:** may be from a live or deceased adult or from a deceased pediatric donor

E. **Combined liver-kidney:** Life-saving liver is transplanted first.

III. **Postoperative management and complications**

A. **Location:** transplant surgery ICU or surgical ICU

B. **Volume status and physiology:** Hypotension should prompt evaluation for bleeding.

C. **Coagulopathy:** Approximately 20% of patients have a bleeding complication, often requiring repeat laparotomy and multiple transfusions of blood products to reverse coagulopathy.

D. **Primary nonfunction:** Rare; despite vascular patency, the new liver fails to function and requires urgent retransplantation with another organ.

E. **Hepatic artery or portal vein thrombosis:** also rare, <5% of transplants
   1. **Diagnosis:** Elevated LFTs, especially ammonia, are suggestive; diagnosis is confirmed with US or CT angiography or by re-exploration.
   2. **Treatment:** often requires retransplantation

F. **Biliary complications (including strictures and leaks):** common, ~15% of patients
   1. **Diagnosis:** elevated bilirubin, endoscopic retrograde cholangiopancreatography (ERCP), or bilious drain output
   2. **Management:** includes biliary decompression via stenting or reoperation (Roux-en-Y)

IV. **Outcomes:** One-year patient and graft survival are ~90%.

A. **Long-term outcomes:** vary by cause of disease, with hepatitis C and HCC having high recurrence rates

B. **DCD donor organs:** have more biliary complications and slightly poorer long-term graft

V. **Immunosuppression**

A. **Induction:** Unlike most other solid organ transplants, liver transplants do not receive induction immunosuppression.

B. **Maintenance:** Initially tacrolimus, steroids, and antimetabolites. With hepatitis C or no early rejections, tacrolimus monotherapy may be sufficient long term.

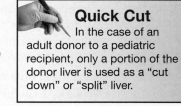

Quick Cut
In the case of an adult donor to a pediatric recipient, only a portion of the donor liver is used as a "cut down" or "split" liver.

Quick Cut
Liver transplants tend to be more resistant to rejection than kidney transplants. In some cases, immunosuppression may be discontinued altogether (tolerance).

VI. **Rejection**

A. **Diagnosis:** Liver rejection may manifest with clinical graft dysfunction or with elevated liver enzymes. Alkaline phosphatase is typically elevated prior to aspartate aminotransferase (AST) and alanine aminotransferase (ALT).

B. **Acute:** indicated by a lymphocytic infiltrate

C. **Chronic:** characterized by fibrosis or paucity of bile ducts

VII. **Alternatives to transplantation:** Few options exist for end-stage liver disease. Patients who are not candidates for organ transplants are generally referred to hospice.

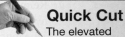

> **Quick Cut**
> The elevated enzyme profile in liver rejection is very similar to and often indistinguishable from recurrent HCV.

> **Quick Cut**
> Hepatocyte transplantation, stem cell technologies, and xenotransplantation are potential future therapies for end stage liver disease.

Kidney Transplantation

I. **Preoperative assessment**

A. **Indications:** Leading etiologies of end-stage renal disease are diabetes, hypertension, and glomerulonephritis.

B. **Contraindications:** specific to kidney transplantation, severe iliac atherosclerosis, and significant abdominal obesity or severe cardiac or pulmonary disease

C. **Donors:** 30% living; 70% deceased donor

II. **Operative strategy:** Figure 23-3

A. **Recipient:** Kidney is transplanted to the extraperitoneal iliac fossa through a curvilinear (Gibson) incision.

1. **Adults:** Donor renal vessels are anastomosed to the common or external iliac vessels.

2. **Children:** Aorta and inferior vena cava may be used.

B. **Urinary drainage:** Ureter is anastomosed to the bladder.

C. **Recipient nephrectomy:** indicated for chronic persistent pyelonephritis, persistent upper tract stones, vesicoureteral reflux, severe unmanageable high-renin hypertension, and polycystic kidney disease

> **Quick Cut**
> Kidney transplants are most commonly supplied by the external iliac vessels.

III. **Postoperative management and complications**

A. **Location:** ICU care is usually not required.

B. **Function:** Living donor kidneys should function immediately with a brisk diuresis (up to 1,000 mL/hr) and drop in creatinine.

C. **Delayed graft function (DGF):** Up to 40% of deceased donor kidneys do not function immediately. Management is fluid restriction and dialysis. Function usually returns in 1–2 months.

D. **Oliguria:** rare after living donation and should result in prompt evaluation for obstructive, prerenal, or intrarenal problems (Foley, volume status, thrombosis, acute kidney injury, or rejection)

E. **Vascular complications**

1. **Renal artery thrombosis:** occurs in 1% of transplants

a. **Presentation:** sudden decline in urine output

b. **Diagnosis:** duplex US

c. **Treatment:** requires emergent re-exploration, as it can only be salvaged within minutes of onset

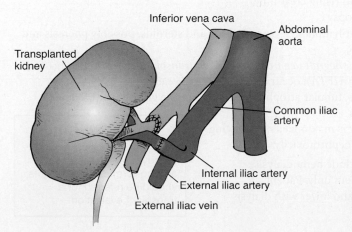

Figure 23-3: The transplanted kidney. (From Snell RS. *Clinical Anatomy by Regions*, 9th ed. Baltimore: Lippincott Williams & Wilkins; 2011.)

2. **Renal artery stenosis:** Presents as uncontrollable hypertension and is diagnosed with duplex US and arteriography. It is managed with operative repair or angioplasty stenting.

3. **Renal artery aneurysm:** Present as pulsatile masses and are diagnosed with duplex US (or by a bruit). Management is surgical repair, stenting, or graft removal and antibiotics (for mycotic aneurysms).

4. **Renal vein thrombosis:** occurs in 1%–4% of transplants.
   a. **Presentation:** graft pain (due to swelling) and hematuria
   b. **Diagnosis:** duplex US
   c. **Management:** Immediate surgical exploration. Partial venous thrombosis can be managed with anticoagulation.

F. **Ureteral obstruction:** occurs in 1%–9% of transplants
   1. **Presentation:** oliguria or polyuria with rising creatinine
   2. **Diagnosis:** hydronephrosis
   3. **Treatment:** initially, a retrograde ureteral stent or a nephrostomy tube, followed by surgical revision via ureteroneocystostomy or ureteroureterostomy

G. **Urinary leaks and fistulas:** occurs 5–7 days after transplantation
   1. **Presentation:** elevated creatinine and a perinephric fluid collection
   2. **Diagnosis:** confirmed with pyelograms or nuclear medicine scans
   3. **Treatment:** similar to that for ureteral obstruction discussed earlier

H. **Lymphoceles:** occur in less than 5% of recipients and appear as a perinephric lymph collection
   1. **Presentation:** decreased urine output and/or rising creatinine and ipsilateral leg edema
   2. **Diagnosis:** US (fluid collection with or without hydronephrosis)
   3. **Management:** percutaneous or laparoscopic drainage

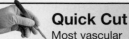

Quick Cut
Most vascular complications require urgent or emergent intervention by open or endovascular techniques.

Quick Cut
Lymphocele can be distinguished from urinoma by sending a fluid sample for creatinine level and culture. Lymphocele has a low creatinine (equal to serum); urinoma has high creatinine.

V. **Outcomes:** Kidney transplant outcomes have improved over the last several decades.
   A. **Recipients of living donor kidney:** One-year survival approaches 98%–99% and graft half-life is 17 years.
   B. **Recipients of deceased donor kidney:** One-year survival is 91% with graft half-life of 10 years.

VI. **Immunosuppression**
   A. **Induction:** Not required but decreases early rejection and is almost universally used. Basiliximab, thymoglobulin, and alemtuzumab are leading induction agents.
   B. **Maintenance:** generally tacrolimus, steroids, and mycophenolate, with an early steroid taper

VII. **Rejection**
   A. **Acute rejection:** mostly occurs 1 week–3 months after transplantation; in ~10%–15% of patients, within the first 6 months after transplant
      1. **Presentation:** low urine output and rising creatinine
      2. **Diagnosis:** made with a kidney biopsy
      3. **Management:** pulse steroids or antilymphocyte sera for ACR and steroids, possibly pheresis and IVIG or other treatments for AMR
   B. **Chronic rejection:** known as *chronic allograft nephropathy* (*CAN*), *transplant glomerulopathy* (*TG*), and *interstitial fibrosis/tubular atrophy* (*IFTA*); occurs over months to years
      1. **Presentation:** glomerular sclerosis, tubular atrophy, duplication of the glomerular basement membrane, and interstitial fibrosis
      2. **Treatment:** No cure, but longevity is maximized by adjusting immunosuppression to minimize nephrotoxicity.

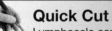

Quick Cut
Because survival improves with transplantation, all long-term dialysis patients should be referred for a transplant evaluation.

VIII. **Alternatives to transplantation:** Include hemodialysis, peritoneal dialysis, or medical management only. Patient survival is greatest with transplantation and lower with dialysis (10%–20% annual mortality rates).

Pancreatic and Islet Transplantation

I. Preoperative assessment

A. Indications: Solitary pancreas transplants are performed mainly for patients with brittle type 1 diabetes (defined by hypoglycemic unawareness) and occasionally for patients after total pancreatectomy for chronic pancreatitis or trauma or as part of a multivisceral transplant.

B. Contraindications: specific to pancreas transplant, insulin requirement greater than 100 units/day indicating high insulin resistance, severe iliac atherosclerosis, BMI greater than 30 kg/m^2, and poor cardiovascular health

C. Donors and outcome: Graft outcomes affected by donor age, BMI, cause of death, and the appearance of the pancreas. Worse outcomes are seen with donor BMI greater than 30 kg/m^2, age older than 50 years, and death due to cerebrovascular accident.

II. Operative strategy

A. Simultaneous pancreas-kidney (SPK): Both kidney and pancreas are obtained from a single donor and transplanted into the recipient with the advantages of better outcomes than pancreas-alone transplant and only one operation needed.

B. Pancreas after kidney (PAK): living donor kidney transplant followed months later by deceased donor pancreas transplant

1. **Advantages:** can avoid dialysis if a live donor is available and maximizes patient survival, which depends on a functioning kidney

2. **Disadvantages:** Rejection of pancreas may occur without rejection of kidneys, delaying detection, and requires two operations.

C. Pancreas transplant alone (PTA): Indicated for brittle diabetics without significant nephropathy. There is no mortality benefit, but PTA significantly improves quality of life.

D. Simultaneous pancreas and live donor kidney (SPLK): Patient may receive a living donor kidney and a deceased donor pancreas during the same operation, if the living donor is willing to be "on call."

E. Venous drainage: Portal vein is anastomosed either to the recipient vena cava or iliac vein (systemic drainage) or to a mesenteric vein branch (portal drainage).

F. Arterial supply: Pancreatic blood supply is from the celiac axis (splenic artery) and superior mesenteric artery (SMA) (inferior pancreaticoduodenal arteries). In back table preparation, the internal and external branches of the donor iliac artery Y graft are anastomosed to the splenic artery and SMA. The common iliac Y graft is then anastomosed to the recipient iliac artery.

G. Exocrine drainage: Donor duodenum is anastomosed to the recipient jejunum (enteric drainage) or bladder (bladder drainage).

III. Postoperative management and complications

A. Graft thrombosis: Presents as sudden rise in glucose, is diagnosed by duplex US, and treated by excision of the graft. Temporary anticoagulation is frequently used to prevent this complication or to treat partial vein thromboses.

B. Postoperative hemorrhage (either intraperitoneal or from a staple line): can occur in up to 20% of cases

C. Anastomotic leaks (from the duodenal anastomosis or staple lines): Difficult to repair. Treatment includes IV antibiotics and antifungals, bowel rest, and anastomotic revision (possibly to Roux-en-Y drainage). It may require allograft pancreatectomy.

IV. Outcomes: One-year graft survival for SPK is 90%, PAK 85%, and PTA 85%.

V. Immunosuppression

A. Induction: Decreases early rejection. Thymoglobulin, alemtuzumab, and basiliximab are leading induction agents.

B. Maintenance: generally tacrolimus, steroids, and mycophenolate, with an early steroid taper

VI. Rejection: no reliable markers; suspected by elevated amylase or lipase (sometimes elevated glucose but often this is a sign of irreversibility)

    A. Diagnosis: can only be made by biopsy

    B. Treatment: similar to rejection of kidney transplants

VII. Alternatives to transplantation

    A. Islet transplantation: Islets are isolated by enzymatically digesting the pancreas and are infused through the portal or mesenteric vein and embolize to the liver (Fig. 23-4).

        1. Indications: same as whole pancreas transplant

        2. Donors: more lenient criteria (older and more obese patients are acceptable)

        3. Mortality: close to zero; still requires immunosuppression

        4. Insulin dependence: at highest volume centers, 80%–90% at 1 year but only 20% at 5 years

        5. Sensitization: Islet transplants can sensitize patients, making future kidney or pancreas transplants very difficult to match.

    B. Insulin therapy: can be given by individual injections or management using an insulin pump and glucose sensor

> **Quick Cut**
> Islet cell transplants do not function as well or last as long as solid pancreas transplants.

Small Bowel and Multivisceral Transplantation

I. Indications: Patients with short bowel syndrome (SBS) (less than 200 cm of functioning small bowel) from congenital abnormalities, Crohn disease, mesenteric thrombosis, trauma, or desmoid tumors. Most patients are on long-term total parenteral nutrition (TPN) and lose access, have line sepsis, or develop cholestatic liver disease due to TPN.

II. Operative strategy

    A. Small bowel only

        1. Venous outflow: may be portal or systemic

        2. GI anastomosis: performed in side-to-side fashion

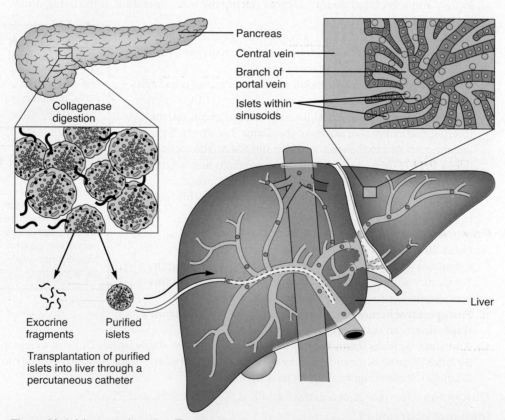

Figure 23-4: Islet transplantation. The pancreas is procured as a whole organ from the donor. The islets are isolated from the pancreas and are purified and infused into a cannula placed in a branch of the recipient's portal vein. (From Mulholland MW, Maier RV, Lillemoe KD, et al. *Greenfield's Surgery: Scientific Principles and Practice*, 4th ed. Philadelphia: Lippincott Williams & Wilkins; 2006.)

    3. Ileostomy: end or loop ileostomy

    4. Feeding access: with jejunostomy or gastrostomy

  B. Multivisceral transplant: Can include liver/small bowel or liver/pancreas/small bowel. Donor small bowel is procured with preservation of vessels (either SMA/superior mesenteric vein or aorta and vena cava).

III. Postoperative management and complications: include bleeding, thrombosis, anastomotic leaks, stomal problems, and sepsis

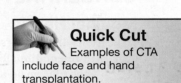

> **Quick Cut**
> Graft-versus-host disease is more common in small bowel transplants due to the large amount of lymphoid tissue present.

  A. Emergency re-exploration: high rate after transplant

  B. PTLD: secondary to EBV

  C. Graft function: monitored by absorption studies and direct biopsy

IV. Outcomes: improved quality of life compared to dependence on TPN

  A. Patient survival: 1-year, 75%; 3-year, 55%–80%

  C. Three-year graft survival: 62%

V. Immunosuppression: Induction therapy is commonly used with two or three drug maintenance regimens.

VI. Rejection: very common (acute rejection in 30%–55%); diagnosed by malabsorption and ileal biopsy

VII. Alternative to transplantation: TPN

Composite Tissue Allograft and Vascularized Composite Allograft Transplants

I. Definition: Composite tissue techniques involve transplantation of multiple tissue types (e.g., muscle, bone, vessels, nerves, and skin) in a functional unit. Composite tissue allograft (CTA) requires more specialized surgery and immunosuppression than does solid organ transplant.

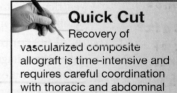

> **Quick Cut**
> Examples of CTA include face and hand transplantation.

II. Indications: Face: patients with severe facial deformities due to trauma or burns. Hand: amputees

III. Operative strategy: Skin, subcutaneous tissues, bones, muscles, nerves, and vessels need to be recovered together.

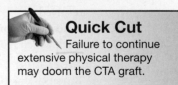

> **Quick Cut**
> Recovery of vascularized composite allograft is time-intensive and requires careful coordination with thoracic and abdominal recovery teams.

IV. Postoperative management and complications: include bleeding, thrombosis, and rejection

  A. Extensive therapy (physical, occupational, swallow, or speech): will be required

  B. Graft function: monitored by function (degree of active and passive joint movement) and appearance

V. Outcomes

  A. Face transplants (partial or whole): Approximately 25 have been performed, with four recipient deaths.

  B. Hand transplants: have been performed with some success, but there are high costs, rehabilitation requirements, uncertain long-term outcome, and side effects resulting from immunosuppression

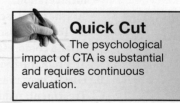

> **Quick Cut**
> Failure to continue extensive physical therapy may doom the CTA graft.

> **Quick Cut**
> The psychological impact of CTA is substantial and requires continuous evaluation.

VI. Immunosuppression: Induction therapy is commonly used with two or three drug maintenance in a variety of regimens.

VII. Rejection: common; diagnosed by skin biopsy

VIII. Alternatives to transplantation: amputation of limbs with use of prosthetics or nonfunctional coverage of open areas by reconstructive surgery (tissue flaps and skin grafts)

Chapter 24

Pediatric Surgery

Clint D. Cappiello, Alexis D. Smith, and Eric Strauch

INTRODUCTION

Pediatric surgery is a distinct specialty because infants and children have both different pathology and a different physiologic response than adults.

> **Quick Cut**
> Remember that children are not just small versions of adults.

CONGENITAL HERNIAS

Inguinal Hernia

I. **Incidence:** occurs in 1%–4% of all children

A. Presentation: Right side ~60%, left side 30%, and bilateral 10% of the time; male-to-female ratio ranges from 3:1 to 10:1.

B. Premature infants: Incidence is up to 10× greater.

C. Increased: in patients with hydrocephalus who are treated with ventriculoperitoneal (VP) shunts, in patients with connective tissue disorders, and in infants and children on peritoneal dialysis

[handwritten margin note:] R side > L side / M > F / *more common in premies / → greater risk of incarc. (2-5x)

> **Quick Cut**
> Repair of an inguinal hernia remains the most common general surgical procedure in children.

II. **Clinical presentation:** Figure 24-1

A. Age: Often diagnosed in infancy, and ~35% of patients present before age 6 months.

B. Classic history: mass or bulge in the groin, scrotum, or labia, which usually occurs during times of increased abdominal pressure and usually disappears after straining or crying has resolved

C. If no mass is present: Physician can feel the thickened spermatic cord, which represents the nondistended hernia sac.

> **Quick Cut**
> Unlike in adults, a congenital inguinal hernia results from a patent processus vaginalis, not a breakdown in the inguinal floor.

III. **Incarceration**

A. Boys: Risk associated with a hernia is the chance of intestinal incarceration.

    1. **Intestinal ischemia and obstruction:** can occur

    2. **Testicular ischemia:** Entrapped bowel becomes edematous and compresses the spermatic vessels.

    3. **Prematurity:** Risk of incarceration in a premature infant is 2–5× higher than in the older child.

B. Girls: Ovarian incarceration can occur as well as incarceration of the intestine.

> **Quick Cut**
> A nonreducible hernia is incarcerated and warrants emergent surgical intervention.

C. Treatment: reduction of the incarcerated hernia, hydration of the patient, and herniorrhaphy

[handwritten margin note:] Tx: / reduction / hydration / herniorrhaphy

    1. **Premature infant:** hernia repaired during the admission in the first 24–48 hours

    2. **Approach:** Reduction is performed with or without sedation by gentle, continuous pressure on the incarcerated intestine.

    3. **If hernia does not reduce:** Most hernias will reduce, but if not, emergent repair, evaluation of the intestine, and resection of necrotic intestine needs to be performed.

> **Quick Cut**
> In infants younger than age 1 year, the risk of incarceration doubles with delaying repair.

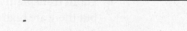

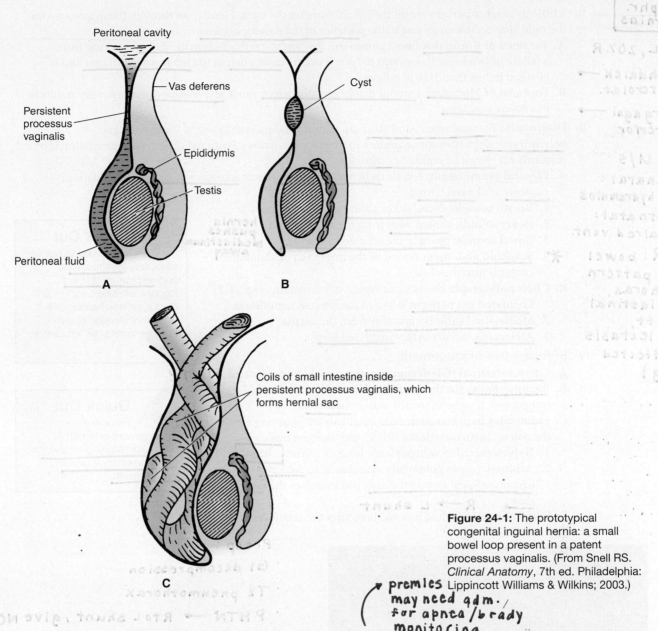

Figure 24-1: The prototypical congenital inguinal hernia: a small bowel loop present in a patent processus vaginalis. (From Snell RS. *Clinical Anatomy*, 7th ed. Philadelphia: Lippincott Williams & Wilkins; 2003.)

IV. Herniorrhaphy: A hernia should be repaired soon after it is diagnosed, unless a major medical reason prohibits. In most children, the hernia can be repaired with outpatient surgery. Premature infants may have apnea and bradycardia after surgery and require overnight admission for monitoring.

   A. Procedure: Open herniorrhaphy in the child consists of identifying the sac, dissecting the spermatic structures free, and ligating the sac high at the internal ring of the inguinal canal. Floor repair is rarely needed.

   B. Laparoscopy: Laparoscopic herniorrhaphy has also gained popularity. Laparoscopic evaluation of the contralateral side can also be performed.

   C. Complications: damage to the vas deferens, vascular injury to the testes, recurrence, and iatrogenic cryptorchidism

   D. Recurrence rate: reported to be 1%, and the highest frequency occurs in premature infants and patients with incarcerated hernias, connective tissue disorders (e.g., Ehlers-Danlos syndrome), or increased intra-abdominal pressure (VP shunts or peritoneal dialysis catheters)

Diaphragmatic Hernias

   I. Definition: Communications through the diaphragm that allow abdominal contents to migrate into the thoracic cavity; incidence is 2.4 in 10,000 live births.

[Handwritten margin notes, left side:]

Diaphr. hernias

80% L, 20% R

* Bochdalek → posterolat.

* Morgagni → anterior

DX: U/S

* prenatal: polyhydramnios

* postnatal: impaired vent.

CXR: bowel gas pattern in thorax, mediastinal shift, atelectasis (unaffected lung)

II. Etiology: Eighty percent are on the left, 20% are on the right. Herniation through the diaphragm on the right side occurs rarely due to the presence of the developing liver.

   A. Foramen of Bochdalek (most common): Posterolateral diaphragmatic defect resulting from a failure of two muscular groups to fuse; it occurs most often in the left hemidiaphragm and is bilateral in less than 10% of infants.

   B. Foramen of Morgagni: anterior diaphragmatic defect; much less common and generally results in less severe problems

III. Diagnosis: Prenatal ultrasound (US) can identify abdominal viscera in the thorax, and polyhydramnios may occur secondary to foregut obstruction. Postnatal diagnosis of herniation is based primarily on impaired ventilatory capacity.

   A. Physical examination: reveals tachypnea, dyspnea, use of accessory muscles for ventilation, cyanosis, and nasal flaring

     1. **Breath sounds:** decreased or absent on the affected side

     2. **Heart sounds:** shifted away from the affected side *[handwritten:] hernia pushes mediastinum away*

     3. **Bowel sounds:** heard in the affected hemithorax

     [handwritten ✱] 4. **Scaphoid abdomen:** caused by the migration of abdominal contents into the chest

   B. Chest radiograph: shows signs typical of herniation (Fig. 24-2)

     1. **Loculated gas pattern:** found in the affected hemithorax

     2. **Mediastinal shift:** occurs away from the hernia

     3. **Atelectasis:** occurs in the unaffected lung

IV. Preoperative management

   A. Gastrointestinal (GI) decompression: should be performed *[handwritten:] NGT?*

   B. Pneumothorax (in the unaffected hemithorax): should be sought and, if present, treated with a chest tube

   C. Pulmonary hypertension: causes right-to-left shunting across the patent ductus arteriosus (PDA) and foramen ovale

     1. **Hypoxemia:** due to hypoplastic lung(s); causes acidosis

     2. **Acidosis:** causes pulmonary vasculature to constrict, which decreases blood flow to the lung and increases the right-to-left shunt *[handwritten:] R → L shunt*

   D. Surgical repair: should proceed only after the infant is stable

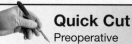

Quick Cut
A right-sided cardiac silhouette (dextrocardia) and respiratory distress signal a left-sided congenital diaphragmatic hernia until proven otherwise, due to bowel entering the left pleural space.

Quick Cut
Preoperative management is aimed at both respiratory insufficiency and pulmonary vascular hypertension.

[Handwritten notes, right side:]

Preop:
- GI decompression
- TX pneumothorax
- PHTN → RtoL shunt, give NO
- Surgical repair
- HFOV: tx hypox., hypercarbia
- ECMO

Op:
[reduce
[repair
[monitor: ABGs, O₂ sat.

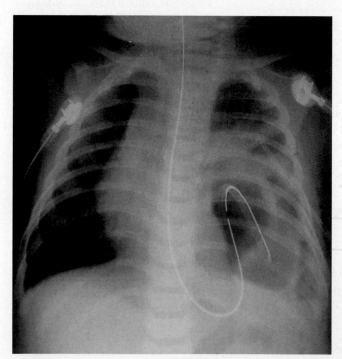

Figure 24-2: Chest radiograph of a newborn with a left congenital diaphragmatic hernia. Mediastinal structures shifted to the right. Abdominal viscera occupy the left hemithorax. Nasogastric tube locates the stomach. (From Mulholland MW, Doherty GM, Maier RV, et al. *Greenfield's Surgery Scientific Principles and Practice*, 4th ed. Philadelphia: Lippincott Williams & Wilkins; 2006.)

E. **High-frequency oscillatory ventilation** (HFOV): for persistent respiratory distress, hypoxemia, and hypercarbia

F. **Nitric oxide (NO):** potent pulmonary vasodilator that is mixed with the gases used in the ventilator to improve hypoxemia by treating pulmonary hypertension

G. **Extracorporeal membrane oxygenation (ECMO):** consider if acidosis with hypoxemia persists

V. **Operative management:** based on the following principles:

A. **Surgical reduction:** Herniated contents are reduced surgically back into the abdomen with a subcostal incision or thoracotomy. Recently, a thoracoscopic approach has been successful.

B. **Repair:** Hernia defect is repaired either primarily or with prosthetic.

C. **Monitoring:** Acid–base balance and respiratory function are monitored carefully; aggressive support is continued as needed.

VI. **Postoperative management:** aimed primarily at maintaining adequate ventilation and perfusion and includes the following:

A. **Respiratory support (on a ventilator):** given as needed, and arterial blood gases are monitored

B. **Atelectasis treatment (of either lung):** Retained secretions are prevented.

C. **Observation for contralateral pneumothorax:** Treat rapidly if it occurs.

D. **Adequate GI decompression:** provided with an intraoperatively placed nasogastric (NG) tube

E. **Intra-abdominal compartment syndrome prevention:** Silo or abdominal patch may be placed because loss of abdominal domain can make primary repair difficult, and the inability to obtain a tension-free closure will result in increased abdominal pressure.

F. **Fluid management:** Critical postoperatively, as patients may be hypovolemic initially. Subsequently, diuretics may be used to avoid fluid overload.

VII. **Prognosis:** depends on preoperative severity and time of presentation

A. **Survival rate:** 60%–90%; long-term mortality is ~10% and is usually secondary to persistent pulmonary hypertension.

1. **Ipsilateral lung:** almost always hypoplastic and does not aid significantly in postoperative respiratory function

2. **Lung development:** If the infant survives, the lung will continue to develop, but a normal complement of alveoli may never be reached.

B. **Pulmonary function:** Approaches normal as survivors reach adulthood. Studies have shown that survivors are expected to develop appropriate exercise tolerance.

VIII. **ECMO patients:** survival rate of 43%–80%; should be considered as a temporary, potentially lifesaving therapy for those for whom no other option is available

Quick Cut
Resolution of respiratory insufficiency depends on the maturity of the contralateral lung and control of pulmonary hypertension.

Quick Cut
The two main types of abdominal wall defects are **gastroschisis** and **omphalocele**. In both, the abdominal contents are outside of the peritoneal cavity; however, presentation and management are considerably different.

ABDOMINAL WALL DEFECTS

Types

Table 24-1: Comparison of Congenital Abdominal Wall Defects

Characteristics	Gastroschisis	Omphalocele
Size of defect	Smaller (<4 cm)	Usually larger (4–12 cm)
Presence of sac	No	Yes, if ruptured sac remnant
Contents of sac	Intestine (midgut)	Intestine (midgut, colon), liver, spleen
Location of defect	Right of umbilicus	Central at umbilicus
Associated anomalies	Rare (intestinal atresia)	Common

Gastroschisis

I. **Clinical features:** usually a small (<4 cm) opening in the abdominal wall, immediately to the right of the cord, which is located in the normal position (Table 24-1)

   A. **Characteristics:** Intestines appear edematous and thickened with a fibrinous peel secondary to the inflammatory response to direct intrauterine exposure to amniotic fluid and postnatal vascular compromise.

> **Quick Cut**
> In gastroschisis, there is no protective sac covering the herniated contents.

   B. **Herniation:** Typically, the entire midgut is herniated; the stomach, urinary bladder, and gonads may also herniate.

   C. **Associated anomalies and syndromes:** Rare; intestinal atresia is the most frequent (10%–15% of cases) anomaly.

II. **Prenatal diagnosis:** most commonly made by prenatal US

III. **Preoperative management:** encompasses three main principles: respiratory support due to infants' prematurity, heat preservation, and fluid resuscitation due to the large surface area of exposed intestines

> **Quick Cut**
> Infants with gastroschisis are more likely to be born premature and often have intrauterine growth retardation with low birth weights.

   A. **Fluids:** Infants are usually hypovolemic and require 125%–150% maintenance intravenous (IV) fluids for adequate resuscitation.

   B. **NG decompression and broad-spectrum antibiotics:** are initiated

   C. **Intestinal ischemia:** may be present due to obstruction of the vascular supply to the intestines

IV. **Operative management:** Emergent; there is no covering of the GI tract to prevent heat and fluid losses. Infants undergo either immediate or delayed primary closure depending on the ability to reduce the herniated viscera.

   A. **Immediate primary closure:** involves decompressing the GI tract and stretching the abdominal wall over the defect with closure immediately after birth

> **Quick Cut**
> Rapid coverage of the exposed viscera with a plastic bowel bag is imperative to protect the bowel and minimize heat and moisture loss.

   B. **Abdominal compartment syndrome:** To avoid this complication, place a preformed Silastic pouch (silo) for temporary coverage. Serial reductions are performed at the bedside until primary closure is feasible (usually in 5–7 days).

Omphalocele

I. **Clinical features:** central abdominal wall defect located at the umbilicus ranging from 2 to 12 cm

   A. **Location:** Most omphaloceles are lateral fold defects that always occur at the umbilicus and are covered with a sac. (See Table 24-1)

   B. **Sac:** Covers the extruding visceral contents (always present); if the omphalocele has ruptured, a sac remnant will be visible. The sac usually contains the liver and midgut.

> **Quick Cut**
> Delayed primary closure is used if there is concern for abdominal compartment syndrome.

   C. **Pentalogy of Cantrell:** Omphalocele may be a constituent; others are diaphragmatic hernia, cleft sternum, absent pericardium, and intracardiac defects.

   D. **Associated anomalies:** trisomies 13 and 18; Beckwith-Wiedemann syndrome; and cardiac, neural tube, and genitourinary malformations

II. **Prenatal diagnosis:** made classically by US, which can also help differentiate an omphalocele from gastroschisis by the presence of a sac

> **Quick Cut**
> Approximately 50% of omphalocele patients have one or more associated anomalies.

III. **Preoperative management:** varies depending on whether the omphalocele sac is intact or ruptured

   A. **All cases:** NG decompression, IV fluid resuscitation, and broad-spectrum antibiotics are instituted in all cases.

   B. **Unruptured omphalocele:** Managed initially nonoperatively; the sac is left intact and protected with a sterile dressing. Workup is initiated for associated defects.

   C. **Ruptured omphalocele:** managed with immediate placement of a silo for temporary coverage of the defect

IV. **Operative management:** Can vary greatly; the choice of procedures includes primary closure, staged repair, or, for an unruptured omphalocele, initial nonoperative management.
   A. **Primary repair:** Can prove to be problematic with larger omphaloceles. If primary repair is attempted, monitoring for intra-abdominal hypertension is essential.
   B. **Staged repair:** Silastic sheeting or preconstructed silo bags can be used to stage the repair. By keeping tension on the prosthetic sac through routine bedside reductions, the abdominal wall can be stretched to accommodate the herniated viscera.
      1. **Closing the defect:** Prosthetic material or biologic mesh can be used.
      2. **Closure:** usually accomplished within 10 days
   C. **Alternative method of treatment:** Cover the defect with skin flaps, leaving the resultant ventral hernia to be repaired later.

V. **Nonoperative management:** Option for patients with associated pulmonary hypoplasia and cardiac anomalies that may not tolerate reduction. Initial nonoperative management acts as a bridge to delayed closure when the infant is more stable.
   A. **Technique:** Sac is coated with silver sulfadiazine (Silvadene) or a silver-impregnated sterile dressing; an eschar forms, with subsequent granulation tissue. The resultant ventral hernia can be repaired later.
   B. **Risks:** sac rupture, requiring subsequent repair in an infected area; sepsis; undiagnosed intestinal atresia; and prolonged hospitalization

Postoperative Management

I. **Muscular paralysis and mechanical ventilation:** may be required until the abdomen stretches enough to accommodate the viscera or a reoperation to loosen the repair

II. **Slow onset of bowel function:** Infants often require parenteral nutrition. Bowel function appears to return faster following repair of an omphalocele.

> **Quick Cut**
> Abdominal compartment syndrome presents with oliguria, ventilatory compromise, decreased venous return, and low cardiac output.

Prognosis

I. **Gastroschisis:** Although more difficult to manage initially, it has few long-term problems.
   A. **Mortality rate:** greatly improved with the use of total parenteral nutrition (TPN) and is now ~5%
   B. **Intestinal strictures:** may develop at evisceration site due to ischemia
   C. **Short-gut syndrome:** may develop if intestinal gangrene is present and an extensive small bowel resection is required

II. **Omphalocele:** Outcome is related to the presence of associated anomalies; overall mortality rate ranges from 20% to 60%.

> **Quick Cut**
> Mortality is related to prematurity, sepsis, associated congenital anomalies, and the viability of the GI tract at the time of surgery.

ESOPHAGEAL ATRESIA AND TRACHEOESOPHAGEAL MALFORMATIONS

Definition

I. **Esophageal atresia (EA) (with or without tracheoesophageal fistula [TEF]):** most common congenital anomaly of the esophagus

II. **Incidence:** Ranging from 1:2,500 to 4,500 live births; there is a wide spectrum of lesions.

III. **Associated anomalies:** high incidence; dictate overall outcomes and survival

Types of Lesions

I. **Pure EA:** proximal and distal blind pouches without a TEF; occurs in 7% of patients (Fig. 24-3)

II. **EA with a proximal TEF:** least common type; occurs in 0.5% of patients

III. **EA (proximal pouch) with a distal TEF:** occurs in 86% of patients

IV. **TEF without atresia (H-type fistula):** occurs in 5% of patients; differs in presentation in that patients tend to present at an older age with recurrent pneumonia

V. **Proximal and distal TEF:** occurs in 1.5% of patients

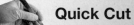

> **Quick Cut**
> Esophageal atresia with proximal pouch and distal tracheoesophageal fistula is the most common variant.

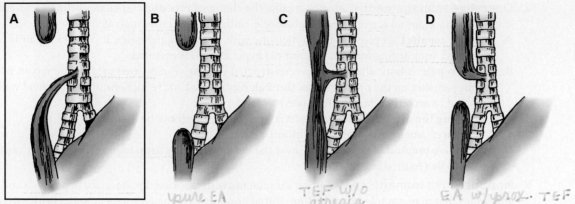

[handwritten annotations: pure EA, TEF w/o atresia, EA w/prox. TEF]

Figure 24-3: Types of esophageal atresia. Atresia with distal tracheoesophgeal fistula (A) is the most common.

[handwritten annotation: EA (prox.) w/distal TEF]

Associated Congenital Anomalies

I. **Cardiovascular anomalies:** Most common; among these, ventricular septal defects (VSDs) and tetralogy of Fallot are most frequent.

II. **VACTERL:** may be fully or partially demonstrated, that is, one or any combination of lesions may occur

Quick Cut
Associated congenital anomalies occur in ~50%–70% of esophageal atresia.

Diagnosis

I. **Physical examination**
  A. **Aspiration of material:** can present as excessive salivation as well as choking and cyanosis with breastfeeding
  B. **Fistula:** can result in pneumonitis and respiratory distress
  C. **Scaphoid abdomen:** accompanies pure atresia due to the lack of distal air in the GI tract

II. **Diagnosis:** Usually made within the first 24 hours after birth. The affected infant classically presents with choking with the first feeding.
  A. **Plain radiographic films (of the chest and the abdomen):** important in establishing the diagnosis
    1. **Chest film:** should confirm the diagnosis by using air as contrast and will demonstrate the blind upper pouch as well as failure of passage by the NG tube
    2. **Gasless abdomen:** characteristic of pure EA
    3. **Long-gap EA:** gap greater than 3 cm between the two ends of the esophagus
  B. **Workup:** Due to high incidence of concomitant congenital defects, thorough workup is warranted preoperatively.
    1. **Physical exam:** focuses on identifying any defects (VACTERL)
    2. **Echocardiography:** best initial screening test for cardiac defects
    3. **Additional testing:** renal ultrasonography and chromosomal analysis

Quick Cut
The **VACTERL** association, a well-recognized anomaly complex, involves **v**ertebral and **a**nal defects, **c**ardiac anomalies, **t**ache**o**esophageal fistula, and **r**enal and **l**imb dysplasia.

Quick Cut
Most esophageal atresias can be diagnosed at the bedside by finding resistance to passage of an NG tube.

Preoperative Management

I. **Decompression of the proximal pouch:** requires a sump tube (Replogle tube) with low, continuous suction

II. **Upright position:** is maintained

III. **Delayed repair:** Placement of a gastrostomy tube prevents further gastric aspiration and provides a route for preoperative feedings with extended delay.

IV. **Long-gap EA:** Stretching the proximal pouch daily shortens the distance between the esophageal ends in preparation for eventual repair.

V. **Broad-spectrum IV antibiotics:** initiated

Operative Management

I. **Primary repair:** Can be undertaken at the time of presentation if the defect measures less than 2 cm and no signs of pneumonitis are present. Broad-spectrum antibiotic therapy is begun.

    A. **Technique:** Extrapleural dissection through the hemithorax opposite the aortic arch is currently favored to prevent empyema from occurring as the result of an anastomotic leak.

        1. **Step 1:** TEF is repaired.

        2. **Step 2:** Primary esophagostomy is performed.

        3. **Step 3:** Dissecting the proximal pouch allows for the adequate length of esophagus necessary to create a tension-free anastomosis.

    B. **Minimally invasive, thoracoscopic EA-TEF repair:** has been proven to be effective and safe and is gaining popularity

II. **Delayed repair:** May be needed if a long-gap EA exists, allowing for growth of the infant and shortening of the gap. Externalized traction sutures may be placed on either end of the esophageal pouches to allow for serial tightening at the bedside over a 10–14-day period in order to approximate the pouches at a quicker rate.

Postoperative Management

I. **Goal:** directed at potential pulmonary and esophageal problems

    A. **Extubation:** done as soon as possible to protect the tracheal repair

    B. **Pulmonary toilet:** necessary to prevent pneumonia or reintubation

    C. **Esophagotracheal suction:** done carefully and with a specifically defined length of tubing to avoid damage to the anastomosis

II. **Survival:** ~85%–95% overall survival, with mortality virtually always related to associated comorbidities

Postoperative Complications

I. **Anastomotic leak:** Due to excessive tension on the anastomosis and ischemia of the esophageal ends; 95% close spontaneously with adequate drainage by a pleural tube and nutritional support.

II. **Anastomotic stricture:** common early complication following TEF repair in as high as 30%–40% of patients

    1. **Cause:** consequence of gastroesophageal reflux (GER), ischemia at the anastomosis, and following an anastomotic leak

    2. **Treatment:** Strictures are treated with serial dilatations.

III. **GER:** most common complication following TEF repair; ~40%–70% of patients

IV. **Recurrent fistulas:** occur in less than 10% of patients and are usually a sequelae of an anastomotic leak but do require a reoperation for ligation of the fistula

Prognosis

I. **Risk stratification:** identifies infants at risk for death and long-term morbidity

II. **Risk factors:** include low birth weight (<1,500 g), major congenital heart disease and other severe associated anomalies, ventilator dependence, and long-gap EA

INTESTINAL MALROTATION

Overview

I. **Definition:** Abnormal placement and fixation of the midgut into the peritoneal cavity. Malrotation can occur independently or can be associated with other malformations, such as diaphragmatic hernia, omphalocele, and gastroschisis (Fig. 24-4).

II. **Normal in utero development:** Midgut develops extra-abdominally then migrates intraperitoneally, where it undergoes a 270-degree rotation.

III. **Displacements caused by malrotation**

    A. **Cecum:** not in the right lower quadrant (RLQ), and the duodenum does not pass posteriorly to the superior mesenteric artery

    B. **Base of the small bowel:** Instead of being fixed from the ligament of Treitz to the cecum in the RLQ, the whole midgut is anchored on the superior mesenteric artery.

    C. **Cecum fixation:** Various stages can be seen, but it is usually fixed to the right upper quadrant (RUQ) with the fibrous bands (Ladd bands) that extend across the duodenum.

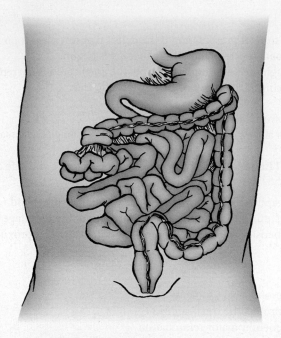

Figure 24-4: Malrotation.

IV. Sequelae

    A. Intestinal obstruction: can result from adhesive bands across the duodenum fixing it to the RUQ; more common in infants and neonates but can occur later in life

    B. Midgut volvulus: More serious than intestinal obstruction; intestine twists on the superior mesenteric vessels, causing obstruction as well as ischemia, potentially leading to gangrene of the entire small bowel.

Clinical Presentation

    I. Bilious vomiting: usual presenting symptom and helps to rule out pyloric stenosis or simple colic

    II. Passage of bloody stool: late occurrence implying ischemia

    III. Appearance: Infant may appear normal, with hemodynamic stability, or may be dehydrated and in shock after the intestine becomes ischemic or necrotic.

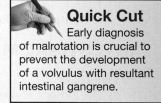

Quick Cut
Bilious emesis in a neonate should prompt a rapid investigation for malrotation and volvulus.

Diagnosis

    I. Radiographs: very useful when making the diagnosis

    A. Plain film: May demonstrate the "double bubble" sign, which is produced by intestinal gas confined to the stomach and duodenum, with small amounts of gas in the residual, unused GI tract. In a newborn with bilious vomiting, this sign is an indication for surgery.

    B. Upper GI series: may demonstrate an abnormally located ligament of Treitz, the presence of the duodenum to the left of midline, a duodenal obstruction, or a "beaked" end in the barium column at the point of the intestinal twist

Quick Cut
Early diagnosis of malrotation is crucial to prevent the development of a volvulus with resultant intestinal gangrene.

    II. Prompt surgical exploration: imperative if the diagnosis of malrotation is suspected but cannot be ruled out

Operative Management

    I. Surgical procedures: vary with the presence or absence of volvulus and the status of the intestine

    A. Simple malrotation: treated by the **Ladd procedure**

        1. Release of adhesive bands and mobilization of the duodenum: Goal is to broaden the mesentery of the intestine as much as possible and to separate the duodenum and ascending colon.

2. **Intestinal obstruction/ischemia prevention:** Cecum is placed in the left upper quadrant and the duodenum in the right lateral abdomen so that both organs will be in favorable positions.

3. **Appendectomy:** Because the appendix may not be in its expected position, this procedure eliminates the potential diagnostic challenge and complications; a future episode of appendicitis may produce.

B. **Malrotation with volvulus:** requires several preliminary steps

1. **Step 1:** counterclockwise detorsion of the midgut volvulus

2. **Step 2:** Bowel is then examined for viability and for areas of necrosis.

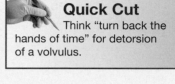

Quick Cut
Think "turn back the hands of time" for detorsion of a volvulus.

a. **Small areas of gangrene:** If present, resection is performed, followed by the Ladd procedure.

b. **Extensive ischemia:** Bowel is untwisted, and the abdomen is closed and re-explored 24 hours later. This second look allows marginally viable tissue to recover, with the hope of minimizing the amount of resection.

II. **Laparoscopic management:** reasonable initial approach

Prognosis

I. **Recurrence (after surgical exploration and a Ladd procedure):** very low (<2%)

II. **Long-term sequelae:** Minimal after repair of **simple malrotation**; however, when **extensive intestinal resection** is required, the result depends strongly on the amount of intestine remaining.

INTESTINAL ATRESIA

Duodenal Atresia and Stenosis

I. **Cause:** May occur because the duodenum fails to recanalize in the early embryonic stages. The lesion may be complex, partial, or in the form of a web.

II. **Associated anomalies**

A. **Trisomy 21:** occurs in 30% of infants with duodenal malformations

B. **Cardiac lesions:** present in many infants (~25%)

C. **Annular pancreas:** ~25%, with the pancreas forming a ring around the duodenum

Quick Cut
Up to 50% of patients with duodenal atresia will have another congenital anomaly of a different organ system.

1. **Cause:** due to failure of the ventral pancreatic bud to completely rotate dorsally

2. **Underlying web/stenosis:** true cause of the obstruction, although the annular pancreas may cause extrinsic compression

III. **Diagnosis:** Prenatal US can diagnose the majority; as with an abdominal radiograph, a double bubble sign is usually present. The **clinical diagnosis** is usually made from two simple findings.

A. **Bilious vomiting:** occurring in a nondistended infant

B. **Double bubble sign (Fig. 24-5):** Paucity of distal gas suggests complete obstruction.

IV. **Preoperative management:** Because these lesions have a high association with other more critical anomalies, stabilization and evaluation can be done before surgery.

A. **Gastric decompression and fluid resuscitation**

B. **Preoperative antibiotics:** administered

V. **Operative management:** Directed at restoring a patent GI tract; repair can be done through a laparotomy or laparoscopy.

A. **Duodenoduodenostomy:** usually can be performed

B. **Duodenojejunostomy:** good alternative if duodenoduodenostomy cannot be done

C. **Tapering duodenoplasty:** may be done first for patients with a dilated, atretic proximal duodenum

D. **Gastrojejunostomy:** contraindicated

E. **Web:** If present, the duodenum is opened at the site of obstruction, the web is excised, and the duodenum is closed transversely. Care must be taken to identify the ampulla of Vater because it is also located on the mesenteric side of the web.

F. **Annular pancreas:** Bypass with duodenoduodenostomy. Annular pancreas is never transected, as the injured duct structures will result in a persistent pancreatic leak.

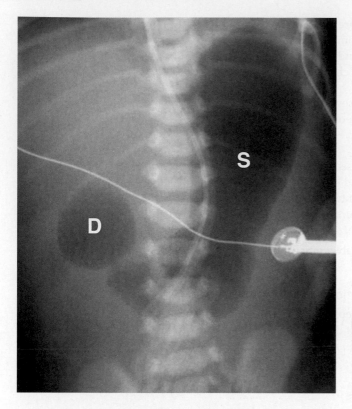

Figure 24-5: Duodenal atresia. Supine radiograph demonstrates gas in the stomach (*S*) and markedly dilated duodenal bulb (*D*), producing the double bubble sign. The remainder of the abdomen is gasless. (From Siegel MJ, Coley BD. *Core Curriculum: Pediatric Imaging*. Philadelphia: Lippincott Williams & Wilkins; 2005.)

    G. Thorough search: done to ensure patency of the entire GI tract because 3.5% of patients have other atresias

    H. NG tube: used for GI decompression

VI. Postoperative management: simple but requires patience

    A. GI decompression: important to protect the suture line and to prevent possible aspiration

    B. GI function: Return is slow.

    C. TPN: Nutritional support is usually needed.

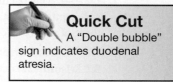

Quick Cut
A "Double bubble" sign indicates duodenal atresia.

VII. Prognosis: Long-term results of surgery are good, with survival approaching 95%. Mortality in these patients is related to prematurity of the infant and to associated anomalies.

Jejunal, Ileal, and Colonic Atresias

I. Cause: In utero vascular accidents result in ischemia of a segment of bowel, with consequent stenosis (5%) or atresia (95%).

    A. Familial intestinal atresias: also exist, with varying patterns of inheritance

    B. Jejunoileal atresias: evenly split between the jejunum and ileum, with the **colon** uncommonly affected

Quick Cut
The severity of the intestinal atresia is related to the size of the vascular arcade that was affected in utero.

II. Associated anomalies: Because they are not embryonic maldevelopments, associated anomalies are much less common; however, ~10% of patients have **cystic fibrosis**.

III. Clinical presentation: Diagnosis is suspected prenatally when there is maternal polyhydramnios or postnatally when an infant develops abdominal distension and bilious vomiting after 24 hours of life or fails to pass meconium. Jaundice may also develop.

    A. Degree of abdominal distention: Varies with the level of the obstruction. Proximal obstructions lead to less distention, whereas more distal lesions produce generalized distention.

    B. Small bowel or colonic atresia: All such patients should have an early evaluation for cystic fibrosis.

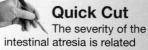

Quick Cut
The passage of meconium does *not* rule out an atresia because the GI tract was intact before the vascular accident.

IV. **Diagnosis:** can be made prenatally with US and fetal magnetic resonance imaging (MRI)
  A. **Abdominal radiographs:** show various degrees of obstruction, depending on the level of the atresia or stenosis; the picture can be confused with meconium ileus
    1. **Differences:** In atresia, air-fluid levels are present; a meconium ileus shows distended bowel and a "soap bubble" appearance.
    2. **Peritoneal calcifications:** suggest intrauterine perforation with meconium peritonitis
  B. **Contrast studies:** helpful in both diagnosis and management
    1. **Contrast enema:** Will reveal colonic lesions; a microcolon suggests the atresia developed early in gestation.
    2. **Rules out:** Hirschsprung disease, meconium ileus, and other congenital disorders, making diagnosis of the atresia more certain

Quick Cut
In intestinal atresia, air-fluid levels are always present on x-ray. Meconium ileus shows only distended bowel.

V. **Preoperative management:** GI decompression and fluid replacement. Gastric losses should be replaced and electrolytes corrected if surgery is to be delayed. Begin broad-spectrum antibiotic therapy.

VI. **Operative management:** Surgery is performed to re-establish intestinal continuity.
  A. **End-to-end intestinal anastomosis:** current **procedure of choice**
    1. **Disadvantage:** may be difficult to accomplish because of the marked size disparity of the bowel—the proximal bowel is dilated, and the distal, unused bowel is small
    2. **Repair tips:** Tapering of the proximal bowel or resection of a limited amount of dilated bowel may aid in the repair.
  B. **GI function:** may be slow to return because the distended bowel has been found to have impaired motility
  C. **NG tube:** placed to allow decompression and prevent aspiration
  D. **Atresia and meconium ileus:** In a patient with both conditions, the distal intestine may contain inspissated small bowel secretions. The site of inspissation should be irrigated with a 4% acetylcysteine (Mucomyst) solution to relieve any potential obstruction.

VII. **Postoperative management:** decompression and patience
  A. **Hyperalimentation:** may be needed until the GI tract recovers
  B. **Malabsorption:** If present, may prolong the recovery time.

VIII. **Prognosis:** Because associated anomalies are few, survival is a function of the prematurity of the infant.
  A. **Survival:** Current results show a survival rate of almost 100%.
  B. **Postoperative complications:** Most common leading to mortality are intestinal obstruction and anastomotic breakdown.

"Apple-Peel" Atresia

I. **Definition:** severe form of small bowel atresia, so named because of its radiographic appearance

II. **Cause:** occurs during a large vascular accident to one or more of the mesenteric arcades in utero

III. **GI function:** In these patients, return is very prolonged, and malabsorption is common.

HIRSCHSPRUNG DISEASE

Overview

I. **Cause:** absence of ganglion cells in the myenteric and submucosal plexus in the intestine
  A. **Ineffective peristalsis:** Affected segment of the bowel is unable to relax.
  B. **Extent:** Usually involves the rectum and extends proximally at varying lengths (short-segment vs. long-segment Hirschsprung); however, the entire colon may be involved and is referred to as **total colonic aganglionosis**.

II. **Incidence:** ranges from 1:4,500 to 7,000 live births
  A. **Classic Hirschsprung disease:** male predominance of 4:1
  B. **Total colonic aganglionosis:** slight male predominance

III. **Genetics:** Approximately 80%–90% of cases are sporadic.
  A. **Inherited familial predisposition:** occurs in ~10% of cases
  B. **RET proto-oncogene mutation:** accounts for the highest proportion of both familial and sporadic cases

Clinical Presentation

I. **Newborns:** classically present with a history of delayed passage of meconium
   A. **Meconium:** usually passed within 24 hours after birth in term infants and within 48 hours in premature infants
   B. **Other signs:** abdominal distention, bilious vomiting, poor feeding, and constipation
   C. **Physical examination:** reveals a distended abdomen
      1. **Loops of stool-filled bowel:** occasionally palpated
      2. **Rectal examination:** often demonstrates a tight anal sphincter with an empty rectal vault

II. **Older children:** constipation, abdominal distention, and failure to thrive

III. **Hirschsprung enterocolitis:** initial clinical presentation of a small percentage of children with Hirschsprung disease who present with profuse diarrhea, abdominal distention, and fever
   A. **Cause:** develops due to intestinal stasis proximal to the aganglionic segment resulting in bacterial overgrowth and translocation
   B. **If suspected:** Contrast enemas for diagnosis should be avoided due to risk of intestinal perforation.
   C. **Treatment:** serial rectal irrigations and IV antibiotics

Quick Cut
The diagnosis of Hirschsprung disease should be suspected in any patient with a history of constipation dating back to the newborn period.

Quick Cut
Classically, an explosion of watery stool occurs with Hirschsprung disease following examination.

Quick Cut
Enterocolitis in Hirschsprung disease can be fatal.

Diagnosis

I. **Initial imaging with upright and decubitus abdominal radiographs:** reveals air-fluid levels and a distended bowel with a paucity of air in the rectum (Fig. 24-6)

II. **Contrast enema:** Next diagnostic study of choice and often facilitates diagnosis; water-soluble contrast is preferred to barium.
   A. **Classic radiographic findings:** narrow, spastic distal intestinal segment with a proximal dilated segment
   B. **Transition zone:** represents the most distal area in which ganglia cells are present
      1. **Location:** most commonly located in the rectosigmoid, but it can occur anywhere in the intestine
      2. **Definition:** Transition zones are less well-defined in short-segment Hirschsprung as well as in total colonic aganglionosis.

III. **Anorectal manometry:** demonstrates elevated resting anal sphincter pressures and an absence of a relaxation reflex

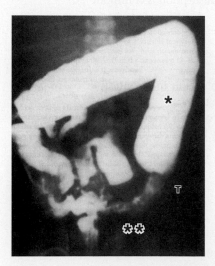

Figure 24-6: Hirschsprung disease. *, dilated normal bowel; T, transition zone; **, aganglionic segment. (From Dudek RW. *BRS Embryology*, 5th ed. Baltimore: Lippincott Williams & Wilkins; 2010.)

IV. **Rectal biopsy:** Specimens are characterized in the absence of ganglion cells and presence of hypertrophied nerve trunks.

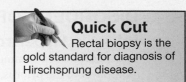

   A. **Bedside suction rectal biopsy:** currently the procedure of choice and confers little risk to the patient
   B. **Considerations:** Although the procedure is simple, it produces small submucosal specimens and requires an experienced pathologist for correct interpretation.

Operative Management

I. **Surgical approach:** Variety; a primary pull-through procedure (one-stage) is the preferred approach, but some infants require an initial diverting colostomy (two-stage procedure) prior to their definitive operation due to enterocolitis or marked dilation of proximal normal colon.

II. **Goals of surgery:** Each operative procedure has three common goals.
   A. **Resect:** involved aganglionic intestine
   B. **Re-establish:** functional GI tract by bringing normal ganglionic bowel to the anus
   C. **Preserve:** sphincter function

III. **Procedures:** Most commonly performed are the endorectal pull-through, Soave, Swenson, and Duhamel, which can be performed either laparoscopically or through an open approach.
   A. **Endorectal pull-through:**
      1. **Step 1:** Rectal mucosa is dissected from the rectal wall transanally up to the peritoneal reflection.
      2. **Step 2:** Abdomen is entered transanally through the rectal wall.
      3. **Step 3:** Proximal normal bowel is pulled through the stripped anorectal segment and is sutured to the anorectal junction.
   B. **Soave procedure:**
      1. **Step 1:** Aganglionic colon is excised to the level of the peritoneal reflection.
      2. **Step 2:** Mucosa is removed in the remaining rectum.
      3. **Step 3:** Proximal normal bowel is pulled through the stripped anorectal segment and is sutured to the anorectal junction.
   C. **Swenson procedure:**
      1. **Step 1:** Involved colon is excised to within 1 cm of the anal mucocutaneous margin.
      2. **Step 2:** Bowel is then sutured to the cuff of distal anorectal segment, thus establishing GI continuity.
   D. **Duhamel procedure:**
      1. **Step 1:** Aganglionic colon is excised to the level of the peritoneal reflection within the abdomen.
      2. **Step 2:** Proximal normal bowel is tunneled between the sacrum and the rectum and is then anastomosed end to side to the low anorectum.

Postoperative Complications

I. **Hirschsprung-associated enterocolitis:** major cause of postoperative morbidity and mortality with incidence rates as high as 30%
   A. **Higher risk:** in patients with an anastomotic stricture, long-segment disease, or total colonic aganglionosis
   B. **Timing:** Usually occurs within the year after the definitive repair; patients present with explosive foul-smelling diarrhea, fever, and abdominal pain and distention.
   C. **Treatment:** Fluid resuscitation, broad-spectrum IV antibiotics, and repeated rectal irrigations with saline. Most cases are managed nonoperatively.

II. **Constipation:** Evaluation of constipation or obstruction includes a rectal exam and contrast enema to evaluate for stricture as well as a suction rectal biopsy to assess for persistent aganglionosis.

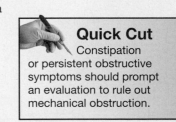

   A. **Anal dilatation:** may be necessary if constipation occurs secondary to the retained aganglionic internal anal sphincter or due to an anastomotic stricture
   B. **Botulinum toxin injection:** may be used when elevated internal anal sphincter tone pressures are documented

III. **Fecal incontinence and diarrhea:** encountered frequently in early postoperative period but improve with bulking agents and usually resolve with time

DISORDERS OF INFANCY

Infantile Hypertrophic Pyloric Stenosis

I. **Definition:** common cause of gastric outlet obstruction in infants due to hypertrophy of the muscular layer of the pylorus, classically causing nonbilious projectile vomiting

II. **Etiology:** Unknown; however, both genetic and environmental factors play a role in the pathophysiology.
   A. **Male-to-female ratio:** 4:1
   B. **Family history:** Offspring of a female with a history of pyloric stenosis have a 10-fold greater chance of developing pyloric stenosis, whereas offspring of a male with a history of pyloric stenosis have a 4-fold greater chance.
   C. **Environmental factors:** breastfeeding, seasonal variability, and erythromycin exposure

III. **Clinical presentation:** Classic presentation is projectile nonbilious vomiting at ages 2–8 weeks.
   A. **Classic derangement:** Vomiting can lead to hypochloremic, hypokalemic metabolic alkalosis.
   B. **Jaundice:** present in 10% of infants

IV. **Diagnosis**
   A. **Physical examination:** Palpation of the enlarged pylorus, also termed "the olive," in the midepigastrium can be diagnostic.
   B. **NG tube:** Complete evacuation of the stomach may aid in finding the mass.
   C. **Ultrasonography:** Standard initial imaging technique; diagnosis is confirmed with a pyloric channel length of 16 mm or greater and a pyloric muscle thickness of 4 mm or greater.
   D. **Upper gastrointestinal (UGI) series:** helpful when US results are equivocal (Fig. 24-7)
      1. **Findings:** elongated pyloric channel with a "string" sign or "railroad track" sign (one to two thin barium tracts, respectively, through the pylorus)
      2. **Slowed gastric emptying of contrast**

V. **Preoperative management:** Correction of the hypokalemic, hypochloremic metabolic alkalosis is (contraction alkalosis) essential prior to anesthesia and surgical correction of pyloric stenosis.
   A. **Goal:** decreasing serum bicarbonate level to less than 30 mEq/L
   B. **Optimal resuscitation:** achieved through IV administration of normal saline boluses and 5% dextrose in 0.45 normal saline containing 20 mEq of potassium chloride at 1.5–2× the normal maintenance rate

Quick Cut
Patience and persistence on physical exam is essential to palpating the enlarged pylorus.

Quick Cut
Surgery for pyloric stenosis should be deferred until the hypochloremic, hypokalemic metabolic alkalosis is corrected: first, restore volume with normal saline, and second, restore potassium as needed.

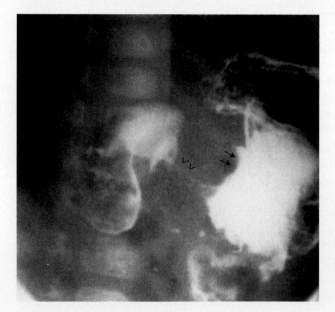

Figure 24-7: The upper GI in this 6-week-old baby shows elongation and narrowing of the pyloric channel (*arrowheads*). On the stomach side, notice the rounded indentation (*arrows*) caused by the very hypertrophied pyloric muscle. This is called the shoulder sign. Together, this combination of signs is diagnostic for pyloric stenosis. (From Erkonen WE, Smith WL. *Radiology 101*, 3rd ed. Philadelphia: Lippincott Williams & Wilkins; 2009.)

VI. Operative management: Surgical procedure of choice is the Ramstedt pyloromyotomy.
   A. Technique: Incision of the serosa is made down the length of the enlarged pylorus to the depth of the mucosa. A complete myotomy is demonstrated through bulging of the submucosa through the divided hypertrophied muscle.
   B. Intraoperative leak test: performed to rule out any perforation
   C. Approach: Pyloromyotomy may be done through an open or laparoscopic approach. Studies have demonstrated equal efficacy and complication rates.

VII. Postoperative management: Patient may be started on feedings of glucose and water or an electrolyte infant formula (e.g., Pedialyte) 4–6 hours after surgery.
   A. Complications: Vomiting occurs in 50%–80% of patients postoperatively because of gastric atony or acute gastritis but is usually self-limited and can be minimized with slow advancement of feedings.
      1. Duodenal perforation: If recognized intraoperatively, handled by a simple repair and omental patch, NG decompression for 24–48 hours, and antibiotics; unrecognized duodenal perforation can result in significant morbidity and mortality.
      2. Incomplete pyloromyotomy: Frequent vomiting beyond 1 week may indicate an incomplete pyloromyotomy; treatment is repyloromyotomy.

VIII. Prognosis: Long-term studies indicate no sequelae such as ulcer disease, food intolerance, or hiatal hernia occurring after a pyloromyotomy for infantile hypertrophic pyloric stenosis. In addition, no problems with growth and development occur.

Biliary Atresia

I. Definition: Disease process that results in progressive inflammatory destruction of the bile ducts and occurs in ~1 in every 20,000 births. If untreated, the disease progresses to cirrhosis of the liver and is the most common indication for liver transplantation in the pediatric U.S. population.

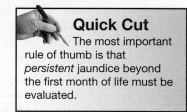

Quick Cut
Untreated biliary atresia leads to cirrhosis in 3–4 months.

II. Etiology: Unknown; however, both environmental (viruses) and hereditary factors have been implicated to cause the final common pathway of biliary inflammation, luminal obliteration, and fibrosis.

III. Classification: three types
   A. Type I: atresia restricted to the common bile duct (~12%)
   B. Type II: level of atresia within the common hepatic duct (~3%)
   C. Type III: atresia at the porta hepatis (most common ~85%)

IV. Clinical presentation: Infants usually present with persistent jaundice and pale acholic stools.
   A. Laboratory studies: reveal conjugated hyperbilirubinemia
   B. Liver function studies: may or may not be abnormal, depending on the degree of liver damage from cholestasis

Quick Cut
The most important rule of thumb is that *persistent* jaundice beyond the first month of life must be evaluated.

V. Diagnosis: Workup is designed to differentiate true anatomic obstruction of the biliary tree from other causes of hyperbilirubinemia.
   A. TORCH (toxoplasmosis, **o**thers, **r**ubella, **c**ytomegalovirus, and **h**erpes simplex virus): antibody titers
   B. Serum electrophoretic patterns: examined for alpha-1 antitrypsin deficiency
   C. Ultrasonography: Biliary atresia is suspected if the gallbladder or ducts are not visualized.
   D. Hepatobiliary scintigraphy: Nuclear scans using technetium-99m (^{99m}Tc)–labeled iminodiacetic acid derivatives look for biliary excretion into the GI tract. Failure of the isotope to appear in the intestine within 24 hours is suggestive of biliary atresia.
   E. Percutaneous liver biopsy: Predominant finding commonly seen in biliary atresia is bile ductular proliferation and inflammation.
   F. Diagnostic laparotomy or laparoscopy: Perform if biliary atresia cannot be ruled out by aforementioned methods.
      1. Intraoperative cholangiography: If normal patent biliary system is demonstrated, a **wedge biopsy** of the liver is taken and the surgical procedure is ended.
      2. If patency cannot be demonstrated: Porta hepatis is explored to find the atretic duct and proceed with a biliary drainage procedure.

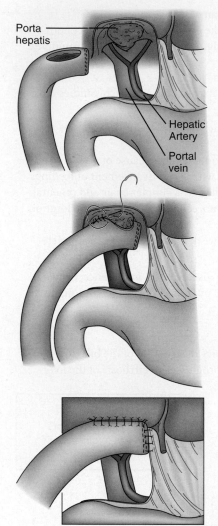

Porta
hepatis

Hepatic
Artery

Portal
vein

Figure 24-8: Kasai procedure for biliary atresia, with Roux limb. (From Blackbourne LH. *Advanced Surgical Recall*, 2nd ed. Baltimore: Lippincott Williams & Wilkins; 2004.)

VI. Treatment
A. Hepatic portoenterostomy (Kasai procedure): standard operation and mainstay of initial operative interventions (Fig. 24-8)

B. Goal: Excise all extrahepatic biliary remnants in order to complete a wide anastomosis of jejunum to the porta hepatis (portoenterostomy) to allow for drainage of the biliary ductules and restore biliary drainage of the liver.

VII. Prognosis: Currently, without surgical intervention, biliary atresia is fatal from cirrhosis resulting in end-stage liver disease.
A. Native liver function: ~40% of patients 10 years after Kasai portoenterostomy

B. Liver transplantation: necessary in 60% of patients for long-term survival

1. **Donor pool:** Four percent mortality rate has been noted while on the transplantation list; however, the use of living-related liver transplant and split-liver deceased donor transplant has increased the donor pool in infants and children.

2. **2.5-year survival rates:** ~85%

> **Quick Cut**
> Biliary atresia patients account for more than 50% of all pediatric liver transplant patients.

Necrotizing Enterocolitis
I. Definition: devastating disease of the neonatal intestinal tract
II. Etiology: Likely multifactorial, and several hypotheses exist. It is believed that the immature intestine suffers from decreased barrier function; when coupled with aberrant microbial colonization and

ischemic injury, the resultant exuberant immune response leads to necrotizing enterocolitis (NEC). The current theory revolves around an imbalance between intestinal immunity, enterocyte barrier function, and altered microbial flora leading to increased permeability.

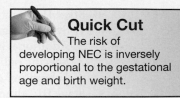

Quick Cut

The risk of developing NEC is inversely proportional to the gestational age and birth weight.

III. **Epidemiology:** Prematurity and low birth weight are the most commonly associated risk factors.
   A. **Estimated prevalence:** ~7% in extremely low- and very-low-birth-weight infants
   B. **Mortality risk:** 20%–30% in these infants, with the highest risk among infants requiring surgery

IV. **Clinical presentation:** usually occurs within the first 2 weeks of life
   A. **First signs:** usually intolerance to formula and abdominal distention, with the passage of heme-positive stools
   B. **Associated perinatal problems:** premature rupture of the membranes, prolonged labor, amnionitis, respiratory distress, apneic episodes, cyanosis, or delivery room resuscitation
   C. **Physical exam findings:** correlate with the extent of the disease
      1. **Mild NEC:** Benign exam may be found.
      2. **More severe NEC:** Abdominal distention and tenderness will increase with severity of the disease.
      3. **Necrotic or perforated intestine:** often results in abdominal mass or abdominal wall erythema

V. **Diagnosis**
   A. **Laboratory findings:** leukopenia, thrombocytopenia (both associated with gram-negative sepsis), anemia, hyponatremia, metabolic acidosis, and coagulopathy
   B. **Abdominal radiographs (anteroposterior and left lateral decubitus):** Facilitate diagnosis and are used to monitor the patient's clinical course. Findings include the following.
      1. **Distended, edematous intestines**
      2. **Intramural air (pneumatosis intestinalis):** Figure 24-9
      3. **Portal venous gas**
      4. **Isolated persistent distended loop of bowel or "fixed loop":** persists over serial radiographs
      5. **Free intraperitoneal air:** suggests intestinal perforation

VI. **Treatment:** based on **Bell's stages**
   A. **Stage I:** mild systemic signs
      1. **Mild systemic signs:** apnea, bradycardia, temperature instability
      2. **Mild intestinal signs:** abdominal distention, increased gastric residuals, bloody stools
      3. **Radiologic signs:** nonspecific or normal

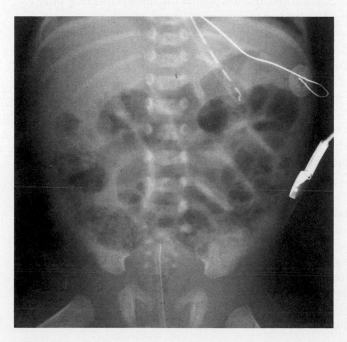

Figure 24-9: Necrotizing enterocolitis. Multiple loops of distended bowel have bubbly and linear radiolucencies in the bowel wall (pneumatosis intestinalis). (From Brant WE, Helms CA. *Brant and Helms Solution.* Philadelphia: Lippincott Williams & Wilkins; 2006.)

B. Stage II: definitive disease
1. **Systemic signs:** mild to moderate
2. **Additional intestinal signs:** absent bowel sounds, abdominal tenderness
3. **Specific radiologic signs:** pneumatosis intestinalis, portal venous gas
4. **Laboratory changes:** metabolic acidosis, thrombocytopenia

C. Stage III: advanced disease
1. **Severe systemic illness:** hypotension, sepsis
2. **Additional intestinal signs:** abdominal distention, peritonitis
3. **Severe radiologic findings:** pneumoperitoneum
4. **Additional laboratory changes:** metabolic and respiratory acidosis, disseminated intravascular coagulopathy

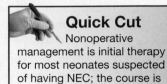

Quick Cut
Nonoperative management is initial therapy for most neonates suspected of having NEC; the course is usually 7–14 days.

VII. Medical management: GI decompression, parenteral antibiotic therapy, fluid resuscitation, and TPN

VIII. Operative management: Approximately 40% of patients require surgery for NEC complications.

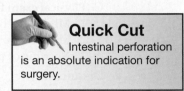

Quick Cut
Intestinal perforation is an absolute indication for surgery.

A. Abdominal radiograph: Can usually document with a cross-table lateral or left lateral decubitus position; films are obtained every 4–6 hours or as clinically indicated.

B. Treatment: Resection of the involved intestine; GI tract is diverted with a proximal enterostomy and mucous fistula. The stomas should be placed to prevent tension on the inflamed mesentery.

C. Isolated perforation or limited disease: Primary anastomosis of the normal bowel is performed in neonates, with relatively stable physiology and no evidence of coagulopathy or sepsis.

D. Severely ill patient (or in the extremely low birth weight infant [<1,000 g]): Major procedure may not be tolerated; placement of peritoneal drains (using local anesthesia) at the bedside can be performed.

IX. Postoperative management: Includes continued medical management of the primary disease as well as routine postsurgical care; infant is treated with antibiotics, GI decompression, and TPN.

A. Disease progression: Requires further surgery for additional perforations. Recurrent NEC occurs in ~4%–6% of patients.

B. Oral feedings: Delayed until after the acute disease resolves and clinical evidence suggests return of bowel function. Dietary adjustments may be necessary until the mucosa has regenerated and undergone functional maturation.

C. Enterostomy: Can be closed during the initial hospitalization or after discharge. Operating prior to 4 weeks postoperatively may prove difficult secondary to inflammation and adhesions.

D. Stoma management: Can be difficult; early recognition and treatment of these complications are necessary to prevent further complications.
1. **Local problems:** include prolapse, degeneration of the surrounding skin, or mucosal irritation
2. **Physiologic problems:** Include fluid losses, electrolyte abnormalities, and intolerance of the diet. A proximal ostomy will be the most difficult to manage in terms of output and physiologic derangement.

E. Strictures: with subsequent intestinal obstruction occurs in ~30% of cases
1. **Timing:** usually occurs 3–6 weeks after the acute episode
2. **Treatment:** resection and primary anastomosis once the patient is prepared nutritionally for surgery

X. Prognosis

A. Mortality rate: Significantly different between neonates treated with medical versus surgical management (67% vs. 30%); overall mortality increases with decreasing birth weight.

B. Long-term morbidity: Related to the length and function of the remaining intestine and other comorbidities related to prematurity after recovery from NEC.
1. **Extensive bowel resection:** Patient may develop short-bowel syndrome.
2. **Comorbidities:** intraventricular hemorrhage, chronic pulmonary insufficiency, and associated cardiac problems
3. **Neurodevelopmental problems:** found in ~50% of patients

XI. Prevention: Although several modalities have been studied and evaluated as possible adjuncts for the prevention of NEC, currently the only recommendations with evidence of both safety and efficacy are breast milk and nonaggressive enteral nutrition. It has also been shown that prenatal maternal glucocorticoids decrease the rate of NEC development in premature neonates.

SOLID TUMORS

Wilms Tumor

> **Quick Cut**
> The two most common solid tumors of childhood are Wilms tumor and neuroblastoma. Although other tumors occur (e.g., rhabdomyosarcoma, Ewing tumor, osteogenic sarcoma, various brain tumors), Wilms tumor illustrates the multidisciplinary approach that is currently used in the management of tumors that occur in childhood.

 I. **Definition:** Involves either the entire kidney or a part of it; bilateral involvement occurs in 4%–13% of cases.

 II. **Etiology:** Mesodermal, mesonephric, and metanephric origins have been proposed.

 III. **Incidence:** An estimated 500 new cases of Wilms tumor occur each year in the United States. Wilms tumors account for more than 90% of all pediatric renal tumors.

 IV. **Clinical presentation:** Asymptomatic flank mass is usually discovered by the parents or during a routine physical examination. The mass is smooth, lobulated, and commonly mobile.
   A. **Other symptoms:** abdominal pain, hematuria, and anorexia
   B. **Hypertension:** occurs in ~10% of patients secondary to activation of the renin–angiotensin system
   C. **Mean age at diagnosis:** 3 years
   D. **Males:** Tumor may invade the spermatic vein, leading to a varicocele.
   E. **Cardiac dysfunction:** Tumor can extend into the right atrium via the inferior vena cava.

 V. **Associated anomalies:** individual congenital anomalies or part of a syndrome
   A. **WAGR syndrome:** Wilms tumor, aniridia, genitourinary malformation, and mental retardation
   B. **Beckwith-Wiedemann syndrome:** congenital growth dysregulation with visceromegaly, macroglossia, omphalocele, and hyperinsulinemic hypoglycemia at birth

 VI. **Diagnosis:** Imaging studies to aid in the diagnosis of Wilms tumor should define the nature of the abdominal mass, the organ of origin, the status of the contralateral kidney, the presence of tumor in the renal vein or vena cava, and the presence or absence of distal metastases
   A. **Chest computed tomography (CT) scan:** will reveal metastasis to the lung, which is the most common site
   B. **Ultrasonography with a Doppler examination:** can identify the organ of origin, the opposite kidney, and the presence of renal vein or vena cava involvement
   C. **CT scan:** can identify the organ of origin if there is bilateral kidney involvement
   D. **MRI:** avoids radiation exposure but has not been shown to be superior to CT imaging

 VII. **Staging**
   A. **Stage I:** Tumor is limited to the kidney and is completely excised; the surface of the renal capsule is intact. The tumor was not ruptured before or during removal. There is no residual tumor apparent beyond the margins of resection.
   B. **Stage II:** Tumor extends beyond the kidney but is completely removed. There is regional extension of the tumor (i.e., penetration through the outer surface of the renal capsule into the perirenal soft tissues). Vessels outside the kidney substance are infiltrated or contain tumor thrombus.
   C. **Stage III:** Residual nonhematogenous tumor is confined to the abdomen. Lymph nodes on biopsy are found to be involved in the hilus, the periaortic chains, or beyond. There has been diffuse peritoneal contamination by tumor, such as spillage or tumor beyond the flank. Implants are found on the peritoneal surface, and the tumor extends beyond the surgical margins either microscopically or grossly. The tumor is not completely resectable because of local infiltration into vital structures.
   D. **Stage IV:** Hematogenous metastases can occur with deposits beyond stage III (e.g., lung, liver, bone, or brain).
   E. **Stage V:** Bilateral renal involvement is evident at diagnosis. An attempt should be made to stage each side according to the aforementioned criteria on the basis of the extent of disease before a biopsy.

Table 24-2: Wilms Tumor Survival Rates

Wilms Tumor 4-Year Survival Rate		
Stage	FH	UFH
I	99%	83%
II	98%	81%
III	94%	72%
IV	86%	38%
V	87%	55%

FH, favorable histology; UFH, unfavorable histology.
From American Cancer Society. Survival rates for Wilms tumor by stage and histology. American Cancer Society Web site. http://www.cancer.org/cancer/wilmstumor/detailedguide/wilms-tumor-survival-rates. Accessed February 14, 2015.

VIII. Management: involves a multidisciplinary approach

    A. Surgery: Mainstay of treatment; timing depends on tumor stage.

        1. Operation includes: exploratory laparotomy, examination of the opposite kidney, resection of the tumor, and periaortic node dissection or sampling

        2. Vena caval extension: Requires the removal of the tumor thrombus. This operation may require a cardiopulmonary bypass to assist in the resection.

    B. Chemotherapy: critical for cure

    C. Radiotherapy: Used to treat extensive disease (stages III–V); complications include secondary cancers in children; interference with growth and development of bones, joints, and muscles; radiation pneumonitis; radiation enteritis; and cardiotoxicity.

IX. Prognosis: Survival is related to stage, response to treatment (stages IV and V patients), loss of heterozygosity, and the histology of the tumor, which is reported as favorable (FH) and unfavorable (UFH) and dictates treatment protocols. Current 4-year survival rates by stage and histology are shown in Table 24-2.

> **Quick Cut**
> Because of the good prognosis with Wilms tumor, even in the setting of extensive disease, it is acceptable to resect other organs.

Study Questions for Part VI

Directions: *Each of the numbered items in this section is followed by several possible answers. Select the ONE lettered answer that is BEST in each case.*

Questions 1–2

A 35-year-old man has right-sided serous otitis media and a right upper neck mass.

1. It is most important to evaluate this patient for which of the following?

   A. Cancer of the right ear
   B. Cancer of the right tonsil
   C. Cancer of the right maxillary sinus
   D. Cancer of the nasopharynx
   E. Hodgkin lymphoma

2. Which of the following will be the primary treatment for this tumor?

   A. Local excision to negative margins
   B. Wide local excision and radical neck dissection
   C. Neoadjuvant chemotherapy followed by resection of residual tumor
   D. Unilateral radiotherapy with combined chemotherapy
   E. Bilateral radiotherapy

3. A 65-year-old man is found to have a small invasive squamous cell carcinoma of the right vocal cord. The right vocal cord is paralyzed, and a lymph node in the right anterior neck is 4 cm in diameter. Optimal treatment of the primary tumor should include which of the following?

   A. Total laryngectomy
   B. Vertical hemilaryngectomy
   C. Supraglottic (horizontal) laryngectomy
   D. Right cordectomy
   E. Chemotherapy

Questions 4–5

A 55-year-old woman presents with complaint of a mass overlying the angle of the right mandible. She says the mass has been slowly enlarging over the past 2–3 years and that the mass is painless. On physical examination, it is firm and overlies the angle of the right mandible and the area between the angle and the tragus of the ear. Neurologic examination of the head and neck is completely normal.

4. Which of the following does this mass most likely represent?

   A. Mucoepidermoid cancer of the parotid gland
   B. Acute parotitis
   C. Benign mixed tumor of the parotid gland (pleomorphic adenoma)
   D. Malignant mixed tumor of the parotid gland
   E. Hemangioma of the parotid gland

5. What will be the optimal treatment for this lesion?

   A. Radiation therapy
   B. Total parotidectomy with preservation of the facial nerve
   C. Total parotidectomy including resection of the facial nerve
   D. Superficial parotidectomy
   E. Enucleation

6. A 9-year-old girl presents with drainage from the midline neck. There is some surrounding cellulitis and an apparent 2-cm mass that elevates with swallowing. The most appropriate definitive management of this condition is:

   A. Antibiotics alone
   B. Thyroid scanning
   C. US-guided aspiration
   D. Complete surgical excision
   E. Radioiodine therapy

7. A 71-year-old man presents with mild hearing loss and tinnitus of the right ear. His symptoms are new and not particularly troubling to him. MRI demonstrates a solid lesion in the internal auditory canal. The most appropriate management is:

   A. Surgical resection
   B. Radiation therapy
   C. Observation
   D. Fine-needle aspiration
   E. Radiofrequency ablation

8. A 60-year-old man has a smoking history of 80 pack-years and presents with a lesion on the tongue. The biopsy is consistent with squamous cell carcinoma. A full workup demonstrates a 1.5-cm solid lesion in the left upper lobe of the lung but is otherwise negative. The most appropriate management is:

   A. Radiation therapy
   B. Chemotherapy only
   C. Radical surgical resection
   D. Surgical resection and chemotherapy
   E. Referral to hospice care

9. A 37-year-old man undergoes Roux-en-Y gastric bypass for morbid obesity. He recovers uneventfully and is discharged home the following day. He returns on postoperative day 6 with abdominal pain, tachycardia, and low-grade fever. His abdominal exam is unremarkable, and his abdominal CT scan shows significant inflammation in the upper abdomen with some free fluid. The best initial treatment is:

   A. Acid reduction with proton pump inhibitors
   B. Loperamide
   C. Increased pain control with oral narcotics
   D. Diagnostic laparoscopy
   E. Nonsteroidal anti-inflammatory drugs

10. Which of the following patients meets criteria for bariatric surgery?

    A. 15-year-old boy with body mass index (BMI) 39.9 kg/m^2
    B. 25-year-old woman with BMI 33 kg/m^2 and allergic asthma
    C. 35-year-old man with BMI 38 kg/m^2 and a deviated septum
    D. 45-year-old woman with BMI 39 kg/m^2, diabetes mellitus, and degenerative joint disease
    E. 79-year-old man with BMI 39.9 kg/m^2

11. A 60-year-old woman is taken to the operating room for a laparoscopic cholecystectomy. After insufflation of the abdomen with CO_2, her respiratory rate increases dramatically and she becomes hypotensive with decreased cardiac output. The most likely reason for this acute event is:

    A. Acidosis secondary to carbon dioxide
    B. Pneumothorax
    C. Volume depletion
    D. Oversedation with narcotics
    E. Decreased sympathetic activity

12. A 35-year-old man undergoes laparoscopic ventral hernia repair with lysis of adhesions. The procedure is uneventful, and he is admitted to the hospital for recovery. After 3 days, he develops a newly distended abdomen, abdominal pain, and hypotension that does not respond to 1 L of normal saline. The most likely explanation is:

A. Myocardial infarction
B. Missed enterotomy
C. Acidosis secondary to pneumoperitoneum
D. Deep venous thrombosis
E. Gas bloat syndrome

13. A 25-year-old woman presents with a 2-cm palpable left neck nodule. She is asymptomatic but is anxious about the lump in her neck. She visits her primary care physician, who orders a US, which demonstrates a solid lesion. She presents to your office for evaluation. The most appropriate means of diagnosis is:

A. Computerized tomography of the neck
B. Magnetic resonance angiography (MRA)
C. Fine-needle aspiration
D. Incisional biopsy
E. Excisional biopsy

14. The American Cancer Society (ACS) recommends routine screening for all of the following *except*:

A. Mammography for breast cancer
B. Pap smear for cervical cancer
C. Prostate-specific antigen (PSA) for prostate cancer
D. Colonoscopy for colon cancer
E. Fecal occult blood testing for colon cancer

15. A new chemotherapeutic agent is developed to treat advanced lung cancer. The company begins a large trial of 1,000 patients comparing the efficacy of the new medication versus a leading medication that has been in use for the last 5 years. This trial can best be described as:

A. Phase 0
B. Phase I
C. Phase II
D. Phase III
E. Double-blind, randomized controlled trial

16. A 22-year-old man is shot in the chest. He presents to the emergency department with incoherent mumbling but his eyes open to vocal commands and no response to painful stimuli. What is his Glasgow Coma Scale score?

A. 6
B. 8
C. 10
D. 12
E. 14

17. The same patient in question number 8 has a systolic blood pressure of 60 mm Hg, a thready pulse, and has some blood bubbling from a hole in his lateral left chest. The most important initial maneuver is:

A. Endotracheal intubation
B. Administration of 1 L of crystalloid
C. Occlusive dressings to the wound
D. Blood sample for cross match
E. Examination of the pupils

18. After stabilization, the patient's hemodynamics improve but do not normalize. The patient is also difficult to ventilate. Chest x-ray shows collapse of the lung on the left side and shift of the mediastinal structures to the right. The next best maneuver is:

A. Administration of 100% oxygen
B. Operative thoracotomy
C. Chest tube insertion
D. Needle decompression of the left chest
E. Administration of surfactant

19. A 27-year-old woman with end-stage renal disease secondary to glomerulonephritis undergoes renal transplantation in the right iliac fossa. Two months after operation, she develops some edema of the right leg along with decreased urine output. CT scan demonstrates a fluid collection near the kidney, and an aspiration of the collection shows a creatinine level equal to serum. The best next step in management is:

A. Diagnostic laparoscopy and internal drainage
B. Open operation and ureteral revision
C. Pulsed corticosteroids
D. Blood transfusion
E. Percutaneous drainage

20. A 42-year-old man with insulin-dependent diabetes mellitus undergoes pancreas transplantation. After good initial results, at postoperative day 4, he develops increasing glucose levels requiring insulin. The best initial means of diagnosis is:

A. CT scan with contrast
B. MRI-guided biopsy
C. Urine culture
D. Serum antibody levels
E. Retroperitoneal US

21. A 33-year-old man has a kidney transplant. One month later, he presents with decreased urine output and increased serum creatinine. A renal biopsy is performed, which is consistent with acute rejection. The best initial treatment is:

A. Decreased immunosuppressant levels
B. Transplant nephrectomy
C. Plasmapheresis
D. Pulsed corticosteroids
E. CT scan with IV contrast

22. A 4-week-old male infant presents to the emergency department with a 3-day history of vomiting. The family reports that he had an uneventful birth history and was developing normally. The emesis has been nonbilious, quite forceful, and occurring immediately after feedings. On physical examination, you feel a firm mass in the epigastric region. The best course of action is:

A. Immediate laparotomy
B. Fluid resuscitation and semiurgent operation
C. Laparoscopic pyloromyotomy
D. NG decompression
E. Hydroxy iminodiacetic acid (HIDA) scan and liver function tests

23. A newborn girl presents with a mass at the umbilicus. She is in no distress. Immediately to the right of the umbilical cord, an apparent loop of bowel is exposed to the air. The best initial treatment for the management of this patient is:

    A. Application of silver sulfadiazine
    B. Echocardiography
    C. Immediate operation with primary abdominal wall closure
    D. Sterile dressing and repair prior to discharge
    E. Skin grafting

24. A 2-day-old female infant has not yet passed meconium. There is no relevant maternal or birth history. On examination, her abdomen is soft but distended, and vital signs are normal. Rectal examination is performed, and the rectal vault appears empty, but following withdrawal of the finger, a rush of stool emerges. The best diagnostic test for this patient is:

    A. Abdominal x-ray
    B. Computerized tomography of the abdomen
    C. Genetic analysis for CFTR
    D. Contrast enema with barium
    E. Rectal biopsy

25. In which of the following situations would the best results be obtained for an emergency department thoracotomy?

    A. Cardiac arrest in a construction worker after falling from a scaffold eight stories high
    B. Cardiac arrest following a motor vehicle accident with expulsion of the individual from the car
    C. Cardiac arrest following a gunshot wound to the abdomen
    D. External cardiac massage that has failed after more than 10 minutes in a trauma patient
    E. Cardiac arrest following a stab wound to the chest

26. A 21-year-old male is brought to the emergency room after an assault with a baseball bat. He has suffered obvious head trauma. He opens his eyes spontaneously, does not speak but makes incomprehensible sounds, and localizes to pain. What is his Glasgow Coma Scale score?

    A. 8
    B. 9
    C. 10
    D. 11
    E. 12

Questions 27–28

A 50-year-old man is brought to the emergency department immediately after suffering full-thickness burns over the entire surface of both upper extremities and the anterior chest and abdomen. His weight is approximately 155 lb. Initial fluid resuscitation has been started with lactated Ringer solution.

27. The initial resuscitation rate should be approximately which of the following?

    A. 300 mL/hr
    B. 600 mL/hr
    C. 900 mL/hr
    D. 1,200 mL/hr
    E. 1,500 mL/hr

The patient responds to treatment.

28. After 8 hours, the fluid rate should be changed to which of the following?

A. 300 mL/hr
B. 600 mL/hr
C. 900 mL/hr
D. 1,200 mL/hr
E. 1,500 mL/hr

29. A 2,600-g newborn without any obvious anomalies turns blue during her first feeding. An attempt at passing an oral gastric tube to decompress the stomach is unsuccessful. Which of the following statements is correct?

A. The most likely form of tracheal esophageal malformation is a blind pouch without a tracheal fistula.
B. No further workup for other anomalies is indicated owing to the normal appearance of the patient.
C. Because the orogastric tube does not pass, it should be removed to prevent gagging.
D. Primary repair can be undertaken if the defect is less than 2 cm in length.
E. If the lung fields are clear to auscultation after the cyanotic episode, an immediate chest radiograph would not aid in the newborn's management.

30. Which of the following statements about laparoscopic surgery is true?

A. Due to the minimally invasive nature of laparoscopy, preoperative evaluation of patients is less critical than for laparotomy.
B. Routine use of orogastric tubes and urinary catheters is unnecessary during advanced laparoscopic procedures.
C. The abdomen is always prepared and draped for potential laparotomy.
D. Antithromboembolic pumps are not needed during laparoscopic procedures, as the risk of deep venous thrombosis is less than for laparotomy.
E. Spinal anesthesia is sufficient for most advanced laparoscopic procedures.

31. Which of the following physiologic changes occurs as a result of carbon dioxide pneumoperitoneum?

A. Decreased pulmonary compliance due to diaphragm elevation and increased abdominal pressure
B. Metabolic alkalosis from systemic absorption of carbon dioxide
C. Increased cardiac output as a result of increased venous return
D. Decreased systemic vascular resistance
E. Decreased mean arterial pressure

32. A 32-year-old woman undergoes a laparoscopic cholecystectomy for biliary colic. Forty-eight hours after the operation, she complains of fever and RUQ pain. Laboratory studies reveal an elevated white blood cell count as well as an elevated total bilirubin. Which of the following is not part of the initial management?

A. CT scan of the abdomen
B. HIDA biliary scan
C. Surgical exploration
D. Endoscopic retrograde cholangiopancreatography (ERCP)
E. Broad-spectrum antibiotics

33. Which of the following is true about pediatric hernias?

A. The incidence is roughly equal in males and females, with males becoming more common as age increases.
B. Congenital pediatric hernias are bilateral 50% of the time.
C. Inguinal hernias often close spontaneously in children, and repair should be delayed until 2 years of age.
D. Incarcerated hernias in children should never be reduced. Emergency repair is mandatory.
E. Right-sided inguinal hernias are twice as common as left-sided inguinal hernias.

34. A victim of a motor vehicle accident who was thrown from the vehicle is brought to the emergency department. The patient is unconscious and hypotensive. He is found to have a dilated left pupil, decreased breath sounds over the right chest, a moderately distended abdomen, an unstable pelvis, and severe bruises over the thighs. After resuscitation with 2 L of crystalloid and 2 units of type-specific packed red blood cells, the patient remains hypotensive with a systolic blood pressure in the low 80's. What is the least likely explanation for this patient's hypotension?

A. External blood loss
B. Bleeding into the chest
C. Retroperitoneal bleeding
D. Severe closed head injury
E. Femoral fractures

35. An adult male is brought to the emergency department for evaluation and treatment following injury in a house fire. The patient was found in a closed room. He has singed facial hair and full-thickness burns over approximately 30% of his body surface area. All of the following are important in his initial stabilization and treatment *except* which?

A. Endotracheal intubation
B. IV fluid resuscitation
C. Insertion of a ureteral catheter
D. Tetanus toxoid administration
E. Systemic antibiotics

36. With the increasing use of US, prenatal diagnosis of abdominal wall defects is becoming more common. You are asked to consult a family with this prenatal diagnosis. Which of the following points and discussion is not true?

A. Closure may require more than a single operation.
B. If gastroschisis is strongly suspected, amniocentesis is essential to rule out chromosomal abnormalities.
C. TPN is frequently used.
D. The outcome of this category of patient is related both to the integrity of the GI tract or to associated anomalies.
E. One of the primary goals of treatment with abdominal wall defects is to protect the exposed contents of the abdomen.

37. Disadvantages of laparoscopy when compared with laparotomy include all of the following *except* which?

A. Difficulty controlling severe bleeding
B. Poorer visualization of the operative field
C. Greater difficulty placing sutures
D. Loss of tactile sensation
E. Higher operating room costs

38. Laparoscopic cholecystectomy is indicated for all of the following conditions *except* which?

A. Biliary dyskinesia
B. Initial treatment in patients with severe cholangitis
C. Acute cholecystitis
D. Symptomatic cholelithiasis
E. Biliary pancreatitis

QUESTIONS 39–43

For each clinical situation, match the appropriate diagnosis.
    A. Acute tubular necrosis
    B. Hyperacute rejection
    C. Graft versus host disease
    D. Acute rejection
    E. Chronic rejection

39. Occurs when there is cross-match incompatibility

40. Usually a temporary condition or poor renal function that lasts from 1–14 days related to preservation, ischemia, and reperfusion of the transplanted kidney

41. Can usually be successfully treated with high doses of immunosuppression, such as methylprednisolone

42. More prevalent in small bowel transplantation than in other organ transplants related to the large amount of lymphoid tissue associated with the graft

43. Slow decline in renal function over months or years resulting from humoral and cellular events that are generally not treatable or reversible

Questions 44–45

For each question, match the appropriate immunosuppressive agent.
    A. Corticosteroids
    B. Tacrolimus
    C. Cyclosporine
    D. Antithymocyte globulin
    E. Mycophenolate

44. A calcineurin inhibitor that became the mainstay of immunosuppressive regimens in the 1980s and continues as the basis of many immunosuppressive regimens with toxicities that include hypertension, gingival hyperplasia, and nephrotoxicity

45. An antimetabolite used as part of triple immunosuppression therapy

Questions 46–49

Match the GI anomaly with the listed statement.
    A. Malrotation
    B. Duodenal atresia
    C. Small bowel (jejunal and ileal) atresia
    D. Imperforate anus

46. While considering a vascular accident, there is an associated finding of cystic fibrosis in a patient with this GI problem.

47. Although part of the VACTERL complex, it is associated more commonly with renal malformations.

48. Complete intestinal necrosis is the most feared complication.

49. There is a high association with trisomy 21.

Answers and Explanations

1–2. The answers are 1-D (Chapter 18, Nasopharynx Cancer, Clinical Evaluation, I–II) **and 2-E** (Chapter 18, Nasopharynx Cancer, Treatment and Prognosis, I–II). The two most common presenting symptoms of cancer of the nasopharynx are enlarged posterior cervical lymph nodes and unilateral serous otitis media. Cancer of the right ear, right tonsil, or right maxillary sinus or Hodgkin lymphoma generally do not cause otitis media and usually occur in an older age group. Hodgkin lymphoma will lead to serous otitis media only if Waldeyer ring involvement has led to eustachian tube dysfunction, which is a rare occurrence.

Bilateral radiotherapy is the primary treatment for all epithelial nasopharyngeal tumors.

3. The answer is A (Chapter 18, Larynx Cancer, Treatment and Prognosis, IV). Any carcinoma of the vocal cord that leads to fixation of the cord or of the hemilarynx is at least T3. Massive involvement of surrounding soft tissues will make the tumor stage T4. The presence of a single ipsilateral lymph node greater than 3 cm but less than 6 cm in diameter makes the stage of the neck node N2a. Multiple small lymph nodes on the same side of the neck as the primary tumor are classified N2b, and lymph nodes involving the opposite side of the neck change the staging to N3.

T3 tumors cannot be adequately treated with partial laryngectomy in most cases; total laryngectomy is required. Radiation therapy is used postoperatively as a planned combined treatment in most cases. Chemotherapy is used for inoperable cases or in experimental protocols.

4–5. The answers are 4-C (Chapter 18, Parotid Neoplasms, Benign, I–II) **and 5-D** (Chapter 18, Evaluation and Management of Parotid Masses, Surgical Management, I). The history given is most consistent with a benign neoplasm of the parotid gland. Benign mixed tumors are the most common benign tumors of the salivary glands. Benign salivary tumors account for 60% of all parotid tumors. Malignant tumors, such as a mucoepidermoid cancer, usually grow more rapidly and are more often associated with facial nerve paralysis. The absence of pain makes acute parotitis unlikely. Hemangiomas of the parotid gland are much rarer than benign mixed tumors.

The optimal treatment for a benign mixed tumor is removal of the tumor with a margin of normal parotid gland. This usually can be accomplished with a superficial parotidectomy. Although these tumors often appear to shell out, removal by simple enucleation results in a very high recurrence rate. Excision of the entire gland with or without the facial nerve is indicated for malignant tumors. Radiation therapy does not have a role in the management of this lesion.

6. The answer is D (Chapter 18, Congenital Masses, Lesions of Thyroid Origin, II, D). The patient is presenting with signs and symptoms of a thyroglossal cyst. If there is initial infection, antibiotics are used to temporize. Definitive management is complete surgical excision, including a portion of the hyoid bone.

7. The answer is C (Chapter 18, Acquired Lesions, Peripheral Nerve Tumors, II D). The patient presents with an acoustic neuroma, a subtype of schwannoma. As these are slow-growing tumors, the most appropriate management is expectant, with observation. Should the lesion become more symptomatic, surgical resection or radiation may be indicated.

8. The answer is B (Chapter 18, Malignant Lesions of the Head and Neck, Treatment, III C). The patient has evidence of metastatic disease and is a candidate for palliative therapy only. Metastatic disease is a contraindication to surgery. Radiation therapy may be useful for control of primary disease, or in the setting of multiple primary lesions in the same vicinity, but is generally avoided in this setting. Hospice care is reserved for those who are at imminent risk of demise.

9. The answer is D (Chapter 19, Complications III Gastric bypass A 2). In the postoperative patient, physical examination is relatively unreliable. Patients may present with marginal ulceration, for which the treatment is acid suppression, but typically develop pain weeks after the operation if routine acid suppression is not provided. Antidiarrheals are not indicated for pain, and further narcotic therapy is only useful if the patient has had inadequate pain control at home.

10. **The answer is D** (Chapter 19, Patient Selection, I–II). BMI ≥ 40 kg/m^2 is the conventional threshold for bariatric surgery. In adolescents, a higher cutoff is used, and careful consideration must be given to the elderly. Patients with BMI 35–39.9 kg/m^2 with medical comorbidities related to obesity are also candidates for bariatric surgery.

11. **The answer is A** (Chapter 20, General Principles, Physiologic Changes Associated with Pneumoperitoneum, I–II). The patient's distress is related to the pneumoperitoneum. Insufflation of gas into a vein may result in air embolus, and absorption of CO_2 can cause a clinically significant acidosis. Pneumothorax may occur with malposition of the needle but is unlikely. Volume deficits usually do not produce such a dramatic picture. Sedation diminishes the respiratory rate, and sympathetic activity is not typically changed by abdominal surgery.

12. **The answer is B** (Chapter 20, Selected Laparoscopic Procedures, Laparoscopic Ventral Hernia Repair, IV C). The patient has signs and symptoms of peritonitis consistent with a delayed perforation. The injury may have been partial thickness at time of operation and evolved over the ensuing 2 days. Myocardial infarction is possible but should cause chest pain and is less likely in a young patient. Pneumoperitoneum is essentially completely resorbed over the first 2 postoperative days and would not contribute to an acute event. deep venous thrombosis should produce swelling in the leg or respiratory difficulty if a pulmonary embolism develops. Gas bloat may produce abdominal distension but is uncommon in this setting.

13. **The answer is C** (Chapter 18, Neck cancer, II B). A solid, palpable neck lesion should have fine-needle aspiration. Incisional and excisional biopsy are premature as the lesion may require more extensive margins or neck dissection. CT is a useful adjunct, but the initial diagnosis is best achieved through FNA. MRA will not provide useful information at this point.

14. **The answer is C** (Chapter 21, Screening and Diagnosis, Overview, I D). ACS guidelines are based on both the test characteristics (the likelihood of cancer detection) as well as the likelihood of impacting the patient's course and treatment. Among these listed, PSA has not shown a demonstrable survival benefit for mass screening purposes.

15. **The answer is D** (Chapter 21, Research and Training, Clinical Trials, I C). This is a phase III study, comparing a new treatment to standard of care. A phase 0 study is an informal term used to describe pharmacokinetic studies. Phase I tests the safety of a medication. Phase II trials investigate a clinical effect. No mention is made of this trial design, so randomization of patients is possible but not definitive. Similarly, blinding the subjects and the providers to intervention is a technique that is not explicit from the question.

16. **The answer is B** (Chapter 22, Trauma, Patient Evaluation, II A 4). Eyes: 3 for response to voice. Verbal: 2 for incomprehensible sounds. Motor: 1 for no response to pain.

17. **The answer is A** (Chapter 22, Trauma, Patient Evaluation, II A). The primary survey (ABCs) begins with airway assessment. The patient is in extremis, and intubation should be the first priority. Volume resuscitation should also begin promptly, along with the secondary survey assessing for injuries. Pupillary exam is appropriate to help determine neurologic status but should wait.

18. **The answer is D** (Chapter 22, Specific Injuries, Pneumothorax and Hemothorax, I B). The patient has a tension pneumothorax, and the best initial maneuver is needle decompression via the second interspace. Once released, the patient should have a chest tube placed for ongoing treatment. Increased oxygen levels will not resolve the condition, and thoracotomy is overaggressive and not sufficiently prompt to address tension pneumothorax. There is no role for surfactant in the management of the adult trauma patient.

19. **The answer is A** (Chapter 23, Organ-Specific Considerations, Kidney Transplantation, III H 3). The patient is presenting with a symptomatic lymphocele. The best management is internal drainage, which can be performed with minimally invasive techniques. A urinoma should have a markedly elevated creatinine level. The patient does not show signs of rejection, so corticosteroids are contraindicated. If the patient has a hematoma, evacuation would be reasonable, but ongoing

transfusion is not. For lymphocele, percutaneous drainage results in unacceptably high rates of recurrence.

20. **The answer is E** (Chapter 23, Organ-Specific Considerations, Pancreatic and Islet Transplantation, III A). The patient may have a catastrophic vascular event. The initial maneuver is to rule out vascular events by US. CT scan cannot assess the inflow and outflow adequately, and nonspecific findings would lead to other diagnostic modalities. Biopsy is not specific enough to yield a diagnosis. Urine culture would not be useful, even in cases of bladder drainage. Antibody levels are not useful.

21. **The answer is D** (Chapter 23, Organ-Specific Considerations, Kidney Transplantation, VII). For acute rejection, high-dose corticosteroids with a taper is the treatment of choice. Occasionally, cyclosporine toxicity may cause decreased graft function, but this is not consistent with the biopsy results. Nephrectomy is the last resort, when the graft is unsalvageable. Plasmapheresis only has role for preformed antibodies or hyperacute rejection. Additional contrast will not provide a diagnosis and may allow further renal injury.

22. **The answer is B** (Chapter 24, Disorders of Infancy, Infantile Hypertrophic Pyloric Stenosis, V). The infant presents with classic signs and symptoms for hypertrophic pyloric stenosis. The initial management should be correction of electrolyte abnormalities—as the infant is expected to have hypochloremic, hypokalemic metabolic alkalosis—then operation for pyloromyotomy. Immediate laparotomy is indicated for questions of ischemia, not present in this case. NG decompression is unnecessary, as this represents a high obstruction. Liver scanning and biochemical profile is indicated in cases of jaundice only.

23. **The answer is C** (Chapter 24, Abdominal Wall Defects, Gastroschisis, IV). The patient is presenting with gastroschisis. As this represents a congenital evisceration, emergent surgery is indicated. Unlike omphalocele, there is no role for nonoperative management. Further, because the risk of major cardiac anomalies is low, operation should not be delayed in search of other defects. Silver sulfadiazine is useful for nonruptured omphalocele. Inguinal hernias should be repaired prior to discharge. Skin grafting is rarely indicated in abdominal wall closure.

24. **The answer is E** (Chapter 24, Hirschsprung Disease, Diagnosis, IV). The history is consistent with Hirschsprung disease. There is aganglionosis of a portion of colon, resulting in the inability to pass stool. Abdominal plain films may reveal obstruction and air-fluid levels but are nonspecific. CT may also reveal distended loops but does not provide conclusive diagnosis. Cystic fibrosis may be associated with intestinal atresia but more typically small bowel. Contrast enema certainly suggests the diagnosis, but water-soluble agents are preferred. Rectal biopsy remains the gold standard of diagnosis.

25. **The answer is E** (Chapter 22, Trauma, Resuscitative Thoracotomy, V). Emergency department thoracotomies should only be performed by trained personnel and for specific indications. The best results and the highest salvage rates have been obtained with emergency thoracotomy following cardiac arrest from penetrating injury to the chest (patient E). In general, major blunt trauma (patients A and B) and failed external cardiac massage lasting for 10 minutes (patient D) are relative contraindications. A patient whose heart stops after a gunshot wound to the abdomen (patient C) has likely exsanguinated and will not benefit from an emergency thoracotomy.

26. **The answer is D** (Chapter 22, Fig. 22-1). He receives 4 points for eye opening, 2 for best verbal response, and 5 for best motor response.

27-28. **The answers are 27-B and 28-A** (Chapter 22, Burns, Burn Injury, III). The burn involves approximately 36% of the body surface area (BSA). According to the Parkland formula, 4 mL/kg of body weight/% BSA burned of lactated Ringer solution should be administered during the first 24 hours. Half of this amount should be given during the first 8 hours after injury and the remainder over the next 16 hours.

29. **The answer is D** (Chapter 24, Esophageal Atresia and Tracheoesophageal Malformations, Operative Management, I). A primary repair at time of presentation can be undertaken if

the defect is less than 2 cm in length. A blind proximal pouch with a distant TEF is the most common type of malformation. There is a 40% incidence of associated anomalies in one or more other organ systems. Decompression of the proximal pouch is important to reduce aspiration. A radiograph can help to demonstrate the anatomy.

30. **The answer is C** (Chapter 20, Selected Laparoscopic Procedures, Laparoscopic Cholecystectomy, III). Because all laparoscopic procedures have the potential to be converted to laparotomy, preoperative preparation must be as thorough as for open abdominal surgery. The bladder and stomach are decompressed with a urinary catheter and an orogastric tube, respectively, to avoid injury during creation of the pneumoperitoneum. Prophylaxis against deep venous thrombosis is necessary, as risk factors for that condition are inherent in laparoscopy. General anesthesia is needed for the vast majority of advanced laparoscopic procedures; spinal anesthesia cannot achieve a high enough level without respiratory embarrassment.

31. **The answer is A** (Chapter 20, General Principles, Physiologic Changes Associated with Pneumoperitoneum, IV). Physiologic changes associated with carbon dioxide pneumoperitoneum are complex and interdependent, but several generalizations can be made. Pulmonary compliance is decreased from diaphragmatic elevation and increased intra-abdominal pressure. Hypercarbia causes acidosis, not alkalosis. Cardiac output is usually decreased due to decreased venous return, and blood pressure and systemic vascular resistance are increased.

32. **The answer is C** (Chapter 20, Selected Laparoscopic Procedures, Laparoscopic Cholecystectomy, III B 1). Bile duct injuries or bile leaks after laparoscopic cholecystectomy should not initially be managed by surgical exploration. Resuscitation, antibiotics, and appropriate imaging to define the anatomy of the problem are the first steps.

33. **The answer is E** (Chapter 24, Congenital Hernias, Inguinal Hernias, I). Sixty percent of pediatric inguinal hernias are right sided, 30% are left sided, and 10%–15% are bilateral. The male-to-female ratio is 6:1. Inguinal hernias do not close spontaneously like umbilical hernias and should be repaired when diagnosed. Incarcerated hernias are managed with reduction followed by hydration and repair.

34. **The answer is D** (Chapter 22, Trauma, Shock, II B). Multiple trauma patients with hypotension and hypovolemic shock are rarely, if ever, hypotensive secondary to head injury. The treating physician must look for another cause of hypotension, which is almost always blood loss. The blood loss can be from five different areas: (1) external blood loss from lacerations or an open wound (details should be obtained from the rescue workers at the scene of the accident); (2) intrathoracic blood loss; (3) intra-abdominal blood loss; (4) retroperitoneal bleeding almost always associated with pelvic fractures; and (5) bleeding into the thighs secondary to femur fractures, which can cause shock. In the patient described, the closed head injury would be the least likely mechanism for this continued hypotension.

35. **The answer is E** (Chapter 22, Burns, Inhalation Injury, I). The patient described is at a high risk for suffering an inhalation injury. Delayed airway obstruction can develop rapidly during the first 24–48 hours after injury. It is best to perform endotracheal intubation early before respiratory problems develop, as later intubation can be difficult. Vigorous IV fluid resuscitation is indicated for all patients who have full-thickness burns involving more than 20% BSA. Because urine output must be followed very closely, an indwelling ureteral catheter is mandatory in the management of these patients. Tetanus toxoid with or without hyperimmune immunoglobulin should be given if the patient's tetanus immunization status is not current. Systemic antibiotics are usually not indicated in the initial management of burn patients.

36. **The answer is B** (Chapter 24, Abdominal Wall Defects). The general category of abdominal wall defects consists of gastroschisis and omphaloceles. The primary goal of treatment is to protect the exposed or potentially exposed GI tract. This is done either by abdominal wall closure, scarification of the omphalocele sac, or covering with Silastic or silicon material with staged reduction and closure. Although coverage is complete and the GI tract is functional, nutrition is usually accomplished by TPN. The outcome for the patient is dictated by the integrity and viability of the GI tract (gastroschisis) or associated anomalies (omphalocele). Chromosomal abnormalities may be present in patients with omphaloceles but not with gastroschisis.

37. The answer is B (Chapter 20, General Principles, Advantages and Disadvantages of Minimal Access Surgery). It is generally agreed that improved visualization of the operative field due to magnification and improved light delivery to remote areas of the abdomen are an advantage of laparoscopy over laparotomy. Difficulty controlling severe bleeding, greater difficulty placing sutures, loss of tactile sensation, and higher operating costs are clear disadvantages of laparoscopy as compared with laparotomy.

38. The answer is B (Chapter 20, Selected Laparoscopic Procedures, Laparoscopic Cholecystectomy, I). Laparoscopic cholecystectomy is indicated for most symptomatic biliary conditions, including biliary colic, acute cholecystitis, biliary dyskinesia, and biliary pancreatitis, after resolution of pancreatitis. However, initial therapy for cholangitis is hydration, broad-spectrum antibiotics, and drainage of the common bile duct. Cholecystectomy is performed at a later time after resolution of sepsis.

39–43. The answers are 39-B, 40-A, 41-D, 42-C, and 43-E (Chapter 23, Overview, Rejection, I, II, IV). Hyperacute rejection occurs when the serum of the recipient has preformed antidonor antibodies. Before transplantation, the recipient's blood is examined for the presence of cytotoxic antibodies specifically directed against antigens on the donor's T lymphocytes (cross-match test). Hyperacute rejection cannot be treated but can be avoided. Kidney transplants are occasionally associated with a period of acute tubular necrosis, which is a temporary condition thought to be related to conditions that occur during obtaining and preserving the kidney. It occurs rarely in living donor transplants. High doses of immunosuppression—either methylprednisolone or antithymocyte globulin or OKT3—are used to treat acute rejection. This diagnosis is usually made via the detection and workup of graft dysfunction and may include a biopsy. Acute rejection can be treated and is reversible. Chronic rejection usually has an insidious onset and is multifactorial, involving both cell-mediated and humoral arms of the immune system. In lung transplantation, it is known histologically as bronchiolitis obliterans. Generally, there is no known effective therapy. Because the small bowel is rich in lymphoid tissue, graft versus host disease has become more prevalent in this group of recipients than in other organ transplants. This is caused by the proliferation of donor-derived immunocompetent cells with a number of clinical presentations, including skin rash.

44–45. The answers are 44-C and 45-E (Chapter 23, Overview, Immunosuppression, I, Table 23-1). Calcineurin inhibitors block the calcineurin-dependent pathway of helper T-cell activation and include cyclosporine and tacrolimus, which are both used in maintenance immunosuppressive regimens. Cyclosporine became the mainstay of immunosuppressive regimens in the early 1980s and is now in a new formulation known as Neoral. Associated side effects include nephrotoxicity, hypertension, tremor, and hirsutism. Tacrolimus, which was introduced more recently, is also a profound inhibitor of T-cell function, with many similar side effects as cyclosporine. Corticosteroids inhibit all leukocytes and have numerous side effects, including excessive weight gain, diabetes, and cushingoid facies. Mycophenolate is an antimetabolite that impairs lymphocyte function by blocking purine biosynthesis via inhibition of the enzyme inosine monophosphate dehydrogenase.

46–49. The answers are 46-C, 47-D, 48-A, and 49-B (Chapter 24, Intestinal Atresia). GI anomalies vary greatly. The difference between duodenal atresia and the other small bowel atresias is a developmental (duodenal) accident versus a vascular accident (jejunum and ileum). Therefore, chromosomal abnormalities (most commonly, trisomy 21) appear with duodenal problems. The exception to this general rule is the associated incidence of cystic fibrosis with small bowel atresias. Malrotation, although it causes an obstruction, may also pose a vascular problem. This is related to the midgut volvulus, which can cause total ischemia to the intestine. Renal malformations occur in 40% of the imperforate anus, either as a VACTERL complex or related to the disease itself (urethral fistula).

Part VII

Surgical Subspecialties
Chapter Cuts and Caveats

CHAPTER 25

Urologic Surgery:

◆ Acute vesical outlet obstruction may represent an emergency: Acute urinary retention is best treated by catheter drainage, either a Foley catheter or suprapubic tube.

◆ Perineal infection may spread among fascial planes rapidly, leading to death. The question of Fournier gangrene should prompt immediate imaging and broad-spectrum antibiotics.

◆ Trauma to the GU tract is common. After trauma, blood at the meatus in a male is a sign of urethral injury and requires imaging prior to catheterization. Most renal trauma can be managed nonoperatively. Most ureteral trauma requires reconstruction.

◆ Benign prostatic hypertrophy is common in elderly men and is typically treated medically initially. Symptoms include hesitancy, frequency, and decreased power of the urinary stream. Those that do not respond may undergo trans-urethral surgery.

◆ Most testicular tumors are of germ cell origin (deriving from the cells that make up the reproductive system). They typically metastasize to the para-aortic lymph nodes. Early detection through self-examination may improve survival.

CHAPTER 26

Plastic and Reconstructive Surgery:

◆ The "reconstructive ladder" provides a guide to the optimal management of wounds and soft tissue defects. Simpler solutions such as local rearrangements are tried first, followed by local flaps, then "free flaps." The higher on the ladder, the more difficult the procedure and the greater the likelihood of complications.

◆ Flaps may include fascia, muscle, or both. Free flaps are more complicated and have higher failure rates than pedicled flaps.

◆ Infected wounds do not support skin grafts.

◆ Wounds reach most of their ultimate strength by 6 weeks postoperation, which reaches a maximum of 80% of the integrity of nonwounded tissue.

◆ Immediate breast reconstruction does not change outcomes in early-stage breast cancer.

◆ Reconstructive surgical techniques can be used as adjuncts in abdominal wall reconstruction (complex hernias) as well as defects of the chest wall.

◆ Melanoma is an invasive skin cancer. It is staged by depth, using the Breslow system of absolute distance in millimeters. Treatment is generally surgical with wide excision. Adjuvant therapy is used for advanced disease.

CHAPTER 27

Neurosurgery:

- The skull is a rigid container with fixed volume, so increases in volume (bleed, tumor, cerebral edema) necessarily cause an increase in pressure.
- $CPP = MAP - ICP$.
- Epidural hematomas usually arise from trauma to the middle meningeal artery and present with a lucid interval between bouts of decreased consciousness. Unilateral papillary dilatation often signifies significant cerebral compression. Treatment of significant hematomas is evacuation.
- Spinal cord injury results in motor and sensory deficits below the level of the lesion. They also may have loss of sympathetic tone (spinal shock). Treatment is largely supportive once spinal stabilization has taken place.
- Symptomatic aneurysms should be treated by open surgery or endovascular occlusion.

CHAPTER 28

Orthopedics:

- Compartment syndrome may follow fractures and crush injuries, is most likely to develop in the leg, and needs prompt decompression to minimize disability. Pressure may be measured directly within each fascial compartment.
- Open fractures require antibiotics and urgent operative debridement and stabilization.
- Osteomyelitis is usually treated with long-term antibiotics.
- All patients with knee dislocations require a peripheral pulse exam and ABI due to the risk of popliteal artery injury.
- Bony tumors usually represent metastasis rather than primary malignancies.

Urologic Surgery

Jessica Felton, Daniel Reznicek, and Andrew Kramer

UROLOGIC EMERGENCIES

Acute Urinary Retention
I. **Definition:** abrupt inability to pass urine, typically associated with lower abdominal and suprapubic discomfort; usually requires **greater than 200 mL** of urine in the bladder
II. **Cause:** In men, more commonly due to obstruction in the urethra or prostate. In women, a neurogenic bladder component is often present.
III. **Treatment:** must be addressed promptly by either a urethral catheter or suprapubic tube placement

Priapism
I. **Definition:** unwanted erection present for **more than 4 hours** in the absence of sexual excitation
II. **Types (two)**
  A. **Low flow (ischemic; most common):** Patients have pain, rigid corpus cavernosa, and little or no arterial inflow.
  B. **High flow (nonischemic; less common):** Partial, nonpainful erections are nonemergent and usually associated with prior trauma.
III. **Diagnosis:** Physical exam findings and intercavernosal arterial blood gases help differentiate between low- and high-flow priapism.
IV. **Treatment**
  A. **First-line treatment:** For ischemic priapism, aspiration of the corporal blood reduces the pressure and removes the anoxic blood.
  B. **Other:** saline irrigation, sympathomimetic injections, and surgical intervention involving shunts created between the corpus cavernosum and spongiosum
V. **Risk factors**
  A. **Hematologic disorders:** Sickle cell disease is responsible for up to one third of all cases. Other hematologic disorders such as leukemia and thalassemia may also precipitate priapism.
  B. **Medications:** Trazodone, hydralazine, and cocaine are commonly tested. Many other medications may also cause priapism.
  C. **Neurogenic:** Spinal cord injuries, neuropathies, and even spinal anesthesia can cause priapism.

Testicular Torsion
I. **Presentation:** usually presents as sudden onset of pain with associated nausea and vomiting, often in males age younger than 25 years
II. **Physical findings:** pain to palpation and loss of the cremasteric reflex
III. **Diagnosis:** Always include a scrotal ultrasound in any patient in whom torsion is suspected due to the small window of opportunity to save a torsed testicle (Fig. 25-1).
IV. **Treatment:** immediate surgical exploration, detorsion of the affected side, and bilateral orchidopexy

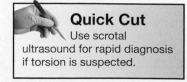

Quick Cut
Use scrotal ultrasound for rapid diagnosis if torsion is suspected.

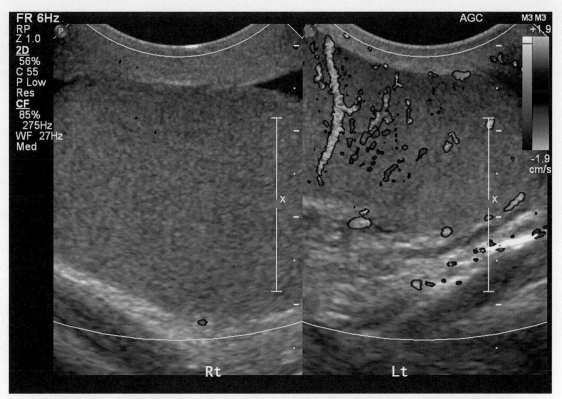

Figure 25-1: Scrotal ultrasound performed on a 17-year-old male with acute right scrotal pain for 3 hours. Doppler demonstrates adequate flow in the left testicle and lack of flow on the right consistent with testicular torsion.

Obstructive Uropathy

I. **Emergent:** when urinary tract obstruction (e.g., stone) is causing sepsis or worsening renal function

II. **Treatment:** Upper urinary tract obstruction requires drainage and may include a ureteral stent or percutaneous nephrostomy tube.

Paraphimosis

I. **Definition:** Foreskin is retracted over the glans and cannot be reduced to its normal position.

II. **Physiology:** Entrapped skin ring leads to increasing edema of the glans distally and may cause arterial occlusion and necrosis.

III. **Treatment:** Reduction can be attempted after squeezing the glans firmly for 5 minutes to reduce swelling and then quickly pulling the foreskin forward. Alternatively, a dorsal slit can be performed, which releases the skin ring with an incision.

Fournier Gangrene

I. **Definition:** necrotizing fasciitis or the perineum and genitalia

II. **Physical findings:** Patients have pain out of proportion to the extent of infection. Crepitus, cellulitis, necrosis, and foul-smelling lesions are usually present.

III. **Diagnosis:** If in doubt, order a computed tomography (CT) scan rather than ultrasound because CT will demonstrate air tracking through the tissue planes.

IV. **Treatment:** Broad-spectrum antibiotics and early wide debridement of necrotic tissue are required. Most commonly, it is a mixed infection with gram-positive, gram-negative, and anaerobic bacteria.

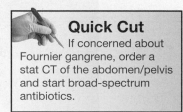

Quick Cut
If concerned about Fournier gangrene, order a stat CT of the abdomen/pelvis and start broad-spectrum antibiotics.

URINARY TRACT STONES

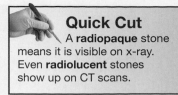

Quick Cut
A **radiopaque** stone means it is visible on x-ray. Even **radiolucent** stones show up on CT scans.

Types of Urinary Calculi

I. **Calcium oxalate stones (most common):** radiopaque and most commonly idiopathic, but other disorders such as hyperparathyroidism, renal tubular acidosis, and chronic diarrheal states can also cause calcium oxalate stones (Fig. 25-2)

II. **Uric acid stones:** radiolucent stones caused by insulin resistance, dietary purine excess, and gout

III. **Cystine calculi:** faintly radiopaque and rare
   A. **Cause: Cystinuria** is an autosomal recessive disorder that causes a defect in renal tubular reabsorption of four amino acids: cystine, ornithine, arginine, and lysine. Only cystine forms calculi.
   B. **Prevention:** Overhydration and urine alkalinization to pH 7.5 are the most effective preventive measures. Oral cystine-binding drugs, such as d-penicillamine or alpha-mercapto-propionylglycine, also help.

IV. **Struvite calculi:** Radiopaque stones usually related to chronic urinary tract infections (UTIs) with urea-splitting bacteria, which maintain alkaline urine. *Proteus* is the most common causative bacteria.

Clinical Presentation

I. **Pain:** Most frequent symptom caused by ureteral obstruction. The site of pain is related to the location of the obstructing calculus (e.g., flank pain, lower abdominal pain, testicular pain, or vulvar pain).

II. **Other symptoms:** hematuria (visible or microscopic), nausea and vomiting, and irritative bladder symptoms (e.g., from a ureterovesical junction calculus)

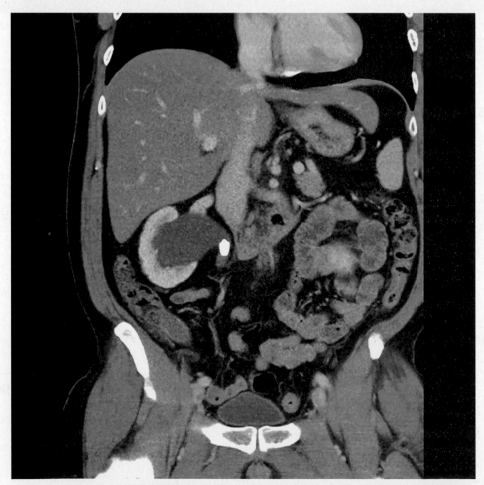

Figure 25-2: CT scan performed on a 44-year-old male with right-sided abdominal pain and gross hematuria. CT scan demonstrated an obstructing stone near the ureteropelvic junction and hydronephrosis.

Diagnosis

I. **Physical examination:** Patients are usually uncomfortable and have costovertebral angle tenderness.

II. **Urinalysis:** Hematuria is usually present; a uric acid stone is unlikely to be found in a patient with a urine pH of 6.5 or higher.

III. **Noncontrast abdominal/pelvic CT:** diagnostic test of choice

IV. **Ultrasonography:** Can be useful in pregnant females or children to avoid radiation exposure. It defines hydronephrosis or an acoustic shadow from a calculus but is much less sensitive than CT. Often used in conjunction with a plain abdominal x-ray.

V. **Cystourethroscopy with retrograde pyelography:** may be needed to confirm calculus presence and reveal its location if imaging studies are not definitive

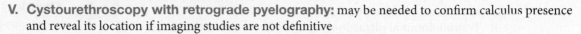
Quick Cut
Patients with urinary calculi often have writhing pain and have difficulty lying still, which differs from peritonitis and acute abdomen in which pain is exacerbated by movement.

Treatment

I. **Observation:** Reserved for stones with reasonable likelihood of spontaneous passing, which is related to stone size and obstruction site. Encourage adequate hydration, using a urine strainer, controlling pain, and an alpha blocker to reduce ureteral spasm and improve stone passage rate.

II. **Surgical procedures:** Advances in endoscopic techniques, extracorporeal shock wave lithotripsy (ESWL), and endourology successfully allow most calculi to be removed without open surgical procedures.

A. **Ureteroscopy and/or stent placement:** Transurethral approach into the ureter to stent the kidney and allow the stone to pass or a ureteroscope may be used to treat the stone directly.

   1. Calculi can be basketed and removed intact or fragmented with lasers.

   2. Stent is often left in the ureter after stone manipulation to alleviate obstruction from edema.

B. **Percutaneous nephrolithotomy (PCNL):** Nephrostomy tube tract in the flank is best suited for large calculi that can be fragmented and removed using ultrasonic, electrohydraulic, or laser lithotriptors.

C. **ESWL:** External energy source is focused by fluoroscopic or ultrasound guidance on a calculus to provide a high-pressure zone that can fragment the calculus. The gravel-like fragments pass through the ureter.

D. **Complications:** bleeding, perinephric hematoma, "steinstrasse" (gravel causing ureteral obstruction), and hypertension

E. **Contraindications:** coagulopathy, antiplatelet medications, or infection

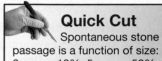
Quick Cut
Spontaneous stone passage is a function of size: 6 mm = 10%, 5 mm = 50%, 4 mm = 90%

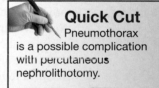
Quick Cut
Pneumothorax is a possible complication with percutaneous nephrolithotomy.

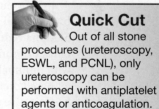
Quick Cut
Out of all stone procedures (ureteroscopy, ESWL, and PCNL), only ureteroscopy can be performed with antiplatelet agents or anticoagulation.

BENIGN PROSTATIC DISORDERS

Benign Prostatic Hyperplasia

I. **Definition:** Benign prostatic hyperplasia (BPH) is a benign enlargement of the prostate gland that occurs commonly in aging men.

A. **Histology:** Changes include stromal and epithelial hyperplasia in the transition (periurethral) zone, which can compress the prostatic urethra and obstruct urinary flow.

B. **Clinical sequela: Lower urinary tract symptoms (LUTS)** occur in a subset of patients with histologic BPH. Obstruction is thought to be due to both prostate size and urethral tone.

II. **Diagnosis:** Can only be definitely made with prostatic tissue evaluated by a pathologist; however, presumptive BPH can be diagnosed based on the patient's irritative or obstructive symptoms and findings on digital rectal examination (DRE).

III. Symptoms

A. Obstructive voiding symptoms: tend to respond best to treatment
1. Diminished force of urinary stream despite a full bladder
2. Hesitancy in initiating flow
3. Sense of incomplete emptying
4. Intermittency or "double voiding"
5. Urinary retention

B. Irritative voiding symptoms: thought to be caused by detrusor instability from chronic obstruction and include frequency, urgency, nocturia, and dysuria

IV. Physical examination and diagnostic testing

A. Gland palpation: to assess size, consistency, and presence or absence of induration on DRE

B. Transabdominal ultrasonography or direct catheterization: to assess residual urine volume in the bladder

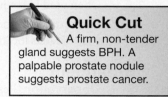

Quick Cut
A firm, non-tender gland suggests BPH. A palpable prostate nodule suggests prostate cancer.

C. Pressure flow studies: Significant bladder contraction but decreased force of stream suggest obstruction due to the prostate. Absence of force suggests an intrinsic detrusor insufficiency.

V. Treatment: Medical therapy remains the first-line treatment for presumed BPH. If medical treatment fails, many surgical options for removing the transition zone tissue of the prostate remain.

A. Indications for treatment: Most men initiating treatment do so for relief of symptoms rather than any absolute indication. Absolute indications for intervention include the following.
1. Urinary retention
2. Significant or recurrent gross hematuria not due to other causes
3. Bladder calculi
4. Bilateral hydroureteronephrosis with renal insufficiency secondary to bladder outlet obstruction
5. Repeated UTIs caused by urinary stasis

B. Medical therapy: Relieves symptoms in men with mild to moderate disease. Although objective improvement may be minimal, if symptomatic improvement occurs, treatment is successful.

1. **Selective alpha-1 sympatholytics:** block alpha-1 receptors in the prostatic capsule and bladder neck area, reducing outlet resistance and improving symptoms

   Quick Cut
   Selective alpha-1 sympatholytics include tamsulosin, terazosin, alfuzosin and reduce prostatic resistance to urinary flow.

   a. **Mild to moderate LUTS:** These are the most commonly used first-line treatment with good symptomatic improvement.
   b. **Principal side effect:** orthostatic hypotension

2. **5-Alpha reductase inhibitors:** block intraprostatic conversion of testosterone to dihydrotestosterone (DHT), reducing prostatic size and improving symptoms with minimal side effects
   a. Based on the principle that prostatic growth is androgen dependent
   b. Objective symptom improvements have been modest, and a trial of 3–6 months may slightly be required to determine efficacy.
   c. These agents reduce the risk of acute urinary retention and the need for transurethral resection of the prostate (TURP).

3. **Combination therapy (e.g. 5-alpha reductase inhibitor plus alpha sympatholytics):** has been shown in randomized controlled trials to be superior to single-agent therapy for disease progression prevention

C. Surgical therapy
1. **TURP:** provides reliable and immediate improvement in both symptoms and voiding dynamics
   a. **Procedure:** Wire loop attached to an electrocautery unit is used to resect tissue under direct cystoscopic vision. Regional anesthesia is commonly used.
   b. **Complications:** bleeding, infection, retrograde ejaculation, bladder neck contracture, urethral stricture, and impotence (rarely)
   c. **Transurethral incision (TUI):** may be appropriate for patients who have small glands and is associated with a lower incidence of bladder neck contracture and retrograde ejaculation

Table 25-1: Diagnostic Features of Prostatitis/Chronic Pelvic Pain Syndrome

Type of Prostatitis	Symptoms	Systemic Signs	Increased WBCs in EPS	Positive Culture
Acute bacterial prostatitis	Yes	Yes	Yes	Yes
Chronic bacterial prostatitis	Yes	No	Yes	Yes
Nonbacterial prostatitis	Yes	No	Yes	No
Prostadynia	Yes	No	No	No

WBC, white blood cell count; EPS, expressed prostatic secretions.

2. **Open prostatectomy (enucleation):** usually reserved for patients with glands greater than 60 g or in whom other pathology exists (e.g., vesical calculus or bladder diverticulum requiring repair)
3. **Minimally invasive prostatic surgical options:** have evolved dramatically and include techniques such as microwave therapy, laser ablation, and transurethral needle ablation (TUNA)

Nonbacterial Prostatitis

I. **Definition:** Benign inflammation that may be bacterial or nonbacterial. Patients tend to be younger than those presenting with BPH, and symptoms tend to be more irritative and painful rather than obstructive (Table 25-1).

II. **Symptoms:** Often synonymous with "male pelvic pain syndrome," creating an array of symptoms ranging from urinary frequency, urgency, perineal pain, and dysuria. The hallmark symptom is **pain**.

III. **Treatment:** although no clear standard-of-care treatment exists, many use a combination of antibiotics, alpha blockers, muscle relaxants, and biofeedback

Quick Cut
With prostatitis, it is important to rule out acute bacterial infection. Acute bacterial prostatitis is always associated with a UTI and requires antibiotics. Constitutional symptoms such as fever and chills are usually present.

GENITOURINARY MALIGNANCIES

Prostate Tumors

I. **Epidemiology and diagnosis:** Prostate cancer is the most common noncutaneous cancer among men worldwide. The current lifetime risk of prostate cancer for men living in the United States is approximately one in six.
A. **Present screening modalities:** DRE and prostate-specific antigen (PSA) test
   1. **DRE:** traditional cancer detection method, assessing for induration, or a "nodule," in the prostate and should be performed yearly
   2. **PSA level:** PSA is a serine protease that serves to liquefy semen after ejaculation.
      a. **Roles:** diagnostic and in following response to cancer treatment
      b. When combined with DRE, determination of the PSA level improves the ability to detect cancers. It has a high specificity, but low sensitivity and is good for ruling out those who do not have cancer (low false-positive rate).
B. **Prostate biopsy:** Office-based procedure performed with transrectal ultrasound (TRUS) guidance in men who have a suspicious DRE and/or an elevated level of PSA. Risks include bleeding (urinary tract or rectal) and infection. Significant complications occur in less than 0.5%–1% of men.

II. **Treatment**
A. **Expectant management (two types)**
   1. **Watchful waiting: Noncurative** treatment; goal is to **limit morbidity** from disease or therapy.
      a. Treatment is delayed until symptoms become evident, at which time androgen deprivation therapy (ADT) is initiated.
      b. Usually for patients expected to live less than 5 years who may develop local symptoms but will not die from the disease

2. **Active surveillance:** Selective delayed definitive (**curative intent**) therapy; this approach carefully monitors the patient with cancer with frequent PSAs and biopsies with the goal of undergoing curative therapy when the risks of cancer exceed the risks of treatment (usually low-risk prostate cancers in healthier patients).

B. **Surgery:** Radical prostatectomy is a treatment for locally confined tumors in appropriate surgical candidates. There has been a dramatic shift from open radical retropubic prostatectomy to minimally invasive techniques, such as laparoscopic and robotic-assisted laparoscopic prostatectomy.

C. **Radiation:** Radiation can include implantation of radioactive pellets (brachytherapy) or external beam radiation.

D. **ADT:** Either surgical or chemical is effective. Androgens fuel prostate growth; therefore inhibiting them prevents prostate cancer growth. Common medications used include gonadotropin-releasing hormone agonists (leuprolide, goserelin) and androgen receptor antagonists (bicalutamide, flutamide).

> **Quick Cut**
> The only two curative therapies for prostate cancer are radiation (either external beam or brachytherapy) and surgery.

III. **Prognosis**
A. **Survival:** Median survival with metastatic disease is 2–2.5 years. Men who have a good biochemical response (PSA nadir less than 4 ng/mL) have a longer survival than those with poor biochemical response (PSA nadir greater than 4 ng/mL).

B. **Hormone refractory disease:** Disease progression after androgen ablation therapy. Survival averages 12–18 months.
1. **Chemotherapy:** To date, no therapies are consistently effective, but several chemotherapy agents are approved with modest efficacy (mitoxantrone, docetaxel).
2. **Other:** Immunologic agents have also been developed, and **sipuleucel-T** was the first therapeutic vaccine to be U.S. Food and Drug Administration (FDA) approved for the treatment of any cancer.

Bladder Carcinoma

I. **Epidemiology and Diagnosis**
A. **Incidence:** In the United States, greater than 70,000 new cases per year are diagnosed. Men are more commonly affected than women (3:1).
B. **Age:** generally, a disease of the elderly; median age 67–70 years
C. **Risk factors:** occupational exposure to aniline dyes, aromatic amines, and naphthylamine; cigarette smoking; phenacetin (analgesic) abuse; chronic inflammation; *Schistosoma haematobium* cystitis; history of cyclophosphamide treatment; and history of pelvic irradiation
D. **Clinical presentation:** Painless hematuria is the most common (85%) presenting symptom. Bladder irritability with urinary frequency, urgency, and dysuria is commonly associated with diffuse carcinoma in situ or invasive cancer.

> **Quick Cut**
> Painless hematuria is the most common presenting symptom of bladder cancer.

E. **Diagnosis:** Cystoscopy and urine cytology are the mainstay of detection.

II. **Treatment**
A. **Superficial transitional cell tumor** (nonmuscle invasive)
1. **Complete transurethral resection:** The tumor is resected in superficial and deep components. Deep resection is performed to define if muscle-invasive disease is present. All visible tumors should be resected.
   a. **Random bladder and prostatic urethral biopsies:** Can determine the multifocal extent of disease. Pathologic evaluation includes grade of lesion (low or high grade), evidence of invasion into the lamina propria or muscle, and carcinoma in situ (CIS) in random bladder biopsies.
   b. **Serial endoscopic and cytologic follow-up:** Should be done at regular intervals; 70% of patients develop recurrences.
2. **Intravesical adjuvant chemotherapy:** may reduce recurrence rate to 30%–45%
   a. **Thiotepa:** alkylating agent
   b. **Mitomycin C:** inhibits DNA synthesis (alkylating agent)
   c. **Doxorubicin:** inhibits DNA synthesis (anthracycline antibiotic)

3. **Bacillus Calmette-Guerin (BCG):** attenuated strain of *Mycobacterium bovis* that has a stimulatory effect on immune responses and is the only intravesicular agent to reduce the risk of **progression** to muscle-invasive disease

4. **Alpha interferon:** immune modulator

B. **CIS:** Despite its lack of invasion, CIS represents a **high-grade lesion**, with a 50% chance of developing into invasive carcinoma.

1. **Initial treatment:** Intravesical BCG is usually given in 6 weekly instillations.

2. **Maintenance therapy:** Repeat induction course with incomplete response (normal follow-up cystoscopy, biopsies, and cytology) to earlier discussion.

C. **Muscle-invasive disease** (invasion into muscularis propria)

1. **Radiation therapy:** relatively ineffective (20% long-term survival)

a. Newer investigational uses of radiation therapy involve attempts at bladder preservation through combination protocols using systemic chemotherapy plus radiation therapy.

b. Radiation therapy prior to radical cystectomy has not improved survival or decreased the incidence of local recurrence.

2. **Radical cystectomy**

a. **In men:** Pelvic lymphadenectomy with cystoprostatectomy is performed. Urethrectomy is performed with tumor involvement of the prostatic urethra.

b. **In women:** Anterior pelvic exenteration is often performed, in which the bladder, urethra, uterus, fallopian tubes, ovaries, and anterior vaginal wall are removed.

3. **Urinary diversion:** required once the bladder is removed and can be done in several ways

a. **Conduits:** can be created using ileum or transverse colon and allow urine to passively drain into an external collection device on the abdominal wall

b. **Continent diversion:** creation of an intra-abdominal urine reservoir, which requires drainage by passing a catheter through a stoma on the abdominal wall

c. **Neobladder formation:** Using the small bowel (ileum) or colon, allows men to void via urethra. Preliminary results among women are fair, with high rates of incontinence.

III. **Prognosis:** varies dramatically between superficial carcinoma (85% of cases) and muscle-invasive carcinoma (15% of cases)

A. **Organ-confined lesions:** Five-year survival is 70%–75% after radical cystectomy for invasive disease.

B. **Metastatic cancer:** 50–70% of patients have a partial or complete response to systemic therapy for metastatic disease. Only ~10% are durable responses (>3 years), and 5-year survival rate is 5%–20% for metastatic cancer.

Renal Pelvis and Ureter Transitional Cell Carcinoma

I. **Epidemiology and diagnosis:** uncommon, usually unilateral tumor (bilateral in 2%–5%)

A. **Risk factors:** similar to bladder lesions, with addition of Balkan nephropathy

B. **Progression:** Only 2%–4% of people with bladder transitional tumors will develop upper tract lesions; ~50% of people presenting with an upper tract transitional tumor will develop a bladder lesion.

C. **Signs and symptoms:** gross hematuria, microscopic hematuria, and flank pain caused by an obstruction

D. **Diagnosis:** CT scan, retrograde pyelography, and ureteroscopy are effective (Figs. 25-3 and 25-4).

II. **Treatment**

A. **Nephroureterectomy**

1. **Traditional radical treatment:** removal of the kidney, entire ureter, and a cuff of bladder at the ureteral orifice

2. **Conservative excision:** may be appropriate for low-grade, low-stage ureteral tumors and involves tumor excision with primary ureteroureterostomy or ureteral reimplantation (into the bladder) for distal ureteral lesions

B. **Endoscopic treatment:** Newer equipment has allowed for endoscopic ureteral resection of low-grade and low-stage tumors. The role is still evolving but is currently reserved for patients with low-grade papillary tumors in solitary renal units or for patients whose health precludes major surgical intervention.

III. **Prognosis:** Depends largely on stage. When completely resected, prognosis remains good. However, upper tracts transitional cell carcinoma (TCC) can quickly become high stage due to its ready ability to invade through the thin wall of the ureter, renal pelvis, and beyond.

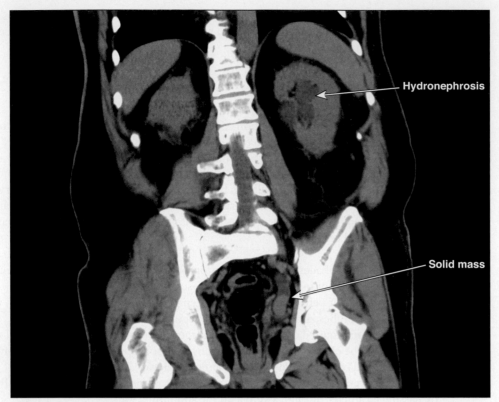

Figure 25-3: A 71-year-old male presented with gross hematuria. CT scan here without contrast demonstrates left-sided hydroureteronephrosis. In the distal left ureter, a dense mass appears to be causing the hydronephrosis. Final pathology demonstrated urothelial carcinoma.

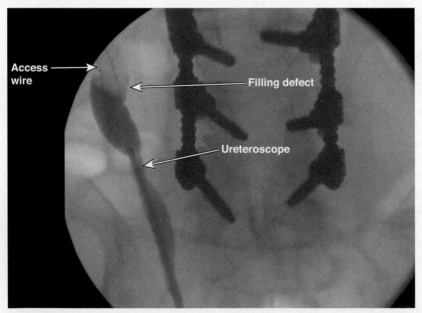

Figure 25-4: This retrograde ureterogram was made by injecting contrast up the ureter with a ureteroscope. Contrast does not fill up the entire ureter because it contains a mass. The U-shaped defect is also referred to as a *goblet sign*. In an obstructing stone, the ureter would spasm around the filling defect. Here, the ureter is dilated in the area of the mass.

Renal Cell Carcinoma

I. **Epidemiology:** ~65,000 new cases per year
  A. **Incidence:** more common in men than in women and has a peak incidence in the fifth to seventh decades of life
  B. **von Hippel–Lindau disease (VHL):** associated with renal cell carcinoma

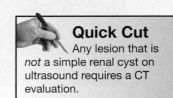

> **Quick Cut**
> The renal cell carcinoma classic triad of pain, hematuria, and flank mass is now very uncommon with the advent of frequent CT scans—greater than 50% are now found incidentally.

II. **Clinical presentation and diagnosis:** commonly discovered during radiographic studies for other complaints (incidental)
  A. **Paraneoplastic syndromes:** occur in ~20% and include Stauffer syndrome (nonmetastatic hepatic dysfunction), hypercalcemia (unclear etiology), hypertension, erythrocytosis, and endogenous pyrogen production
  B. **Imaging:** often used in the evaluation, workup, and diagnosis
    1. **Ultrasonography:** useful for differentiating a simple renal cyst (i.e., absence of internal echoes; a smooth, thin wall; and an acoustic shadow arising from the edges) from a complex or solid lesion

> **Quick Cut**
> Any lesion that is *not* a simple renal cyst on ultrasound requires a CT evaluation.

    2. **CT scan with intravenous (IV) and oral contrast:** Most cost-effective diagnostic and staging modality; evaluates local tumor, venous extension, regional lymph nodes, and liver metastases. Noncontrast CT scans often miss large renal lesions (Fig. 25-5).
    3. **Magnetic resonance imaging:** may be of benefit in those who cannot have contrast and may help define involvement of the renal vein
    4. **Percutaneous aspiration and biopsy:** Historically contraindicated due to the possibility of tumor tracking but is now becoming more common. Biopsy is a reasonable method of diagnosis for patients with metastatic disease for tissue confirmation.

III. **Treatment**
  A. **Radical nephrectomy (open or laparoscopic):** Surgical removal of the ipsilateral adrenal gland, kidney, and investing adipose tissue and fascia. Regional lymphadenectomy may also be performed.
  B. **Cardiopulmonary bypass:** May be required when renal cell carcinoma invades the renal vein and inferior vena cava and extends to the right atrium. Although this is rare, surgical treatment to excise the tumor is more extensive.

IV. **Prognosis**
  A. **Stage I:** Five-year cancer-specific survival rate is greater than 90%.
  B. **Stage II:** Five-year survival rate is 75%–80%.
  C. **Stage IV:** Median survival is 16–20 months, and the 5-year survival rate is less than 10% for patients with distant metastases.

Testicular Tumors

I. **Definition:** Ninety-five percent of all testicular tumors are **germ cell tumors (GCTs)**.
  A. **Non-GCTs:** rare; include sex cord, sex stromal, lymphomas, and other rare tumors
  B. **GCTs:** Major tumors are **seminomatous** and **nonseminomatous** tumors. Nonseminomatous germ cell tumors (NSGCTs) include embryonal carcinoma, teratoma, choriocarcinoma, and yolk sac tumors, alone or in combination. Secondary tumors include lymphomas.

II. **Epidemiology**
  A. **Cryptorchidism (undescended testis):** increases testicular malignancy risk
  B. **Incidence:** Although testis tumors are generally uncommon, they are the *most common* malignancy in men ages 20–34 years.
  C. **Tumor type:** age dependent
    1. **Yolk sac tumors and teratomas:** common in infants
    2. **All cell types:** seen in young adults
    3. **Seminoma:** more common in men ages 35–60 years
    4. **Lymphomas:** predominate in men age greater than 60 years

> **Quick Cut**
> Testicular cancer is most common malignancy in men age less than 35 years.

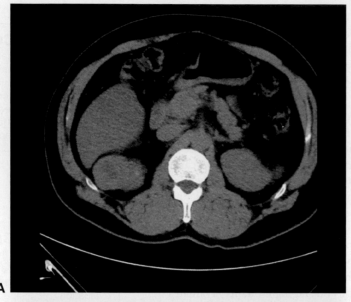

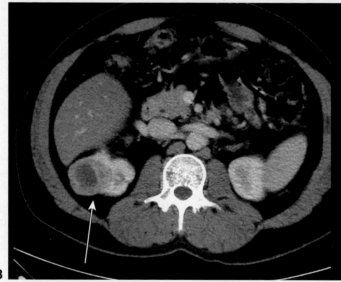

Figure 25-5: **A:** CT scan without contrast demonstrates a normal-appearing right kidney. **B:** Portal venous phase demonstrates a large posterior lesion with solid and cystic components, consistent with renal cell carcinoma.

III. **Clinical presentation and diagnosis:** Painless testicular swelling or enlargement is the classic presenting sign, often diagnosed by self-exam.

A. **Pain (13%–49%):** suggests hemorrhage or infarction and may be confused with epididymitis

B. **Physical examination:** may reveal a firm, nontender, or mildly tender distinct mass or diffuse testicular swelling

C. **Reactive hydrocele:** occurs in 5%–10% of cases

D. **Ultrasonography:** Gold standard in diagnosis. It is very sensitive in determining the size, location, and echogenicity of palpable testicular abnormalities, particularly if a hydrocele limits the physical examination.

E. **Alpha-fetoprotein (AFP), beta-human chorionic gonadotropin (HCG), and lactate dehydrogenase (LDH):** Serum marker levels are useful for diagnosis, for following the response to treatment, and for identifying recurrent disease.

1. **AFP:** may be elevated in patients with yolk sac tumors, embryonal carcinoma, and (rarely) in teratomas

2. **Beta-HCG:** Elevation may accompany choriocarcinoma, embryonal carcinoma, and seminomas. Seminomas do not elaborate AFP; therefore, an elevation confirms a nonseminomatous component.

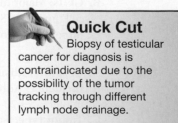

Quick Cut
Biopsy of testicular cancer for diagnosis is contraindicated due to the possibility of the tumor tracking through different lymph node drainage.

IV. **Treatment:** Varies with cell type and disease stage. Initial treatment is surgical exploration via an inguinal approach to avoid potential contamination of scrotal lymphatic draining during tumor manipulation.
   A. **Seminoma:** uniquely radiosensitive and chemosensitive
      1. **Low-stage seminoma:** Postorchiectomy treatment options include close observation, single-agent carboplatin therapy, or radiation therapy. Survival approaches 100%.
      2. **High-stage seminomas:** Current recommendations include up to four courses of chemotherapy with cisplatin, etoposide, and bleomycin.
         a. **Postchemotherapy radiation:** Sometimes considered for patients with a residual retroperitoneal mass.
         b. **Prognosis:** Sixty-seven percent complete response rate to chemotherapy and an overall survival rate of 72% can be expected.
   B. **NSGCTs**
      1. **Low-stage NSGCT:** Treatment involves inguinal orchiectomy followed by either modified retroperitoneal lymphadenectomy (RPLND), primary chemotherapy, or by an intense surveillance protocol.
         a. **Surveillance:** Generally reserved for compliant patients at low risk of micrometastatic disease. Risk factors of the primary testis tumor favoring RPLND include an embryonal carcinoma component, vascular or lymphatic invasion, and extension into peritesticular structures.
         b. **RPLND (~30% of stage I patients):** Surgical removal of specific high-risk lymphatic tissue. Most patients with micrometastases receive two cycles of adjuvant platinum-based chemotherapy.
         c. **Survival:** approaches 92% for both groups
      2. **High-stage NSGCT:** Patients with minimal nodal involvement radiographically or failure to normalize markers postorchiectomy should undergo either RPLND or chemotherapy alone. Intermediate prognosis tumors have 5-year survival of 80%; poor prognosis tumors have a 5-year survival of 48%.

> **Quick Cut**
> Seminomas are common between ages 35 and 60 years, are uniquely radio- and chemosensitive, and confer great long-term survival if diagnosed early.

MALE ERECTILE DYSFUNCTION

Penis

I. **Anatomy**
   A. **Penile erectile tissue:** contained within three **erectile bodies**: two dorsally situated **corpora cavernosa** and one ventrally located **corpus spongiosum**
   B. **Urethra:** lies within the corpus spongiosum, which consists of cavernous, expansible spaces
   C. **Tunica albuginea:** Thick, fibrous tissue layer surrounding each of the three corpora. The fascia of the tunica around the cavernosa is much thicker, which helps support the increased pressure in the corpus spongiosum spaces.

Penile Erection and Detumescence

I. **Hemodynamics:** Arterial flow increases, and increased venous resistance also contributes.

II. **Neurophysiology:** Cavernous nerves mediate neurovascular interaction.
   A. **Erections with genital stimulation:** require only an intact sacral reflex
   B. **Parasympathetic nervous system:** primary importance; nitric oxide (NO) released from nonadrenergic, noncholinergic neurons and the endothelium leads to vascular and corporal smooth muscle relaxation

Diagnosis

I. **History:** very important when evaluating the cause of erectile dysfunction
   A. **Nature of onset and problem duration:** Important; psychogenic impotence may be abrupt in onset with a life stress.
   B. **Interview with sexual partner:** may prove beneficial
   C. **Nocturnal or early morning erections:** may suggest a psychogenic cause
   D. **History of pelvic trauma (including vascular or neurogenic injury):** important to discern
   E. **Risk factors:** diabetes, hypertension, smoking, heart disease, and hypercholesterolemia

II. **Physical examination:** Special emphasis on the neurologic and vascular examination. The penis should be examined for plaques and the testes for size and consistency.

III. **Laboratory tests:** testosterone level and serologic tests for systemic disease (e.g., anemia, renal insufficiency)

IV. **Diagnostic tests:** not indicated in every patient
   A. **Nocturnal penile tumescence:** Measurements are taken of nocturnal erections occurring during rapid eye movement sleep. Gauges are placed on the flaccid penis at bedtime and attached to a monitor overnight that evaluates the number, duration, and rigidity of erections.
   B. **Intracorporeal injections of vasoactive substances (e.g., papaverine, phentolamine, and prostaglandin E):** Used to elicit an erection. Response with a normal erection eliminates a significant venous leak etiology for erectile dysfunction.
   C. **Duplex sonography evaluation:** provides an objective measure of arterial penile blood flow and a relative assessment of venous drainage
      1. **Cavernosal arteries:** evaluated for increased width and flow after intracorporeal vasoactive injection
      2. **Venous outflow:** Should diminish during erections; if venous outflow is still high on duplex study, suspect a venous leak.

V. **Treatment**
   A. **Counseling:** required for men with a significant psychogenic component
   B. **Oral therapy:** has revolutionized treatment
      1. **Selective phosphodiesterase type 5 inhibitors:** enhance erection through the NO/cyclic guanosine monophosphate (cGMP) pathway
      2. **Three agents have been FDA approved:** sildenafil, vardenafil, and tadalafil
   C. **Vacuum erection device:** External pump mechanism that draws blood into the penis to obtain an erection. The blood is retained by the placement of a constricting rubber ring at the base of the penis.
   D. **Vasoactive intracorporeal injections:** self-administered, with risks composed of bruising, mild scar formation, or priapism
   E. **Penile implant:** Device surgically implanted into the corpora cavernosum. Several styles exist that are either malleable or inflatable.
      1. **Risks:** infection associated with the prosthetic material
      2. **Mechanism:** Inflatable prostheses have two chambers in the corpus cavernosum, with a reservoir in the retropubic space (of Retzius) and a pump in the scrotum. Saline is inserted into the reservoir at the time of the procedure and stays in circuit between the cylinders and reservoir for the life of the device, regulated by the pump in the scrotum.
      3. **Satisfaction:** approaches 95%

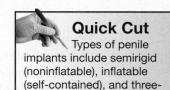

Quick Cut
Types of penile implants include semirigid (noninflatable), inflatable (self-contained), and three-piece inflatable.

VOIDING DYSFUNCTION

Definitions

I. **Voiding:** complex act involving detrusor contraction with sphincteric relaxation (the micturition reflex), which is coordinated in the pontine micturition center and controlled by cerebral input

II. **Dysfunction:** Lesions occurring throughout the nervous system often profoundly affect voiding.
   A. **Hyperreflexia (bladder overactivity):** produced by upper motor neuron lesions (suprasacral)
   B. **Areflexia (bladder flaccidity):** produced by lower motor neuron lesions (sacral nerve roots or cauda equina)

Quick Cut
Hyperreflexia is an exaggerated reflex response, whereas *areflexia* is the absence of a reflex response.

Diagnosis

I. **History:** Detailed historical information regarding frequency, urgency, nocturia, sensation of fullness, straining, incontinence, erectile function, bowel habits, paralysis, paresthesias, history of neurologic and vertebral disease, pelvic surgery, and trauma as well as a review of medications are vital parts of diagnosis.

II. **Physical examination:** Assessment of sensation; motor function; and reflexes of the lower extremities, perineum, and rectal areas is done. Anal sphincter tone should also be assessed, as should the **bulbocavernosal reflex** (contraction of the anal sphincter with compression of the glans or clitoris or with traction on an indwelling urethral catheter).

III. **Urodynamic studies**
   A. **Filling cystometry:** Creation of a pressure–volume curve during bladder filling. Normal bladder sensation, high compliance (accommodation to increasing volumes with minimal increase in pressure), and the absence of uninhibited contractions during filling comprise a normal study.
   B. **Voiding phase:** Assesses flow rate, contractility, and vesical pressure during voiding. Postvoid residual urine is recorded.
   C. **Electromyelography (EMG) of the striated sphincter:** Demonstrates sphincteric function and determines if appropriate sphincter relaxation occurs with voiding. Denervation of the sphincter may be elicited.

> **Quick Cut**
> Urodynamics are helpful for determining bladder function (i.e., capacity, compliance, and contractility), sphincter function, outlet resistance, and flow rate.

Voiding Dysfunction Patterns

I. **Detrusor hyperreflexia (hypertonic neurogenic bladder):** occurs with suprasacral lesions and is characterized by diminished bladder capacity and uninhibitable detrusor contractions
   A. **Presenting symptoms:** Irritative, such as urgency and frequency. If intravesical pressures become elevated, vesicoureteral reflux and upper tract deterioration may occur.
   B. **Treatment:** anticholinergics, intermittent bladder catheterization, and (sometimes) surgical bladder augmentation

II. **Detrusor areflexia (atonic bladder):** occurs with lesions of the sacral cord, nerve roots, or cauda equina, resulting in loss of the sacral reflex arc
   A. **Symptoms:** Increased capacity, decreased intravesical pressure, absence of efficient bladder contractions, and urinary retention with overflow incontinence may result.
   B. **Treatment:** Medical therapy is generally ineffective. Catheterization (indwelling or intermittent) and urinary diversion are often used.

III. **Detrusor external sphincter dyssynergia (DSD):** This condition results from lesions of the spinal cord and may occur alone or may complicate a hyperreflexic or atonic picture.
   A. **Pathophysiology:** involves contraction of the external sphincter during bladder contraction, causing a "functional" outlet obstruction with poor emptying and high detrusor pressures which may cause kidney damage
   B. **Treatment:** medication to promote urinary retention (anticholinergics) and intermittent catheterization

Voiding Dysfunction in Specific Diseases

I. **Spinal cord injury:** Suprasacral lesions usually cause hyperreflexia with DSD, and sacral lesions usually cause areflexia.

II. **Cerebrovascular accidents:** Result in loss of cortical inhibition with detrusor hyperreflexia, manifested by urgency with urge incontinence. DSD is not featured, and patients often contract the sphincter voluntarily.

III. **Parkinson disease:** causes detrusor hyperreflexia, resulting in urgency, frequency, incontinence, and failure of the external sphincter to relax, which may complicate the picture

IV. **Multiple sclerosis:** Leads to voiding dysfunction in 50%–80% of those affected. Most commonly, urgency, frequency, and incontinence are seen; occasionally, retention. Urodynamic studies reveal detrusor hyperreflexia in most cases.

V. **Myelodysplasia:** various abnormal conditions of vertebral development that affect spinal cord function, of which myelomeningocele is most common
   A. **Findings:** poorly compliant bladder with high intravesical pressure, weak detrusor contractions, and DSD
   B. **Management:** anticholinergic agents to diminish bladder pressures and intermittent catheterization to overcome failure of the bladder to empty

VI. **Lumbar disc disease:** Causes detrusor acontractility and decreased sphincteric activity; obstructive voiding symptoms predominate. Urinary retention may occur.

VII. **Diabetic neuropathy:** autonomic neuropathy manifested by diminished bladder sensation, increased capacity, decreased contractility, and elevated postvoid residual volume

Incontinence

I. **Definition:** Leakage of urine should be first classified based on history. The etiologies are manifold, and the treatment should be directed toward eliminating the underlying cause or mitigating the incontinence.

> **Quick Cut**
> Types of urinary incontinence include stress, urge, overflow, and total.

II. **Classifications:** four types
   A. **Stress urinary incontinence:** leakage of urine during Valsalva or increased abdominal pressure
      1. **Incidence:** Although it is more common in women after childbirth and age causing progressive laxity in the pelvic floor, men also may develop it after radical prostatectomy or pelvic radiation.
      2. **Treatment:** may be behavioral (including fluid management and Kegel exercises), medical, and surgical (i.e., urethral slings and other procedures to strengthen the pelvic floor)
   B. **Urge incontinence:** Urine leakage due to detrusor overactivity, which may be idiopathic or have an underlying neurologic basis relating to a pre-existing disease state. Treatment is often medical; first-line therapy is often anticholinergic agents.
   C. **Overflow incontinence (also known as paradoxical incontinence):** With urinary retention, the addition of even small quantities of increased volume in the bladder cause urine leakage. Some patients do not realize they are in retention with large volumes of urine in the bladder. In these patients, only discovery by bladder scan or catheter placement of a full bladder is overflow incontinence even suspected.
   D. **Continuous incontinence:** Due to a urinary fistula that bypasses the urethral sphincter. In females, it may be due to an ectopic ureter that enters in the urethra or a vesicovaginal fistula. Unless the communication between the urinary tract and the outside is repaired, it will continue indefinitely. A temporizing measure may be diverting the urine via nephrostomy tubes, ureteral stents, or urethral catheterization. The fistula is bypassed or the urine is diverted away from it; patients may achieve dryness until the fistula is repaired.

Treatment

I. **Pharmacologic treatment:** allows manipulation of bladder contractility (via cholinergic receptors in the bladder) and changes in outlet resistance (via alpha-adrenergic receptors in the bladder neck, prostatic capsule, and urethra)

II. **Catheterization**
   A. **Indwelling catheter:** may have an additional channel to allow infusions such as water or saline to flush clots or topical agents
   B. **Intermittent catheterization:** Frees the patient from continuous appliance usage and lowers the incidence of UTIs, meatal erosion, urethral stricture, and epididymitis. Patients develop bacterial colonization, which requires no treatment unless symptoms of infection occur.

III. **Urinary diversion (away from the bladder):** Forming an ileal conduit or catheterizable reservoir may be necessary in patients with recurrent urosepsis or renal insufficiency caused by a detrusor problem.

IV. **Bladder augmentation:** Increasing capacity and decreasing intravesical pressure may be required in patients with hyperreflexia or in those with small and contracted, poorly compliant bladders secondary to long-standing neurologic disease (e.g., myelomeningocele), radiation cystitis, or chemically induced bladder fibrosis. Intermittent catheterization is usually required.

Autonomic Dysreflexia

I. **Definition:** outpouring of sympathetic activity in response to afferent visceral stimulation in patients with spinal cord injuries with lesions above T6

II. **Effects:** Bladder, urethral, or rectal stimulation may produce profound hypertension, bradycardia, diaphoresis, headache, and piloerection in these patients.

III. **Treatment:** Withdrawal of the stimulant and medication directed at the hypertensive crisis. Prophylaxis with various medications (e.g., chlorpromazine, nifedipine) is sometimes useful in affected patients who require urologic manipulation.

UROLOGIC TRAUMA

Blunt Trauma

I. **Evaluation:** Need for radiographic assessment in patients with urologic trauma is based on the mechanism of injury, vital signs, physical examination, and urinalysis.

  A. **Gross hematuria (or microhematuria and a systolic blood pressure [SBP] less than 90 mm Hg):** requires radiographic evaluation of the kidneys

  B. **Microhematuria (in patients who have always had an SBP less than 90 mm Hg):** does not require a radiographic evaluation unless clinical suspicion is high based on the mechanism of injury (e.g., fall from a height, direct blows, high-speed motor vehicle crashes)

  C. **Penetrating trauma (regardless of the degree of hematuria):** requires an evaluation

II. **Radiographic tests:** CT scan of the abdomen and pelvis, cystogram, retrograde urethrogram, and renal angiography are possibilities.

Renal Injuries

I. **Classification:** Renal injuries are grades 1 through 5.

  A. **Grade 1 (contusion):** no obvious parenchymal injury, but subcapsular hematoma is possible

  B. **Grade 2 (minor lacerations):** superficial cortical disruptions that do not involve the collecting system and are less than 1 cm

  C. **Grade 3 (major lacerations):** deep corticomedullary lacerations that do not involve the collecting system but are greater than 2 cm

  D. **Grade 4 (deep lacerations):** involve the collecting system or cause urinary extravasation

  E. **Grade 5:** defined as either an avulsion of the renal hilum or a shattered kidney

II. **Radiographic assessment**

  A. **Abdominal/pelvic CT scan:** first-line test performed to rule out renal injury

  1. **Dry CT:** done first to help demonstrate stones

  2. **Early venous phase and 10-minute delayed images:** Done next; the delayed phase helps define the ureteral anatomy.

  B. **Renal arteriography:** generally reserved for patients with possible vascular injuries that are not elucidated on the CT scan and may require embolization

III. **Treatment**

  A. **Nonoperative:** Contusions, minor lacerations, and some major lacerations can be managed with bed rest, serial hematocrit evaluation, and hydration. Ureteral stenting may be required in cases of ongoing urinary extravasation.

  B. **Angiography and embolization:** can control most renal bleeding

  C. **Surgical exploration:** Debridement of nonviable renal tissue, closure of the collecting system, coverage of the injury with perinephric adipose tissue, and drainage of the retroperitoneum. Stents are usually not needed.

IV. **Renal trauma complications**

  A. **Post-traumatic hypertension:** uncommon but may occur in 5%–10% of patients and is mediated by renin owing to ischemic tissue

  B. **Associated injuries:** more common in patients with penetrating rather than blunt trauma

  1. **Blunt trauma:** Right renal injuries are associated with liver trauma, and left renal injuries are associated with splenic injuries.

  2. **Penetrating trauma:** Bowel lacerations, pancreatic injury, and other vascular injuries occur.

> **Quick Cut**
> Typically, only grade 5 renal injuries require open surgical exploration and only in the setting of an unstable patient (they have a high risk of associated intra-abdominal injuries). The remaining renal injuries can be managed non-operatively, with occasional stenting of grade 4 renal injuries.

> **Quick Cut**
> Initial identification of associated injuries with appropriate treatment will prevent many complications of renal trauma.

Ureteral Injuries

I. **Etiology:** Ureteral injuries are caused primarily by penetrating trauma or iatrogenic injury.

    A. **Deceleration injuries:** may result in avulsion of the ureteropelvic junction, especially in children

    B. **Blast effect from gunshot wounds:** Bullet may not have directly transected the ureter, but thermal damage to surrounding structures results from the bullet wound, and the precarious nature of the ureter's blood supply make it susceptible to collateral damage.

II. **Radiographic assessment:** CT initially identifies injury site; **intraoperative retrograde pyelogram** can further delineate the injury.

III. **Treatment**

    A. **Complete ureteral transections:** should be explored and repaired

    B. **Partial injuries (or suspected devitalization from blast effect):** should undergo initial attempts at stenting, either anterograde or retrograde, prior to attempting open repair

Bladder Trauma (Lower Urinary Tract)

I. **Etiology:** Blunt bladder trauma is frequently associated with pelvic fractures. Rupture can be extraperitoneal or intraperitoneal, depending on the location of the tear.

    A. **Extraperitoneal:** Majority of bladder injuries (80%); these ruptures have a much better prognosis and are easier to manage.

    B. **Intraperitoneal:** These 20% are due to the continuity of the bladder dome with the peritoneum, whereas the rest of the bladder is extraperitoneal or pelvic. Associated urethral injuries should always be considered as a possibility.

II. **Evaluation**

    A. **Retrograde urethrogram (RUG):** Blood at the urethral meatus, an elevated prostate gland on DRE, or a mechanism of injury possibly causing a urethral tear should prompt an RUG before bladder catheterization.

    B. **Plain film cystography:** Drainage and oblique films are necessary. A **cystogram** involves maximally (400–500 mL) filling the bladder to determine extravasation of contrast medium (e.g., CT or plain film).

Quick Cut
The prognosis of intraperitoneal bladder perforations in general is much worse, but this may be due to the much higher likelihood of associated injuries to vital intraperitoneal structures.

III. **Treatment:** For intraperitoneal bladder injuries, treatment is immediate surgery, whereas for extraperitoneal injuries, treatment is a long-term Foley catheter in the urethra.

Urethral Injuries

I. **Evaluation:** Examination and radiographic assessment are described earlier. A high index of suspicion should be maintained, because passage of a urethral catheter may significantly worsen a mild urethral injury by theoretically turning a small laceration into a complete avulsion or disruption.

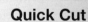

Quick Cut
Always perform an RUG before inserting a Foley catheter in someone with a history of trauma and blood at the urethral meatus.

II. **Treatment**

    A. **Penetrating anterior urethral injuries:** Should be explored, debrided, and repaired primarily; a urethral catheter should be left in place after repair.

    B. **Complete prostatomembranous urethral disruptions (from blunt trauma):** require open suprapubic tube placement

        1. **Attempts at primary repair:** not warranted

        2. **Attempts at "realignment" (over a urethral catheter or with flexible cystoscopes):** may be indicated

        3. **Follow-up open repair of post-traumatic strictures:** should occur 3–6 months after the injury

Penile Injuries

I. **Fracture of the erect penis:** Caused by direct blunt trauma that significantly buckles the corpus cavernosum, resulting in a tear of

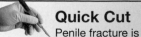

Quick Cut
Penile fracture is most commonly associated with sexual activity.

the tunica albuginea overlying the corpora cavernosa. Urethral tears are associated in some penile fracture cases (20%) and should always be ruled out by an RUG.

A. **Physical findings:** ecchymosis, swelling, and deviation of the penis

B. **Diagnosis:** usually made based on physical examination and the patient's history, which usually includes the penis buckling during sexual activity, followed by rapid detumescence, sharp pain, and immediate bruising and swelling

C. **Treatment:** operative repair and closure of any cavernosal tear

    1. **Surgical exploration:** to prevent scarring of the corpus cavernosum and subsequent Peyronie disease (abnormal penile curvature)

    2. **Urethrogram with repair of the urethral injury:** may be necessary

II. **Penetrating penile trauma:** Evaluated and treated similarly to a fractured penis. All such injuries should be explored and repaired.

Testicular Trauma

I. **Blunt trauma:** Testicular rupture is the primary injury that requires surgical repair; testicular ultrasound is the gold standard when making this diagnosis.

A. **Evaluation:** Physical examination is integral and can reveal a large hematocele. Extrusion of the seminiferous tubules from the confines of the tunica albuginea of the testis can be found with ultrasound or surgical exploration.

B. **Treatment:** Repair involves debriding extruded or nonviable seminiferous tubules and closure of the overlying tunica albuginea of the testicle.

II. **Penetrating trauma:** Physical examination and ultrasound may prove helpful. All suspected testicular or spermatic cord injuries should be explored.

Plastic and Reconstructive Surgery

Niluka A. Wickramaratne, Helen G. Hui-Chou,
Devinder Singh, and Tripp Holton

OVERVIEW

Background

I. **Definition:** Plastic surgery is a broad field that encompasses the reconstruction of body parts altered by birth defects, trauma, oncologic resections, and advanced age.

II. **Effect of war:** The field truly emerged during the 20th century, when the burden of patients deformed by war was met by the advances in anesthesia, aseptic techniques, and antibiotics.

Quick Cut
"Plastic" originates from the Greek word "plastikos," which means to mold and reshape.

Notable Figures

I. **Sushruta (circa 600 BCE, India):** known for writing the *Sushruta Samhita* (Sanskrit: *Sushruta's Compendium*), a text describing his many surgical techniques, including the first total nasal reconstruction

II. **Gasparo Tagliacozzi (1545–1599, Italy):** developed the Tagliacozzi flap, a tubed, pedicled medial arm flap used for nasal reconstruction (Fig. 26-1)

III. **Sir Harold Gilles (1882–1960, New Zealand):** First modern plastic surgeon; he coined the reconstructive term to "replace like with like."

IV. **Joseph E. Murray (1919–2012, United States):** Only plastic surgeon to win a Nobel prize; he became interested in transplantation immunology when studying skin allografts in burn patients and was the first surgeon to perform a successful organ transplant in humans.

RECONSTRUCTIVE PLASTIC SURGERY

Wounds and Defects

I. **Reconstructive ladder (Fig. 26-2):** Term used by plastic surgeons to describe the thought process used to approach wounds and defects. They aim to maximize the restoration of form and function while minimizing donor site morbidity. Procedures on the lower rungs tend to be safer and less costly; as the defect becomes larger, more complex, or more critical, the surgeon must adopt a more complex reconstructive procedure.

II. **Negative Pressure Wound Therapy (NPWT):** commonly referred to as a *wound vacuum-assisted closure*; uses suction to

Quick Cut
Surgeons aim to use a procedure from the lowest rung of the reconstructive ladder possible. It is not ideal to walk "down" the ladder.

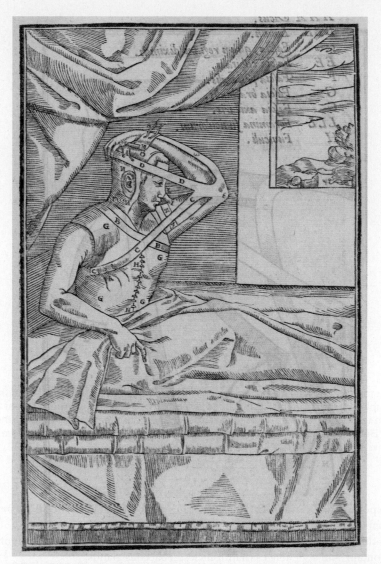

Figure 26-1: The Tagliacozzi flap. One of the seminal descriptions of a flap for nasal coverage, it has become the emblem of plastic surgery.

promote wound healing often on large, chronic wounds, which can be grafted or closed once a granulation bed forms

A. Technique: Wound is dressed with contoured foam, covered with an occlusive dressing, and attached to a pump that applies a controlled level of negative pressure (typically 75–125 mm Hg).

B. "Microdeformation": Mechanical forces speed the healing process by promoting cell migration and proliferation, which accelerates formation of granulation tissue.

III. Skin grafts: used to reconstruct superficial skin wounds too large to close by primary intention and for which secondary healing is inappropriate

A. Wound location: Head and neck wounds often receive full-thickness skin grafts (FTSGs) to match color and texture; defects overlying joints (e.g., the hand) should be treated with FTSGs in order to avoid contractures that limit movement.

B. Underlying structures: Wound bed must contain an adequate blood supply to support graft healing.

   1. Muscle: has a robust blood supply and supports skin grafts very well

   2. Fat: Less vascular; graft has an increased risk of failure.

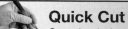

Quick Cut
The negative pressure draws out edematous and infectious fluid from the wound bed, enhancing circulation and decreasing the bacterial burden.

Quick Cut
Once healed, a skin graft replaces the barrier function in the area of the defect.

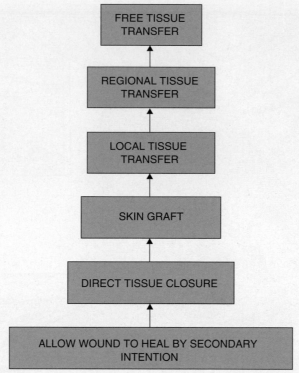

Figure 26-2: The "reconstructive ladder." The progression of techniques is from the most straightforward at the bottom to the most complex at the top. The upper rungs are also accompanied by the greatest risk of complications. In general, surgeons aim to use the lowest rung of the ladder that meets the clinical needs of the patient. (From Thorne CH, Bartlett SP, Beasley RW, et al. *Grabb and Smith's Plastic Surgery*, 6th ed. Baltimore: Lippincott Williams & Wilkins; 2006.)

3. **Exposed bone/tendon/cartilage (lacking periosteum, peritendon, or perichondrium):** cannot support grafts

C. **Split-thickness skin grafts (STSGs):** Contain the epidermis and a portion of the dermis. They do not contain skin appendages (hair follicles, sebaceous glands, sweat glands), which are located in the deep dermis and/or subcutaneous tissue.

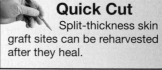
Quick Cut
Split-thickness skin grafts cannot secrete skin oils, sweat, or grow hair.

1. **Advantages:** Large supply of donor areas (renewable supply as the site re-epithelializes) and decreased primary contracture; meshing can increase surface area and allow drainage of fluid that may otherwise separate the graft from the wound bed.

2. **Disadvantages:** cosmetically (aesthetically) inferior, decreased durability, variable pigmentation, and increased secondary contracture

Quick Cut
Split-thickness skin graft sites can be reharvested after they heal.

3. **Common donor sites:** Abdomen, buttocks, and thighs, which provide a large amount of skin. Even the scalp can serve as a donor site.

D. **FTSGs:** Contain the epidermis, dermis, and variable amounts of subcutaneous fat. The donor site must be closed primarily or with an STSG, and, thus, they are usually taken from areas with redundant skin. The graft will retain its normal hair growth, secretions, and pigmentation once healed in the recipient site.

1. **Advantages:** cosmetically superior (even compared to a nonmeshed STSG), less secondary contracture, and increased durability

2. **Disadvantages:** limited donor sites and increased primary contracture

3. **Common donor sites:** Postauricular and supraclavicular skin provides an excellent match for facial defects. Other common FTSG donor sites include the medial arm, medial forearm, and groin crease.

E. **Graft healing:** Adherence of the graft is very important for survival. Occurs in three phases.

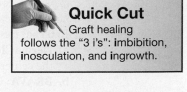

Quick Cut
Graft healing follows the "3 i's": imbibition, inosculation, and ingrowth.

  1. **Plasmatic imbibition (days 1–2):** Nutrients are absorbed passively from the blood supply in the recipient wound bed.
  2. **Inosculation (day 3):** formation of anastomotic connections between the capillaries in the recipient bed and vessels in the dermis of the graft
  3. **Angiogenesis (day 5):** ingrowth of new vessels into the graft
F. **Regrowth of the graft's architecture:** occurs at a slower pace, such that eventually, skin appendages, pigmentation, and innervation may return in FTSGs

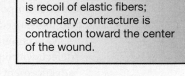

Quick Cut
Primary contracture is recoil of elastic fibers; secondary contracture is contraction toward the center of the wound.

G. **Primary contracture:** immediate reduction in size of the graft after harvesting due to passive recoil of elastic fibers located in the dermis; more common in FTSGs due to a higher concentration of elastin
H. **Secondary contracture:** centripetal contraction toward the center of the wound that occurs after the graft is applied to the recipient site; more common in STSGs likely because they lack the cellular structure and matrix composition found in deeper layers of the dermis
I. **Graft failure:** causes as follows:
  1. **Graft thickness:** In a thicker graft, there are more cells, which means that the graft has a higher metabolic demand.
  2. **Separation of the graft from the wound bed (e.g., excess tension):** disrupts the nutrient supply because initial nourishment of the graft occurs via diffusion

Quick Cut
Wounds must have fewer than 10^5 bacteria per gram of tissue to support a skin graft. Typically, these wounds have good granulation tissue, no necrotic tissue, and no gross purulence.

    a. **Fluid (i.e., blood, serum, or pus) between the graft and the wound bed:** disrupts imbibition
    b. **Shear force and movement between the graft and the recipient bed:** disrupts inosculation/ingrowth
  3. **Infection (e.g., contaminated foreign body):** Infected wounds will not allow skin grafts to adhere; critical bacterial concentration is 10^5 bacteria per gram tissue.

IV. **Other graft types:** as follows:
A. **Fat grafts:** sections of dermal fat can be inlaid into a defect for contouring; often used in breast reconstruction
B. **Tendon grafts:** numerous tendons in the body (e.g., palmaris longus) can be harvested without loss of function; often used to replace damaged tendons in the hand
C. **Cartilage grafts:** Rib, conchal, and septal cartilage grafts can be harvested for ear, nasal, and nipple reconstruction (after mastectomy).
D. **Nerve graft:** Sural nerve grafts are often used to repair peripheral nerve injuries.

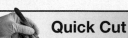

Quick Cut
Nerve regeneration occurs at a rate of 1 mm/day along the graft until reaching the motor endplate.

E. **Vein grafts:** Saphenous vein is often harvested; vein grafts can be used for arterial or venous replacement.
F. **Bone grafts:** Guide regeneration of the native bone along the graft (osteoconduction), unlike vascularized bone flaps where union between the flap and native bone occurs via osteoinduction (recruitment of osteoblasts). Bone autografts can be harvested from sites such as the iliac crest. Cadaveric cancellous bone allograft can also be used.

V. **Tissue expansion:** used to increase the amount of tissue available for local reconstructive procedures by applying mechanical force, which provides a reliable source of tissue with preserved hair and sensation and good color and texture match
A. **Expansion period:** Two properties of skin come into play.
  1. **Biologic creep:** cellular growth and regeneration in response to chronic stretching forces
  2. **Stress relaxation:** principle that the force required to stretch a material a certain length decreases over time
B. **Types:** two broad categories
  1. **Internal tissue expansion:** Silicone reservoir is placed beneath the skin and inflated over time with saline to expand the overlying tissue. Eventually, a fibrous capsule forms around the

expander, containing most of the new vasculature. Common uses include reconstruction of scalp, face and breast defects, and reconstruction after removal of congenital nevi.

2. **External tissue expansion:** uses an external device to apply a constant force on skin
   a. **DermaClose:** uses skin anchors placed around a wound to expand surrounding tissue toward the center
   b. **BRAVA:** Used for breast reconstruction or augmentation; negative pressure provides three-dimensional (3D) tension on the breast.

VI. **Flaps:** units of tissue that are moved or transferred to the recipient site with their own vascular supply (Fig. 26-3)

> **Quick Cut**
> Flaps have their own vascularization; grafts are dependent on the recipient site's blood supply.

A. **Classifications:** by method of transfer, vascular supply, or anatomic components

B. **Local flaps:** used to close cutaneous wounds near the donor site
   1. **Advancement flaps:** Flap is moved forward to fill the defect, without lateral or rotational movement (e.g., V-Y advancement or single pedicle advancement flap).
   2. **Rotation flap:** Semicircular flap rotated on a pivot point to fill an adjacent defect. A backcut (or Burow triangle) is used to facilitate rotation.
   3. **Transposition flap:** rotated on a pivot point to fill a defect contiguous with the base of the flap
      a. **Rhombic flap:** Note that the lesion can be any shape and is excised leaving a rhombic-shaped defect.
      b. **Bilobed flap:** Commonly used for nasal defects; the flap uses two lobes, where the primary lobe is used to fill the defect and the secondary lobe is used to fill the donor site of the primary lobe.

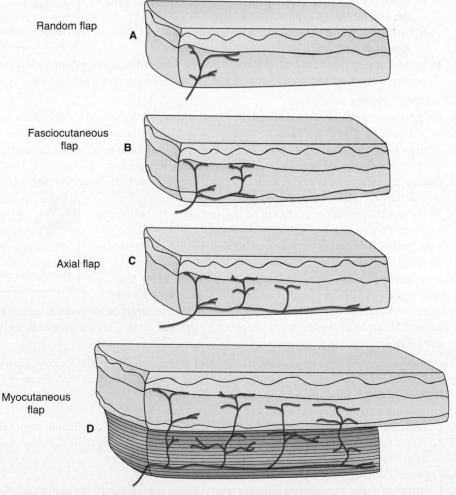

Random flap

Fasciocutaneous flap

Axial flap

Myocutaneous flap

Figure 26-3: Major flap types.

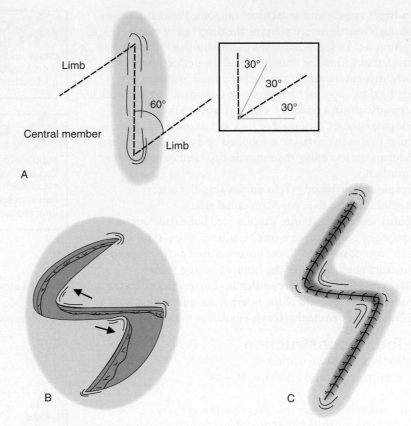

Figure 26-4: Z-plasty. This is a very common plastic surgical technique for local coverage and scar revision.

4. **Z-plasty:** Similar to the transposition flap, two triangular flaps are raised and transposed into the defect created by the other. Used for scar revision (Figure 26-4).
C. **Distant flaps:** Donor site is not adjacent to the recipient site.
   1. **Pedicled:** Flap is still connected to its original vessels.
   2. **Free:** Flap's vasculature is divided from the donor site and reattached at the recipient site using microsurgical anastomosis.
D. **Random flaps:** lack an anatomically defined vascular system and are fed by the dermal–subdermal plexus
E. **Axial flaps:** Based on a defined artery and vein, which originate at the base of the flap and run along its axis. Axial flaps may be distant or locoregional.
F. **Angiosomes:** Units of skin and underlying deep tissue that are supplied by a single source vessel. Source vessels supply the skin and subcutaneous tissue via cutaneous perforator arteries.
G. **Perforator flaps:** Cutaneous flaps that are supplied by one or more perforator arteries. They are named after either their perforator vessel (e.g., deep inferior epigastric perforator flap) or the anatomic region, if the flap can be harvested with multiple perforators (e.g., anterolateral thigh flap).
   1. **Direct cutaneous:** Perforator only pierces the deep fascia, without passing through any other structures.
   2. **Indirect septal and septocutaneous:** Perforator passes through an intermuscular septum before piercing the deep fascia to supply the skin.

Quick Cut
The wider the angles on a "Z" plasty, the longer the final scar length.

Quick Cut
Free tissue transfer has a higher rate of failure and requires longer operating time than pedicled flaps.

Quick Cut
Because a random flap is dependent on vessels entering the base, its width-to-length ratio is limited (typically 1:3).

Quick Cut
The boundaries of skin that can be reliably harvested from a single vessel are defined as an angiosome.

3. **Indirect muscle and musculocutaneous:** Perforator passes through muscle before piercing the deep fascia; more common than septocutaneous perforator flaps and require dissection within the muscle to find the perforating vessels.

H. **Muscle/myocutaneous:** composed of muscle, its fascia, and overlying skin; supplied by at least one dominant vascular pedicle, which is usually in a reliable location relative to the muscle

I. **Fasciocutaneous:** Composed of skin and its underlying fascia; vascular plexus in the fascia is supplied by a perforating artery. These flaps are less bulky than muscle flaps and have less donor site morbidity.

1. **Scapular flap:** based on circumflex scapular artery
2. **Radial forearm flap:** based on radial artery

J. **Osteomyocutaneous/bone:** Vascularized bone flaps can be composed of only bone or a combination of bone, skin, and muscle (composite flap). These are often used as free flaps to reconstruct bony defects of the head, neck, and spine.

1. **Iliac crest flap (deep circumflex iliac artery):** Iliac crest can be harvested alone or with a skin paddle and a segment of the internal oblique muscle.
2. **Fibula flap (peroneal artery):** Fibula can be harvested alone or with a skin paddle.

Head-to-Toe Reconstruction

I. **Cranial/scalp reconstruction**

A. **Layers of the scalp and cranium:** SCALP
1. **Skin**
2. **Subcutaneous tissue:** contains vessels and nerves
3. **Galeal aponeurotic layer:** provides strength; continuous with the frontalis and occipitalis muscles and the temporoparietal fascia laterally
4. **Loose areolar tissue:** subgaleal fascia; provides mobility; contains emissary veins
5. **Pericranium:** adherent to the calvarium

B. **Blood supply (five paired arteries):** supratrochlear, supraorbital, superficial temporal, posterior auricular, and occipital

C. **Soft tissue defects:** Replace "like with like" by using hair-bearing tissue. Treatment options include the following.
1. **Primary closure:** small defects (<3 cm) can be closed primarily
2. **Skin grafting:** often used as a temporizing measure to allow time for tissue expansion
3. **Tissue expansion:** provides a larger amount of scalp tissue with intact sensation and hair growth
4. **Local flaps:** flaps should be based on at least one of the named artery systems
5. **Free tissue transfer:** often required for large defects

D. **Cranial defects:** Treatment must provide structural protection for the brain and should maintain normal shape of the calvarium.
1. **Infection:** If the wound is infected, reconstruction should be delayed until the infection is fully treated.
2. **Treatment options:** include the following:
   a. **Alloplastic materials:** Can be pre-formed using computer-aided design; they are preferred for large defects and are composed of titanium mesh, polymethyl methacrylate (PMMA), or polyether ether ketone (PEEK).
   b. **Autologous bone grafts:** serve as a scaffold for new bone growth from the edges of the defect (osteoconduction)
      (1) **Original bone graft:** If the original bone removed during the craniectomy is preserved (either frozen

Quick Cut
Perforator flaps cause less donor site morbidity because they allow muscle to be preserved.

Quick Cut
The robust blood supply of a myocutaneous flap often allows for successful healing even if the flap is used in an irradiated or infected wound.

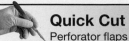

Quick Cut
Remember "S-C-A-L-P" (**s**kin, sub**c**utaneous tissue, galeal **a**poneurotic, **l**oose areolar tissue, and **p**ericranium) for the layers of the scalp.

Quick Cut
Skin grafts on the scalp are susceptible to pressure necrosis, so bolster dressings must be applied with great care.

Quick Cut
Autologous bone is preferred over implants due to a lower infection/extrusion rate.

or placed in the abdominal subcutaneous tissue), it can be used later to reconstruct the defect.

(2) **Other:** split calvarial bone graft (outer table from the parietal bone) or split rib graft

II. Eyelid reconstruction: Eyelid defects commonly occur as a result of oncologic resections (Mohs micrographic surgery) or trauma.

A. **Goals:** Restore eyelid blink function (maintain a functional lacrimal system, which cleans and lubricates the eye), protect the globe (prevent puncture, exposure keratitis, desiccation, etc.), and achieve adequate aesthetic results.

B. **Technique:** Choice depends on the thickness of the defect and the amount of eyelid tissue that is missing.

1. **Partial-thickness loss:** can be closed primarily or with FTSGs, which are used to avoid contracture, which can lead to ectropion

   a. **Skin defects:** best reconstructed with skin grafts from the contralateral eyelid, which provides the best color and thickness match

   b. **Defects of the conjunctiva and tarsal plate:** Although usually occur as part of a full-thickness defect, they may need to be repaired on their own.

2. **Full-thickness defects:** Defects up to 30% of the lid can be closed primarily, but they must be closed in layers to avoid notching. Larger defects are closed with a variety of local flaps.

III. Ear reconstruction:

A. **External ear defects:** arise as a result of trauma, bites, oncologic resections, and congenital malformations

1. **Microtia (congenital hypoplasia):** due to incomplete embryonic development of the ear; may be an isolated defect or associated with other malformations

2. **External ear anatomy:** Pinna can be divided into subunits that define its aesthetic appearance and help guide reconstruction.

   a. **Helix and lobule:** create the overall contour of the ear and are important for projection and the appearance of symmetry with the other ear

   b. **Antihelix and antitragus:** complex cartilaginous folds that give structure and support to the ear

   c. **Conchal complex:** made up of the conchal bowl and cavum conchae; does contain cartilage but is not as important for structural support

3. **Goals of reconstruction:** Replace the cartilaginous framework, recreate 3D morphology, and achieve symmetry with the unaffected side.

B. **Subtotal ear defects:** Defects involving only the skin of the ear can be reconstructed with skin grafts or local skin flaps. Full-thickness defects require reconstruction of both skin and underlying cartilaginous structures. Various chondrocutaneous advancement and rotational flaps have been described.

> **Quick Cut**
> The perichondrium of underlying cartilage must be intact in order for a graft to take.

C. **Total ear reconstruction:** often used for microtia in children and is a multistage procedure

1. **Stage 1:** Costal cartilage (from ribs 6 to 8) is carved to form the framework of the ear, using the contralateral ear as a template to match size and shape.

2. **Stage 2:** Framework is then covered in a pedicled or free temporoparietal fascial flap and inset in the proper location.

3. **Stage 3:** Skin graft is used to cover the fascial flap.

IV. Nasal reconstruction: Nasal defects occur most commonly as a result of trauma or oncologic resection.

A. **Layers:** skin, bone and cartilage, and mucosal lining

B. **Aesthetic subunits (nine):** dorsum, paired sidewalls, tip, paired ala, columella, and paired soft tissue triangles

C. **Goals of reconstruction:** maintain a patent airway, replace all missing layers, and achieve good aesthetic results

D. **Method:** depends on the location, size, and depth of the defect

> **Quick Cut**
> When a defect makes up greater than 50% of a single subunit, it is best to extend the defect and reconstruct the subunit as a whole.

1. **Skin defects:** Small defects in certain locations (e.g., medial canthal region, typically concave areas) heal very well by secondary intention. Various local flaps are used for larger defects or defects in other locations (bilobed, nasolabial, or forehead flaps).

   2. **Lining and structural defects:** Bone and cartilage autografts (conchal or rib cartilage can be harvested) are used to replace midline and alar structures, supporting the soft tissue and restoring projection. Replacing the nasal mucosal lining is very important when reconstructing full-thickness defects. Failure to do so can result in contracture, stenosis of the lumen, exposure and resorption of cartilage or bone grafts, and alar notching.

V. Lip reconstruction: Lip defects are commonly due to tumor resection, congenital clefts, and trauma.
   A. **Lip anatomy:** Skin in the vermilion zone (red zone) is unique so skin grafts cannot be used because of a color and texture mismatch. The epidermis is very thin, allowing the dense capillary plexus to shine through and give the lip its color.
   B. **Goals of reconstruction:** Maintain oral competence, including muscular integrity, sensation, and the aperture of the mouth; preserve normal speech; and achieve good aesthetic results.

> **Quick Cut**
> Microstomia is loss of the aperture of the mouth.

   C. **Method:** Depends on characteristics of the defect, such as size, thickness, and location. In general, local flaps are used to redistribute surrounding lip tissue, which is the only way to replace like with like in the case of vermilion lip tissue.
      1. **Small defects (up to 30%) of the upper or lower lip:** can be closed primarily, depending on their location
      2. **Abbé lip switch flap (two stages):** originally designed to reconstruct the philtrum in bilateral cleft lip defects
         a. **Stage 1:** Full-thickness segment of the unaffected lip (not involving the commissure) is raised (using the labial artery as the pedicle) and rotated into the defect on the other lip.
         b. **Stage 2:** Flap's pedicle is connecting the upper and lower lips and will be divided 2–3 weeks later during the second stage of the procedure. The donor site is closed primarily.

VI. Head and neck: Defects of the aerodigestive tract are usually due to malignancy in the oral cavity. Squamous cell carcinoma is the most common type.
   A. **Functions of the pharynx:** serves as a passageway for food and air, swallowing (propelling food boluses while protecting the airway), and speech (lips and oral cavity shape sounds generated by the vocal cords)
   B. **Goals of reconstruction:** Provide bulk in the oropharynx to eliminate dead space during speech and swallowing, replace the lining of the oral cavity, and restore the continuity of the digestive tract.
   C. **Soft tissue reconstruction:** Although some defects can be reconstructed locally, distant flaps are often necessary to provide adequate bulk. When the defect involves the full circumference of the hypopharynx and esophagus, many of these flaps can be tubed in order to recreate a lumen.
      1. **Pedicled pectoralis major flap:** based on its dominant blood supply, the thoracoacromial artery
      2. **Free flaps:** When used in a tubed configuration, the skin of anterolateral thigh (ALT), radial forearm (commonly used for floor of mouth defects involving the base of the tongue), scapular, and parascapular fasciocutaneous flaps lies on the inside, lining the new lumen. This provides a strong epithelial layer, which protects the flap from food boluses.
      3. **Free jejunum:** Portion of small intestine, oriented in the direction of peristalsis, can be inset with its mesenteric blood supply (See Figure 18-4).
   D. **Bony reconstruction:** Head and neck cancers often require resections that involve the bony skeleton, resulting in large defects of the mandible and midface (maxilla, zygoma, and orbit).
      1. **Goals of reconstruction:** Restore structural support to allow for the normal mechanics of mastication, maintain facial projection, and replace the lining of the oral or nasal cavities.
      2. **Mandibular reconstruction plates:** Can be used on their own to bridge a defect in the mandible without replacing the bony segment. High failure rates result from the metal plate eventually extruding through the soft tissue of the mouth or face, or the plate itself may fracture after some time due to the forces of mastication.
      3. **Nonvascularized bone grafts:** Segments of autologous bone grafts can be harvested from various sites (iliac crest, scapula, rib, fibula, and radius) and fixed using metal plates. Only used for small defects (6 cm or less). High failure rate due to resorption and infection because they rely on the surrounding vascular bed for survival. Must be done delayed.
      4. **Vascularized bone flaps:** Segment of bone is harvested with its blood supply. The free fibula flap (peroneal artery and vein) is most commonly used for mandibular reconstruction. These have better success rates than bone grafts or reconstruction plates. The flap vessels are usually anastomosed to the facial artery and vein using microsurgery.

VII. Breast reconstruction: Reconstruction after surgical resection is an important part of breast cancer treatment. The type of reconstruction used depends on characteristics of the defect (size of the defect—i.e., mastectomy or lumpectomy, quality of skin flaps after the mastectomy) and other patient factors (e.g., patient preference, size of the contralateral breast, medical comorbidities, body habitus).

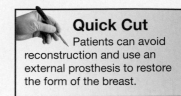

> **Quick Cut**
> Patients can avoid reconstruction and use an external prosthesis to restore the form of the breast.

- **A. Timing:** depends on patient preference, tumor biology, and the need for adjuvant radiation therapy
  1. **Immediate:** usually done in early-stage cancers (stages I and II), when radiation therapy is not expected
     a. **Advantages:** better cosmetic result (mastectomy skin can be used, skin is not contracted, premastectomy landmarks are available), single-stage procedure, and easier access to recipient vessels when free tissue transfer is performed
     b. **Disadvantages:** If postoperative radiation is required, it can cause skin changes (shrinkage, contracture, firmness and pigment changes), fat necrosis, and deformity, and wound healing complications may delay further adjuvant therapy.
  2. **Delayed-immediate:** Performed in patients at a somewhat increased risk of requiring adjuvant radiation therapy. A tissue expander is placed at the time of mastectomy and filled as appropriate. If radiation is required, it can be deflated and refilled after the therapy. Definitive reconstruction is performed once therapy is complete.
     a. **Advantages:** allows for skin preservation even with radiation
     b. **Disadvantages:** Two stages are required.
  3. **Delayed:** Reconstruction is performed well after the mastectomy (months to years later).
     a. **Advantage:** Postoperative radiation will not affect the reconstruction. (months to years later)
     b. **Disadvantages:** Two-stage procedure, cosmetically inferior, and reconstruction may be more difficult and recipient vessels may be difficult to find due to scarring.
- **B. Types:** include oncoplastic breast reduction, implant-based, and autologous tissue transfer
  1. **Oncoplastic breast reduction:** involves performing adjacent tissue transfer, most commonly in the form of a reduction mammoplasty at the same time as breast conserving therapy (BCT)
     a. **Indications:** best in patients who require fairly large lumpectomies
     b. **Advantages:** allows the plastic surgeon to rearrange breast tissue to fill the defect while still maintaining symmetry and cosmesis

> **Quick Cut**
> Symmetry can be achieved by reduction in the contralateral breast.

  2. **Tissue expander:** Placed under the pectoralis major at the time of the mastectomy for a delayed-immediate reconstruction. After the expansion process is finished, the tissue expander is removed and replaced with an implant, or an autologous tissue transfer is done to reconstruct the breast.
  3. **Saline:** silicone shell filled with saline solution (physiologic)
     a. **Advantages:** low capsular contracture rates, leaks are safely absorbed by the body, and easier to adjust for size
     b. **Disadvantages:** Wrinkling; leakage will cause complete deflation.
  4. **Silicone:** silicone shell filled with silicone filler
     a. **Advantages:** more natural feel than saline; less wrinkling
     b. **Disadvantages:** Higher contracture rates; rupture can cause local inflammation and granuloma formation.
  5. **Autologous tissue transfer:** Involves using either pedicled or free flap. Choice of flap depends on the size of the breast, prior surgeries (which limit the availability of donor sites), and any medical comorbidities.
     a. **Transverse rectus abdominis muscle (TRAM):** based on the superior epigastric artery (Fig. 26-5)
        (1) **Disadvantage:** not commonly performed due to high donor site morbidity (hernia, abdominal wall weakness, and larger potential areas of fat necrosis)
        (2) **Donor site:** May require mesh reconstruction; concurrent abdominoplasty is performed to close the site.

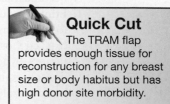

> **Quick Cut**
> The TRAM flap provides enough tissue for reconstruction for any breast size or body habitus but has high donor site morbidity.

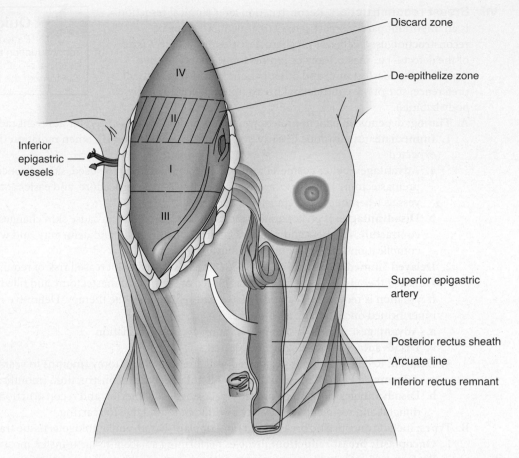

Figure 26-5: The transverse rectus abdominis muscle (TRAM) flap. The TRAM is a pedicled flap, based on the superior epigastric artery. (From Jaffee RA, *Anesthesiologist's Manual of Surgical Procedures*, 5th ed. Baltimore: Lippincott Williams & Wilkins; 2014; reproduced with permission from Spear SL. *Surgery of the Breast: Principles and Art*. Philadelphia: Lippincott-Raven; 1998.)

    b. Latissimus dorsi: based on the thoracodorsal artery
      (1) Advantages: can be used for reconstruction of small/medium breast and/or in conjunction with an implant
      (2) Donor site: Long-term morbidity is low, although seroma formation is common.
    c. Abdominally based flaps: Free flaps using an abdominal skin paddle are desirable because the donor incision can be closed with a concurrent abdominoplasty and include the free TRAM and deep inferior epigastric perforator, which involves dissecting within the rectus to find the perforator, without taking any muscle.
    d. Recipient vessels: Free flaps include internal mammary vessels and thoracodorsal vessels (less common).

VIII. Breast deformities: include gynecomastia, macromastia, and tuberous breast
    A. Gynecomastia: enlargement of breast tissue in males
      1. Etiology: due to an excess of estrogens relative to androgens; may be due to underlying disease (e.g., cirrhosis, hypothyroidism, adrenal and testicular tumors, hypogonadism, Klinefelter syndrome) or certain drugs (e.g., marijuana, anabolic steroids, spironolactone, ketoconazole, cimetidine, or puberty)

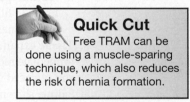

Quick Cut
Free TRAM can be done using a muscle-sparing technique, which also reduces the risk of hernia formation.

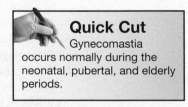

Quick Cut
Gynecomastia occurs normally during the neonatal, pubertal, and elderly periods.

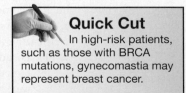

Quick Cut
In high-risk patients, such as those with BRCA mutations, gynecomastia may represent breast cancer.

2. **Treatment:** Idiopathic gynecomastia should be observed initially because it often regresses.
   a. **Medical:** Aromatase inhibitors (tamoxifen) decrease peripheral conversion of androgens to estrogens.
   b. **Surgical:** includes suction lipectomy or surgical excision
B. **Macromastia:** excessive enlargement of the female breasts
   1. **Etiology:** due to an abnormal growth response to normal circulating amounts of estrogen that causes large increases in fibrous and fatty tissue but a relatively small increase in glandular tissue
   2. **Symptoms:** neck, back, and shoulder pain; intertriginous rashes, infections, and maceration at the inframammary fold (IMF)
   3. **Treatment:** surgical
      a. **Reduction mammoplasty:** Goal is to relieve symptoms by reducing breast volume and reposition the nipple–arcolar complex (NAC) at or above the level of the IMF through many possible techniques. The NAC is left on a dermoglandular pedicle, which preserves blood supply and innervation. Pedicle design and skin patterns are generally independent of each other.
         (1) **Pedicle designs:** inferior, superior, central, and medial pedicles
         (2) **Skin patterns:** inverted T (Wise pattern), vertical, and circumareolar
      b. **Suction lipectomy:** used as an adjunct for contouring

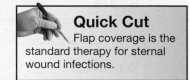

> **Quick Cut**
> Lipectomy alone will not address breast projection or nipple position.

C. **Tuberous breast:** abnormal breast development, resulting in narrow breast base, high IMF, and large areola due to herniation of the breast parenchyma into the areolar space
   1. **Location:** usually bilateral but may be unilateral
   2. **Treatment:** external tissue expansion with fat grafting to increase breast volume; surgery to expand the base of the breast, reduce the size of the areola, and correct the nipple location

IX. **Chest wall:** Defects arise as a result of trauma, tumor resections, infections, radiation damage, and congenital conditions.
   A. **Mediastinitis:** Infection of the sternal wound is a life-threatening complication of cardiac procedures and requires complex flap reconstruction.
   B. **Structures:** Pleural lining is important for maintaining an airtight seal over the lungs, which prevents pneumothorax and fistulas; ribs are important for skeletal structure and support, protection of vital organs, and proper breathing mechanics; and the sternum is the point of articulation for the ribs and clavicles.

> **Quick Cut**
> Removal of all devitalized or infected tissue and hardware is key to the success of the subsequent reconstruction.

   C. **Goals of reconstruction:** Restore stability and structure of the ribs and chest wall, obliterate dead space, and restore the pleural lining.
   D. **Structural defects:** Reconstruction of rib defects is indicated when four or more ribs are involved and the defect is longer than 5 cm, as these will result in paradoxical motion and poor breathing mechanics.
      1. **Soft tissue flaps:** Bridging the space left by the missing ribs or sternum can provide enough stability to allow for normal breathing.
         a. **Tensor fascia latae flap:** provides strong fascia
         b. **Thick muscle flaps:** such as the rectus abdominis myocutaneous flap
      2. **Alloplastic materials:** used when more support is needed (typically for lateral chest rib cage rather than sternum)
         a. **Polypropylene or polytetrafluoroethylene mesh:** can be used for semirigid fixation
         b. **PMMA:** even more rigid; can be embedded within mesh layers for additional support
   E. **Sternal wounds:** Vacuum-assisted closure is often used as a bridge to definitive reconstruction; pedicled flaps bring well-vascularized tissue into the wound, which speeds healing. The sternum does not require rigid fixation or bony union.

> **Quick Cut**
> Flap coverage is the standard therapy for sternal wound infections.

      1. **Pectoralis flap:** Considered the workhorse for sternal wounds; the pectoralis major has two vascular systems: the dominant thoracoacromial artery and a set of segmental perforators from the internal thoracic artery (ITA) (also called the *internal mammary*).

2. **Pectoralis turnover flap:** Based medially on the segmental perforators from the ITA; the pectoralis muscle is separated from its humeral attachment laterally, and the thoracoacromial pedicle is divided at the clavicle; the muscle is flipped medially and inset into the wound.

> **Quick Cut**
> Coronary artery bypass grafting usually involves harvesting the left ITA; in these patients, the pectoralis turnover flap may be limited to the right side.

3. **Unilateral advancement flap:** Based on the thoracoacromial artery pedicle; the muscle is divided from its medial attachments and advanced further medially into the sternal wound.
4. **Rectus abdominis muscle flap:** based on the superior epigastric artery
5. **Omental flap:** Based on the either the left or right gastroepiploic artery; typically avoided in patients with previous abdominal surgeries due to damage or scarring of the omentum. There is a potential risk of infectious spread between the mediastinal and peritoneal cavities or herniation of abdominal organs into the chest.

X. **Abdomen:** Techniques are as follows.
   A. **Panniculectomy:** resection of hanging skin and fat of the low abdomen typically done via a waistline incision (distinguished from abdominoplasty, as there is no dissection above the umbilicus and no umbilical transposition); may also be done with a fleur-de-lis pattern, which adds a vertical midline incision and is designed to resect tissue in the vertical and horizontal directions

> **Quick Cut**
> The indication for panniculectomy is generally to improve hygiene and to limit intertrigo (rashing of skin folds).

   B. **Abdominal wall reconstruction:** Mainstay is component separation.
      1. **Technique:** Incise the external oblique fascia and divide the underlying muscle, which allows the midline rectus muscle to be advanced toward the midline for closure under less tension. Many surgeons will augment this closure with biologic or permanent mesh placed deep to the repair (sublay) or on top of the repair (onlay).
      2. **Advantages:** Spares innervation to the rectus muscles (innervation lies in the deeper internal obliques) as well as the blood supply, which runs within the rectus (a communication of deep inferior epigastric vessels and the internal mammary or superior epigastric vessels).

XI. **Lower extremity:** Techniques are as follows.
   A. **Groin coverage for vascular grafts:** Typically accomplished with the rotation of regional pedicled muscle flaps. Use of the adjacent sartorius muscle is often the first choice. Each patient's anatomy must be determined, as blood supply to the muscle of choice may have been excluded by vascular disease or bypasses.
   B. **Trauma:** Mainstay of coverage for open wounds of the knee and upper one third of the leg includes use of the medial and lateral gastrocnemius muscles as well as the soleus; lower one-third wounds are very challenging to reconstruct and most require free flap coverage.

WOUND HEALING AND DISEASES OF SKIN AND SOFT TISSUE

Phases of Wound Healing
I. **Inflammatory:** Platelets secrete inflammatory mediators, attracting neutrophils and macrophages.
II. **Proliferative:** Fibroblasts enter the wound and lay down collagen, resulting in granulation tissue; epithelialization occurs.
III. **Maturation:** Collagen cross-linking, collagen remodeling, and myofibroblasts cause wound contraction.

> **Quick Cut**
> By 6 weeks postinjury, the wound will reach its ultimate strength: 80% of the original.

Scars
I. **Hypertrophic scars:** within the border of scar
II. **Keloids:** exceed border of scar, often pedunculated

Wounds
I. **Acne inversa (formerly hidradenitis suppurativa):** Infection of the subcutaneous tissue in areas of skin bearing apocrine sweat glands (typically in the axilla or groin). Treatment involves antibiotics, incision and drainage, and excision with either primary closure or skin grafting.

Table 26-1: Stages of Pressure Ulcers

Stage	Characteristics
I	Intact skin with nonblanchable redness of a localized area
II	Partial-thickness loss of dermis presenting as a shallow open ulcer with a red pink wound bed
III	Subcutaneous fat is visible.
IV	Full-thickness tissue loss with exposed bone, tendon, or muscle

II. **Pressure sores:** evaluation/staging (Table 26-1)
   A. **Management:** Off-load pressure is essential via a specialty bed (low air-loss mattress) and frequent turning protocols; also improve position and treat contractures, optimize nutrition, and manage wound care dressings.
   B. **Types:** Most common sites are sacral, ischial, trochanteric, occipital, heel, etc.

III. **Diabetic foot ulcers:** may be treated by compression or Unna boots; notoriously slow to heal

IV. **Chronic venous stasis:** Characteristic skin changes and edema are managed symptomatically.

Benign Skin Lesions

I. **Cysts:** very common fluid-/matter-filled cavities in the subcutaneous tissues (e.g., epithelial cysts, sebaceous cysts, and epidermal inclusion cysts secondary to puncture of the skin)

II. **Lipomas:** Fat tumors are most commonly found on the neck, shoulders, back, and thighs. Excision is indicated for aesthetic and functional reasons.

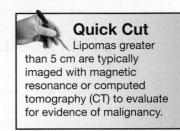

Quick Cut
Lipomas greater than 5 cm are typically imaged with magnetic resonance or computed tomography (CT) to evaluate for evidence of malignancy.

III. **Hemangiomas:** These vascular tumors are the most common tumors of infancy, typically found on the head or neck; they start in the first few weeks of life and tend to grow rapidly over the first year, then involute at a rate of 10% per year.

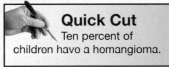

Quick Cut
Ten percent of children have a hemangioma.

   A. **Management:** Can be observed; may also be treated with oral or intralesional corticosteroids (will arrest growth but not reverse it), propranolol, or pulsed dye laser. Surgery is typically reserved for lesions that either threaten airway patency or obstruct the visual field or in highly sensitive cosmetic areas such as the nasal tip. Profound bleeding or ulceration are also indications for excision.
   B. **Kasabach-Merritt syndrome:** features profound thrombocytopenia occurring in conjunction with a hemangioma

IV. **Vascular malformations (VMALs):** May be capillary, venous, lymphatic, or arteriovenous malformations present at birth (helps distinguish them from hemangiomas) that grow proportionally with the child. Angioembolization may be used for treatment, sometimes as an adjunct to en bloc resection.

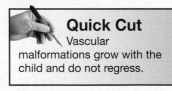

Quick Cut
Vascular malformations grow with the child and do not regress.

Malignant Skin Lesions

I. **Basal cell carcinoma:** commonly occurs on the head and neck; has a pearly appearance with surrounding telangiectasia, and metastasis is rare; treated with Mohs surgery or excision

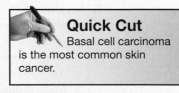

Quick Cut
Basal cell carcinoma is the most common skin cancer.

   A. **Mohs surgery:** involves sequential shavings with immediate pathologic analysis
   B. **Cure rate:** This mapped, layer-by-layer excision with immediate yields excellent cure rates (~95%).

II. **Squamous cell carcinoma:** Exposure to sunlight is the primary risk factor and is associated with premalignant skin lesions and chronic wounds (Marjolin ulcer).
   A. **Presentation:** commonly presents on the lips; often has central ulceration and satellite lesions and may grow rapidly and metastasize via lymphatics and or blood
   B. **Treatment:** can be treated with Mohs or excision

III. **Melanoma:** History of severe sunburns is a known risk factor.
   A. **Presentation:** Lesions look like irregular nevi with asymmetric shape, irregular borders, and changes in size and color.
   B. **Subtypes:** Superficial spreading is the most common; others include nodular, acrolentiginous, and lentigo maligna.
   C. **Staging:** Currently staged using the American Joint Committee on Cancer's tumor-node-metastasis classification. Other classification systems include the following.
      1. **Breslow method:** involved precisely measuring the depth of the tumor in millimeters. Breslow system is preferred.
      2. **Clark classification:** based on histologically determining the deepest level of the skin in which malignant cells are found
   D. **Management:** Excision is the treatment for stages I–III. Stage IV is treated with chemotherapy and radiation. Recommended margins are as follows (based upon Breslow thickness).
      1. **Melanoma in situ (stage 0):** 0.5-cm margins
      2. **Lesions greater than 1.0 mm in thickness:** 1-cm margins
      3. **Lesions >1mm:** 2-cm margins, possible excision of underlying fascia
   E. **Sentinel lymph node (SLN) biopsy:** done to stage nodal disease and determine whether a full lymph node dissection is indicated to remove cancer burden

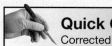
Quick Cut
In malignant melanoma, the depth of lesion in millimeters determines the radial margin in centimeters.

CRANIOFACIAL SURGERY

Pediatric

I. **Cleft lip and cleft palate:** Most common congenital craniofacial anomaly. The primary goal of cleft palate repair is the optimization of normal speech development.

Quick Cut
Corrected too late, the cleft palate will render the patient with hypernasal speech.

   A. **Epidemiology:** Unilateral cleft lips are nine times more common than bilateral. Cleft lips occur twice as commonly on the left as the right.
   B. **Incidence:** 0.3 per 1,000 in African Americans; 1 per 1,000 in Caucasians; 2 per 1,000 in Asians; and 3.6 per 1,000 in Native Americans
   C. **Embryology:** Face forms 4th–10th week of gestation; anomaly develops due to failure of fusion of the two medial nasal prominences of the frontonasal processes to the lateral palatine processes derived from the maxillary prominences.
   D. **Anatomy:** Primary palate is anterior to the incisive foramen and consists of lips, alveolus, and anterior palate; secondary palate is posterior to the incisive foramen and consists of hard and soft palate to the uvula.
   E. **Classification:** described in 1931
      1. **Veau Class I:** isolated soft palate cleft
      2. **Veau Class II:** isolated hard and soft palate
      3. **Veau Class III:** unilateral cleft lip and palate
      4. **Veau Class IV:** bilateral cleft lip and palate
   F. **Treatment:** Requires a multidisciplinary approach; a standard team includes a geneticist, plastic surgeon, otolaryngologist, nutritionist/dietitian, speech pathologist, audiologist, dentist/oral surgeon, nurse, psychologist, and social worker.
   G. **Timing of repairs:** proceeds as follows:
      1. **Age 0–3 months:** presurgical nasoalveolar molding (NAM) or lip adhesion
      2. **Age 3 months:** primary cleft lip repair
      3. **Age 9–18 months:** primary cleft palate repair
      4. **Age 7–9 years:** alveolar bone graft (age of mixed dentition)
      5. **Puberty:** orthodontics
      6. **Adolescence:** open rhinoplasty
      7. **Skeletal maturity:** orthognathic surgery
   H. **Complications:** velopharyngeal incompetence (difficulty in speech), palatal fistulas, and midface hypoplasia (midfacial bony development is retarded by manipulation of these areas during cleft repair)

Adult

I. **Trauma:** Initial management of facial injuries follows basic principles of advanced trauma life support (ATLS) and begins with airway, control of hemorrhage, and evaluation and stabilization of concomitant injuries.

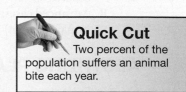

Quick Cut
Facial injuries are rarely life threatening but should alert the examiner to the possibility of airway compromise, cervical spine injuries, or central nervous system injuries.

   A. **Initial evaluation:** history, physical exam, and imaging studies
      1. **Trauma history:** past medical history, allergies, medications, last meal, and mechanism of injury
      2. **Physical exam:** skin and soft tissue from scalp to neck; sensory examination of trigeminal nerve regions of the face and oral cavity; motor examination of the facial nerve, ocular and orbital examination, which is often assisted by ophthalmology to document visual acuity and other injuries to the globe; and intraoral examination of mucosa, dentition, and occlusion of teeth
      3. **Imaging:** Performed to evaluate skeletal abnormalities; CT scans are the most commonly used modality. A panoramic radiograph evaluates the entire mandible, from condyle to condyle, in a single image.
   B. **Types:** mandible (order of most common: angle, condyle, symphysis/parasymphysis), maxilla, nasal bones, and orbital fractures

Quick Cut
Ophthalmologic consultation should be considered in every case of orbital trauma.

      1. **Exam for orbital fractures:** First indication of optic nerve compression may be red color desaturation; direct and consensual pupillary responses; and globe movement.
      2. **Orbital fracture types:** orbital floor, medial orbit, and orbital roof
   C. **Management:** intermaxillary fixation (IMF) and open reduction and internal fixation (ORIF)

HAND SURGERY

Trauma

I. **Fractures:** phalanx (usually treated by alignment then immobilization), metacarpal (boxer's fracture; typically treated with reduction and splinting), carpal (typically managed with casting), and radius/ulna (long bone fractures usually managed with casting)

Quick Cut
Hand fractures are common and require individualized treatment, as function of the hand is critical.

II. **Amputations and replants:** Indications for digital replant include thumb, single digit distal to flexor digitorum superficialis (FDS) insertion, multiple digits, hand amputation through palm, any part in a child, and proximal arm injury with sharp mechanism.
   A. **Contraindications for replant:** single digits proximal to FDS flexor insertion; severely crushed, mangled, or contaminated parts; multiple-level amputation; and multiple trauma or severe medical problems
   B. **Finger reconstruction:** second toe transfer, finger lengthening
   C. **Thumb reconstruction:** lengthening, pollicization, toe-to-thumb transfers

III. **Bite injuries:** Human bites may occur in defensive injury; anaerobic bacteria are common. Dogs and cats are most responsible for animal bites.

Quick Cut
Two percent of the population suffers an animal bite each year.

   A. **Animal bite organisms:** include *Pasteurella* species, *Staphylococcus*, *Streptococcus*, and *Capnocytophaga*
   B. **Treatment for animal bites:** involves aggressive debridement of devitalized tissue, administration of appropriate antibiotics, and tetanus and rabies treatment or prophylaxis

Tumors and Hand Masses

I. **Benign soft tissue masses: Ganglion cysts** are most frequent, causing degeneration of connective tissue in joint capsules or tendon sheaths. Aspiration has high recurrence rate. Surgical excision must remove stalk of ganglion. Other lesions include the following.
   A. **Giant cell tumors:** Likely reaction to injury, with large yellow subcutaneous mass. Treatment is by excision.

B. **Epidermal inclusion cyst:** due to prior implantation of epidermal cells into the dermis; presents as a firm, nontender mass or cyst, and treatment is complete excision

C. **Glomus tumor:** Subcutaneous nodules in subungual region causing cold hypersensitivity and paroxysmal and pinpoint pain. Treat with complete excision.

II. **Malignant soft tissue masses: Squamous cell carcinoma** is most common; usually occurring on the dorsum of the hand in elderly men and with an aggressive metastatic rate. Treat with wide local excision with 5–10-mm margins. Others as follows.

A. **Basal cell carcinoma:** Pearly lesions with ulceration, telangiectasias, and discoloration. Metastasis is uncommon, and treatment is excision of 5-mm margins or Mohs surgery.

B. **Melanoma:** May be visible on skin or subungual. Treatment is wide local excision with margins based on tumor depth or amputation at joint proximal to lesion.

III. **Benign bone tumors:** Enchondroma is most common and is treated with curettage and bone grafting. Osteoid osteoma and osteochondroma are other tumors.

IV. **Malignant bone tumors:** Chondrosarcoma is most common and is treated with en bloc resection with ray amputation for digits. Osteogenic and Ewing sarcoma are others (see Chapter 28).

Infection

I. **Paronychia:** infection where the nail and skin meet; most common infection of the hand

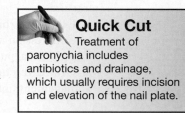

Quick Cut
Treatment of paronychia includes antibiotics and drainage, which usually requires incision and elevation of the nail plate.

A. **Acute:** associated with *Staphylococcus aureus*; treatment with elevation of nail plate and incision into nail fold

B. **Chronic:** usually fungal (*Candida* or atypical *Mycobacterium*); treatment with topical antifungals and eponychial marsupialization (excision of crescent-shaped portion of skin proximal to eponychial fold; wound allowed to close by secondary intention)

II. **Felon:** abscess of pulp of digit

A. **Etiology:** Occurs after puncture wound; *S. aureus* is the most common pathogen.

B. **Treatment:** Open longitudinal incision over pulp in the area of maximal fluctuance; lateral incision over midline may preserve digital arteries; important to divide septa in pulp to allow drainage and packing.

III. **Herpetic whitlow:** Herpes simplex types 1 and 2 infection; clear vesicles may form. Medical treatment with acyclovir; no incision is necessary.

IV. **Flexor tenosynovitis:**

A. **Signs:** (Kanavel's signs) intense pain with any attempt to extend partly flexed finger, finger held in flexion for comfort, uniform swelling involving the entire finger, and percussion tenderness along the course of the tendon sheath

B. **Treatment:** initially antibiotics, splinting, and hand elevation but highly likely to need incision and drainage

V. **Median nerve compression (carpal tunnel syndrome):** typically caused by repetitive motion

A. **Treatment:** initially splinting and avoidance of inciting task; may respond to intracanal injections of steroids

B. **Advanced cases:** may be decompressed with open or endoscopic surgery (release of the transverse carpal ligament)

AESTHETIC PLASTIC SURGERY

Overview

I. **Rationale:** Aesthetic or cosmetic procedures are performed to improve a patient's appearance. Great care must be taken by the plastic surgeon to identify appropriate candidates.

Quick Cut
Aesthetic surgery may be designed to correct a perceived flaw and/or to mitigate effects of aging.

II. **Candidate selection:** As these interventions are truly elective in nature, patients with worrisome medical comorbidities as well as patients suffering from body dysmorphic disorder must be identified. It is incumbent on the surgeon to educate the patient about realistic results and potential risks.

Common Operative Aesthetic Procedures

I. **Breast augmentation:** performed to address micromastia (small breasts)

A. **Treatment:** Patients are counseled about four fundamental options, including size and type of implant (saline or silicone), anatomic position of the implant relative to the pectoralis major muscle (subpectoral or subglandular—on top of the muscle and below the breast gland), and location of incision (four most common access sites are the IMF, periareolar region, axilla, and umbilicus—transumbilical breast augmentation [TUBA]).

B. **Breast ptosis:** Simultaneous assessment of descent of the NAC relative to the IMF must be made. In cases of micromastia with minor ptosis, a subglandular augmentation may rotate the nipple upward and improve or even correct the ptosis.

C. **Complications:** Breast augmentation may be complicated by asymmetry, capsular contracture, diminished nipple sensation, infection, leak or rupture, etc. Due to various issues/complications, the current reoperative rate 3 years after breast augmentation is 13% for saline implants and 21% for silicone.

> **Quick Cut**
> Micromastia is essentially a subjective diagnosis and is identified by the patient.

> **Quick Cut**
> Special mammography techniques (Eklund views) are recommended to maintain sensitivity for cancer surveillance in the reconstructed breast.

II. **Rhinoplasty:** may be approached through either open or closed technique

A. **Historically:** predicated on reduction of the size of various nasal components (classically shaving/reduction of a dorsal hump)

B. **Currently:** Has evolved into a synthesis of reduction and augmentation with careful attention paid to placement of cartilage grafts and suturing techniques to define and augment various aesthetic components of the nose. It is thought that as many as 20% of rhinoplasties require revision.

> **Quick Cut**
> Male and female aesthetic ideals of the nose are quite different.

III. **Blepharoplasty:** Operative rejuvenation of the upper and/or lower eyelids may include a resection or resuspension of the skin and at times the underlying orbicularis oculi muscle.

A. **Fat herniation:** For many patients, the visible deformity of the lower lids is actually through the orbital septum, which may be repositioned, resected, or redraped during skin resection.

B. **Careful preoperative assessment:** Eye-related morbidities such as dry eyes must be assessed. Blepharoplasty may also be a reconstructive operation in the setting of redundant upper eyelid skin (dermatochalasis) leading to impaired visual fields.

> **Quick Cut**
> With all elective cosmetic procedures, careful patient selection is critical.

IV. **Liposuction:** minimal access approach to body contouring whereby the surgeon aspirates and sculpts areas of the patient's undesired fat

A. **Types:** include suction only, power-assisted, ultrasound, and laser forms

B. **Technique:** Surgeon typically starts by infusing tumescent solution into the areas to be liposuctioned. The fluid (saline or lactated Ringer) will often contain epinephrine to decrease blood loss and may contain a local anesthetic such as lidocaine to lessen pain.

C. **Complications:** include lidocaine toxicity, contour deformities or asymmetry, tunneling marks, seroma/hematoma, insufficient or overaspiration, and injury to deep structures (in the case of abdominal liposuction, this includes entry into the peritoneal cavity with possible perforation of bowel)

> **Quick Cut**
> Physiologic complications can arise from massive fluid shifts when liposuction is high volume (5 or more liters of lipoaspirate).

V. **Rhytidectomy (face-lift):** Skin of the face and/or neck is undermined to varying extents, and the underlying superficial musculoaponeurotic system (SMAS) is manipulated (typically elevated or tightened) to correct signs of aging. The skin and SMAS are ideally pulled in different vectors. Evaluation of the aging face and neck generally includes assessment of hairline and style, brow position, crow's feet, nasolabial folds, marionette lines, perioral rhytids (wrinkles), jowling, and whether or not the cervicomental angle is acute or obtuse.

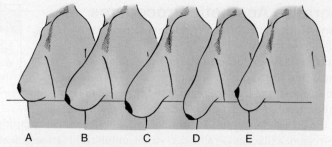

Figure 26-6: Breast ptosis. (From Thorne CH, Bartlett SP, Beasley RW, et al. *Grabb and Smith's Plastic Surgery*, 6th ed. Baltimore: Lippincott Williams & Wilkins; 2006.)

VI. Abdominoplasty: Removes redundant skin and fat from the lower abdomen typically through a hip-to-hip waistline incision. Dissection along the muscular fascia spares the umbilicus, which is transposed through a new midline opening in the abdominoplasty flap, which allows the surgeon to reapproximate the rectus muscles at the midline (linea alba) if previous pregnancy or weight gain has caused a persistent diastasis of the muscles.

VII. Mastopexy: Performed to correct varying degrees of breast ptosis (Fig. 26-6); grade determines extent of invasiveness required for a meaningful correction of the deformity.

> **Quick Cut**
> The ideal breast has all breast tissue including the nipple remaining above the IMF.

    A. Grade 1 ptosis: characterized by a nipple at the IMF
    B. Grade 2 ptosis: has the nipple below the fold
    C. Grade 3 ptosis: has a nipple at the bottom of the breast facing downward when the patient is standing

VIII. Brachioplasty: Excessive skin and fat of the upper arm (elbow to axilla) can be removed but often trades an unsightly excess of loose tissue for a sizeable and difficult to camouflage scar. As with most body aesthetic procedures, it can be enhanced by judicious use of liposuction. A staged approach may be used when significant adipose tissue is present.

> **Quick Cut**
> Contour and appearance surgery comes at the expense of scars, which may be difficult to camouflage.

IX. Chin augmentation: Changing the shape and position of the chin may be done via osteotomies and repositioning of the bony portion of the chin (mandible) or through the use of alloplastic implants (available in a variety of sizes and shapes and must be tailored by the surgeon to address each patient's aesthetic need).

    A. Technique: may be performed through intraoral access or a submental incision
    B. Evaluation: It is critical for the plastic surgeon to evaluate the patient with regard to general facial harmony and specifically, if the chin deformity relates to more complex anatomic deficiencies that must be corrected with orthognathic procedures. The first step would be to assess the patient's dental occlusion.

X. Brow lift: Location and position of eyebrows can affect a patient's appearance.

> **Quick Cut**
> Poor brow shaping and position can make a patient look old or unpleasant.

    A. Ideal position: in males, generally at or just above the superior orbital rim and straight; in females, arching and above the superior orbital rim
    B. Technique: Can be performed endoscopically or via incisions at the hairline or within the frontal hair. During this procedure, certain muscles of the forehead can be excised or transected to improve forehead wrinkling (this wrinkling may also be addressed via botulinum toxin injections).

Body Contouring after Massive Weight Loss

I. Overview: Body contouring/sculpting after massive weight loss (via any combination of diet, exercise, and/or bariatric surgery) often consists of a panel of procedures.

> **Quick Cut**
> Because obese patients are high risk, procedures may be staged to minimize operative times, pain, and blood loss.

    A. Complications: commonly, hematoma and seroma formation, widening of scars, wound healing problems, and infection

B. Patient expectations: Need to be managed starting with the first preoperative assessment. Although some patients may experience amazing results, others will require numerous procedures and have results best appreciated when clothed.

INNOVATIONS AND DEVICES IN PLASTIC SURGERY

Materials

I. **Biologic dermal matrix:** acellular dermal matrix serves as a biologic mesh that may be procured from human (cadaver) or porcine sources; primarily useful as a reinforcement in contaminated fields

II. **Synthetic meshes:** Variety of materials are available to the modern surgeon, varying in composition, arrangement of fibers, pore size, weight, and flexibility.

III. **Bone replacement:** Beyond autograft, cadaveric bone, calcium hydroxyapatite, titanium, and materials such as PEEK or PMMA may be used.

Devices

I. **Laser angiography:** used for intraoperative diagnosis of tissue necrosis and determining viability of skin flaps

II. **Doppler and tissue oximetry:** may also be used to assess tissue perfusion

Surgical Innovations

I. **Vascularized composite allografts (VCAs):** Represent the transplantation of multiple tissue types, including the functional units of hand or face transplant. Although they remain experimental, dozens of VCA have been performed to date.

II. **Bioprosthetics:** artificial materials to replace particular organs or organ functions

III. **Tissue engineering:** Use of cultured cells to recreate a missing or damaged component is still in its infancy.

Chapter 27

Neurosurgery

Kenneth M. Crandall and Charles A. Sansur

ANATOMY

Brain

I. **Skull:** Contains volume of ~1,500 mL comprising the brain (~87%), cerebrospinal fluid (CSF) (~9%), and blood vessels (~4%) in a rigid compartment; normal **cerebral blood flow (CBF)** is ~50 mL/100 g of brain tissue per minute.

II. **Monro-Kellie doctrine:** Under normal conditions, the volume of each of the three brain components is in equilibrium.

> **Quick Cut**
> The Monro-Kellie doctrine assumes that the cranial vault has a fixed maximum volume.

III. **Arterial supply**

  A. **Anterior circulation:** derived from the **internal carotid arteries**, giving rise to the **middle cerebral** and the smaller **anterior cerebral** arteries, which supply the **frontal, temporal**, and **parietal lobes** and the **deep gray matter**

  B. **Posterior circulation:** originates from the vertebral arteries

   1. **Basilar artery:** formed from the vertebral arteries at the caudal margin of the pons

   2. **Branches:** supply the **pons, cerebellum, thalamus**, and divide into the posterior cerebral arteries, which supply the **occipital lobes**

> **Quick Cut**
> The brain is one fiftieth (2%) of body weight but receives one fifth (18%) of the cardiac output.

  C. **Circle of Willis:** Arterial anastomotic circle formed by multiple arteries between the major branches of the anterior and posterior circulations. In the event of a major vessel occlusion, the blood supply to its territory may be supplied by another vessel via the circle of Willis.

IV. **Venous drainage:** All venous blood from the brain uses the internal jugular veins.

  A. **Superficial cerebral veins:** drain the cortex and subcortical white matter into the superior sagittal, transverse, petrosal, or cavernous sinuses

  B. **Deep cerebral veins:** Drain the deeper structures such as the basal ganglia and thalamus. These veins drain into the **great vein of Galen** before emptying into the **straight sinus**.

Spinal Cord

I. **Arterial supply**

  A. **Anterior spinal artery:** originates from the vertebral artery and supplies the anteromedial gray matter

  B. **Posterior spinal artery:** paired; originates from the vertebral artery

  C. **Segmental medullary arteries:** Originate at many levels from branches of the aorta and vertebral arteries. If compromised, spinal cord infarction may result.

> **Quick Cut**
> The artery of Adamkiewicz is a large medullary artery that may be interrupted during aortic surgery.

II. **Venous return:** typically parallels the arterial supply

Cerebrospinal Fluid

I. **Total volume:** Approximately 150 mL, with 25 mL located in the ventricles. CSF is continuously produced, roughly 80% by the choroid plexus, and the rest is secreted in the interstitial spaces of the brain.

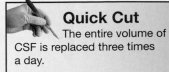
II. **Flow path: CSF flows** from the lateral **ventricles** to the third ventricle through the **foramina of Monro** and reaches the fourth ventricle via the **cerebral aqueduct of Sylvius**. It exits the ventricles to the subarachnoid space through the **foramina of Magendie** (midline) and **Luschka** (lateral).

    A. **Reabsorption:** CSF circulates around the spinal cord and the brain and is reabsorbed into the superior sagittal sinus via the arachnoid villi.

    B. **Arachnoid villi:** act as one-way valves that open at 5 mm Hg

Nervous System Functional Anatomy

I. **Unique pathophysiologic processes:** result from the complexity of the central nervous system's (CNS) functional organization, the rigidity of its bony enclosures, and its responses to injury

II. **Focal lesions:** affect neurologic function by local destruction of nervous tissue; tissue distortion with functional loss attributable to axonal stretching and subsequent synaptic damage; changes in blood flow, causing ischemia or venous congestion; and alterations in the electrical or metabolic activity of a local area, producing an epileptic focus

PATHOPHYSIOLOGY

Intracranial Pressure

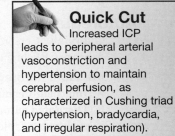
I. **Normal range:** 5–15 mm Hg; problems can develop if the intracranial pressure (ICP) becomes too high or low.

    A. **Compensatory changes:** These must offset a change in any component to maintain a normal ICP.

    B. **Rate of volume change:** has great clinical significance

        1. **Meningioma:** This slow-growing tumor can become quite large before symptoms develop or ICP increases.

        2. **Epidural hematoma:** Small, acute mass lesions can cause tremendous increase in ICP and severe neurologic deficits.

III. **Relationship between ICP and intracranial volume:** described by an exponential curve (Fig. 27-1)

    A. **Beyond the flat portion of the curve:** Intracranial components are no longer able to compensate for changes in volume; therefore, a slight increase in intracranial volume produces a very large increase in ICP.

    B. **Ischemia and herniation:** result when decreases in CSF volume can no longer maintain equilibrium

IV. **Symptoms and signs of increased ICP (intracranial hypertension):** headache, nausea/vomiting, confusion, papilledema, upward gaze paralysis (Parinaud syndrome), cranial nerve (CN) VI palsy, bulging fontanelles and splitting sutures (in infants), lethargy (eventually leading to coma), and Cushing triad (hypertension, bradycardia, and irregular respiration)

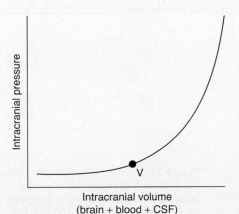

Figure 27-1: This compliance curve represents the pressure–volume relationship within the intracranial space. The ICP stays within normal limits until a critical volume (V) is reached, above which the pressure increases exponentially.

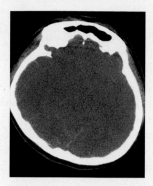

Figure 27-2: Axial CT shows diffuse cerebral edema. (From Castillo M. *Neuroradiology Companion*, 4th ed. Philadelphia: Lippincott Williams & Wilkins; 2011.)

V. ICP measurement

A. Direct: ventriculostomy or intraparenchymal/subarachnoid monitoring devices ("bolts")

B. Indirect: An estimate may be made by **lumbar puncture (LP)**; however, this should be avoided in the presence of space-occupying intracranial lesions due to herniation.

VI. Herniation: When all compensatory mechanisms have been exhausted and the ICP continues to increase, the brain "herniates" or shifts toward the low-pressure compartment (the falx and the tentorium divide the interior of the skull into compartments). Various **herniation syndromes** are recognized.

A. Subfalcine herniation (Fig. 27-2): Displacement from one supratentorial compartment to another may lead to anterior cerebral artery compression and loss of function in the opposite leg and bladder control.

B. Transtentorial (uncal) herniation: most common type of brain herniation

1. **Cause:** occurs when the medial temporal lobe is forced down over the edge of the tentorium leading to midbrain compression

2. **Neurologic signs:** progressive deterioration of consciousness, ipsilateral pupillary dilatation from oculomotor nerve compression, and contralateral hemiparesis as a result of compression of the cerebral peduncles

3. **Hemiparesis:** May be ipsilateral in a minority of cases, whereas pupillary dilatation is ipsilateral in 80%. Thus, pupillary dilatation is more reliable in localizing the lesion.

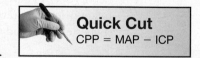

Quick Cut
Progressive deterioration in consciousness and pupillary dilatation is concerning for herniation.

C. Tonsillar herniation (transforamen magnum): Cerebellar tonsils herniate through the foramen magnum resulting in medullary compression, which leads to respiratory depression and death.

Autoregulation

I. Overview: Cerebral blood flow (CBF) versus cerebral perfusion pressure (CPP) is shown in Figure 27-3. **Average CBF:** higher to gray than white matter and is increased in areas of high neuronal activity

II. Pressure autoregulation: maintains CBF over a wide range of MAP (50–150 mm Hg) (see Fig. 27-3)

A. Intact autoregulation: ICP remains stable as blood pressure changes within the limits mentioned earlier.

B. Disrupted autoregulation: from intracranial disease processes such as head injury or tumors

III. CPP: At CPP <50 mmHg, cerebral blood flow is inadequate to provide sufficient oxygen delivery and to sustain normal metabolism.

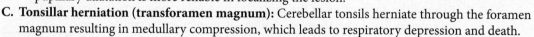

Quick Cut
CPP = MAP − ICP

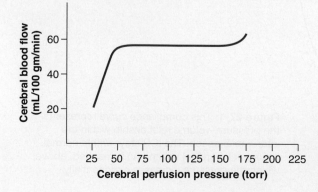

Figure 27-3: Cerebral blood flow versus cerebral perfusion pressure. Due to autoregulation, CBF remains constant for CPP between 50 and 150 mm Hg.

Cerebral Edema

I. **Overview:** The brain reacts to insults by developing edema. The rate of change in edema formation is directly proportional to the neurologic deficits and/or changes in ICP. Acute edema produces more deficits than chronic edema.

II. **Types**

A. **Cytotoxic edema:** Develops from disrupted cellular metabolism with a depletion of glucose and oxygen stores, causing retention of intracellular sodium and water. The blood–brain barrier (BBB) remains intact. Cytotoxic edema is most commonly seen following **infarcts**, cardiac arrest, and in Reye syndrome.

> **Quick Cut**
> Cytotoxic edema is most frequently seen in ischemia. Vasogenic edema is associated with tumors and hemorrhage.

B. **Vasogenic edema:** Results from breakdown of the endothelial tight junctions in the BBB, causing leakage of intravascular proteins and plasma into the extracellular space. This is the most common type of edema seen clinically and may be caused by trauma, brain tumor, infection, and surgery. Steroids may aid in the reduction of vasogenic edema.

EVALUATING THE NEUROSURGICAL PATIENT

Initial Management

I. **Patient's history:** Important; timing of symptoms along with family history of neurologic disease may be the only clues in certain diagnoses.

II. **Vital signs:** All vital signs are controlled by CNS mechanisms. Blood pressure, pulse rate, and respiration can be helpful in localizing a lesion.

A. **Hypertension/bradycardia (Cushing triad):** develops late in brain injury when irreversible neurologic changes may have already occurred

B. **Hypotension:** may be due to loss of vascular tone secondary to loss of sympathetic control, which may be secondary to hypothalamic, medullary, or spinal cord injury (SCI)

> **Quick Cut**
> Patients with intracranial hemorrhage or who require neurosurgical procedures should have coagulation parameters normalized or risk fatal bleeding.

III. **Coagulation status:** Use of antiplatelets or anticoagulants should be assessed along with prothrombin time (PT)/international normalized ratio (INR), partial thromboplastin time (PTT), and platelet levels.

Neurologic Examination

I. **Level of consciousness (LOC):** Should be determined *first*. Patients may present as alert (wide awake), lethargic (sleepy but easily arousable), stuporous (responsive only to noxious stimuli), or unresponsive (no response to noxious stimuli).

> **Quick Cut**
> A detailed neurologic evaluation should be performed on all patients. When this is not possible in emergency situations or in a comatose patient, a brief examination will have to suffice.

II. **Eye examination:** Pupils are examined for their size, symmetry, and reaction to light. Eye position and movements are assessed to aid in localizing the lesion. Funduscopic exam assesses **papilledema**.

A. **Cortical lesion:** Pupil size may be normal, but roving eye movements or gaze deviation are possible.

B. **Midbrain or oculomotor lesion:** may produce a unilateral dilated, nonreactive pupil with the eye deviated downward and outward

C. **Pons lesion:** May be associated with pinpoint pupils (1 mm); however, this can also be seen with narcotic sedation.

> **Quick Cut**
> Brain stem reflexes are very important when examining a comatose patient because the comatose patient cannot provide information on higher levels of function.

III. **Brain stem reflexes:** Check cough, gag, corneal, and oculocephalic (doll's eye) reflexes and the caloric (oculovestibular) response to rule out brain stem damage.

IV. **Motor examination:** In a comatose patient, it may only be possible to assess the response to painful stimuli. **Decorticate (flexor)** or **decerebrate (extensor)** posturing help determine location and severity of injury.

V. **Sensory level determination:** important in spinal cord lesions

VI. Deep tendon reflexes and plantar responses: checked to distinguish a lower motor neuron lesion from an upper motor neuron lesion

HEAD INJURY

Classification

I. **Brain injuries:** occurring after trauma can be classified as the following:

A. **Primary:** occurring instantaneously at the time of impact

B. **Secondary:** resulting from a chain of events triggered by the initial injury by ischemia, hypoxia, and cell-mediated death

II. **Head injuries:** can be categorized as the following:

A. **Closed head injury:** Brain injury with no evidence of scalp laceration or fracture. May result from high speed, nonimpact trauma due to rapid brain acceleration/deceleration.

B. **Blunt head injury:** With or without scalp laceration from impact with a blunt object; all scalp lacerations must be explored if there is a skull fracture present.

C. **Penetrating head injury:** secondary to bullet or knife wound

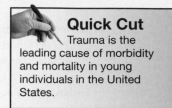

Quick Cut
Trauma is the leading cause of morbidity and mortality in young individuals in the United States.

Quick Cut
In the majority of trauma fatalities, head injury is a primary determinant of outcome.

Initial Management and Assessment

I. **Immediate care:** is not different for head trauma victims from that of any other injured patient and should be in accordance with advanced trauma life support (ATLS) guidelines (see Chapter 22)

II. **Radiographic studies**

A. **Head computed tomography (CT) scans:** Should be performed on all patients with suspected head trauma. Diagnostic findings include the following.

1. **Hematomas:** can be easily diagnosed because of the way blood appears, relative to the brain

a. **Hyperdense:** acute with normal hemoglobin

b. **Isodense:** subacute

c. **Hypodense:** chronic or acute with a low hemoglobin level

2. **Epidural hematomas:** appear as convex (lens-shaped) collections, which typically do not cross suture lines and are usually associated with an overlying skull fracture

3. **Acute subdural hematomas (SDHs):** Have a concavity toward the brain and conform to the shape of the brain surface; they may cross suture lines.

4. **Cerebral edema:** can be assessed by the size of the ventricles, basal subarachnoid cisterns, loss of sulci at the convexity, and degree of midline shift

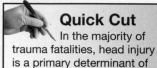

Quick Cut
All trauma patients with a suspected head injury should have head and cervical spine CT scans.

B. **Magnetic resonance imaging (MRI):** can show damage when a CT head scan result is normal in a patient with significant neurologic deficits

1. **Diffuse axonal injury (DAI):** Due to axonal shearing, injuries are imaged better with MRI compared to CT.

2. **Location:** These lesions occur frequently in the corpus callosum, subcortical white matter, and brain stem.

C. **Cervical spine CT scans (with sagittal and coronal reconstructions):** taken to rule out associated spinal injuries

1. **Cervical spine fracture or neurologic deficit referable to the cervical spine:** *absolute contraindication* for immobilization device (cervical collar) removal or performance of flexion/extension views

2. **Flexion/extension views:** In the absence of cervical fracture or cervical spinal cord deficit, these may be required to rule out ligamentous injury.

D. **Cervical spine MRI:** In the patient who has been comatose for longer than 2 weeks, this can be useful to assess for ligamentous injury, disc herniation, or SCI.

Increased Intracranial Pressure Management

I. **Goal:** Reduce CSF, brain, or blood volume within the skull.

A. **Head elevation:** Promotes venous drainage, thereby decreasing ICP. Also, keeping the patient's head straight promotes drainage through the bilateral jugular veins.

B. Hyperventilation: Rapidly helps lower ICP. The cerebral vessels respond quickly to decreasing the arterial Pco_2, causing vasoconstriction; the Pco_2 is maintained between 30 and 35 mm Hg.

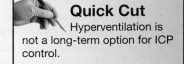

Quick Cut
Hyperventilation is not a long-term option for ICP control.

C. Sedation and paralysis: Blunting the increases in ICP seen with agitation and movement; however, this also compromises the ability to assess the patient's neurologic status. Therefore, short-acting agents such as propofol and fentanyl are recommended. Paralytics may be a last resort.

D. Increasing the serum osmolality (to ~310–320 mOsm): Decreases ICP by pulling fluid out of the brain. Serum osmolality and electrolytes have to be measured every 6 hours.

  1. **Hyperosmolar agents (e.g., mannitol):** Administered intravenously (IV) with a bolus of 1.0 g/kg followed by infusion of 25–50 g every 4–6 hours. Effects can be seen in 5–20 minutes.

  2. **Diuretics:** such as furosemide

  3. **Hypertonic saline:** elevates the patient's sodium (no greater than 155 mEq/L) to pull fluid away from the brain

E. Ventriculostomy: can rapidly decrease a patient's ICP, particularly if hydrocephalus is present, via CSF removal

F. Barbiturates: May be used if all of the previously mentioned efforts fail to lower the ICP. They work by decreasing brain metabolism and therefore intracerebral blood volume; however, they are also associated with hypotension, which can worsen brain injury. Today, they are only given to select patients.

G. Decompressive craniectomy: Removal of part of the skull allows the brain to expand and is used when the aforementioned medical therapies have failed.

II. ICP monitor: Placement is necessary to evaluate the neurologic status and ICP therapy in the unconscious patient.

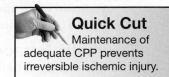

Quick Cut
Maintenance of adequate CPP prevents irreversible ischemic injury.

A. Criteria for placement: Glasgow Coma Scale (GCS) score of 8 or less in a patient with an abnormal head CT *or* GCS less than 8, a normal head CT, age older than 40 years, hypotensive, and/or has decerebrate/decorticate posturing

B. Devices

  1. **Ventriculostomy (intraventricular catheter [IVC] or external ventricular drain [EVD]):** Gold standard, giving the most accurate measurement; allows CSF removal to help lower the ICP. There is a risk of hemorrhage and infection, especially with prolonged use.

  2. **Intraparenchymal monitors/subarachnoid monitors:** Fiber-optic ICP probes useful when a ventriculostomy catheter cannot be placed. Sometimes they screw into the skull via a bolt mechanism. They have a lower risk of infection and parenchymal hemorrhage compared to IVC.

Quick Cut
A ventriculostomy provides constant monitoring of ICP and allows for therapeutic drainage.

III. Consumptive coagulopathy: Severe brain injury causes release of tissue thromboplastin, which activates the extrinsic clotting pathway and can lead to abnormalities in clotting and even disseminated intravascular coagulopathy (DIC). The patient's PT/INR, PTT, and platelet levels should be monitored and corrected accordingly.

IV. Seizure prophylaxis: Risk of post-traumatic epilepsy correlates with severity and location of underlying brain injury.

A. Risk factors: subdural, epidural, or intraparenchymal (contusion) hemorrhages; depressed skull fracture; GCS less than 10; and penetrating brain injury

Quick Cut
Patients with evidence of intracranial hemorrhage should receive seizure prophylaxis for at least 1 week.

B. Phenytoin: Give 1.0 g IV or by mouth as loading dose, followed by 300 mg per day. Dose for children is 10 mg/kg initially, followed by maintenance at ~5 mg/kg per day. Continue for 7 days, unless the patient has had a seizure.

Scalp Injury Management

I. Scalp: Highly vascular; patients can lose large volumes of blood if lacerations are not promptly addressed.

II. Debridement: Thoroughly debride prior to closure, especially if a skull fracture is present.

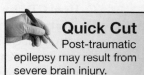

Quick Cut
Post-traumatic epilepsy may result from severe brain injury.

III. **Fractures:** can be classified as follows:
   A. **Linear, stellate, or comminuted:** describe complexity of the fracture line
   B. **Depressed fractures:** have a skull portion that is displaced inward
   C. **Compound fractures:** Overlying scalp is lacerated.
   D. **Basilar fractures:** Traverse the base of the skull; patients may have ecchymosis behind the ear (Battle sign), which may be associated with otorrhea or hemotympanum. Anterior basilar fractures result in periorbital ecchymosis (raccoon's eyes) and possibly rhinorrhea.

IV. **Operative intervention**
   A. **Depressed skull fractures:** May be associated with dural tear and underlying brain damage. Depressed skull fractures greater than 1 cm are usually surgically elevated.
   B. **Compound fractures:** require a thorough debridement and closure to prevent subsequent infection

Traumatic Cerebrospinal Fluid Leaks

I. **Diagnosis:** Assess the fluid for **beta-2 transferrin**; if blood is mixed with the CSF, allow some to drip onto a gauze and assess for the "**halo sign.**"

II. **Post-traumatic CSF fistulas:** Ninety-five percent close spontaneously with conservative management, which includes elevating the head.
   A. **Lumbar CSF drain:** placed in some cases to divert CSF drainage and promote fistula healing
   B. **Craniotomy with closure of the dural defect:** may be necessary if lumbar drainage fails
   C. **Broad spectrum, prophylactic antibiotics:** recommended to prevent associated infection

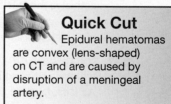

Quick Cut
Most traumatic CSF leaks resolve without surgical intervention.

Traumatic Intracerebral Hemorrhages and Cerebral Contusions

I. **Intracerebral hematomas:** result from vessel tearing in white matter and are due to penetrating trauma or acceleration–deceleration injuries

II. **Cerebral contusions:** Superficial hemorrhages occur when the anterior temporal and frontal lobes strike the rough edges of the tentorium or skull.
   A. **Coup injury:** occurs when the skull strikes the brain underlying the site of impact
   B. **Contrecoup injury:** Occurs directly opposite to the impact site when the brain strikes the inner table of the skull on the opposite side along the force vector. Thus, if a person were struck on the back of the head, the coup injury would be to the occipital lobe and the frontotemporal tips would sustain the contrecoup injury.

III. **Management:** Typically consists of monitoring the patient closely in the intensive care unit (ICU) and repeating the CT scan to assess for changes. Surgical decompression may be necessary when increased ICP becomes refractory to medical management or if the hematoma significantly expands.

Extra-axial Hemorrhages

I. **Epidural hematoma:** collection of blood between the bone and dura, usually of **arterial origin** (high pressure), caused by laceration of the middle meningeal artery with an associated fracture of temporal bone
   A. **Less common etiologies:** Bleeding from the middle meningeal vein or dural venous sinus. Younger patients are at higher risk because their dura are less adherent to the inner table of the skull.

Quick Cut
Epidural hematomas are convex (lens-shaped) on CT and are caused by disruption of a meningeal artery.

   B. **Diagnosis:** Classically, patients present with a **lucid interval**. The patient is knocked out immediately after injury (concussion effect), then regains consciousness but has a headache, and then loses consciousness over minutes to hours as the hematoma expands and creates mass effect (however, this presentation is seen in only 10%–15% of cases).
   C. **Head CT:** characteristic appearance of a convex, lens-shaped high density adjacent to bone
   D. **Treatment:** Very small epidural hematomas without clinical deficits can be conservatively managed with serial CT scans and close clinical observation. Sedation should be minimized because this may alter the patient's neurologic exam. Those that are associated with neurologic deficits or that cause mass effect must be evacuated.

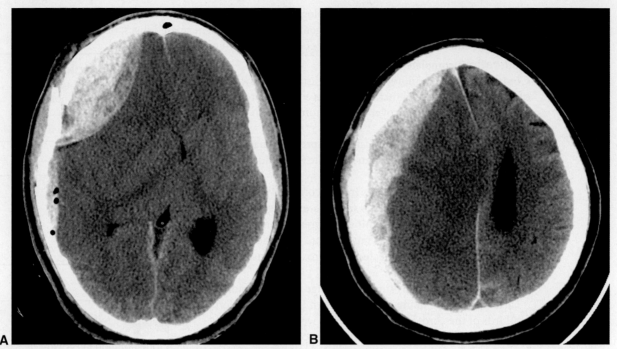

Figure 27-4: Contrast-enhanced CT scan of extra-axial hematomas. **A:** Epidural hematoma. Note the lenticular shape. **B:** Subdural hematoma on the patient's right side. Note the crescent shape of the hematoma. (From Haines DE. Neuroanatomy in Clinical Context. Wolters Kluwer; 2014.)

II. **SDH:** collection of acute or chronic blood that accumulates between the dura and the arachnoid

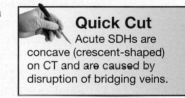

Quick Cut
Acute SDHs are concave (crescent-shaped) on CT and are caused by disruption of bridging veins.

   A. **Etiology:** Typically from disrupted **bridging veins** between the dura and the cortical surface. Older patients are at an increased risk due to brain atrophy causing increased vulnerability to the bridging veins. **Chronic SDH** can also develop from membranes formed from hematoma breakdown.
   B. **Acute SDH:** Presents as an evolving and expanding mass lesion. Often, mental status deteriorates with worsening neurologic deficits.
      1. **Diagnosis:** On CT, a hyperdense concave mass is present between the brain and the skull (Fig. 27-4).
      2. **Treatment:** if decreased mentation or focal neurologic symptoms, usually requires craniotomy and clot evacuation
   C. **Chronic SDH:** often a subtle, slow, progressive deterioration (e.g., headache, hemiparesis, aphasia) over weeks or months, which often presents as dementia in the elderly patient
      1. **Diagnosis:** On CT scan, the concave mass appears either isodense or hypodense depending on the chronicity of the hematoma; 50% are bilateral.
      2. **Treatment:** Can often be treated initially with burr hole drainage of the clot; reaccumulation can require craniotomy for definitive drainage and removal of the membranes.

SPINAL CORD INJURY

Overview

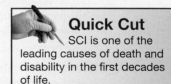

Quick Cut
SCI is one of the leading causes of death and disability in the first decades of life.

   I. **Epidemiology:** 4:1 preponderance of SCI among males to females
      A. **Cause:** Most occur as the result of motor vehicle collisions and falls.
      B. **Incidence:** One million people have traumatic SCI each year in the United States.

II. **Extent of injury:** depends on the morphology and the location of the fracture, the presence of pre-existing degenerative disease (e.g., congenital canal stenosis, herniated discs, or ligamentous hypertrophy), and the patient's age and associated systemic injuries

III. **Classification:** complete or incomplete
   A. **Complete SCIs:** No motor or sensory function below the level of the injury (including rectal). This has a dismal prognosis; 1% exhibit significant recovery if symptoms remain for 24 hours.
   B. **Incomplete SCIs:** Rapid surgical decompression may help restore function in these patients. Specific SCI syndromes include the following.
      1. **Central cord injury:** Results from a concussive blow to the cord, typically in patients with pre-existing stenosis. Deficits in the upper extremities are greater than in the lower extremities and peripheral musculature (e.g., the hands) are usually more severely affected than proximal musculature (e.g., the shoulders).
      2. **Anterior SCI:** Usually involves damage to the anterior spinal artery, resulting in infarction or ischemia of the anterior two thirds of the cord. Significant muscle weakness is seen.
      3. **Brown-Séquard syndrome:** typically occurs from hemisection of the cord after penetrating trauma

Management

I. **Spine immobilization:** Patients should be put in a hard cervical collar and on a hard board in the field *before* the patient is transferred to the hospital.

II. **Proper transfer techniques:** Log-rolling and scoop stretchers while maintaining cervical traction ensure that full spinal precautions are being maintained.

III. **Stabilization:** ATLS protocols (A, B, C, D, E) apply.
   A. **Complete SCI:** Patient may not feel pain associated with a broken limb or with an internal hemorrhage.
   B. **Vital signs:** Observation is critical.
   C. **Cervical or high thoracic SCIs:** Patients may have neurogenic shock secondary to interruption of the sympathetic pathways.
      1. **Signs:** These patients will develop hypotension in association with bradycardia, secondary to unopposed vagal tone.
      2. **Management:** Patients often require volume resuscitation and may also need pressor agents.

IV. **Neurologic evaluation:** Emergency medical personnel may disclose whether the patient ever exhibited motor function.
   A. **Detailed motor and sensory exam:** must be assessed in all four extremities to determine motor and sensory level
   B. **Reflexes:** Sacral reflexes are important because of sparing of the sacral segment of the cord—prognosis for recovery is better if the patient exhibits sacral sparing. Abdominal, cremasteric, and sphincteric reflexes (e.g., bulbocavernosus and anal twitch) must also be assessed.

V. **Radiographic studies:** Patients with suspected injury require cervical spine imaging.
   A. **CT scan:** Sagittal and coronal reconstructions are recommended. Back pain or neurologic symptoms localizing to the thoracic and lumbosacral spine may require additional CT imaging.

Quick Cut
Complete SCI patients have no motor or sensory function below the level of the injury.

Quick Cut
The hallmark presentation of SCI is preservation of light touch, position sense, and vibration.

Quick Cut
The hallmark presentation in Brown-Séquard syndrome is ipsilateral loss of motor function, light touch, and vibration with a contralateral loss of pain and temperature.

Quick Cut
About 15% of patients suffer some improper manipulation of the spine before they arrive at the hospital.

Quick Cut
Methylprednisolone has not been shown to improve outcomes in SCI and is associated with complications.

Quick Cut
Any trauma patient with neck pain, neurologic deficit, or a high-risk mechanism of an injury should be considered to have a cervical cord injury.

    B. **MRI:** If a bony abnormality is identified with CT scan, an additional evaluation with MRI may be necessary, which can reveal spinal cord abnormalities and extra-axial abnormalities (e.g., epidural hematoma, ruptured disc, or ligamentous injury).

    C. **CT myelogram of the spine:** may be necessary in patients with contraindications to MRI (e.g., cardiac pacemaker)

VI. Treatment

    A. **Immobilization:** Nonoperative management is possible if the fracture is not severe, alignment is preserved, and neural elements are not compressed.

      1. **Minor fractures or ligamentous injuries:** hard cervical collar

      2. **More complex fractures:** may heal by the patient wearing a halo device for at least 3 months

    B. **Open reduction and internal fixation:** definitive management for unstable spine fractures

      1. **Immediate surgical intervention:** required in patients with incomplete SCI and in patients who exhibit progressive neurologic deterioration with an MRI scan suggestive of spinal cord or nerve root compression

      2. **Fusion:** allows patients to be more quickly mobilized and rehabilitated, which decreases morbidity from complications secondary to SCI

VII. Complications: Patients with SCIs can suffer from several problems.

    A. **Hypotension:** in the acute setting

    B. **Ileus:** can last 10–14 days

    C. **Renal:** stones, pyelonephritis, and renal failure

    D. **Deep venous thrombosis (DVT):** can lead to pulmonary embolus (PE)

      1. **DVT prophylaxis:** Compression boots are imperative. Often, patients also receive IVC filters.

      2. **Medical:** These patients are also placed on a prophylactic regimen of subcutaneous or low-molecular-weight heparin.

    E. **Infections:** urinary tract infections, pneumonia, and from decubitus ulcers

> **Quick Cut**
> Patients with SCI have many complications, which contribute to morbidity and mortality.

Intracerebral Hemorrhage

I. Hypertensive intracerebral hemorrhage: Also known as *hemorrhagic stroke*, these occur within the brain parenchyma, usually at the site of smaller, perforating arterioles.

    A. **Locations:** basal ganglia, thalamus, cerebellum, and pons

    B. **Diagnosis:** Usually, a history of long-standing hypertension and a relatively sudden onset of focal neurologic deficits, with or without decreased mentation. These patients typically have headache.

> **Quick Cut**
> Intracerebral hemorrhage is less common than ischemic stroke but has a worse prognosis.

      1. **Unenhanced CT scan:** Study of choice; differentiates from ischemic stroke, which may present similarly; however, the treatment is quite different.

      2. **Blood counts and coagulation function:** should be corrected

      3. **Vascular imaging:** May rule out other causes of hemorrhage (vascular malformations, aneurysms). Contrasted MRI will evaluate for tumors and cavernous malformations.

    C. **Treatment:** typically supportive by controlling hypertension and correcting any bleeding disorder to prevent clot expansion and further neurologic decline

      1. **Supratentorial hemorrhages:** Most are associated with significant deficits. Surgery is reserved only for those in reasonable condition with surgically accessible lesions.

      2. **Infratentorial hemorrhages:** frequently require emergent evacuation to prevent brain stem compression

II. Vascular malformations: Typically present with either hemorrhage or seizure. Hemorrhages can present as intracerebral or subarachnoid with acute neurologic changes and headache.

    A. **Types**

      1. **Arteriovenous malformation (AVM):** Most common type; composed of shunts between vessels. Normal brain is not usually seen.

      2. **Telangiectasia:** Capillary tufts are separated by normal brain commonly in the pons; it is unlikely to bleed.

3. **Cavernous malformations (cavernomas):** Packed sinusoidal vessels without normal brain that can occur anywhere in the brain and are often multiple. Familial forms have been documented.
4. **Developmental venous anomalies:** Extensive venous networks and a normal variant of venous drainage. These are benign lesions but may be associated with cavernomas.

B. **Diagnosis**
1. **Noncontrasted CT scan:** first study to order in any patient with acute neurologic changes
2. **Vascular imaging:** Necessary whenever a vascular malformation is suspected. Conventional angiogram is the standard; CT and magnetic resonance angiogram are used more frequently.

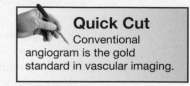

Quick Cut
Conventional angiogram is the gold standard in vascular imaging.

C. **Treatment:** depending on the size and location of the malformation, may include surgery, endovascular embolization, and radiosurgery (or a combination) in addition to the following:
1. **Ventriculostomy:** may be required to control increased mass effect and ICP, especially if blood has leaked into the ventricles and hydrocephalus is present
2. **Hypertension:** should be managed aggressively
3. **Seizure activity:** treated or prophylaxed

III. **Other causes:** Associated with other disease processes, such as a brain tumors (e.g., renal cell carcinoma, melanoma), cerebral vasculitis, anticoagulation therapy, blood dyscrasias (e.g., thrombocytopenia, leukemia), systemic lupus erythematosus, or Sturge-Weber syndrome. Contrasted MRI scan may be helpful.

Subarachnoid Hemorrhage

I. **Cause:** Most commonly caused by head trauma; however, it may also be spontaneous (e.g., aneurysm or AVM).
A. **Spontaneous SAH due to aneurysm rupture:** Usually associated with sudden, severe headache (worst headache of life), vomiting, stiff neck, photophobia, altered mental status, and sometimes a history of an earlier severe so-called "herald headache." Certain aneurysms are associated with specific neurologic findings.
1. **Posterior communicating artery aneurysm:** associated with CN III palsy
2. **Internal carotid–ophthalmic aneurysm:** associated with monocular visual field cut

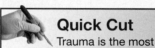

Quick Cut
Trauma is the most common overall cause of subarachnoid hemorrhage (SAH). Aneurysms are the most common cause of spontaneous SAH.

B. **Diagnosis:** CT demonstrates nearly 90% of all SAH. Traumatic SAH is typically seen on the cortical surface, whereas aneurysmal SAH is concentrated in the basilar cisterns (circle of Willis).
1. **Negative CT:** if no mass effect, safe to proceed with LP, which may demonstrate high red blood cell count and xanthochromia
2. **Positive CT or LP:** Angiogram will be needed to determine the number of aneurysms (15% have multiple aneurysms) and whether a correlation exists between aneurysm size/shape and risk of rupture.
3. **Repeat angiogram:** Fifteen percent of patients do not exhibit an angiographically identifiable source of SAH and need another once the subarachnoid blood has dissipated.

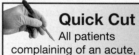

Quick Cut
All patients complaining of an acute, severe headache should be evaluated for SAH with a CT scan.

II. **Types**
A. **Berry aneurysms:** most common; weak areas of the blood vessel wall, typically at a bifurcation
B. **Mycotic aneurysms:** arise secondary to infection, commonly endocarditis
C. **Atherosclerotic aneurysms:** form ectatic or fusiform dilation

III. **Treatment:** Prompt treatment of ruptured aneurysms is required, as they have the propensity to rehemorrhage, particularly in the first 2 weeks.
A. **Craniotomy and surgical clipping:** Standard management of Berry aneurysms. A small metallic clip is placed at the neck to deny flow to the weakened, dilated dome.
B. **Endovascular obliteration:** Fast becoming a main treatment option, particularly in locations difficult to access surgically. Small metal coils are fed into the aneurysm dome through

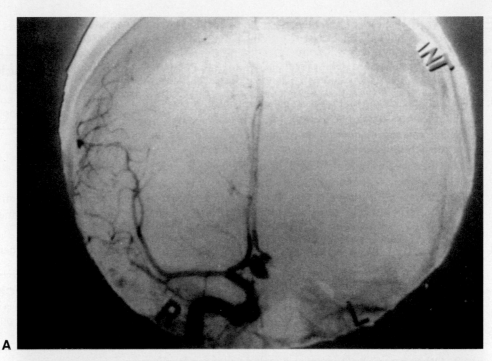

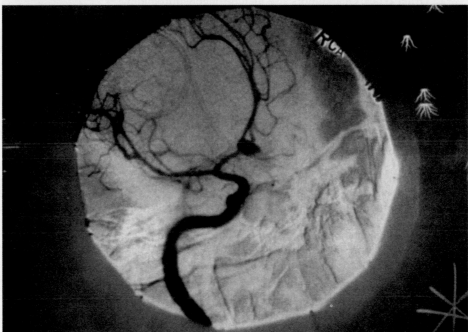

Figure 27-5: Oblique cerebral angiogram. **A:** Right intracranial aneurysm. **B:** After an endovascular coiling of the aneurysm, there is no longer any flow to the aneurysm dome.

angiographically guided microcatheters (Fig. 27-5). The obvious risk of this technique is vessel perforation with catastrophic consequences.

C. ICU: SAH patients require extensive care to address a host of problems, such as hypertension, hyponatremia, cardiac arrhythmias, vasospasm, stroke, and hydrocephalus.

D. Antibiotic therapy: can resolve mycotic aneurysms

IV. Prognosis: Rate of hemorrhage from an unruptured aneurysm is 1%–3% per year; ~10%–15% of patients die before they reach hospital care, and another 40%–50% die during their acute hospitalization. Of those surviving patients, ~50% are able to return to their former lifestyle; the rest survive with impairment.

CENTRAL NERVOUS SYSTEM TUMORS

Overview

I. **Overall incidence:** 10,000–13,000 new brain tumor cases in the United States per year; 4,000 cases of spinal cord tumors

II. **Bimodal distribution:** for the frequency of brain tumors
   A. **First age peak:** occurs in childhood (age 3–10 years)
      1. **Location:** Fifty percent of pediatric brain tumors occur in the posterior fossa, and 50% are supratentorial.
      2. **Common brain tumors in children:** pilocytic astrocytoma, medulloblastoma, craniopharyngioma, and brain stem glioma
   B. **Second age peak:** Occurs in the sixth decade; 75% of adult brain tumors are supratentorial. Common adult brain tumors include metastasis, malignant gliomas, meningiomas, and pituitary adenomas.

III. **Classification:** Nomenclature for CNS is often confusing; most are named based on their cellular origin.
   A. **Glial tumors (gliomas):** constitute nearly 50% of brain tumors; derive from **glial cell lines**
      1. **Histologic grading:** increasing malignancy from low-grade astrocytoma to anaplastic astrocytoma to glioblastoma multiforme (GBM)
      2. **Other types:** Glial tumors also include oligodendrogliomas and ependymomas.
   B. **Nonglial cell tumors: meningiomas** (which arise from arachnoid cells), **schwannomas** (from Schwann cells), **medulloblastomas** (from primitive neuroectodermal remnants), **pituitary tumors** (from hormonal cells in the pituitary gland), **pineal tumors** (often from germ cells), and tumors arising from the blood vessels (**hemangioblastomas** and **metastatic tumors**)

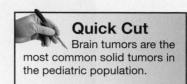

Quick Cut
Brain tumors are the most common solid tumors in the pediatric population.

Quick Cut
GBM is the most common adult primary brain tumor.

Diagnosis

I. **Presentation:** Patients present with symptoms via several mechanisms.
   A. **Mass effect:** Brain and spinal cord are relatively intolerant of space-occupying lesions, which compete with normal tissue within the rigid skull or spinal canal—again, CNS tissues are much more tolerant of slow-growing lesions than rapid volume change.
   B. **Eloquence:** Tumors in eloquent areas of the brain become symptomatic early.
   C. **Blood vessel compression:** May deprive normal areas of the CNS from vital nutrients. Highly metabolic tumors may also "steal" blood from surrounding brain.
   D. **Metabolic impairment:** Chemical messengers produced can interfere with normal "host" brain function.
   E. **Seizures:** caused either by direct mechanical irritation or by affecting normal brain metabolism
   F. **CSF outflow obstruction:** leads to hydrocephalus

Quick Cut
The more eloquent the region where the tumor arises, the more dramatic the patient's symptoms.

II. **Neurologic evaluation:** Look for a history of acute onset or progressive neurologic deficits; asymmetry may aid in localization, and an examination that indicates specific lobar dysfunction is highly suspicious for a focal lesion, such as a brain tumor.

III. **Additional studies:** Required to characterize the lesion. Contrasted CT and MRI scans must demonstrate disruption of the BBB (a frequent manifestation in the vicinity of a tumor).

Specific Brain Tumors

I. **Astrocytomas:** Most common brain tumor in adults; they are slow-growing and infiltrating with poorly defined borders.
   A. **Peak incidence:** during the fourth decade of life
   B. **Clinical presentation:** seizures, headaches, increased ICP, and focal neurologic deficits
   C. **Imaging:** CT and MRI scans show irregular nonhomogeneous enhancement with edema surrounding the tumor (Fig. 27-6).

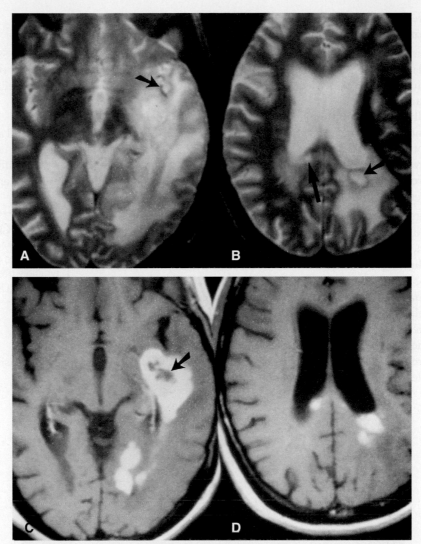

Figure 27-6: A–D: MRI of glioblastoma multiforme. The borders of this lesion enhances brightly with contrast. The *arrows* point to the hypointense core signifies central necrosis (a sign of aggressiveness).

  D. Treatment: chemotherapy as well as the following:
   1. **Aggressive surgical resection:** However, complete resection is nearly impossible given the infiltrative nature of the tumor.
   2. **Radiation therapy:** possibly including high-dose radiosurgery to the site of the tumor
  E. Prognosis: Highly correlated with histologic grade; however, age, comorbidities, and neurologic insult play a role.
 II. **Ependymomas:** generally well-circumscribed tumors that occur in the vicinity of ventricles; may metastasize to other locations through the CSF
  A. Clinical presentation: often includes increased ICP, hydrocephalus, and other focal neurologic symptoms
  B. Imaging: Contrasted MRI or CT scan shows an irregularly enhancing lesion with a well-defined border in the vicinity of the ventricle. Additional imaging of the entire neuraxis is important to rule out metastasis.
  C. Treatment: aggressive surgical resection and radiation
  D. Prognosis: Median survival is 5 years.
 III. **Oligodendrogliomas:** slow-growing gliomas that often have calcification
  A. Clinical presentation: most commonly seizures; often a focal neurologic deficit
  B. Imaging: CT and MRI scans reveal calcified areas in nearly 40%–50%.

    C. Treatment: resection, with or without radiation therapy

    D. Prognosis: Survival rate is 3–10 years depending on grade.

IV. Meningiomas: Arise from the arachnoid layer of the meninges and account for 15% of intracranial neoplasms. Lesions are usually adjacent to the dura with a well-defined border and compress (rather than invade) the brain. Meningiomas are very slow growing and may become incredibly large before producing symptoms.

    A. Clinical presentation: headache, focal neurologic deficits, and seizures

    B. Imaging: CT and MRI scans reveal homogenous, intensely enhancing mass and a well-demarcated border with normal tissue (Fig. 27-7).

    C. Treatment: surgical excision, although stereotactic radiosurgery can be used for difficult to reach lesions

    D. Prognosis: Usually good; however, factors such as location, extent of resection, and grade could create a poorer prognosis.

V. Metastatic tumors: Approximately 20% of cancer patients will develop intracranial metastases, most commonly from the lung, breast, kidney, and melanomas.

> **Quick Cut**
> Metastatic brain tumors are common and typically present as multiple enhancing lesions on MRI.

    A. Clinical presentation: increased ICP, obstructive hydrocephalus, focal neurologic deficit, and spontaneous intracerebral hemorrhage

    B. Imaging: CT and MRI scans reveal multiple well-circumscribed, enhancing masses surrounded by cerebral edema.

    C. Treatment: resection if the lesion is solitary or the histology is in question, steroids, and whole-brain radiation

    D. Prognosis: With treatment, ~50% of patients with a single intracranial metastasis will live for 1 year after diagnosis.

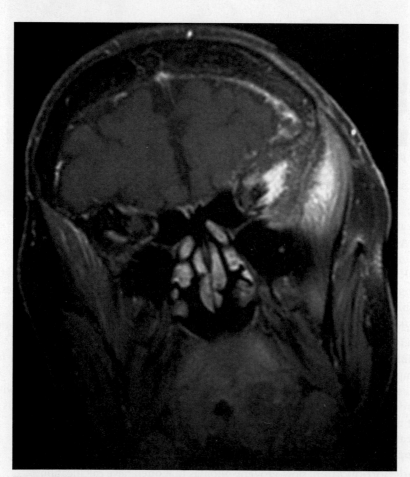

Figure 27-7: T_2-weighted coronal MRI shows left sphenoid wing meningioma. (From Penne RB. *Wills Eye Institute—Oculoplastics*, 2nd ed. Philadelphia: Lippincott Williams & Wilkins; 2011.)

VI. Medulloblastomas: Malignant tumors of the cerebellum and the fourth ventricle from primitive neuroectodermal cells. These tumors present during the first and second decades of life, with a male predominance.
   A. **Clinical presentation:** cerebellar and brain stem dysfunction, hydrocephalus, and increased ICP
   B. **Imaging:** Contrasted CT and MRI scans demonstrate a nonhomogenous, enhancing midline mass usually adjacent to or in the fourth ventricle.
   C. **Treatment:** Extensive surgical resection and radiation therapy to the site and the entire neuraxis to prevent CSF seeding. Radiation therapy cannot always be used in young children, and chemotherapy remains the treatment of choice after surgery.
   D. **Prognosis:** 5–10 year survival but highly dependent on age, extent of resection, and sensitivity to chemoradiation

VII. Hemangioblastomas: most common primary intra-axial tumor in the posterior fossa in adults; can be associated with von Hippel-Lindau disease (along with hemangioblastomas in other organs)

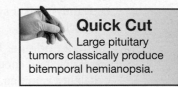

> **Quick Cut**
> Cerebral hemangioblastomas may be associated with von Hippel-Lindau disease.

   A. **Clinical presentation:** Cerebellar dysfunction and possibly hydrocephalus; 10% of patients have erythrocytosis secondary to erythropoietin secretion from the tumor.
   B. **Imaging:** CT and MRI scans usually reveal an enhancing mural nodule within a cyst, and angiography reveals an intense vascular blush.
   C. **Treatment:** Surgical resection is the treatment of choice.
   D. **Prognosis:** generally good

VIII. Vestibular schwannomas (acoustic neuromas): arise from the vestibular portion of CN VIII
   A. **Clinical presentation:** These benign tumors usually present with tinnitus, hearing loss, and evolving unsteadiness. CN VII may be compromised, leading to facial weakness.
   B. **Imaging:** Enhanced CT and MRI scans often demonstrate the acoustic neuroma arising from the internal auditory meatus.
   C. **Evaluation:** Brain stem auditory evoked potentials and audiometric testing are very useful for evaluating these lesions.
   D. **Treatment:** resection, stereotactic radiosurgery, or both
   E. **Prognosis:** Related to tumor size and extent of resection. Both hearing preservation along with facial nerve function are important in determining treatment and prognosis.

Pituitary Tumors

   I. **Clinical presentation:** Pituitary tumors tend to present in several ways.
   A. **Mass effect:** Through compression of the optic chiasm. Classically, the patient presents with bitemporal hemianopsia.
   B. **Endocrinopathy:** Hormonal over- or underproduction causing Cushing syndrome (secondary to excess adrenocorticotropic hormone secretion), acromegaly (secondary to excessive growth hormone secretion), hyperprolactinemia, or hypopituitarism. However, 30% of patients have a nonsecreting adenoma.

> **Quick Cut**
> Large pituitary tumors classically produce bitemporal hemianopsia.

   C. **Apoplexy:** This is an acute hemorrhage into a pituitary tumor. Commonly, these patients will have headache, impaired vision, extraocular muscle dysfunction, and endocrinopathy.

   II. **Diagnostic tests**
   A. **Laboratory analysis:** of the pituitary-related hormones
   B. **Contrasted CT and MRI scans:** demonstrate the tumor along with the surrounding brain structures and bony anatomy

   III. **Treatment**
   A. **Prolactin-secreting adenomas:** Medical therapy, such as **bromocriptine** (a dopaminergic agonist), is the first-line therapy.
   B. **Surgical resection:** Treatment of choice for most non–prolactin-secreting tumors and prolactinomas that are progressively symptomatic despite medical therapy. This is especially true for tumors compressing the optic chiasm with visual field deficits.
      1. **Tumors with little suprasellar extension:** Endoscopic trans-sphenoidal route (nasal or sublabial) can be used.
      2. **Larger tumors:** Craniotomy may be required.

C. Stereotactic radiosurgery: may be used as an adjunct after partial surgical resection and is effective in controlling ~90% of pituitary adenomas that remain after surgery

CONGENITAL NERVOUS SYSTEM LESIONS

Spinal Dysraphism

I. **Spina bifida:** results from failure of the vertebral arches to fuse
  A. **Diagnosis:** It may be totally asymptomatic and be found incidentally on spinal radiograph (spina bifida occulta), or it may be symptomatic.
  B. **Associated congenital anomalies:** can include dermal sinus, diastematomyelia (splitting of the cord into halves), or a tethered spinal cord

II. **Meningocele:** This rare lesion is a saclike posterior midline herniation of the dura mater and is usually not associated with any neurologic deficits. Repair is indicated primarily for cosmetic reasons.

III. **Myelomeningocele:** Herniation of the dura mater and neural elements posteriorly as a result of incomplete closure of the neural tube. This lesion may be associated with hydrocephalus.
  A. **Surgical treatment:** Aimed at closure of the defect. A ventriculoperitoneal (VP) shunt may be necessary if hydrocephalus is present.
  B. **Neurologic defects:** Common; severity is related to the location of the lesion. Higher lesions have a worse prognosis.

> **Quick Cut**
> Spinal dysraphism is usually defective fusion of a raphe and is associated with findings on general physical examination highly suggestive of an underlying abnormality, such as a tuft of hair, nevus, lipoma, abnormal blood vessels, a dimple, or a sinus tract.

Hydrocephalus

I. **Overview:** *Hydrocephalus* literally means "water head," and the abnormality may be congenital or acquired. It is caused by an obstruction to the flow (obstructive hydrocephalus) or reabsorption (communicating hydrocephalus) of CSF.

II. **Etiology:** Most common causes are as follows.
  A. **Complications of intraventricular hemorrhage:** in prematurity
  B. **Aqueductal stenosis**
  C. **Chiari malformation**
    1. **Type I:** Most common; cerebellar tonsils are low lying within the foramen magnum.
    2. **Type II:** associated with myelomeningocele; downward herniation of the fourth ventricle
    3. **Types III and IV:** rare and either cause severe neurologic deficits or are incompatible with life
  D. **Dandy-Walker syndrome:** agenesis of the cerebellar vermis and the foramina of Magendie and Luschka

III. **Clinical findings:** Infants may present with bulging fontanelles, scalp vein dilatation, rapidly increasing head circumference, decreased upward gaze (sun-setting eyes), papilledema, lethargy, irritability, vomiting, and ataxia.

IV. **Treatment:** CT scan or cranial ultrasound (in neonates) shows a dilated ventricular system. MRI may be useful in determining the etiology.
  A. **VP shunt:** Most commonly used method of diverting CSF. Other locations of diversion include the atria of the heart and the pleura.
  B. **Endoscopic third ventriculostomy:** involves the creation of a hole in the floor of the third ventricle, thus diverting the CSF around an obstruction (such as aqueductal stenosis)

> **Quick Cut**
> Ventriculoperitoneal shunting is the most common treatment for hydrocephalus as the peritoneum can reabsorb significant amounts of excess CSF.

FUNCTIONAL NEUROSURGERY

Movement Disorders

I. **Overview:** Many advancements have been made in the treatment of movement disorders (such as Parkinson disease and essential tremor). Initially, lesions were made to destroy the abnormally functioning areas of brain. Today, through deep brain stimulation (DBS), electrodes are placed into the brain and connected to a stimulator to help modulate the abnormal areas.

II. **Parkinson disease:** disorder caused by destruction of dopamine-generating cells in the brain, leading to a malfunction in the basal ganglia
   A. **Presentation:** resting tremor, rigidity, and bradykinesia
   B. **Treatment:** Although there is no cure, symptoms are managed initially using medications, which may have severe side effects. Certain patients are candidates for DBS of the **subthalamic nucleus**. The globus pallidus internus is another therapeutic target but has less of an effect.

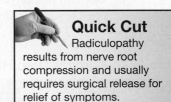

Quick Cut
DBS of the subthalamic nucleus is used in the treatment of Parkinson disease.

III. **Essential tremor:** Characterized by severe intention tremor when a patient tries to perform an action. Similar to Parkinson disease, the symptoms have been significantly improved through DBS (stimulating the ventral intermediate nucleus of the thalamus).

Epilepsy

I. **Etiology:** Recurrent seizures can be a debilitating condition with multiple etiologies.

II. **Treatment:** Mainstay includes antiepileptic drugs, all of which can have serious side effects. Frequently, seizures can become refractory to these medications. Diagnostic tests such as electroencephalography and MRI help determine if there is a particular focus of their seizures, which may respond to surgical resection.

DEGENERATIVE SPINE DISEASE

Overview

I. **Anatomy:** Intervertebral discs contain a soft fibrous center, known as the **nucleus pulposus** surrounded by a tough fibrous layer called the annulus fibrosis.
   A. **Herniated or "slipped" discs:** occur when the nucleus pulposus herniates through a rupture in the annulus fibrosis
   B. **Location:** Typically, the disc herniates either underneath or through the posterior longitudinal ligament. It can then exert pressure on the thecal sac, spinal cord, or, more commonly, one of the nerve roots.

II. **Radiculopathy:** Compression of a nerve root produces symptoms in the dermatomes and muscle groups that the nerve root supplies.

Cervical Disc Herniation

I. **Clinical presentation:** typically presents initially as neck pain, secondary to inflammation of the disc capsule and the adjacent posterior longitudinal ligament
   A. **Pain:** may be located between the scapula, then radiate up into the neck and head (even causing headaches)
   B. **Radicular signs and symptoms:** often accompany cervical disc herniation when nerve root compression occurs and include pain that radiates into the arm, numbness, weakness, and loss of reflexes
   C. **Location:** Most frequently at the C6/C7 level, followed by the C5/C6 level. Each level involved produces classic symptoms based on the nerve roots they compress (Table 27-1).
   D. **Diagnosis:** MRI is helpful in evaluating radiculopathy.

Quick Cut
Radiculopathy results from nerve root compression and usually requires surgical release for relief of symptoms.

II. **Treatment:** Initial management is analgesics, nonsteroidal anti-inflammatory drugs (NSAIDs), muscle relaxants, rest, physical therapy, and steroid injections. If conservative therapy is unsuccessful, surgical decompression and possible fusion may be required.
   A. **Central and lateral herniation:** Anterior approach is used to remove the disc and decompress the spinal cord and nerve roots. The two adjacent vertebral bodies are then fused together. For single-level disease in patients with normal cervical curvature, a **disc replacement** (total disc arthroplasty) may also be performed.
   B. **Far lateral herniation:** Posterior approach is used with laminectomy and foraminotomy. Posterior fusion is sometimes necessary depending on the extent of decompression.

Cervical Spondylosis

I. **Etiology:** caused by progressive degeneration of the discs and ligaments associated with arthritic changes of the joints and osteophyte formation

Table 27-1: Cervical Disc Syndromes

	Disc Space: C4–C5 Nerve Root: C5	Disc Space: C5–C6 Nerve Root: C6	Disc Space: C6–7 Nerve Root: C7	Disc Space: C7–T1 Nerve Root: C8
Sensory loss	Lateral arm	Radial aspect forearm; thumb; index finger web space	Posterior arm; index finger; long finger	Ulnar two fingers; medial forearm
Motor weakness	Shoulder abductors; shoulder external/ internal rotators	Biceps; brachial radialis; supinator/ pronator	C6–C7 wrist extensors; elbow extensors	Finger flexors; ulnar deviator of the hand
Changes in DTRs	Biceps reflex diminished	Biceps and radial reflexes diminished	Triceps reflex diminished	Finger flexor reflex diminished

DTR, deep tendon reflex.
Adapted from Freedman AH, Wilkins RH. *Neurosurgical Management for the House Officer*. Baltimore: Lippincott Williams & Wilkins; 1984.

II. **Clinical presentation:** This degeneration slowly narrows the canal and neural foramina causing gradual compression of the cord and nerve roots. These patients often have disease at multiple levels of the cervical spine.
  A. **Radicular symptom:** caused by the impingement and identical to that seen with disc herniation
  B. **Myelopathy:** Hyperreflexia, gait instability, and difficulty with fine motor tasks results from the gradual narrowing of the canal, compressing the spinal cord.
  C. **Imaging:** MRI helps assess the discs, ligaments, and changes in the spinal cord. CT scans are helpful in evaluating the bony anatomy.

> **Quick Cut**
> Myelopathy results from spinal cord compression.

III. **Treatment:** These patients may also be managed conservatively if there are no motor deficits. If symptoms are debilitating and persist despite these measures, either anterior or posterior surgery may be needed. Surgery could take the form of an anterior fusion, posterior laminectomy with or without fusion, or posterior laminoplasty.

Lumbar Disc Herniation

I. **Overview:** As in the cervical spine, disc herniation represents extrusion of nucleus pulposus through annulus fibrosis. Typically, nerve roots exit through a neural foramen one segment below the herniated disc (L5/S1 disc herniation irritates the S1 nerve root).

II. **Clinical presentation:** Patients usually have a history of back pain along with radicular symptoms, often reporting pain exacerbated by sitting or straining (Valsalva maneuver) See Table 27-2.

Table 27-2: Lumbar Disc Herniation Syndrome

	Disc Space: L1–L2 Nerve Root: L2	Disc Space: L2–L3 Nerve Root: L3	Disc Space: L3–L4 Nerve Root: L4	Disc Space: L4–L5 Nerve Root: L5	Disc Space: L5–S1 Nerve Root: S1	Disc space: S1–S2 Nerve Root: S2–S3
Distribution of sensory loss	Anterior thigh; inguinal ligament	Anterior thigh	Anterior thigh; medial leg to the medial malleolus	Lateral leg; dorsum of foot to big toe	Lateral leg; foot to small toe; sole of foot	Buttocks; perineal region; genitalia
Motor weakness	Hip flexion; hip abduction	Hip abduction; knee extension	Knee extension; foot inversion	Foot and toe extension	Foot and toe flexion	Intrinsic muscles of the foot
Reflex changes	—	—	Decreased knee jerk	Decreased or absent knee jerk	Decreased or absent ankle jerk	Sphincteric dysfunction

Adapted from Freedman AH, Wilkins RH. *Neurosurgical Management for the House Officer*. Baltimore: Williams & Wilkins; 1984.

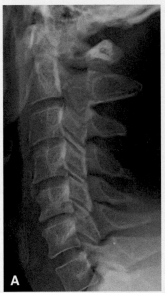
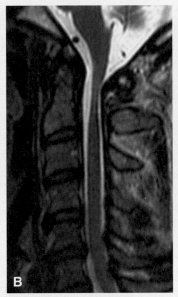
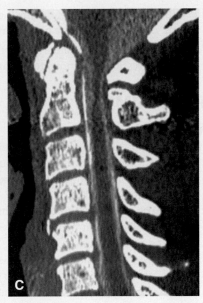
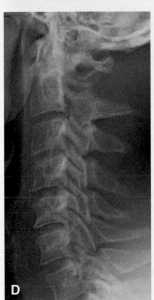
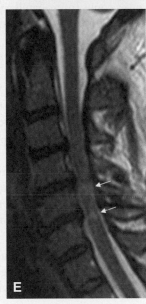

Figure 27-8: A–D: Spinal cord signal changes. **A,B:** A 32-year-old man with a 12-year history of progressive upper and lower extremity myelopathy. Magnetic resonance imaging (MRI) demonstrated congenital anomalies at C1–C2, with associated hypertrophy of the ligamentum flavum causing severe dorsal spinal cord compression. **C:** Computed tomographic myelogram demonstrates abnormal bony projections on the ventral surfaces of the C1 and C2 laminar arches, causing compression. He underwent posterior decompression of C1 and C2 **(D)** with excellent improvement in symptoms. **E:** A 52-year-old woman with bilateral hand clumsiness. Sagittal MRI demonstrates patchy spinal cord signal changes at C5 and C6 *(arrows)* along with spondylotic cord compression. (From Bridwell KH, DeWald RL. *Textbook of Spinal Surgery*, 3rd ed. Philadelphia: Lippincott Williams & Wilkins; 2011.)

III. **Physical examination:** Reveals intense lumbosacral spasm. Frequently, a positive "straight leg raising" sign, as well as radicular signs and symptoms, are present.

IV. **Treatment:** Patients are first treated conservatively.
   A. **Imaging:** If symptoms do not improve, MRI can determine nerve root compression (Fig. 27-8). If an MRI cannot be obtained, CT myelography is an alternative.
   B. **Discectomy:** typically needed through a posterior approach if the pain does not respond to conservative management or the patient has significant neurologic deficits

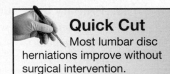

Quick Cut
Most lumbar disc herniations improve without surgical intervention.

Lumbar Spondylosis

I. **Overview:** Chronic degeneration can cause arthropathy, disc degeneration, and ligamentous hypertrophy leading to narrowing of the canal.

II. **Clinical presentation:** The patient describes back and leg pain that is aching in nature, exacerbated by prolonged standing or walking, and ameliorated by sitting (**neurogenic claudication**). More severe central stenosis can present as **cauda equina syndrome**, with significant leg weakness, saddle anesthesia, and bowel/bladder dysfunction.

Quick Cut
Cauda equina syndrome is a neurosurgical *emergency* requiring prompt decompression.

III. **Diagnosis:** MRI scan remains the best technique to visualize the discs, ligaments, and nerve roots. CT scan is used to assess the bony anatomy.

IV. **Treatment:** Conservative therapy is again the primary treatment. As the disease progresses, surgical decompression by laminectomy (and usually fusion) may be required.

SPINE TUMORS

Overview

I. **Classification:** Generally, by their location being intramedullary (intrinsic to the spinal cord), extramedullary, intradural, or extradural. Similar to the brain, they are further classified based on their histologic cell of origin.

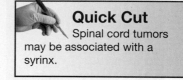

Quick Cut
Spinal cord tumors may be associated with a syrinx.

   A. **Intramedullary tumors:** intrinsic to the spinal cord and typically present with gradually progressive neurologic deficits and myelopathy
      1. **Astrocytomas:** All grades, as in the brain, can also occur within the spinal cord. Most frequently, they occur in the cervical or thoracic regions and may be associated with a syrinx.
      2. **Ependymomas:** Often occur in the cervical spine and can also be associated with a syrinx. A second group of ependymomas involves conus (myxopapillary ependymoma).
   B. **Intradural, extramedullary tumors:** produce symptoms through nerve root compression (causing radiculopathy and myelopathy)
      1 **Meningiomas:** most frequently occur in the thoracic spine and are managed similarly to their intracranial counterparts
      2. **Schwannomas:** Arise from Schwann cells, which are associated with the nerve roots. These present as dumbbell-shaped tumors protruding throughout the neural foramen (they can be intradural or extradural). Often, schwannomas may be multiple.

II. **Diagnosis:** usually established by neurologic examination and then proceeding with radiographic studies
   A. **MRI scan with and without contrast:** study of choice for all tumors
      1. **Intramedullary tumors:** present as an enhancing mass expanding the spinal cord
      2. **Intradural and extradural lesions:** typically enhance and compress the spinal cord
   B. **CT scan:** can be helpful in assessing bony anatomy particularly in metastatic disease (which has a propensity to invade bone)

III. **Metastatic tumors:** Most commonly encountered **extradural spinal column** tumor, typically originating from the vertebral body; they most frequently are associated with primary tumors from lung, breast, and prostate. These tumors are best treated aggressively with decompression and fusion (in most cases) often followed by radiation.

IV. **Primary bone tumors:** Although rare, en bloc resection of these lesions is curative and should be recommended when possible. Radiation and chemotherapy also play a role in postoperative management.

PERIPHERAL NERVES

Carpal Tunnel Syndrome

I. **Etiology:** results from **median nerve** entrapment as it traverses under the **carpal ligament** at the wrist

II. **Presentation:** Patients typically present with hand pain and numbness over the palmar thumb and first two digits. Weakness, particularly with thumb opposition may also be present.

III. **Diagnostic studies:** can include electromyography (EMG)/nerve conduction velocity (NCV) abnormalities and physical exam findings, such as a **Tinel sign** (pain with percussion of the carpal ligament)

IV. **Treatment:** Conservative management with wrist splints is first attempted and patients with continued symptoms may require surgical decompression of the nerve by cutting the carpal ligament.

Quick Cut
Carpal tunnel syndrome produces median nerve neuropathy.

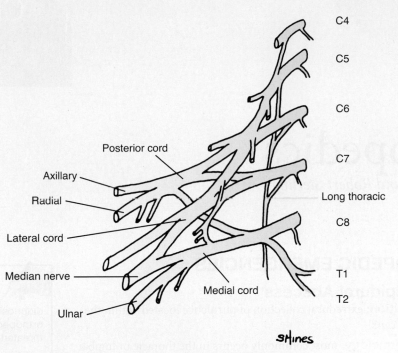

Figure 27-9: Simplified diagram of the brachial plexus.

Cubital Tunnel Syndrome

I. **Etiology:** results from **ulnar nerve** entrapment as it traverses the cubital tunnel in the elbow

II. **Presentation:** Patients present with pain and numbness on the ulnar surface of the hand along with hand weakness.

III. **Diagnosis and treatment:** Diagnostic workup is similar to that for carpal tunnel syndrome and treatment involves decompressing the nerve in the cubital tunnel.

Brachial Plexus

I. **Anatomy:** exceedingly complex anatomic structure that involves a transition from the cervical roots (C5–T1) into the axilla and four main nerves—musculocutaneous, axillary, median, and ulnar (Fig. 27-9)

II. **Clinical presentation:** Injuries can result from trauma or neoplasia. Most typically, brachial plexopathy is seen in the setting of trauma where the neck is severely stretched and avulsion injury occurs to the plexus (tearing the nerve roots from the spinal cord).

III. **Evaluation:** Includes physical exam along with extensive EMG/NCV studies. Can involve a CT myelogram and an MRI to evaluate the nerve roots and brachial plexus.

IV. **Treatment and prognosis:** Nerve root avulsions generally have a very poor prognosis. With residual motor and sensory function, the patient has an excellent chance of regaining function of the nerve root. However, if the nerve root is severed, then the patient may need a nerve transposition to restore function. Furthermore, a dorsal root entry zone (DREZ) procedure may need to be performed to treat pain.

Chapter 28

Orthopedics

Oliver Tannous and Robert Sterling

ORTHOPEDIC EMERGENCIES

Spinal Epidural Abscess

I. **Definition:** extradural collection of purulence located within the spinal canal

II. **Epidemiology:** most commonly occurs in the thoracic or lumbar spine

A. **Risk factors:** intravenous (IV) drug abuse, immunodeficiency (HIV, immunosuppressive medications, end-stage renal disease), prior spinal osteomyelitis or discitis, recent spine surgery, or recent systemic infection; may spread hematogenously or locally

B. **Most common organisms:** *Staphylococcus aureus* and gram-negative rods

III. **Diagnosis:** Symptoms include bowel/bladder incontinence, local or radicular pain, saddle anesthesia, and lower extremity (LE) weakness. Thoracic abscess patients may present with myelopathic symptoms (wide-based spastic gait, dermatomal chest pain, LE spasticity, or paraparesis).

A. **Physical exam:** LE weakness, absent rectal tone and/or volition, LE clonus, or positive Babinski reflex

B. **Imaging:** Magnetic resonance imaging (MRI) is the test of choice. Computed tomography (CT) myelogram is the next best imaging modality if an MRI is contraindicated.

IV. **Treatment:** In the presence of neurologic deficits, **emergent spinal canal decompression and evacuation** of the abscess is indicated. A small abscess without neurologic deficit may be treated with a course of IV antibiotics and bracing with frequent clinical follow-up.

> **Quick Cut**
> Without rapid diagnosis and treatment, orthopedic emergencies threaten life or limb function.

> **Quick Cut**
> MRI with gadolinium is the most sensitive imaging modality to differentiate abscess from cerebrospinal fluid.

Pelvic Ring Injuries with Hemodynamic Instability

I. **Types:** Injuries that disrupt the sacroiliac (SI) joint can cause hemorrhage from the pelvic venous plexus. Fractures into the greater sciatic notch can lacerate the superior gluteal artery.

II. **Diagnosis:** anteroposterior (AP) pelvic x-ray demonstrating pubic symphysis widening (Fig. 28-1) or SI joint widening, persistent hemodynamic instability not attributable to another cause after initial management with pelvic compression binder, expanding pelvic hematoma seen on CT scan, or active bleeding seen on pelvic arteriogram

III. **Initial management:** includes aggressive fluid resuscitation, application of a **pelvic binder** centered on the greater trochanters, intra-abdominal source of hemorrhage ruled out, and emergent pelvic stabilization of a hemodynamically unstable patient

A. **External pelvic fixation:** decreases pelvic volume to improve tamponade

B. **Pelvic angiogram with embolization of actively bleeding vessels:** if external fixation and fluid replacement fail

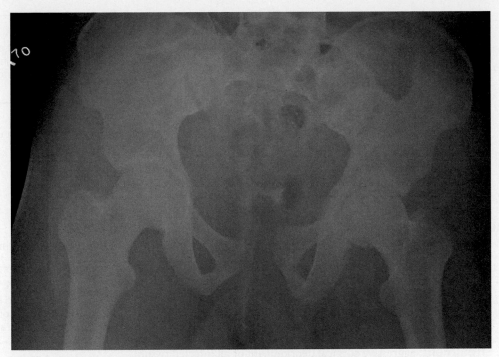

Figure 28-1: Pubic symphysis widening in a pelvic ring injury.

IV. **Definitive stabilization:** occurs semi-electively after the patient stabilizes
  A. **Closed/open reduction of the SI joint, sacrum, or posterior ilium:** undertaken with internal fixation
  B. **Open reduction and internal fixation (ORIF):** of the anterior ring or continued external fixation is achieved (Fig. 28-2)

Compartment Syndrome

  I. **Definition:** Increased interstitial fluid pressure within an osseofascial compartment. This causes microcirculatory compromise, leading to necrosis of the muscle within the compartment and dysfunction of the nerves.

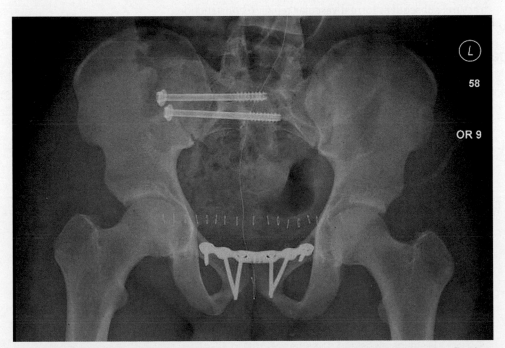

Figure 28-2: AP pelvic x-ray showed plating of the symphysis and sacroiliac joint screw fixation.

II. **Causes:** fracture, crush injuries, arterial injury, tight cast/dressing, burns, gunshot injury, intramuscular hematoma

III. **Diagnosis** primarily clinical
A. **Pain:** escalating pain in the extremity in spite of increasing pain medication administration, pain out of proportion to the injury, pain with passive stretch of the myotendinous units within the compartment, pain and tenseness on palpation (less reliable finding)
B. **Intracompartmental pressure measurement:** used when clinical exam is unclear or in unreliable/unconscious patients
1. **Absolute pressure measurement:** greater than 30 mm Hg
2. Pressure less than 30 mm Hg below the diastolic blood pressure

IV. **Treatment:** emergent surgical release of all involved compartments

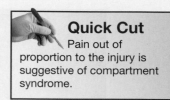

Quick Cut
Pain out of proportion to the injury is suggestive of compartment syndrome.

Necrotizing Fasciitis

I. **Definition:** rapidly ascending infection caused by group A *Streptococcus* that can lead to limb loss and death if treatment is delayed

II. **Diagnosis:** progressive soft tissue infection that may have crepitus

III. **Imaging:** X-ray with subcutaneous air; CT scan can aid in diagnosis by showing abscess and/or gas in the soft tissues; MRI can demonstrate fasciitis.

IV. **Treatment:** aggressive surgical debridement of all infected tissue and parenteral antibiotics

Quick Cut
Air in the soft tissues may be detected on physical exam or on plain radiographs.

Fractures and Dislocations Associated with Vascular Injury

I. **Common sites include the following:** distal femur, proximal tibia, supracondylar humerus (primarily in children), knee dislocations

II. **Diagnosis:** Suspicion is based on proximity with clinical signs of vascular injury suggested by ankle-brachial indices (ABIs) less than 0.8 (Table 28-1) and require arterial duplex ultrasonography or CT angiography; or intraoperative angiogram.

III. **Treatment:** placement of a temporary vascular shunt followed by orthopedic stabilization of the fracture; subsequent formal vascular repair/reconstruction

IV. **Outcome:** amputation rate near 100% if warm ischemia time exceeds 6 hours

Quick Cut
Fractures and dislocations associated with vascular injury constitute limb-threatening injuries.

Scapulothoracic Dissociation

I. **Definition:** traumatic dissociation of the scapula from the thorax

II. **Presentation:** usually seen on chest x-ray as lateral displacement of the scapula (Fig. 28-3)
A. **Vascular injuries:** occur in up to 90% of cases and often include the subclavian or axillary arteries
B. **Brachial plexus injuries:** present in up to 95% of cases

III. **Outcomes:** flail extremity rate of 50%, amputation rate of 20%, and mortality rate of 10%

Table 28-1: Physical Signs of a Major Arterial Injury

Absent or comparably weak pulses
Distal cyanosis
Expanding hematoma
Pulsatile bleeding
Comparably cold extremity
Distal paralysis and paresthesias
Bleeding not controlled with direct pressure

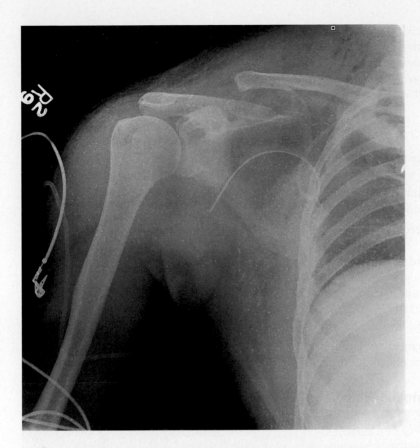

Figure 28-3: X-ray showing lateral displacement of the scapula indicative of scapulothoracic dissociation.

ORTHOPEDIC URGENCIES

Open Fracture

I. **Definition:** any fracture that has been exposed to the external environment, usually not only through the skin but also through hollow visceral organs (Fig. 28-4)

II. **Management:** Splinting is done initially with removal of gross contamination and placement of sterile dressings.

A. **Medical:** Administration of a first-generation cephalosporin (vancomycin in patients who are allergic to penicillin). Use of an

> **Quick Cut**
> Urgencies are not immediately life or limb threatening, but significant delay in diagnosis and treatment can result in loss of limb or joint function and prolonged treatment.

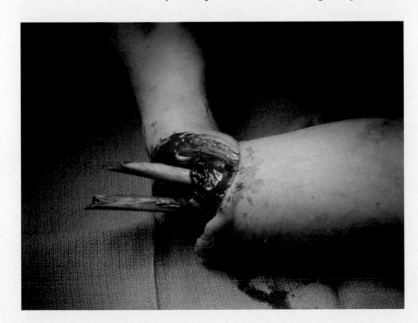

Figure 28-4: Open forearm fracture with both radius and ulna exposed.

aminoglycoside and penicillin should be considered for patients with large wounds or for those with soil or farm contamination. Tetanus prophylaxis is administered.

B. Definitive: Definitive irrigation and debridement are performed in the operating room with stabilization.

> **Quick Cut**
> Open fracture requires urgent treatment to decrease the risk of osteomyelitis.

Septic Arthritis

I. Presentation: rapid onset of atraumatic pain in a joint

II. Etiology: Typically hematogenous origin; immunocompromised patients are at increased risk.

III. Physical examination: joint effusion, exquisite tenderness to palpation, and severe pain with minimal motion of the joint

IV. Diagnosis: confirmed by needle aspiration with synovial fluid analysis (Table 28-2)

> **Quick Cut**
> Septic arthritis requires urgent treatment to prevent postinfectious arthritis.

A. Synovial fluid white blood cell (WBC) count: More than 50,000 with greater than 90% polymorphonuclear leukocytes (PMNs) suggest the diagnosis.

B. Crystals: Fluid must be inspected for crystals; an acute gout flare can have an exceptionally high WBC count with mostly PMNs.

C. Differential diagnosis: includes aseptic arthritis (rheumatoid, psoriatic, etc.) and gout

V. Treatment: Surgical debridement and lavage of the joint (open or arthroscopic). Antibiotic therapy should not be instituted before obtaining adequate specimens for a culture and sensitivity.

Table 28-2: Examination of the Synovial Fluid

	Normal	Group I Noninflammatory	Group II Inflammatory	Group III Septic
Gross appearance	Transparent, clear	Transparent, yellow	Opaque or translucent, yellow	Opaque, yellow to green
Viscosity	High	High	Low	Variable
White cells/mm³	<200	<2,000	5,000–75,000	>50,000, often >100,000
Polymorphonuclear leukocytes	<25%	<50%	>50%, <90%	>95%
Culture	Negative	Negative	Negative	Often positive
Glucose (mg/dL)	Almost equal to blood	Almost equal to blood	>25, lower than blood	>50, lower than blood
Associated conditions	—	Degenerative joint disease Trauma* Neuropathic arthropathy* Hypertrophic osteoarthropathy† Pigmented villonodular synovitis* SLE† Acute rheumatic fever† Erythema nodosum	Rheumatoid arthritis Connective tissue diseases (SLE, PSS, DM/PM) Ankylosing spondylitis Other seronegative spondyloarthropathies (psoriatic arthritis, Reiter syndrome, arthritis of chronic inflammatory bowel disease) Crystal-induced synovitis (gout or pseudogout) Acute rheumatic fever	Bacterial infections Compromised immunity (disease-or medication-related) Other joint disease

*May be hemorrhagic.
†Group I or II.
SLE, systemic lupus erythematosus; PSS, progressive systemic sclerosis; DM/PM, dermatomyositis/polymyositis.
Reprinted with permission from Rodnan GP, Schumacher HR. Examination of synovial fluid. In: *Primer on Rheumatic Diseases*, 8th ed. Atlanta: Atlanta Arthritis Foundation; 1983:187.

Hip Dislocation

I. **Presentation:** History of moderate to severe trauma to the extremity and inability to move the hip. Most dislocations are posterior and the leg is internally rotated at the hip and shorter than the contralateral limb.

II. **Diagnosis:** Pelvic or hip x-ray demonstrates the dislocation (Fig. 28-5); CT scan can demonstrate femoral head or acetabular fracture.

III. **Treatment:** Expedient reduction under general anesthesia; CT scan to evaluate for femoral head or acetabular fracture after reduction.

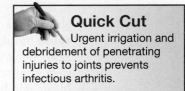

Quick Cut
Urgent reduction of hip dislocation decreases the risk of femoral head osteonecrosis.

Penetrating Injuries to Joints

I. **Diagnosis:** Intra-articular injection of sterile saline at a point distant to the laceration with leak at the injury site aids in the diagnosis.

II. **Treatment:** formal irrigation and debridement (open or arthroscopically) to prevent infectious arthritis

Quick Cut
Urgent irrigation and debridement of penetrating injuries to joints prevents infectious arthritis.

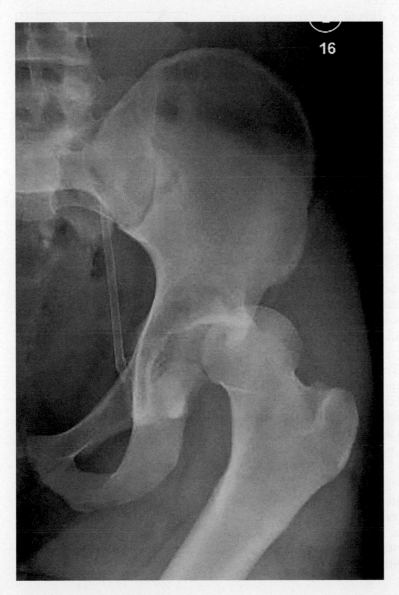

Figure 28-5: X-ray demonstrating posterior hip dislocation.

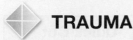

TRAUMA

Overview

I. **Advanced trauma life support (ATLS):** In the management of trauma patients, it is important to remember ATLS guidelines with strict adherence to the ABCs (airway, breathing, circulation; see Chapter 22).

II. **Extent of injury to the musculoskeletal system:** varies according to the patient's age, the direction of the energy causing the trauma, and the magnitude of the trauma

> **Quick Cut**
> Orthopedic injuries are more likely to be limb threatening than life threatening.

   A. **Patient's age:** suggests the weak link in the musculoskeletal system
      1. **In skeletally immature patients:** Weak link is the growth plate at the ends of the long bones.
      2. **Young but skeletally mature patients (16–50 years of age):** may be more likely to sustain ligamentous injuries because the relative strength of the mature bone exceeds that of the supporting soft tissues
      3. **In late middle-aged or elderly patients (with significant osteopenia):** Injuries to the ligaments are uncommon; fractures of the metaphyseal portions of long bones are prevalent (i.e., distal radius, hip). The metaphyseal area is at risk because the likelihood of osteopenia is much greater in this metabolically active area.
   B. **Direction of the trauma:** may determine which structures are injured (e.g., knee-dash injury that occurs in motor vehicle collisions frequently causes fractures of the patella and femur as well as posterior hip fractures or dislocations)

> **Quick Cut**
> Patterns of injury may occur, leading to predictable groups of damage based on the mechanism of injury.

   C. **Magnitude of the trauma:** related to the energy imparted ($E = \frac{1}{2} mv^2$), where m = mass and v = velocity
      1. **High-energy injuries (e.g., in motor vehicle accidents):** tend to cause comminuted, complex skeletal injuries, which may be open fractures
      2. **Low-energy injuries:** frequently occur in the elderly or during sports and are more likely to cause simple, isolated injuries of ligaments, muscles, or bones

Fracture

I. **Description:** Radiographic appearance may give insight into the type of trauma that produced a particular fracture. Other descriptors are as follows.
   A. **Location:** may be the diaphysis (shaft), the metaphysis (juxta-articular), or through the joint surface (articular)
   B. **Orientation:** may be transverse, oblique, spiral, segmental, comminuted, or incomplete such as greenstick in the growing skeleton (Figs. 28-6 and 28-7)
   C. **Displacement:** may be expressed in terms of bone diameters (e.g., 1 bone diameter of displacement = 100% displacement) in shaft fractures and in millimeters of step-off in articular fractures (e.g., tibial plateau fractures)
   D. **Impaction:** frequently occurs in the proximal humerus and may indicate stability
   E. **Angulation:** should use the apex of the fracture as a point of reference (i.e., apex dorsal)
   F. **Rotation:** often best assessed clinically but may be appreciated on radiograph
   G. **Open or closed:** open, or compound (old terminology), indicates a soft tissue injury in the region of the fracture with exposure to the external environment
      1. **Communication:** All wounds in the proximity of fractures should be assumed to communicate with it.
      2. **Classification:** Gustilo classification (Table 28-3)

II. **Stress fracture:** Implies a fracture resulting from abnormal stresses on normal bone (fatigue fracture) or normal stresses on abnormal or osteopenic bone (insufficiency fracture). Osteoporosis is a common cause of an insufficiency fracture.
   A. **Common sites in patients with normal bone:** tarsal bones (calcaneus), metatarsals, and tibial shaft
   B. **Common sites in patients with osteopenic bone:** femoral neck, foot, pelvis, and vertebrae

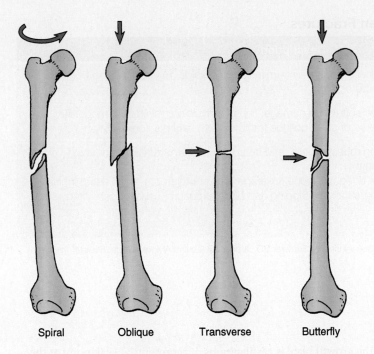

Figure 28-6: Long bone fracture patterns. (Redrawn with permission from Rang M. *Children's Fractures*, 2nd ed. Philadelphia: JB Lippincott; 1983:5.)

Spiral Oblique Transverse Butterfly

C. **Diagnosis:** Plain radiographs are helpful if reactive healing has occurred.
   1. **Bone scans:** quite sensitive but not specific
   2. **MRI:** Very sensitive and has increased specificity if a linear signal change is present; T2 image will most commonly demonstrate edema in the area of fracture.

III. **Pathologic fractures:** occurring in a weakened bone due to metabolic bone disease or a tumorous condition (i.e., a primary bone malignancy, myeloma, or metastatic disease)

IV. **Impending pathologic fractures:** Lytic defect in bone, often due to a metastasis, weakens the bone but has not yet caused a fracture. Prophylactic stabilization is often performed to prevent a fracture.

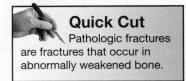

Quick Cut
Pathologic fractures are fractures that occur in abnormally weakened bone.

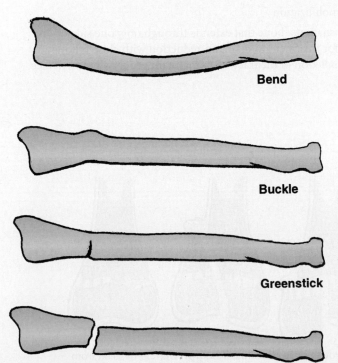

Bend

Buckle

Greenstick

Figure 28-7: Fracture patterns in children. (Redrawn with permission from Rang M. *Children's Fractures*, 2nd ed. Philadelphia: JB Lippincott; 1983:2.)

Table 28-3: Gustilo Classification of Open Fractures

Grade	Description
Grade 1	Skin opening of 1 cm or less, quite clean; most likely from inside to outside; minimal muscle contusion; simple transverse or short oblique fractures
Grade 2	Laceration >1 cm long, with extensive soft tissue damage, flaps, or avulsion; minimal to moderate crushing components; simple transverse or short oblique fractures with minimal comminution
Grade 3	Extensive soft tissue damage including muscles, skin, and neurovascular structures; often a high-velocity injury with a severe crushing component • *3A*: Extensive soft tissue laceration, adequate bone coverage; segmental fractures, gunshot injuries • *3B*: Extensive soft tissue injury with periosteal stripping and bone exposure; usually associated with massive contamination • *3C*: Vascular injury requiring repair

Reprinted with permission from Behrens F. Fractures with soft tissue injuries. In: Browrer BD, Jupiter JB, Levine AM, et al, eds. *Skeletal Trauma*, Philadelphia: WB Saunders; 1992:313.

Fractures in Children

I. **Growth plate fractures:** Because the growth plate is cartilaginous, it represents a weak point at the ends of the bone.
   A. **Classification:** Salter-Harris classification (Fig. 28-8)
   B. **Types:** All types of growth plate fractures may be associated with growth arrest, and the parents should be advised of this.
      1. **Types 1 and 2:** Do well with closed reduction and cast immobilization; however, some may require pin or screw fixation. Growth arrest is unlikely.
      2. **Types 3 and 4:** Frequently require open reduction and fixation because they are intra-articular fractures; they are at greatest risk of causing growth arrest.

II. **Buckle (or torus) fractures:** incomplete fractures that occur in the metaphysis of bones adjacent to (but not involving) the growth plate (Fig. 28-9)
   A. **Most common site:** distal radius
   B. **Treatment:** often require only cast immobilization

III. **Greenstick fractures:** Fractures in the shaft of a bone that extends through only one side or one aspect of the cortex. Casting is employed for treatment to maintain reduction with close follow-up, as reangulation can occur and require completion of the fracture to maintain proper alignment (see Fig. 28-9).

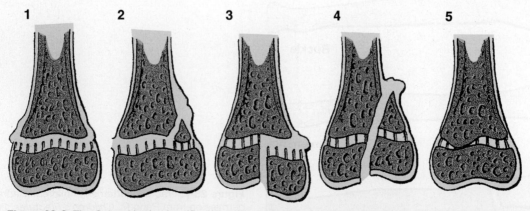

Figure 28-8: The Salter-Harris classification of growth plate fractures. (Redrawn with permission from Salter RB, Harris WR. Injuries involving the epiphyseal plate. *J Bone Joint Surg.* 1963;45A:587.)

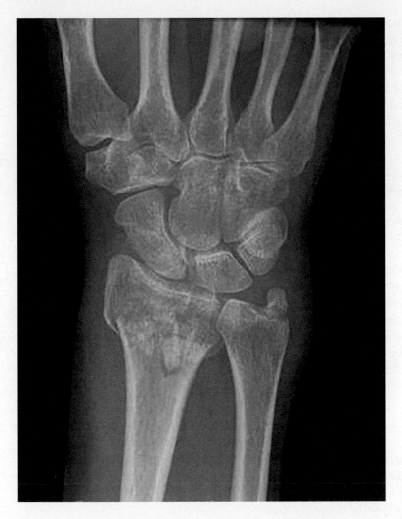

Figure 28-9: X-ray showing extra-articular distal radius fracture.

IV. **Child abuse fractures:** Careful history obtained from the child's parents, caregiver, and siblings, as well as a complete physical examination, is important when differentiating fractures caused by accidents from those caused by child abuse.

A. **Common presentation:** spiral long bone fractures in the absence of a consistent injury history

B. **Diaphyseal femur fracture:** Any child younger than 36 months with this fracture should be evaluated for child abuse.

C. **Multiple fractures of varying age and stage of healing:** often diagnostic of child abuse

D. **Radiograph skeletal survey should be performed:** AP projection of the trunk and extremities plus anterior, posterior, and lateral views of the skull

V. **Supracondylar fractures of the humerus:** Careful neurovascular examination must be done before and after any attempts at reduction are made.

A. **Displaced fractures:** require urgent attention due to the potential for compression or entrapment of the brachial artery that can lead to limb ischemia and compartment syndrome

B. **Treatment of nondisplaced fractures:** long-arm casting for 4–6 weeks

C. **Treatment of displaced fractures:** closed (occasionally open) reduction with pin stabilization and long-arm casting with pin removal in 4–6 weeks

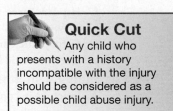

Quick Cut
Any child who presents with a history incompatible with the injury should be considered as a possible child abuse injury.

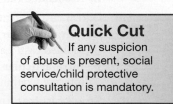

Quick Cut
If any suspicion of abuse is present, social service/child protective consultation is mandatory.

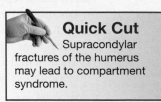

Quick Cut
Supracondylar fractures of the humerus may lead to compartment syndrome.

VI. **Fractures of both forearm bones**
  A. **Age younger than 10 years:** closed reduction and molded plaster immobilization with close observation acutely for compartment syndrome
  B. **Age older than 10 years:** Attempt closed reduction, but ORIF may be necessary. Remodeling of the diaphysis is minimal after age 10 years so anatomic reduction is necessary.

VII. **Distal radius fractures:** Distal radial metaphysis is a frequent site for buckle fractures; distal radial epiphyseal plate is a frequent site for growth plate fractures (which, if displaced, should have a closed reduction under anesthesia with cast immobilization).

VIII. **Femur fractures**
  A. **Children age younger than 6 months:** most often treated with Pavlik harness or early spica casting
  B. **Children age 7 months–5 years:** Postfracture overgrowth is common so 1–2-cm shortening is accepted.
    1. **Overlap less than 2–3 cm:** treatment with spica casting
    2. **Overlap greater than 3 cm:** surgical treatment with flexible nails or external fixation to maintain length
  C. **Children age 5–11 years:** Surgical treatment with flexible intramedullary nails is indicated.
  D. **Children age older than 11 years:** Surgical treatment with flexible intramedullary nails, rigid intramedullary nail, or submuscular plating is indicated.

IX. **Fractures of the tibia:** associated with compartment syndromes
  A. **Examination:** All patients with tibia fractures should be examined for any skin disruption, and the neurovascular status of the leg should be evaluated and documented.
  B. **Treatment:** Managed in children with plaster immobilization. If open wounds are present, external fixation allows access for wound care.

Fractures in Adults

I. **Fractures of the distal radius, proximal humerus, hip, and spine:** all common in elderly persons with osteoporosis
  A. **Distal radius fracture:** See section III below.
  B. **Proximal humerus fractures:** Early motion after callus development is essential to decrease shoulder stiffness.
    1. **Simple fractures:** sling and swathe immobilization
    2. **Comminuted fractures:** ORIF or prosthetic replacement
  C. **Hip fractures: ORIF or arthroplasty is associated with better long-term** function and patient survival.
  D. **Osteopenic compression fractures of the spine:** Managed with bracing for 3–4 months. Metastatic disease should be ruled out as a cause.

II. **Humeral shaft fractures:** Isolated fracture is usually treated with a sling and humeral fracture brace.
  A. **Fracture in conjunction with multiple trauma (LE fractures or ipsilateral forearm fractures):** usually treated with surgical fixation to enable upper extremity (UE) weight bearing for crutch/walker use
  B. **Associated radial nerve palsy:** often recovers spontaneously

III. **Distal radius fractures**
  A. **Extra-articular fractures (see Fig. 28-9):** Treated by closed reduction and immobilization in a well-molded cast; fracture comminution may necessitate surgical fixation.
  B. **Intra-articular fractures:** treated by reduction and stabilization with pinning, external fixation, or internal fixation to restore the joint anatomy

IV. **Scaphoid fractures:** often occurs in the young, as energy sustained from a fall is transferred to the scaphoid and resisted by the distal radius (Fig. 28-10)
  A. **Diagnosis:** Wrist pain, especially in the anatomic snuffbox after a fall on an outstretched wrist, should arouse suspicion of this carpal bone injury.
  B. **Treatment:** Healing is often delayed owing to a precarious blood supply to the bone, which is largely covered with articular cartilage.
    1. **Nondisplaced fractures:** thumb-spica casting
    2. **Displaced fractures:** surgical open reduction and fixation

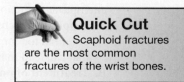
Quick Cut
Scaphoid fractures are the most common fractures of the wrist bones.

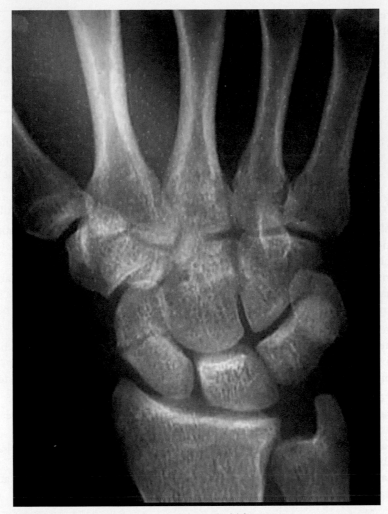

Figure 28-10: X-ray demonstrating scaphoid fracture.

V. Boxer's fractures (fracture of the fourth or fifth metacarpal neck): from a closed fist striking on the ulnar side of the hand
   A. Angular deformity: well tolerated up to 40 degrees in the fourth metacarpal neck and 60 degrees in the fifth
   B. Malrotation: poorly tolerated as it causes the fingers to overlap
   C. Treatment: casting unless severe angulation or malrotation is present

VI. Spinal fractures: Initial evaluation and treatment includes evaluation for neurologic injury with a complete motor, sensory, and reflex examination; complete spinal CT is indicated to rule out these fractures. All patients suspected of having a spinal injury should be immobilized on a long spine board with a cervical collar and head blocks.

> **Quick Cut**
> All unconscious patients involved in motor vehicle or motorcycle accidents should be assumed to have a spinal injury until proven otherwise.

   A. Cervical spine fractures: frequently associated with quadriplegia and frequently multiple levels of injury
   B. Thoracic spine fractures: Simple compression fractures often in elderly osteopenic patients secondary to minimal trauma (e.g., coughing) may be due to metastatic disease; high-energy mechanisms are associated with more complex fracture can result in paraplegia.
   C. Lumbar spine fractures
      1. Presentation: L1–L2 mixed neurologic can be seen from injury to the conus medullaris (upper motor neuron) or cauda equina (lower motor neuron); below L2, typically involves only nerve roots.

2. **Treatment:** Urgent decompression of neural elements in patients with incomplete or progressive neural deficits or injuries at the level of the cauda equina is the optimal approach.

   a. **Steroids:** If begun within 3 hours of injury, continue for 23 hours. If begun 3–8 hours postinjury, continue for 48 hours. After 8 hours, steroids do not improve return of function.

   b. **Spinal stabilization:** Performed to prevent worsening of a neural deficit and restore alignment. Patients with complete quadriplegia or paraplegia should also be considered as candidates for spinal stabilization with instrumentation on a less urgent basis to allow early rehabilitation.

VII. Pelvic fractures: See "Pelvic Ring Injuries with Hemodynamic Instability" earlier.

VIII. Femoral shaft fractures: Early stabilization decreases pulmonary complications.

  A. Traction (on a short-term basis): if the patient is too critically ill for surgery (e.g., severe coagulopathy, marked elevation of intracranial pressure)

  B. External fixation: Indicated for initial stabilization of the fracture in an unstable trauma patient. Formal stabilization should be performed as soon as the patient's condition is stable.

  C. Intramedullary stabilization: treatment of choice for isolated femoral shaft fractures (Fig. 28-11)

IX. Tibial fractures

  A. Isolated closed fracture treatment: Plaster immobilization and early weight bearing; intramedullary nail fixation can facilitate early return to ambulation.

  B. Multiple injuries or open tibial fracture treatment: intramedullary rods; external fixation

X. Ankle fractures:

  A. Lateral malleolus fracture alone: Cast treatment is the mainstay; surgical treatment if the ankle mortise is wide on initial x-rays.

  B. Medial malleolus fracture alone: often a vertical or oblique fracture, which leaves the ankle unstable; surgical treatment with reduction and fixation

  C. Medial malleolus and lateral malleolus fracture: Surgical reduction and fixation is indicated to maintain fracture reduction (Figure 28-12).

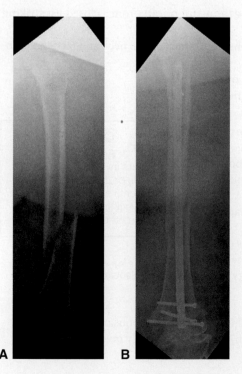

A   B

Figure 28-11: Midshaft spiral femur fracture and image after intramedullary nail placement.

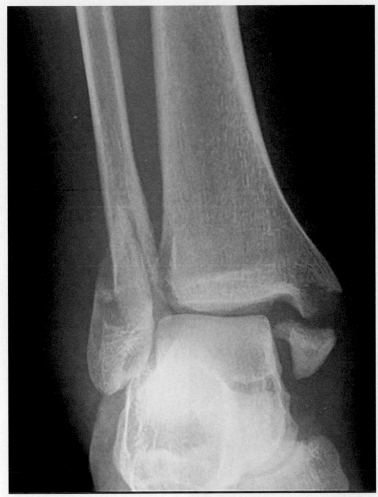

Figure 28-12: Ankle fracture involving both medial and lateral malleoli.

XI. Calcaneus fractures: often due to axial loading (during a motor vehicle accident or fall from a height); may be associated with a contralateral ankle or vertebral fracture
  A. CT scan: performed to characterize the fracture pattern due to the complex osteology of the calcaneus
  B. Poor prognostic factors: age older than 50 years, manual labor, worker's compensation, bilateral calcaneal fractures, smokers, or peripheral vascular disease
  C. Treatment: casting for stress fractures, nondisplaced fractures, high-risk patients; surgical reduction and fixation for displaced or impacted fractures (often delayed [7–10 days] to allow swelling to decrease)

Dislocations
  I. Shoulder: especially common in young adults and result in labral tear
    A. Presentation: Frequently recur in patients age younger than 40 years. In patients age older than 40 years, a tear of the rotator cuff should be suspected. May have associated **axillary nerve palsy**.
    B. Management: Immediate reduction and sling immobilization; early physical therapy. Arthroscopic labral repair is indicated for recurrent dislocators or high-demand athletes.
  II. Hip: See "Hip Dislocation" earlier.
  III. Knee: implies severe ligamentous injury around the knee and dislocations should raise awareness for potential popliteal artery injury (Fig. 28-13)
    A. Etiology: Ligamentous knee injuries occur most commonly in sports-related activities. Total ligamentous disruptions and dislocations are usually the result of violent injuries.

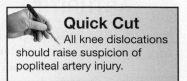

Quick Cut
All knee dislocations should raise suspicion of popliteal artery injury.

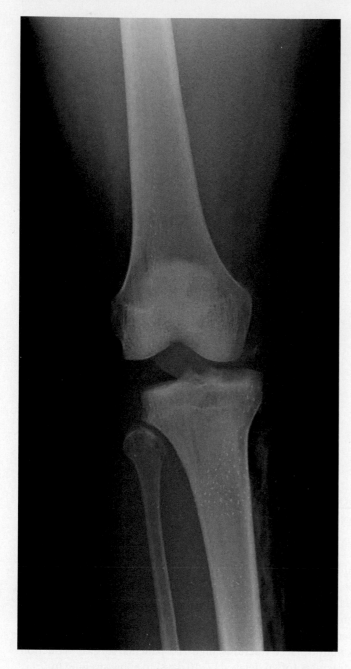

Figure 28-13: AP knee x-ray demonstrating joint space widening (especially laterally) with subluxation consistent with multiple ligament injuries.

    B. Management: First step is to evaluate the neurovascular status of the LE. Then, the ligaments and capsule around the knee are evaluated. Gentle reduction of the joint should be performed.

        1. ABI: All patients with knee dislocations require a pulse evaluation and documentation of the ABI. A patient with an abnormal ABI requires formal angiographic evaluation of flow through the popliteal artery.

        2. Delayed ligamentous reconstruction: performed after the appropriate vascular intervention to restore knee stability

ARTHRITIS

Classification

    I. Primary osteoarthritis: Primary pathology is in the articular cartilage.

        A. Most common sites: hip, knee, and spine

        B. Heberden nodes: often seen on physical exam

II. Post-traumatic arthritis: isolated joint degeneration following trauma to that joint

III. Rheumatoid arthritis and its variants: include the autoimmune group of inflammatory diseases in which the hyaline articular cartilage is secondarily attacked by a local invasive pannus that primarily involves the synovium

IV. Crystal deposition diseases: Include **gout** and **calcium pyrophosphate deposition disease**. These diseases usually present as an isolated hot, inflamed joint.

V. Infectious arthritis: See "Septic Arthritis" earlier.

Nonoperative Management

I. Pharmacologic management: maximized by consultation with a rheumatologist
- **A. Nonsteroidal anti-inflammatory drugs (NSAIDs):** especially important in osteoarthritis, which can be treated conservatively for years. Crystalline and degenerative joint diseases require NSAIDs during acute flare-ups, but the natural history of these diseases is not altered by long-term management with these drugs.
- **B. Corticosteroids:** used in rheumatoid and osteoarthritis to reduce inflammation; used systemically in multiple joint or generalized disease; used locally by injection into a single joint in patients with degenerative or post-traumatic rheumatoid arthritis
- **C. Disease-modifying antirheumatic drugs (DMARDs):** First line of treatment for rheumatoid arthritis and should be initiated on initial diagnosis. May result in disease remission and significant improvement in long-term outcomes.
- **D. Biologic agents (tumor necrosis factor antagonists and interleukin receptor antagonists):** second-line agents and used in combination with DMARDs when first-line treatment is ineffective

II. Exercise and splinting: Have an important place after the acute joint inflammation has been controlled. A full range of joint motion and muscle strength is maintained by exercising the joint through a painless arc of motion. Splinting in a functional position prevents establishment of contractures.

III. Injection (of corticosteroid, directly into symptomatic joints): can be an effective measure to provide temporary relief of symptoms

Operative Management

I. Osteotomy: Correction of malalignment may alter the mechanics enough to give significant relief from pain. The disease process must not have completely destroyed the joint for osteotomy to be successful.
- **A. Goal:** Osteotomy is designed to transfer weight bearing onto relatively normal articular surface in the setting of noninflammatory arthritis.
- **B. Temporizing measure:** Osteotomy about the hip and knee can be performed in patients too young to consider arthroplasty but who wish to preserve motion.

II. Arthrodesis: Commonly used in the small joints of the wrist, hand, foot, and ankle. Arthrodesis of the shoulder, hip, and knee are less well tolerated.
- **A. Technique:** Joint surfaces are excised and the bones on each side heal together in a fixed position.
- **B. Indications:** pain relief
- **C. Results:** very durable and long lasting

> **Quick Cut**
> Any patient who has a high functional demand should be considered for arthrodesis rather than for arthroplasty.

III. Arthroplasty (total joint replacement): Relieves pain, preserves motion, and is the most common surgical treatment for arthritis. It can be used for joints destroyed by any of the arthritides, but major joints such as the hip, knee, shoulder, and elbow are common sites.
- **A. Indications:** pain relief predominantly in patients who are usually older and less active
- **B. Postinfectious arthritis:** relative contraindication because of the increased risk of infection around the implant
- **C. Outcome:** Typical "life expectancy" for a hip or knee arthroplasty implant is ~20 years, depending on the functional requirements and weight of the patient. Failure is at a rate of ~1% per year.

◆ INFECTIONS

Acute Osteomyelitis

I. **Clinical presentation:** Hematogenous osteomyelitis is common in childhood.

    A. **Children:** In the metaphysis of children's bones, there is a unique capillary venous sinusoid underneath the growth plate. Minor trauma predisposes to sludging and allows minor bacteremic conditions to initiate an infection.

    B. **Progression:** Infection can track beneath the periosteum. Loss of blood supply devitalizes the bone, and the resulting necrotic bone is called a *sequestrum*. The elevated periosteum lays down extensive new bone, which is termed an *involucrum*.

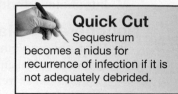

Quick Cut
Sequestrum becomes a nidus for recurrence of infection if it is not adequately debrided.

    C. **Septic arthritis:** can result if the metaphysis is intra-articular, such as in the case of the hip or shoulder, allowing eruption of the infection out of the medullary space to enter into the synovial cavity

II. **Pediatric etiology**

    A. **Neonates:** *S. aureus* and gram-negative rods predominate

    B. **Young children (age 2–5 years):** frequently caused by *Haemophilus*, *Staphylococcus*, and *Streptococcus* species

    C. **Older children (age 5 years or older):** *S. aureus* is the predominant causal organism.

    D. **History:** Child with a history of minor trauma who does not improve must be considered to have possibly developed osteomyelitis. A child's refusal to bear weight on an extremity demands a workup for osteomyelitis or septic arthritis.

III. **Adult etiology:** Patient whose immune system is suppressed and patients with sickle cell disease are predisposed to osteomyelitis from hematogenous spread of unusual organisms.

    A. **Gram-negative infections:** Patients with immunosuppression and IV drug users are susceptible particularly to *Pseudomonas aeruginosa*.

    B. *Salmonella*: Patients with sickle cell anemia have a particularly high incidence of this type of osteomyelitis.

    C. *Gonococcal* septic arthritis: most common organism in adolescent, sexually active patients

IV. **Diagnosis:** Careful physical examination, complete blood count (CBC), sedimentation rate, and bone scan help to confirm the diagnosis. Needle aspiration of the affected bone or joint is the definitive diagnostic test.

V. **Treatment:** Includes appropriate IV antibiotics and surgical drainage. Initial antibiotic treatment should be selected to cover the most likely causes of organisms and should always include coverage for *Staphylococcus*.

Chronic Osteomyelitis

I. **Etiology:** Uncommon; however, it is seen in patients who have had severe open fractures, in immunosuppressed patients, and in patients with pressure ulcerations secondary to paraplegia.

II. **Clinical presentation:** Osteomyelitis involving the bony cortex is a particularly difficult problem. WBCs, as well as antibiotics, have only limited access to the site of infection.

    A. **Early treatment:** Attempts to cure chronic osteomyelitis involve a thorough debridement of infected nonviable bone (sequestrum), open wound care, and a prolonged course of IV antibiotics.

Quick Cut
Cortical bone has minimal vascularity and is even less well vascularized in the face of osteomyelitis.

    B. **Late treatment:** After all devascularized bone and soft tissue have been removed, and once a stable wound base has been established, the overlying soft tissue and bone defect need to be addressed.

        1. **Flaps:** Bone defect can be packed with antibiotic-impregnated beads (frequently, tobramycin or gentamicin beads) followed by rotational or free vascularized tissue coverage. Later, the flap can be elevated, the beads can be removed, and cancellous autografting can be performed.

2. **Ring:** A ring external fixator may be used to transport bone to fill defects. Occasionally, the wounds can be left open during transport, and they will close spontaneously once the defect is closed.
3. **Grafts:** Use of vascularized bone grafts, such as the free vascularized fibula or fibular transposition graft, is an option for large bone defects.

TUMORS

Primary Bone Tumors

I. **Clinical presentation:** Patients with a neoplastic bone lesion present with pain, swelling, or occasionally, a pathologic fracture. This applies to bony metastases as well as for *primary* tumors of bone.

II. **Diagnosis:** In addition to differentiating a primary tumor from a metastatic lesion of bone, some metabolic processes, such as hyperparathyroidism and infection, must be carefully considered.

A. **Physical examination:** demonstrates the tumor mass

B. **Plain radiographs:** often suggest the etiology and nature of the bone lesion based on its location, appearance, and the response of the surrounding normal bone (Fig. 28-14)

1. **Malignancy:** expected if the films show a large tumor, aggressive destruction of bone, ineffective reaction of the bone to the tumor, and extension of the tumor into soft tissue

2. **Benign lesions:** expected if the films show a small, well-circumscribed lytic lesion; thick, sclerotic rim of reactive adjacent bone; and no extension into soft tissue

III. **Workup:** Includes a CT scan and MRI of the involved extremity to stage the tumor and delineate its extent and anatomic relationships. A technetium-99m (^{99m}Tc) scan is helpful in determining metastatic involvement of distant parts of the skeleton.

A. **Suspected malignancy:** CT scan of the chest is important to rule out pulmonary metastases.

B. **Biopsy:** should be performed after staging has been completed and should be planned so that the incision can be excised with a definitive resection

>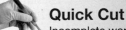
> **Quick Cut**
> Bony lesions may result from primary tumors, metastases, or metabolic processes.

> **Quick Cut**
> Incomplete workup or a poorly planned biopsy of a primary bone tumor may prove fatal for the patient or result in loss of limb.

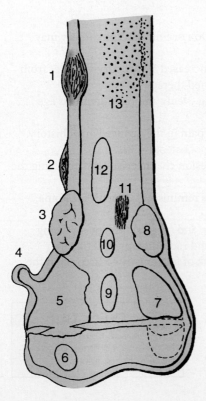

Figure 28-14: Schematic of the distal femur. Numbered sites represent tumor locations: (*1*) cortical fibrous dysplasia and adamantinoma, (*2*) osteoid osteoma, (*3*) chondromyxoid fibroma, (*4*) osteochondroma, (*5*) osteosarcoma, (*6*) chondroblastoma, (*7*) giant cell tumor, (*8*) nonossifying fibroma, (*9*) enchondroma or chondrosarcoma, (*10*) bone cyst or osteoblastoma, (*11*) fibrosarcoma or malignant fibrous histiocytoma, (*12*) fibrous dysplasia, and (*13*) Ewing sarcoma or other small round tumors. (Redrawn with permission from Moser RP, Madewell JE. An approach to primary bone tumors. *Radiol Clin North Am*. 1987;25[6]:1079–1080.)

IV. Treatment: Surgical treatment continues to be the mainstay of management for both benign and malignant tumors of the extremities. The surgical margin varies significantly with the aggressiveness of the lesion.

    A. Benign tumors: can be treated by intralesional or intracapsular excision of the tumor with or without chemical cautery, electrocautery, or cryotherapy and with or without bone grafting of the defect

    B. Malignant tumors: require at least a 2-cm margin

    C. Metastases: Isolated pulmonary metastases of sarcoma should be considered for surgical resection because the literature shows that this occasionally results in a cure and certainly a prolonged life span in these patients.

V. Adjuvant therapy for malignant tumors: Radiotherapy and chemotherapy may have important roles as adjunctive therapy in anticipation of limb-sparing procedures.

    A. Radiation: Some tumors (e.g., Ewing tumors) are very sensitive to radiotherapy. Some protocols include radiation therapy initially, but in general, radiation therapy is not an important part of the protocol.

    B. Chemotherapy: Ewing tumors are well known to be very sensitive to various chemotherapeutic regimens. Osteosarcoma is sensitive to some chemotherapeutic agents, and presurgical treatment can lessen the size of the tumor.

VI. Types of primary bone tumors:

    A. Osteosarcoma: More than 60% of patients with these tumors are age 10–20 years.

      1. Clinical presentation: Sixty percent occur about the knee at either the distal femur or the proximal tibia. Typically, pain and tumefaction is present.

      2. Imaging: Radiographically, the lesion is commonly lytic, but it may be a characteristically blastic lesion of the bone and produce a classic sunburst appearance. MRI and CT scans show that the lesion is ill defined with soft tissue extension.

      3. Histology: Tumor may be predominantly fibrogenic, chondrogenic, or osteogenic; each of the three cell types predominates in approximately equal numbers.

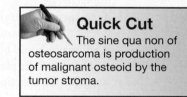

Quick Cut
The sine qua non of osteosarcoma is production of malignant osteoid by the tumor stroma.

      4. Treatment

        a. Neoadjuvant chemotherapy (given before surgery): Can narrow surgical margins and facilitate limb salvage. A high tumor kill rate observed in the resected specimen correlates favorably with long-term survival.

        b. Surgical resection: Cornerstone of management; amputation or limb salvage surgery may be required.

        c. Adjuvant chemotherapy: has a beneficial effect and has increased 5-year survival rates from 10% to 20% with surgery alone to almost 60% with combined therapy

    B. Ewing sarcoma: disease of childhood and adolescence, occurring evenly among individuals age younger than 20 years

      1. Clinical presentation: Typically, significant tumefaction and pain in the involved area; history, physical examination, and radiographic findings mimic those of osteomyelitis.

      2. Imaging: Radiologically, the lesion is seen to be a lytic bone lesion characteristically involving the diaphysis with some periosteal reaction.

      3. Histology: Small round cells, which may form pseudorosettes reminiscent of neuroblastoma. Chromosomal translocation t11:22 is associated.

      4. Treatment: Relative roles of chemotherapy, radiation therapy, and surgical therapy are being evaluated. These tumors are sensitive to both chemotherapy and radiotherapy, and together these modalities have a significant cure rate. Patients are at risk of forming osteosarcoma in the radiated bone during early adulthood.

    C. Multiple myeloma: most common primary malignancy of bone that occurs in patients who are 30 years and older with a peak incidence at age 50–60 years

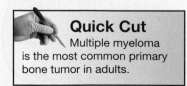

Quick Cut
Multiple myeloma is the most common primary bone tumor in adults.

      1. Clinical presentation: Characterized by overproduction of monoclonal immunoglobulins or immunoglobulin subchains (Bence Jones, or M, protein); initial presentation is often a pathologic fracture, frequently of the spine or long bones.

2. **Diagnosis:** should be suspected when lytic lesions are found in a patient with anemia, elevated sedimentation rate, and elevated serum calcium levels
   a. **Labs:** Diagnosis can be made by serum or urine electrophoresis or immunophoresis in 95% of cases, but 5% of patients with myeloma are nonsecretors of M protein.
   b. **Biopsy of the bone marrow:** To identify secreting and nonsecreting tumors and to show plasma cells replacing the marrow. The percentage of bone marrow replacement offers some prognostic information.
   c. **Plain radiography:** reveals punched-out lytic lesions, with little adjacent reactive bone, that occur frequently in the spine, pelvis, proximal femur, and skull
   d. **Bone scans:** Typically "cold" in the absence of pathologic fracture; skeletal survey is indicated to evaluate for other bony lesions.
3. **Treatment:** combination of chemotherapy and radiation therapy with palliative surgical fixation of pathologic fractures to improve the patient's quality of life

VII. **Metastatic disease:** Tumors metastatic to the skeleton are significantly more common than primary musculoskeletal tumors. Primary tumors that most commonly metastasize to bone include carcinomas of the breast, lung, prostate, thyroid, and kidney, or indeed, almost any type of tumor.
   A. **Diagnosis:** Most bony metastatic disease presents with pain in the involved bone. Metastatic bone disease may be the initial presentation of a malignancy.
      1. **Radiographs:** Show most bone lesions to be lytic. With some breast tumors and most prostatic tumors, the bone lesion has a blastic appearance.
      2. **Bone scans:** Helpful when a single symptomatic lytic lesion is found on initial radiographs. If the bone scan shows multiple lesions, the likelihood of metastatic disease is high.
      3. **Skeletal metastases of unknown origin:** best worked up with a history and physical examination; blood tests including CBC, thyroid-stimulating hormone, and calcium level; urine analysis; whole-body bone scan; plain radiographs of the chest and the involved bone; and a CT scan of the chest, abdomen, and pelvis
   B. **Treatment:** radiation therapy
      1. **Prophylactic bone fixation:** indicated when a bone lesion places the bone at significant risk of fracture without treatment
      2. **Pathologic fractures:** generally should be fixed internally using a combination of metal implants plus methylmethacrylate bone cement to manage bone loss

ADULT ORTHOPEDICS

Shoulder and Elbow

I. **Rotator cuff tear:** Rotator cuff consists of the supraspinatus, infraspinatus, teres minor, and subscapularis muscles. Acute tears occur in overhead throwing athletes or patients age older than 40 years with shoulder dislocation. Chronic degenerative tears are usually seen in patients older than 60 years.
   A. **Symptoms:** include shoulder pain exacerbated by overhead activity, night pain, and shoulder weakness
   B. **Diagnosis:** MRI is the imaging of choice to confirm clinical suspicion for rotator cuff tears. Ultrasound may be an effective alternative but is dependent on the comfort level of the user.
   C. **Treatment:** Physical therapy, NSAIDs, and steroid injection are the first line; arthroscopic rotator cuff repair is indicated for failed conservative treatment.

II. **Anterior shoulder instability:** Most common cause is an anterior shoulder dislocation.
   A. **Associated lesions:** Bankart (tear of the anterior labrum) and Hill-Sachs (impaction of the posterior humeral head onto the anterior glenoid) lesions
   B. **Recurrence:** high rate—up to 90% in first-time dislocators age younger than 25 years

III. **Lateral epicondylitis:** tendinosis (tendon degeneration) of the origin of extensor carpi radialis brevis (ECRB) tendon at the lateral epicondyle of the humerus; most common cause of elbow pain and attributed to overexertion of the forearm with repetitive wrist extension and forearm pronation/supination
   A. **Presentation:** elbow pain exacerbated by resisted wrist extension and gripping activities
   B. **Physical exam:** reveals tenderness to palpation of the origin of ECRB on the lateral epicondyle

C. Treatment: Activity modification, physical therapy, NSAIDs, and steroid injections. A proximal forearm band may help alleviate symptoms, as it offloads tension from the ECRB tendon. Surgical debridement of the tendon is warranted in patients refractory to aforementioned management after several months of symptoms.

Hand

I. **Carpal tunnel syndrome:** compression of the median nerve at the wrist; most common UE compressive neuropathy, affecting up to 10% of the population
   A. **Symptoms:** numbness and paresthesias in the median nerve distribution
   B. **Physical exam:** may reveal thenar atrophy and positive Tinel sign at the wrist (tapping above the carpal aggravates symptoms)
   C. **Diagnosis:** Clinical; nerve conduction velocity (NCV) and electromyography (EMG) may help confirm the diagnosis.
   D. **Treatment:** Wrist splinting, activity modification, or steroid injection into the carpal tunnel. If this fails, surgical release of the transverse carpal ligament is indicated.

> **Quick Cut**
> Carpal tunnel syndrome is initially managed by rest and splinting.

II. **Trigger finger:** Clicking and catching of the flexor tendons at the A1 pulley (annular ligament at the metacarpophalangeal joint). Symptoms respond well to steroid injection. Surgical release of the A1 pulley indicated for failed injections.

III. **Paronychia:** infection at the nail fold; most common hand infection
   A. **Acute infection:** occurs secondary to trauma such as nail biting or manicure; most commonly *S. aureus*
   B. **Chronic infection:** occurs with prolonged exposure to water or chemicals; most commonly *Candida albicans*
   C. **Treatment:** removal of the nail plate, irrigation, and antibiotics/antifungals

IV. **Flexor tenosynovitis:** infection of the synovial sheath of the flexor tendons of the hand
   A. **Symptoms:** Kanavel signs found on exam
   B. **Treatment:** incision and drainage of the flexor tendon sheath; IV antibiotics and observation of clinical improvement

> **Quick Cut**
> Kanavel signs are:
> - flexed posture of the affected finger
> - pain with passive stretch of the digit
> - sausage-like swelling
> - tenderness to palpation over the flexor tendon
> - and possible spread by communication with the synovial sheaths of the thumb and small finger.

V. **Ganglion cyst:** mucin-filled cyst that involves a joint or tendon sheath usually caused by trauma or degeneration; commonly occurs at the dorsal or volar wrist
   A. **Presentation:** Appears as a firm, well-circumscribed mass that transilluminates over a light source. Symptoms may include pain that radiates to the fingers with wrist motion or direct trauma to the cyst.
   B. **Treatment:** Observation; aspiration has a high recurrence rate. Surgical cyst resection indicated for failed observation and persistent pain.

Hip

I. **Trochanteric bursitis:** Pain over the lateral aspect of the hip thought to be due to inflammation in the bursa between the greater trochanter and the iliotibial band. Tendinosis of the gluteus medius and minimus tendons is often the primary cause of trochanteric bursitis.
   A. **Symptoms:** Include lateral hip pain that may radiate to the buttocks, groin, or lower back. Pain is exacerbated by stair climbing or rising from a seated position. Patients often complain of inability to sleep on the affected side.
   B. **Physical exam:** reveals tenderness to palpation over the trochanter and pain with resisted abduction
   C. **Treatment:** NSAIDs, physical therapy, and steroid injection are often effective.

Knee

I. **Anterior cruciate ligament (ACL) tear:** ACL is the major ligament that stabilizes the tibia from translating anteriorly beneath the femur. Most common mechanism is a noncontact pivoting injury; patients feel a "pop" in the knee and often results in acute hemarthrosis.
   A. **Physical exam:** reveals a positive Lachman test (increased anterior tibial translation with the knee flexed to 30 degrees)

B. Treatment: Nonoperative treatment with activity modification and physical therapy is acceptable for low-demand patients. ACL reconstruction indicated for active patients who want to return to sports and those with persistent instability.

II. **Posterior cruciate ligament (PCL) tear:** PCL stabilizes the tibia from posterior translation beneath the femur. It is injured with a posteriorly directed force onto the tibia such as a dashboard injury.
   A. Physical exam: reveals a positive posterior drawer test
   B. Treatment: Bracing is indicated for low-demand patients. PCL reconstruction is indicated for PCL injuries combined with other ligamentous injury.

III. **Medial collateral ligament (MCL) tear:** MCL stabilizes the knee against valgus stress; most commonly injured ligament of the knee. Treatment is physical therapy and bracing for partial tears. Operative repair or reconstruction for complete tears or combined ligamentous injuries.

IV. **Lateral collateral ligament (LCL) tear:** LCL stabilizes the knee against varus stress; injury of the LCL is usually combined with other ligamentous injuries. Treatment is physical therapy and bracing for partial tears. Operative repair or reconstruction for complete tears or combined ligamentous injuries.

V. **Meniscal tear:** variable etiology, location, and morphology
   A. Classification: degenerative, traumatic, or both
   B. Location: may occur in the medial (most common) or lateral compartments
   C. Involvement: may involve the lateral one third (vascularized), middle one third, or inner one third (avascular) zones of the meniscus
   D. Tear pattern: may be vertical, horizontal, radial, bucket-handle, parrot beak, or complex
   E. Presentation: medial or lateral-sided joint pain with mechanical symptoms (clicking or locking of the knee)
   F. Physical exam: may reveal an effusion, joint line tenderness, and a positive McMurray test
   G. Treatment: NSAIDs and physical therapy; surgical treatment for mechanical symptoms (catching/locking) or persistent pain
      1. **Partial meniscectomy:** for tears not amenable to repair
      2. **Meniscal repair:** for tears in the peripheral (vascular) zone
      3. **Meniscal transplantation:** option for young patients with normal mechanical alignment of the knee and no full-thickness cartilage defects

VI. **Quadriceps and patellar tendon tear:** most often occurs in middle-aged and older patients, especially those with diabetes mellitus or renal disease
   A. Physical examination: Mild swelling and tenderness; patient is unable to initiate extension against gravity with the knee at 90 degrees of flexion.
   B. Treatment: surgical repair

Foot and Ankle

I. **Ankle sprains:** typically inversion injuries that involve the anterior talofibular ligament (ATFL) and less frequently the calcaneofibular ligament (CFL)
   A. Treatment: rest, ice, compression, and elevation (RICE)
   B. Functional mobilization: achieved with a stirrup brace with weight bearing as tolerated

II. **Achilles tendon disruptions:** usually young to middle-aged patients who typically feel a sharp pain or hear an audible "pop"
   A. Physical examination: Thompson test is performed with the patient prone and the examiner squeezing the calf looking for plantar flexion of the foot. Greatly decreased or absent flexion is a positive sign of rupture.
   B. Treatment: controversial
      1. **Casting:** yields higher rerupture rates
      2. **Surgical treatment:** increased infection rate at the site

Study Questions for Part VII

Directions: *Each of the numbered items in this section is followed by several possible answers. Select the ONE lettered answer that is BEST in each case.*

1. A 47-year-old patient with a history of left-sided nephrectomy for trauma 20 years ago presents with right flank pain and hematuria. Laboratory studies reveal a creatinine of 2.5 mg/dL. Which of the following is the appropriate management plan?

   A. Hydration overnight, followed by repeat evaluation of serum creatinine
   B. Intravenous pyelography (IVP)
   C. CT scan of abdomen and pelvis with oral and IV contrast
   D. Ultrasonography followed by urgent cystoscopy
   E. Percutaneous nephrostomy tube placement

2. Which of the following are potential sequelae of benign prostatic hyperplasia?

   A. Bladder stone formation
   B. Recurrent urinary tract infections secondary to prostatitis
   C. Prostate cancer
   D. Bladder cancer
   E. Organic impotence

3. A 68-year-old man undergoes a CT scan of the abdomen as part of the evaluation for some mild abdominal tenderness after a motor vehicle collision. The scan reveals no evidence of trauma, but a 4-cm solid left renal mass is noted. There is evidence of thrombus in the inferior vena cava. Which of the following treatments is *not* indicated?

   A. Preoperative chemotherapy and radiation to downstage tumor
   B. Resection of the left adrenal gland
   C. Resection of the para-aortic lymph nodes
   D. Resection of the left kidney
   E. Incision of vena cava and removal of thrombus

4. A 23-year-old man has a solid mass in his left testis. When it is removed, the pathology reveals an embryonal carcinoma with a teratoma. A CT scan of the chest and abdomen reveals 8 cm of lymphadenopathy in the periaortic nodes. What is the recommended treatment?

   A. Modified nerve-sparing retroperitoneal lymph node dissection
   B. Full bilateral retroperitoneal lymph node dissection
   C. Chemotherapy with paclitaxel (Taxol), gemcitabine, and cisplatin
   D. Chemotherapy with cisplatin, etoposide, and bleomycin
   E. Chemotherapy plus retroperitoneal radiation

5. Which testicular cancer cell type is extremely radiosensitive?

   A. Embryonal carcinoma
   B. Yolk sac tumor
   C. Seminoma
   D. Choriocarcinoma
   E. Teratocarcinoma

6. A 21-year-old male patient is brought to the emergency department for evaluation after a motor vehicle accident. As part of this secondary survey, the patient is found to have blood at the urethral meatus. What is the next maneuver?

A. Foley catheter insertion followed by cystogram
B. Urethrogram
C. IVP
D. CT scan
E. Diagnostic peritoneal lavage

Directions: *The group of items in this section consists of lettered options followed by a set of numbered items. For each item, select the lettered option(s) that is(are) most closely associated with it. Each lettered option may be selected once, more than once, or not at all.*

7. A 70-year-old man presents to the outpatient clinic with complaints of difficulty in voiding. He reports some hesitancy in initiating flow, as well as a sense of incomplete emptying. He has not had any fever or chills and complains of only a mild dull pain in the lower midline. What is the most likely source of his symptoms?

A. Simple urinary tract infection
B. Pyelonephritis
C. Prostatic cancer
D. Benign prostatic hyperplasia
E. Ureteral stones

8. The patient has normal vital signs and no pain on physical examination. Ultrasound examination in the previous patient demonstrates 150 mL of urine remaining in the bladder following voiding. The best initial treatment for the management of this patient is:

A. Narcotics
B. Ciprofloxacin
C. Tamsulosin (Flomax)
D. Cystoscopy
E. Open prostatectomy with lymph node dissection

9. A 34-year-old man is involved in a motorcycle crash and sustains significant damage to legs and skin. He has a large skin defect over the majority of the back of the hand. The most appropriate definitive management for this patient is:

A. Split-thickness skin grafting
B. Primary closure
C. Biologic dressing
D. Vacuum-assisted closure
E. Full-thickness skin grafting

10. A 9-year-old boy falls off his bicycle, strikes the edge of a curb, and shears off a portion of his upper lip. On examination, he is hemodynamically stable without evidence of any internal injury. The right upper lip has a large flap that is nearly transected and ischemic and approximately 20% of the overall lip length. After debridement of devitalized tissue, the best management for this defect is:

A. Healing by secondary intention
B. Primary closure
C. Nasolabial rotational flap
D. Buccal flap
E. Free flap from LE

11. A 27-year-old man is struck on the side of the head during a company softball game. The patient complains of headache, has had two episodes of emesis, and is somewhat lethargic. The most likely source of his problems is:

    A. Elevated intracranial pressure
    B. Contrecoup injury
    C. Cranial nerve V injury
    D. Cranial nerve VII injury
    E. Basilar skull fracture

12. The same patient from question number 11 was initially briefly unconscious at the scene then regained consciousness. Although under evaluation, his mental state deteriorates. The most likely explanation for this is:

    A. Subdural hemorrhage
    B. Subarachnoid hemorrhage
    C. Epidural hematoma
    D. Basilar skull fracture
    E. Inner ear disruption

13. A 30-year-old woman is stabbed in the back and presents to the emergency department in a highly anxious state. Her heart rate is 120 beats per minute and her blood pressure is 100/50 mm Hg. On exam, she does not have motor function in her right leg, which is also numb. On the left leg, she does not react to painful stimuli and is insensate to temperature. The most likely etiology of her problem is:

    A. Central cord syndrome
    B. Neurogenic shock
    C. Anterior spinal cord injury
    D. Diffuse axonal injury
    E. Hemisection of the spinal cord

14. A 20-year-old man is in a motor vehicle collision and has a fracture of the left tibia. On exam, he has a nondisplaced fracture and terrible pain in the leg, which seems to be getting worse despite narcotic pain medication. The pulse in the leg is present but diminished relative to the other side. The patient also complains of numbness in the affected foot. The best initial treatment is:

    A. Fluid resuscitation
    P. Parenteral narcotics
    C. Operative release of the compartments of the leg
    D. External fixation
    E. CT angiography

15. An 18-year-old girl falls from atop a piece of furniture onto a hard surface but stops her fall on an outstretched hand. She only complains of pain in her wrist. What is the most likely injury?

    A. Distal radial fracture
    B. Distal ulnar fracture
    C. Lunate bone fracture
    D. Scaphoid bone fracture
    E. Boxer's fracture

16. A 25-year-old man has been playing basketball when another player fell atop his knee. He felt a popping sensation, followed by acute pain. On exam, the lower leg moves forward freely at the knee joint. The patient has a weakly palpable pulse in the leg, and the ABI is 0.6 (and 1.0 on the unaffected side). The most appropriate next step is:

    A. Angiography
    B. Knee brace immobilization
    C. Urgent arthroscopy
    D. Heparinization
    E. Serial pulse examinations

17. A 47-year-old woman is undergoing a left mastectomy for a large breast cancer. Postoperative chemotherapy is planned. Which of the following is not true?

A. A tissue expander can be placed at the time of the initial operation to provide reconstruction.
B. A latissimus dorsi flap can provide adequate tissue for reconstruction.
C. Reconstruction must be delayed until after treatment for the primary tumor is complete.
D. A contralateral reduction mammoplasty can provide symmetry.
E. Nipple reconstruction is typically performed as a separate procedure.

18. A 68-year-old woman has a Mohs excision on the tip of her nose. A full-thickness skin graft with a tie-over dressing is used. On the fifth postoperative day, the dressing is removed, and the graft is pink. What is the most likely reason for this?

A. Imbibition
B. Inosculation
C. Infection
D. Fibrination
E. Collagenesis

19. Which of the following is the best treatment for melanoma?

A. Surgical excision
B. Chemotherapy
C. Radiation therapy
D. Immunotherapy
E. Regional hyperthermic perfusion

20. A 21-year-old male suffers a severe comminuted fracture of the right LE with considerable soft tissue loss after a motorcycle accident. He has exposed bone and tendon in his wound after external fixation. Which is the appropriate management?

A. Split-thickness skin graft
B. Full-thickness skin graft
C. Allograft followed by full-thickness skin graft
D. Z plasty
E. Muscle flap

21. The son of a 74-year-old woman calls her primary care physician for advice. He says that his mother has been complaining of headache and vertigo for several hours and is vomiting. Apart from a deep venous thrombosis in her left leg 2 months ago, she has been healthy. They shared dinner the night before, and she had been fine. She now is asking for a prescription for the same motion sickness pills that she used to help her son when she drove him to camp. What should the physician do?

A. Call in a prescription for droperidol.
B. Make arrangements to see the patient in clinic tomorrow.
C. Make arrangements to see the patient in clinic today.
D. Recommend that the patient be taken to the emergency department in an ambulance.
E. Order a ventilation/perfusion scan to rule out pulmonary embolism.

22. Which of these statements is true?

A. Brain metastases occur more frequently than primary brain tumors.
B. The Cushing response is the tachycardia and hypertension seen with mass lesions of the pituitary.
C. The Cushing response is bradycardia and hypotension seen with terminal brain herniation.
D. The Cushing response is the maintenance of cerebral perfusion pressure against variations in systemic blood pressure.
E. Primary brain tumors are more common than metastatic brain tumors.

Questions 23–24

A 38-year-old previously healthy female presents with a single partial seizure. Physical examination is unremarkable. A CT head scan shows a lesion that enhances with contrast measuring 1.5 × 1 cm in the tip of the right temporal lobe surrounded by a rim of local edema.

23. What is the best way to proceed?

    A. Stereotactic needle biopsy
    B. Open biopsy
    C. Tumor resection
    D. Electroencephalography (EEG)
    E. Brain MRI, chest radiograph

24. If this patient's lesion is resected and it turns out to be a glioblastoma, which of the following is true?

    A. The patient's median expected survival is 2 years.
    B. Additional surgery is not meaningful.
    C. The patient's prognosis is unchanged by radiation therapy.
    D. Age is an important prognostic factor for this tumor.
    E. The clinical presentation of the tumor was uncommon for this patient.

25. Which of the following major joint dislocations constitutes the direst surgical emergency?

    A. Hip dislocation
    B. Knee dislocation
    C. Shoulder dislocation
    D. Elbow dislocation
    E. Subtalar dislocation

26. A 37-year-old intoxicated man is struck by the bumper of a car while he is crossing the street. He sustains a comminuted closed proximal one-third tibia and fibula fractures. The fractures are stabilized with an external fixator 1 hour after the man arrives at the trauma bay. Approximately 2 hours after surgery, he has a severe pain that is not controlled by IV morphine. The physical examination demonstrates 2+ dorsalis pedis and posterior tibial pulses, increased swelling of the leg, decreased sensation and paresthesias of the first web space, and exquisite pain with active and passive motion of the toes. What should be the next step in treatment?

    A. Four compartment fasciotomies of the leg
    B. Femoral angiography with runoff
    C. Elevation of the leg above the heart
    D. Continued observation
    E. Repeat plain radiographs of the leg

27. Which of the following describes the most appropriate treatment regimen for a newly diagnosed primary osteogenic sarcoma of the distal femur?

    A. Above-knee amputation and chemotherapy
    B. Radiation therapy
    C. Limb salvage surgery with marginal excision
    D. Neoadjuvant and adjuvant chemotherapy with surgical excision
    E. A combination of chemotherapy and radiation therapy

28. A patient is involved in a high-speed motor vehicle collision. The patient has a Glasgow Coma Scale (GCS) score of 7 on arrival. Which of the following is not urgently indicated?

    A. Emergent intubation
    B. Placement of an intraventricular catheter
    C. Nasogastric tube to prevent aspiration
    D. Spinal cord immobilization
    E. Urgent CT scan of the brain

Answers and Explanations

1. **The answer is D** (Chapter 25, Urologic Emergencies, Obstructive Uropathy, and Urinary Tract Stones, Treatment). An obstruction calculus in a patient with a single kidney represents an indication for emergency surgery. Hydration alone is insufficient and may lead to permanent renal impairment. Radiographic studies with IV contrast may cause nephrotoxicity with impaired renal function. Percutaneous nephrostomy tube placement should be reserved for cases in which cystoscopy and retrograde pyelography and stent placement fail.

2. **The answer is A** (Chapter 25, Benign Prostatic Disorders, Benign Prostatic Hyperplasia, V A 3). Bladder stone formation due to urinary stasis is a known sequelae of benign prostatic hyperplasia (BPH), and with severe obstructive symptoms, patients can have bilateral hydroureteronephrosis and renal failure, commonly known as obstructive azotemia. Recurrent prostatitis is caused by bacterial or nonbacterial infection of the prostate and has no correlation with BPH. Bladder and prostate cancer or organic impotence are not directly associated with BPH.

3. **The answer is A** (Chapter 25, Genitourinary Malignancies, Renal Cell Carcinoma, III). Renal cell carcinoma is very chemotherapy resistant. A left radical nephrectomy includes the left kidney, adrenal gland, and investing and fascia as well as a regional lymphadenectomy. Removal of tumor thrombus from the inferior vena cava is indicated.

4. **The answer is D** (Chapter 25, Genitourinary Malignancies, Testicular Tumors, IV B). Men with metastatic nonseminomatous testicular carcinoma, and in this case with bulky retroperitoneal disease, are best treated initially with systemic chemotherapy. The agents of choice are cisplatin, etoposide, and bleomycin.

5. **The answer is C** (Chapter 25, Genitourinary Malignancies, Testicular Tumors, IV A). Seminomas are uniquely radiosensitive among testicular tumors. Other nonseminomatous tumors, on the other hand, respond to chemotherapy and are generally radioresistant.

6. **The answer is B** (Chapter 25, Urologic Trauma, Bladder Trauma [Lower Urinary Tract], II A). The finding of blood at the urethral meatus or an elevated prostate gland suggests a urethral tear. Passage of a Foley catheter may exacerbate a urethral tear. IVP and CT scan detect injuries to the kidney, ureters, and bladder but not injuries to the urethra. The patient must have a carefully performed urethrogram before any other urologic manipulation.

7. **The answer is D** (Chapter 25, Benign Prostatic Disorders, Benign Prostatic Hyperplasia, III). Benign prostatic hyperplasia is a common condition that presents with signs and symptoms due to the mechanical impingement of the urethra. Common symptoms include obstructive symptoms, such as those described in the question earlier, as well as irritative symptoms, such as frequency, urgency, nocturia, and dysuria. Physical exam demonstrates an enlarged, firm gland, and diagnosis may be confirmed on biopsy.

8. **The answer is C** (Chapter 25, Benign Prostatic Disorders, Benign Prostatic Hyperplasia, V). The initial treatment of benign prostatic hypertrophy is medical. Alpha blockade, such as with tamsulosin, is appropriate. Narcotics are useful in the management of kidney stones. Antibiotics are appropriate for urinary tract infection and suspected bacterial prostatitis. Cystoscopy is an excellent diagnostic maneuver for lesions of the bladder. Prostatectomy is typically reserved for cases of malignancy.

9. **The answer is E** (Chapter 26, Reconstructive Plastic Surgery, Wounds and Defects, III A). After initial debridement and wound care to minimize contamination, the definitive management of a functional area across a joint is full-thickness skin grafting. Split-thickness grafts are contraindicated due to the risk of contracture and reduced mobility. Primary closure is a great technique for small defects but produces too much tension in areas of substantial loss. Vacuum-assisted closure suffers the same risk of loss of function, and biologic dressings probably have their greatest use as temporary closure in burn patients.

10. **The answer is B** (Chapter 26, Reconstructive Plastic Surgery, Head-to-Toe Reconstruction, V). Lip defects that are up to one third of the lip length are amenable to primary closure. Secondary intention produces significant deformity. Local flaps are unacceptable cosmetically, and free flaps from dissimilar areas have no role in reconstruction.

11. **The answer is A** (Chapter 27, Pathophysiology, Intracranial Pressure, IV). The patient is displaying classic signs of elevated intracranial pressure, including headache, nausea, and decreased levels of consciousness. Contrecoup injury may occur opposite the site of direct injury but in and of itself does not explain the patient's symptoms. Trigeminal and facial nerve injuries are uncommon and do not lead to the listed symptoms. The mechanism of injury is highly unlikely to damage the base of the skull.

12. **The answer is C** (Chapter 27, Head Injury, Extra-axial Hemorrhages, I D). The patient had a "lucid interval" typical of the arterial injury associated with epidural hematomas. Subarachnoid hemorrhage usually produces a "thunderclap" headache that does not remit, and subdural hematomas produce chronic, progressive symptoms. Basilar skull fracture may produce characteristic bruising patterns on the face and head.

13. **The answer is E** (Chapter 27, Spinal Cord Injury, Overview, III B 3). Brown-Séquard syndrome, or hemisection of the spinal cord, typically results from penetrating trauma, with loss of motor function and sensation to light touch and vibration ipsilaterally, with loss of pain and temperature sensation contralaterally. Central cord lesions typically affect upper extremities more than lower. The patient does not meet parameters for shock. Anterior spinal cord problems lead to muscle weakness but preservation of sensation. Diffuse axonal injury leads to difficulty with mentation rather than focal sensory defects.

14. **The answer is C** (Chapter 28, Orthopedic Emergencies, Epidural Abscess, IV). The patient is presenting with early signs and symptoms of compartment syndrome. It would be reasonable to measure compartment pressures, but the treatment is emergent decompression. Overly aggressive fluid resuscitation may worsen the symptoms, and narcotics may only mask the pain leading to worsening necrosis. External fixation is a good option if an open fracture is present but will not address this patient's problems.

15. **The answer is D** (Chapter 28, Trauma, Fractures in Adults, IV). The scaphoid bone is the most commonly injured bone of the wrist, typically injured during a fall. This represents an urgent situation, as the blood supply to this region is notoriously tenuous. Radiographs should be obtained immediately. If the fracture is nondisplaced, a thumb-spica cast is appropriate; displaced fractures require operative fixation.

16. **The answer is A** (Chapter 28, Trauma, Dislocations, III B 1). A knee dislocation places the popliteal artery at risk. The priority is on diagnosis, with a formal angiogram for patients with an abnormal ABI. A knee brace may be used but is insufficient to address the limb-threatening injury to the artery. Arthroscopic surgery may help with the ligaments but again ignores the vasculature. Heparin is not indicated until a diagnosis is made.

17. **The answer is C** (Chapter 26, Head-to-Toe Reconstruction, Breast Reconstruction, VII A). Breast reconstruction can be performed either at the time of mastectomy or as a delayed procedure. Timing is not dependent on adjuvant treatment.

18. **The answer is B** (Chapter 26, Reconstructive Plastic Surgery, Wounds and Defects, III E 2). Skin grafts are initially held in place by fibrin bonds. Imbibition is from passive movement of nutrient to the graft from the donor tissue. When inosculation, or vascular budding, occurs, the graft turns pink from return of circulation to the graft.

19. **The answer is A** (Chapter 26, Wound Healing and Diseases of Skin and Soft Tissue, Malignant Skin Lesions, III D). Surgical excision remains the definitive treatment for melanoma. All of the other options are adjuvant treatments.

20. **The answer is E** (Chapter 26, Reconstructive Plastic Surgery, Head-to-Toe Reconstruction, XI A). Bone denuded of periosteum and tendons does not support skin grafts. These areas require muscle flaps for coverage.

21. **The answer is D** (Chapter 27, Spinal Cord Injury, Intracerebral Hemorrhage, I B). The patient has symptoms referable to the central nervous system. Her age makes stroke likely. Having had a recent venous thrombosis, she will likely be on anticoagulant therapy. Thus, a hemorrhage should be suspected. There is no information about motor weakness; therefore, the cerebellum is a more likely location than the cerebrum. The vertigo also implicates the cerebellum. The posterior fossa is a very tight compartment, intolerant of mass effects. Uncontrolled hypertension leads to progression of clot size and is the mechanism for rapid symptom progression and death. Even without clot growth, there is a risk for development of hydrocephalus. The patient needs to be evaluated emergently, her blood pressure normalized if elevated, and a CT scan performed to look for the suspected cerebellar hemorrhage. She will then need either surgery or observation in the intensive care unit. Pulmonary embolism is far less likely than stroke and usually presents with dyspnea. Thus, the ventilation-perfusion scan is not indicated. The son is not vomiting, so the food they had shared is unlikely to be causing her symptoms. Droperidol is given intravenously and would be of little use to the patient at home even if all she really needed was an antiemetic.

22. **The answer is A** (Chapter 27, Pathophysiology, Intracranial Pressure, IV). The Cushing response is the combination of bradycardia and hypertension. Metastatic cancers greatly outnumber primary brain neoplasms. Even if only one fifth of cancers cause brain metastases, these still outnumber primary tumors.

23. **The answer is E** (Chapter 27, Central Nervous System Tumors, Specific Brain Tumors, I B). Late-onset seizure should be considered to be caused by a brain tumor until proven otherwise. CT head scan appearance is only suggestive of etiology; it cannot be fully depended on to distinguish between primary tumors and metastases. MRI can reveal additional small lesions often not visible on CT. Multiple lesions would suggest metastases rather than primary tumor, as primary parenchymal tumors are usually but not always solitary. A lesion found on chest radiograph suggests a brain metastases because primary brain tumors do not spread to the lungs. If MRI shows multiple lesions, the surgeon can target the safest one for biopsy. If there is only one lesion, suggesting a primary brain neoplasm, its location in the tip of the nondominant hemisphere allows for radical resection.

24. **The answer is D** (Chapter 27, Central Nervous System Tumors, Specific Brain Tumors, I B). Younger patients with glioblastomas tend to survive longer than the elderly, and supratentorial location is more common than infratentorial location in adults. The median expected survival for a patient with a glioblastoma is 1 year. Aggressive cytoreductive surgery improves survival. The difficult issue is the postoperative quality of life. Survival is improved by radiation, although the time gained is weeks or months, not years. The tumor was located in the anterior temporal lobe where seizures are a common presentation.

25. **The answer is B** (Chapter 28, Trauma, Dislocations, III). Dislocation of the knee is accompanied by a 30%–33% incidence of injury to the popliteal vasculature (and nerve). A pre- and postreduction neurovascular examination is mandatory, and any suggestion of altered perfusion (ABI <0.9, decreased pulses, signs of ischemia) requires an evaluation of the vascular supply distal to the knee. Frank tears or intimal injuries can occur. Dislocation of the hip can lead to avascular necrosis of the femoral head, especially if reduction is delayed for longer than 12 hours; however, this injury is not limb threatening. Shoulder dislocation is associated with axillary nerve trauma and rotator cuff tears in older people. Simple (no fracture) elbow or subtalar dislocations tend to be stable following reduction.

26. **The answer is A** (Chapter 28, Orthopedic Emergencies, Compartment Syndrome, III). Compartment syndrome is common after high-energy trauma, particularly that which has a component of crushing injury. The diagnosis is made clinically by pain out of proportion to that expected from the injury and pain with passive stretch of muscles in the involved compartment. Intracompartmental pressure monitoring can be used to confirm the diagnosis or to make it in an obtunded patient. Femoral angiography would be indicated if vascular injury were suspected. Elevation of the leg can actually exacerbate compartment syndrome by decreasing the arterial inflow pressure if elevation is excessive. Plain radiographs and continued observation are not indicated because excessive delay in treatment can result in irreversible ischemia. Fasciotomies must be performed to relieve the compartment syndrome.

27. The answer is D (Chapter 28, Tumors, Primary Bone Tumors, VI A 4). Primary osteogenic sarcoma occurs most frequently in adolescence and young adulthood and appears most commonly about the knee (distal femur and proximal tibia). The combination of neoadjuvant (before surgery) and adjuvant chemotherapy, with surgical resection to achieve at least a wide (2-cm cuff of normal tissue) surgical margin, has increased the 5-year disease-free survival rate to more than 60%. Radiation is not indicated when clean surgical margins are obtained.

28. The answer is C (Chapter 27, Head Injury, Initial Management and Assessment, Increased Intracranial Pressure Management). A GCS less than 8 requires intubation and intracranial pressure monitoring. Spinal cord immobilization should be practiced for all trauma patients. A CT scan will greatly aid diagnosis. Although gastric decompression may be part of this patient's management, this is a secondary concern. In fact, placement of a tube before imaging may complicate a basilar skull fracture.

Grade "A" Cuts: Useful Surgical Knowledge Pairings by System

 ASSOCIATIONS WITH HIGH VALUE FOR THE SURGICAL STUDENT

Cardiovascular	Think
Aortic dissection—proximal (type A)	Surgery
Aortic dissection—distal (type B)	Blood pressure control
Deep venous thrombosis (DVT)/pulmonary embolism (PE)	Best strategy is prevention
Transient ischemic attack and carotid lesion	Endarterectomy
Completed stroke	Usually no surgery
Abdominal aortic aneurysm >5 cm	Repair
Abdominal aortic aneurysm (AAA) and pain	Rupture; emergent repair
Aortic graft and gastrointestinal (GI) bleed	Rule out (R/O) aortoenteric fistula
Aortic graft and fever	R/O graft infection
Aortoiliac occlusive disease	Impotence, buttock claudication
Extremity rest pain or tissue loss	Urgent revascularization
Ankle-brachial index (ABI) 0.4–0.7	Claudication
ABI <0.4	Rest pain
Extrinsic coagulation cascade	Prothrombin time, blocked by warfarin
Intrinsic coagulation cascade	Partial thromboplastin time, blocked by heparin
Popliteal aneurysms	Limb-threatening (thrombosis)
Femoral aneurysms	Not limb-threatening
Iliac veins	Have no valves
Virchow triad	Stasis, intimal injury, hypercoagulability

Esophagus

Esophagus	Think
Dysphagia	Must do endoscopy, R/O cancer
"Bird's beak" esophagram	Achalasia
Nissen fundoplication	Treats gastroesophageal reflux disease (GERD), not Barrett dysplasia
Poor peristalsis and GERD	Consider Nissen with caution, may have dysphagia
High-grade Barrett	25% risk of carcinoma
Cancer in Barrett	Curative by resection
Esophageal cancer	EUS to stage; early disease is resectable
Zenker diverticulum	Cricothyroidotomy
Esophageal perforation	Diversion, tube thoracostomy
Esophageal perforation	Most commonly iatrogenic
Alkali injury	Liquefaction necrosis
Histologic layer absent in esophagus	Serosa
Scleroderma	Avoid surgery

Stomach/Duodenum

Stomach/Duodenum	Think
Gastric varices	Splenic vein thrombosis
Nonhealing gastric ulcer	Resection of ulcer, R/O cancer
Bleeding ulcer	Endoscopic intervention
Anterior duodenal ulcer	Perforates, patch with omentum
Posterior duodenal ulcer	Bleeds, high rebleed rate
Gastrointestinal stromal tumor (GIST)	Resection +/− imatinib
Mucosa-associated lymphoid tissue lymphoma	Treat *Helicobacter pylori* (antibiotics)
Ulcer and high gastrin levels	Zollinger-Ellison syndrome
Severe obesity (body mass index $>40 \text{ kg/m}^2$)	Bariatric surgery
Most feared bariatric surgery complication	Anastomotic leak
Gastric cancer	Surgery for R0 and R1 nodal disease
Nutritional deficiencies after bariatric surgery	Vitamin B_{12}, Ca, Fe, fat-soluble vitamins
Four major gastric arteries (two gastric, two gastroepiploic)	Only one of four necessary to preserve viability of stomach
Most important stimulus for secretin release	Gastric acid
Most important stimulus for gastrin release	A meal
Most important stimulus for parietal cell	Acetylcholine, histamine, gastrin

Liver

Liver	Think
Cyst—simple	No surgery
Cyst with internal echo	Bacterial abscess
Cyst with "anchovy paste"	Amebic abscess
Cyst with calcifications	*Echinococcus*
Abscess etiology	Bacteremia, GI perforation, intravenous drug abuse
Solid mass—most common benign lesion	Hemangioma
Solid mass—most common cancer	Metastasis
Solitary colorectal metastasis	Positron emission tomography to prove isolated, then resection
Hepatic adenoma	Has risk of rupture, often surgery

Focal nodular hyperplasia (FNH)	Central stellate scar on computed tomography (CT)
Focal nodular hyperplasia	No surgery
Alpha-fetoprotein	Hepatocellular carcinoma
Bleeding esophageal varices	Endoscopic banding
Refractory bleeding esophageal varices	Transjugular intrahepatic portosystemic shunt
High MELD score for end stage liver disease	Serious liver failure (think transplant)
Bleeding with cirrhosis	Low factors II, VII, IX, X, and platelets
Replaced right hepatic artery	Arises from SMA

Biliary-Pancreas / Think

Jaundice—painful	Gallstones
Jaundice—painless	Cancer
Primary sclerosing cholangitis	Ulcerative colitis
Mucosal gallbladder cancer	Curable with cholecystectomy
Cholangiocarcinoma	Usually not resectable
Ampullary cancer	Often curative resection is possible
Fever, jaundice, right upper quadrant pain	Cholangitis
Gallbladder wall edema and gallstones	Acute cholecystitis
Acute pancreatitis etiology	Gallstones or alcohol
Chronic pancreatitis	Ductal stricture ("chain of lakes") and calcification
Pancreatic pseudocyst	Most resolve; otherwise cyst—gastrostomy
Pancreatic pseudocyst	Communicates with pancreatic duct
CA 19-9	Pancreatic cancer marker

Small Intestine / Think

Small bowel obstruction (SBO) and hernia	Surgery
SBO most common cause in the United States	Adhesions
Closed loop obstruction	Surgical emergency
Acute abdomen	Almost always surgical
Meckel diverticulum	Bleed (heterotopic gastric mucosa)
Intussusception in adults	Polypoid mass as lead point; resect
Crohn disease	Creeping fat, transmural inflammation, perianal disease
Crohn disease with bleed, stricture, perforation, or fistula	Surgery
Carcinoid of the small bowel	Obstruction, bleeding; more aggressive
Carcinoid of the appendix	Curable with resection, less aggressive

Colon / Think

Cecal volvulus	Left upper quadrant distended loop, surgical resection
Sigmoid volvulus	Right upper quadrant loop, decompression, then surgery
Volvulus	"Bent inner tube" sign on x-ray
Retrocecal appendix	20% occurrence, no McBurney tenderness
Vascular watershed areas	Splenic flexure, rectosigmoid
Bloody diarrhea after AAA repair	Colonoscopy—assess for ischemic colitis (IMA injury)
Clostridium difficile colitis	Diagnosis: polymerase chain reaction or pseudomembranes Surgery if refractory to antibiotics (metronidazole)

Ulcerative colitis	Increased risk of colon cancer over time
Ulcerative colitis	Toxic megacolon risk, pseudopolyps, no skip lesions
Ulcerative colitis	Cured by total proctocolectomy
Ulcerative colitis	Sequence: inflammation-dysplasia-cancer in flat areas
Colon cancer	Sequence: APC + KRAS mutations-adenomatous polyp-cancer
Colon cancer	Stage III gets adjuvant chemotherapy
Colon cancer	5% incidence of second primary lesion
Rectal cancer	Radiation sensitive
Rectal cancer	Neoadjuvant sometimes used—stage III
Anal cancer	Definitive treatment is medical (not surgery)
Pneumaturia	Fistula to bladder from diverticulitis
Diverticular bleeding	Usually stops spontaneously

Endocrine/Breast

Think

Multiple endocrine neoplasia (MEN) 1	Pancreas, pituitary, parathyroid lesions
MEN 2A	Medullary carcinoma of the thyroid (MTC), pheo, parathyroid hyperplasia
MEN 2B	MTC, pheo, marfanoid habitus
Thyroid nodule	Fine-needle aspiration (FNA)
Papillary cancer	95% 5-year survival with thyroidectomy, spreads by lymph nodes
Follicular cancer	80% 20-year survival with thyroidectomy, blood-borne spread
Medullary thyroid carcinoma	Poor prognosis, total thyroidectomy
Primary hyperparathyroidism	Single adenoma, resection
Secondary hyperparathyroidism	Hyperplasia of all glands in renal failure
Primary hyperaldosteronism	Look for aldosterone-producing adrenal adenoma.
Thymectomy	May cure myasthenia gravis
Pheochromocytoma	Adrenal medulla; alpha block before surgery
Ductal carcinoma in situ	Resection and radiation therapy
Lobular carcinoma in situ	Marker for increased risk of bilateral breast cancer
Partial mastectomy (lumpectomy)	Equivalent survival to mastectomy
Inflammatory breast cancer	Intradermal metastases, initial chemoradiation
Bloody nipple discharge	Intraductal papilloma
Nonresolving breast abscess	Breast cancer
Winged scapula after axillary dissection	Long thoracic nerve injury

Pediatrics

Think

Abdominal wall defect—gastroschisis	No associated anomalies, operate
Abdominal wall defect—omphalocele	High associated anomalies, identify before repair
Most common esophageal atresia	Proximal pouch with distal tracheoesophageal fistula
Ileocolic intussusception	Currant jelly stools, reduce with enema
Malrotation	Bilious vomiting
Pyloric stenosis	Projectile vomiting
Duodenal atresia	Double bubble sign, duodenal bypass

Jejunal atresia	In utero vascular accident; resection
Hirschsprung disease	No meconium in 24 hours, rectal biopsy
Midline neck mass	Thyroglossal duct cyst

Trauma — Think

Trauma	Think
Cushing triad in traumatic brain injury	Bradycardia, hypertension, irregular respiration
Closed head injury	Increases sympathetic tone
Spinal cord injury	Decreases sympathetic tone
Penetrating neck trauma	Zone II—OR; zone I or III—imaging before therapy
Rapid deceleration injury	Aortic tear at ligamentum arteriosum
Initial wound healing	Type III collagen predominates
Initial wound	Po_2 at center of wound is zero
Electrical burn	Can underestimate injury; rhabdomyolysis
Carbonaceous sputum	Inhalational injury; intubate
Circumferential burn	Escharotomy (possible extremity ischemia)
Only burn antibiotic to penetrate eschar	Mafenide
Unconscious patient neck clearance	Clinical exam unreliable, use CT
Blood at meatus	Urethral injury; urethrogram
Most sensitive sign of renal trauma	Hematuria
Most common form of shock	Hypovolemia
Most common organ damaged in blunt trauma	Spleen; usually nonoperative salvage
Splenectomy	Vaccinate: *Haemophilus influenzae*, pneumococcus, meningococcus
Most sensitive tissues to pressure	Skin > fat > muscle

Other Pairings — Think

Other Pairings	Think
Endoscopic ultrasound; good for	Rectal, prostate, pancreatic, esophageal cancer staging
CT with intravenous contrast; good for	Vascular tumors; necrotic pancreas; abscess ("rim-enhancing"); "blush" equals bleeding
CT with oral contrast; good for	Bowel versus abscess
CT chest; good for	Esophageal injury/leak, coin lesion, PE
Focused assessment with sonography for trauma (FAST); good for	Abdominal trauma, pericardial effusion (fluid = bleeding in trauma)
Endoscopic retrograde cholangiopancreatography (ERCP); good for	Common bile duct stones, bile leak, pancreatic ductogram (pseudocyst) Carries a 2% incidence of pancreatitis
Ultrasound; good for	DVT (duplex), visceral vessel assessment
Tagged red blood cell scan; good for	GI bleeding, hepatic hemangioma (magnetic resonance imaging [MRI] and CT angiography also diagnostic)
Technetium-99 scan; good for	Thyroid, Meckel, biliary tree
Hepatic iminodiacetic acid scan (HIDA); good for	Acute cholecystitis, biliary dyskinesia
Suspected spinal cord injury	CT for bony injury MRI for ligamentous injury
Rapid correction of hyponatremia	May cause central pontine myelosis
Order of cell arrival in wound	Polymorphonuclear leukocyte, macrophage, lymphocyte, fibroblast

Chronic wounds	Pressure sores, diabetic foot ulcer, venous leg ulcers
Reverse steroid effect on wound healing	Vitamin A
Keloid	Grows beyond border of original scar
Warfarin-induced skin necrosis	Protein C deficiency
Catheter-related bloodstream infections	Coag-negative *Staphylococcus*
Spontaneous bacterial peritonitis	Gram-negative bacteria
Infection with lactation	*Staphylococcus aureus*
Acute sialadenitis	*S. aureus*
Small intestinal cell fuel	Glutamine
Colonocyte fuel	Short-chain fatty acids
Short-chain fatty acids	Acetate, butyrate, propionate
Major histocompatibility complex II	Antigen-presenting cells (macrophages, dendritic cells), endothelium

Index